Back Pain: Assessment and Treatment

Back Pain: Assessment and Treatment

Edited by Angus Sanders

hayle
medical

New York

Hayle Medical,
750 Third Avenue, 9th Floor,
New York, NY 10017, USA

Visit us on the World Wide Web at:
www.haylemedical.com

ISBN: 978-1-63241-482-3

Trademark Notice: Registered trademark of products or corporate names are used only for explanation and identification without intent to infringe.

Cataloging-in-Publication Data

Back pain : assessment and treatment / edited by Angus Sanders.
    p. cm.
Includes bibliographical references and index.
ISBN 978-1-63241-482-3
1. Backache. 2. Backache--Treatment. 3. Backache--Diagnosis.
4. Backache--Treatment--Evaluation. I. Sanders, Angus.
RD771.B217 B33 2018
617.564--dc23

Table of Contents

Preface..IX

Chapter 1   **The Effectiveness of Pilates Exercise in People with Chronic Low Back Pain**.................................1
Cherie Wells, Gregory S. Kolt, Paul Marshall, Bridget Hill,
Andrea Bialocerkowski

Chapter 2   **The Association between the History of Cardiovascular Diseases and Chronic
Low Back Pain in South Koreans**...15
In-Hyuk Ha, Jinho Lee, Me-riong Kim, Hyejin Kim, Joon-Shik Shin

Chapter 3   **Return to Work Coordination Programmes for Work Disability:
A Meta-Analysis of Randomised Controlled Trials**..23
Stefan Schandelmaier, Shanil Ebrahim, Susan C. A. Burkhardt,
Wout E. L. de Boer, Thomas Zumbrunn, Gordon H. Guyatt, Jason W. Busse,
Regina Kunz

Chapter 4   **Diaphragm Postural Function Analysis using Magnetic Resonance Imaging**...................36
Pavel Vostatek, Daniel Novák, Tomas Rychnovský, Šarka Rychnovská

Chapter 5   **Ultrasonographic Assessment of Enthesitis in HLA-B27 Positive Patients with
Rheumatoid Arthritis, a Matched Case-Only Study**..49
Antonio Mera-Varela, Aida Ferreiro-Iglesias, Eva Perez-Pampin,
Marisol Porto-Silva, Juan J. Gómez-Reino, Antonio Gonzalez

Chapter 6   **How well do Randomized Trials Inform Decision Making: Systematic
Review using Comparative Effectiveness Research Measures on Acupuncture
for Back Pain**..55
Claudia M. Witt, Eric Manheimer, Richard Hammerschlag, Rainer Lüdtke,
Lixing Lao, Sean R. Tunis, Brian M. Berman

Chapter 7   **Influence of Control Group on Effect Size in Trials of Acupuncture for Chronic
Pain: A Secondary Analysis of an Individual Patient Data Meta-Analysis**.....................65
Hugh MacPherson, Emily Vertosick, George Lewith, Klaus Linde,
Karen J. Sherman, Claudia M. Witt, Andrew J. Vickers

Chapter 8   **Incomplete Reporting of Baseline Characteristics in Clinical Trials: An
Analysis of Randomized Controlled Trials and Systematic Reviews Involving
Patients with Chronic Low Back Pain**..73
Maria M. Wertli, Manuela Schöb, Florian Brunner, Johann Steurer

Chapter 9   **Adherence of French GPs to Chronic Neuropathic Pain Clinical Guidelines:
Results of a Cross-Sectional, Randomized, "e" Case-Vignette Survey**............................82
Valéria Martinez, Nadine Attal, Bertrand Vanzo, Eric Vicaut, Jean Michel Gautier,
Didier Bouhassira, Michel Lantéri Minet

Chapter 10   **Velocity of Lordosis Angle during Spinal Flexion and Extension**...93
Tobias Consmüller, Antonius Rohlmann, Daniel Weinland, Claudia Druschel,
Georg N. Duda, William R. Taylor

Chapter 11   **Predictors of Occurrence and Severity of First Time Low Back Pain Episodes:
Findings from a Military Inception Cohort**...100
Steven Z. George, John D. Childs, Deydre S. Teyhen, Samuel S. Wu,
Alison C. Wright, Jessica L. Dugan, Michael E. Robinson

Chapter 12   **Soft Tissue Artefacts of the Human Back: Comparison of the Sagittal
Curvature of the Spine Measured using Skin Markers and an Open
Upright MRI**...109
Roland Zemp, Renate List, Turgut Gülay, Jean Pierre Elsig, Jaroslav Naxera,
William R. Taylor, Silvio Lorenzetti

Chapter 13   **A Meta-Analysis of Core Stability Exercise versus General Exercise for
Chronic Low Back Pain**..117
Xue-Qiang Wang, Jie-Jiao Zheng, Zhuo-Wei Yu, Xia Bi, Shu-Jie Lou, Jing Liu,
Bin Cai, Ying-Hui Hua, Mark Wu, Mao-Ling Wei, Hai-Min Shen, Yi Chen,
Yu-Jian Pan, Guo-Hui Xu, Pei-Jie Chen

Chapter 14   **Flexion Relaxation and its Relation to Pain and Function over the Duration
of a Back Pain Episode**...124
Raymond W. McGorry, Jia-Hua Lin

Chapter 15   **Predictors for Half-Year Outcome of Impairment in Daily Life for Back Pain
Patients Referred for Physiotherapy: A Prospective Observational Study**...................132
Sven Karstens, Katja Hermann, Ingo Froböse, Stephan W. Weiler

Chapter 16   **Threshold of Musculoskeletal Pain Intensity for Increased Risk of
Long-Term Sickness Absence among Female Healthcare Workers in
Eldercare**..139
Lars L. Andersen, Thomas Clausen, Hermann Burr, Andreas Holtermann

Chapter 17   **Assessing Sleep Disturbance in Low Back Pain: The Validity of Portable
Instruments**...145
Saad M. Alsaadi, James H. McAuley, Julia M. Hush, Delwyn J. Bartlett,
Zoe M. McKeough, Ronald R. Grunstein, George C. Dungan II, Chris G. Maher

Chapter 18   **Evaluation of the Validity of Job Exposure Matrix for Psychosocial Factors
at Work**...152
Svetlana Solovieva, Tiina Pensola, Johanna Kausto, Rahman Shiri,
Markku Heliövaara, Alex Burdorf, Kirsti Husgafvel-Pursiainen, Eira Viikari-Juntura

Chapter 19   **Disrupted TH17/Treg Balance in Patients with Chronic Low Back Pain**.................161
Benjamin Luchting, Banafscheh Rachinger-Adam, Julia Zeitler, Lisa Egenberger,
Patrick Möhnle, Simone Kreth, Shahnaz Christina Azad

Chapter 20   **Preoperative MRI Findings Predict Two-Year Postoperative Clinical Outcome
in Lumbar Spinal Stenosis**...171
Pekka Kuittinen, Petri Sipola, Ville Leinonen, Tapani Saari, Sanna Sinikallio,
Sakari Savolainen, Heikki Kröger, Veli Turunen, Olavi Airaksinen, Timo Aalto

Chapter 21   **Do Abnormal Serum Lipid Levels Increase the Risk of Chronic Low Back
Pain? The Nord-Trøndelag Health Study**..177
Ingrid Heuch, Ivar Heuch, Knut Hagen, John-Anker Zwart

Chapter 22   **Clinical Significance of Tumor Necrosis Factor-α Inhibitors in the Treatment
of Sciatica**..185
Yun Fu Wang, Ping You Chen, Wei Chang, Fi Qi Zhu, Li Li Xu, Song Lin Wang,
Li Ying Chang, Jie Luo, Guang Jian Liu

Chapter 23   **Percutaneous Resolution of Lumbar Facet Joint Cysts as an Alternative
Treatment to Surgery**..198
Feng Shuang, Shu-Xun Hou, Jia-Liang Zhu, Dong-Feng Ren, Zheng Cao,
Jia-Guang Tang

Chapter 24   **A 35-Year Trend Analysis for Back Pain in Austria: The Role of Obesity**....................207
Franziska Großschädl, Wolfgang Freidl, Éva Rásky, Nathalie Burkert,
Johanna Muckenhuber, Willibald J. Stronegger

Permissions

List of Contributors

Index

Preface

This book has been an outcome of determined endeavour from a group of educationists in the field. The primary objective was to involve a broad spectrum of professionals from diverse cultural background involved in the field for developing new researches. The book not only targets students but also scholars pursuing higher research for further enhancement of the theoretical and practical applications of the subject.

Back pain is caused by irritation, strain and damage that is caused in the region where the spinal muscles, tendons, nerves and discs interconnect. This book discusses the pathophysiology for assessment as well as treatment procedures for back pain. Strain and stress caused to the body as well as injuries to the spine can cause back pain. Physical therapy, medication and surgery are some of the treatments that are available for this disorder. The topics included in this book on back pain are of utmost significance and bound to provide incredible insights. With state-of-the-art inputs by acclaimed experts of this field, this book targets students and professionals.

It was an honour to edit such a profound book and also a challenging task to compile and examine all the relevant data for accuracy and originality. I wish to acknowledge the efforts of the contributors for submitting such brilliant and diverse chapters in the field and for endlessly working for the completion of the book. Last, but not the least; I thank my family for being a constant source of support in all my research endeavours.

Editor

The Effectiveness of Pilates Exercise in People with Chronic Low Back Pain

Cherie Wells[1,2]*, **Gregory S. Kolt**[2], **Paul Marshall**[2], **Bridget Hill**[3], **Andrea Bialocerkowski**[4]

1 Faculty of Health, University of Canberra, Bruce, Australian Capital Territory, Australia, 2 School of Science and Health, University of Western Sydney, Campbelltown, New South Wales, Australia, 3 Epworth HealthCare, Richmond, Victoria, Australia, 4 Griffith Health Institute, Griffith University, Gold Coast, Queensland, Australia

Abstract

Objective: To evaluate the effectiveness of Pilates exercise in people with chronic low back pain (CLBP) through a systematic review of randomised controlled trials (RCTs).

Data Sources: A search for RCTs was undertaken using Medical Search Terms and synonyms for "Pilates" and "low back pain" within the maximal date range of 10 databases. Databases included the Cumulative Index to Nursing and Allied Health Literature; Cochrane Library; Medline; Physiotherapy Evidence Database; ProQuest: Health and Medical Complete, Nursing and Allied Health Source, Dissertation and Theses; Scopus; Sport Discus; Web of Science.

Study Selection: Two independent reviewers were involved in the selection of evidence. To be included, relevant RCTs needed to be published in the English language. From 152 studies, 14 RCTs were included.

Data Extraction: Two independent reviewers appraised the methodological quality of RCTs using the McMaster Critical Review Form for Quantitative Studies. The author(s), year of publication, and details regarding participants, Pilates exercise, comparison treatments, and outcome measures, and findings, were then extracted.

Data Synthesis: The methodological quality of RCTs ranged from "poor" to "excellent". A meta-analysis of RCTs was not undertaken due to the heterogeneity of RCTs. Pilates exercise provided statistically significant improvements in pain and functional ability compared to usual care and physical activity between 4 and 15 weeks, but not at 24 weeks. There were no consistent statistically significant differences in improvements in pain and functional ability with Pilates exercise, massage therapy, or other forms of exercise at any time period.

Conclusions: Pilates exercise offers greater improvements in pain and functional ability compared to usual care and physical activity in the short term. Pilates exercise offers equivalent improvements to massage therapy and other forms of exercise. Future research should explore optimal Pilates exercise designs, and whether some people with CLBP may benefit from Pilates exercise more than others.

Editor: François Hug, The University of Queensland, Australia

Funding: The authors have no support or funding to report.

Competing Interests: The authors have declared that no competing interests exist.

* Email: Cherie.Wells@canberra.edu.au

Introduction

Chronic low back pain (CLBP) is defined as pain for more than twelve weeks in the posterior lumbar region between the twelfth ribs and inferior gluteal folds [1]. CLBP is highly prevalent and associated with significant levels of disability [2–4]. As a consequence, CLBP places a large social and economic burden on society [2–4].

Pilates exercise is a commonly prescribed to people with CLBP [5–7]. Pilates exercise is named after its founder, Joseph Pilates, who developed a series of exercises in the 1920s to encourage physical and mental conditioning [8,9]. Core stability, strength and flexibility are emphasised in Pilates exercise, as is control of movement, posture, and breathing [9]. All of these aspects of Pilates exercise may benefit people with CLBP as exercises with

similar features have been successful in reducing pain and improving functional ability [10–12].

When treating people with CLBP, it has been suggested in a Delphi survey that supervised Pilates exercise sessions should be undertaken 2–3 times per week for 3–6 months, and be supplemented by home exercises [13]. Individualised supervision has been advised in the first 2 weeks, but thereafter group sessions of up to 4 clients per therapist [13]. The use of specialised Pilates exercise equipment with spring resistance, such as a Reformer, has also been recommended for people with CLBP [13,14].

Despite the popularity of Pilates exercise in treating people with CLBP, its effectiveness in people with CLBP is yet to be established [15]. Six systematic reviews have investigated the effectiveness of Pilates exercise in people with CLBP, and a protocol for a Cochrane review has also been published [6,7,16–20]. Completed reviews, though, report different findings [6,7,16–

20]. Several reviews report a decrease in pain, but not all report improvements in functional ability [6,16–18]. Other reviews report no improvement in pain or functional ability or inconclusive findings [7,13,19]. The small number and mixed methodological quality of primary studies has made reporting of credible results difficult [15]. Several reviews have also conducted meta-analyses in the presence of significant clinical heterogeneity, resulting in misleading findings [15].

Recently, several randomised controlled trials (RCTs) have been published that are relevant to evaluating the effectiveness of Pilates exercise in people with CLBP [21–26]. The majority of these RCTs have not been included in prior reviews, so incorporating this new evidence in an updated systematic review is indicated. Given there is now a moderate volume of evidence available, it is also appropriate that this new systematic review includes only RCTs. This will ensure this review represents a high level of evidence and increases the credibility of results [15,27,28].

The aim of the following systematic review is to provide an update on the effectiveness of Pilates exercise in reducing pain and improving functional ability of people with CLBP based on the highest level and quality of research evidence available [28].

Materials and Methods

Study Design

A systematic review was undertaken to locate, evaluate and summarise findings from RCTs that have investigated the effectiveness of Pilates exercise in people with CLBP. A systematic review was chosen over a narrative review as it limits bias and error in the selection and appraisal of evidence [29,30]. In this systematic review, a comprehensive search of the literature was undertaken to answer a focused question, the methodological quality of primary studies was appraised, and findings were synthesised to address the study aim [29,30].

Search Strategy

A comprehensive literature search for evidence was undertaken on the 1st May, 2014 using 10 databases: Cumulative Index to Nursing and Allied Health Literature, Cochrane Library, Medline, Physiotherapy Evidence Database, ProQuest: Health and Medical Complete, Proquest: Nursing and Allied Health Source, Proquest: Dissertation and Theses, Scopus, Sport Discus, and Web of Science. To ensure relevant trials were not overlooked, the maximal date range available in each database was used. Medical Subject Headings terms of "Pilates", "Pilates method", and "Low Back Pain" and synonyms for low back pain were inputted in the title, abstract, and as able, the keyword fields to identify relevant evidence (Table 1).

Preliminary searching revealed that expanding the literature searches to include "exercise", "motor control", or "core stability" did not identify any additional Pilates specific exercise studies, nor did changing the Boolean operator to "or". Removing "low back pain" also did not identify any additional studies. Once RCTs were selected for inclusion, their reference lists were searched for additional, relevant studies that met inclusion criterion [16–19,24–29]. In addition, reference lists of previous systematic reviews of this topic were searched to ensure relevant studies were not missed [6,7,15–19].

Selection of Evidence

Selection of relevant studies was based on the study's title and the abstract, and as required, the full document. Two independent reviewers selected the evidence according to the selection criteria (CW, BH). Any disagreements were resolved through discussion with a third reviewer (AB). To be considered in this systematic review, studies needed to:

1. Be published in the English language, as access to interpreters was not available.

2. Be published in full so that the methodological quality of the study could be assessed alongside results. Abstracts were excluded as they contained insufficient data to enable analysis of methodological quality [31].

3. Be RCTs to limit the risk of bias in findings regarding efficacy [26]. If studies reported that they were RCTs but did not describe the randomisation procedure they were included in this review. If, however, studies reported that they were RCTs, but described a pseudo-random technique of allocating participants to groups, such as alternative allocation, they were excluded from this review [27,28].

4. Assess the effectiveness of Pilates exercise where the term "Pilates" was used to describe the type of prescribed exercise being investigated. Exercises described as "motor control" or "lumbar stabilisation" did not suffice for Pilates. This is because Pilates may include other features apart from motor control and lumbar stabilisation [9].

5. Include participants with CLBP, that is, localised pain in the lumbar region of more than 3 months in duration [1]. If studies only included participants with low back pain of less than 3 months duration, they were excluded. This is because people with CLBP respond differently to treatment compared to those with acute or subacute symptoms [32]. If studies included participants with acute or subacute low back pain and CLBP, the study was included as findings were still considered relevant.

6. Use outcome measures with appropriate psychometric qualities that evaluate pain and/or functional ability in people with CLBP [33]. For example, the Visual Analog Scale and Numerical Rating Scale for pain, and the Oswestry Disability Questionnaire and Roland Morris Disability Questionnaire for functional ability. RCTs with outcome measures for pain and/or functional ability that did not have sufficient validity, reliability, or responsiveness were excluded to avoid imprecise measurements of treatment effect [33].

Appraisal of Evidence

The methodological quality of included RCTs was evaluated by two independent reviewers using the McMaster Critical Review Form for Quantitative Studies (CW, BH) [34]. This critical appraisal tool was utilised because it is comprehensive in assessing methodological quality of quantitative evidence [35]. This critical appraisal tool also has good inter-rater reliability [36–38]. To confirm the reliability of scoring in this review, the percentage agreement and kappa score between the two reviewers was calculated [39]. Any disagreements between reviewers were resolved through discussion with a third reviewer (AB).

The McMaster Critical Review Form for Quantitative Studies directs reviewers to consider 16 items of methodological quality relating to the study's purpose, literature review, design, sample, outcomes, intervention, results and conclusions [34]. Guidelines for the appraisal of evidence in this review were created to assist reviewers in consistently evaluating methodological quality (Table 2). These were based on guidelines provided by the authors of the McMaster appraisal tool [34,38].

If RCTs met each criterion outlined in the appraisal guidelines, they received a score of "one" for that item, or, if they did not

Table 1. Search Strategy.

Database	Date Range	Key Words	Fields
Cochrane Library	1800–2014	(low back pain OR dorsalgia OR *spin* pain OR backache OR lumbago) AND (pilates OR pilates method)	Title, Abstract or Keyword
Cumulative Index to Nursing and Allied Health Literature	1970–2014	(low back pain OR dorsalgia OR *spin* pain OR backache OR lumbago) AND (pilates OR pilates method)	Title, Abstract, or Word in Subject Heading
Medline-	1928–2014	(low back pain OR dorsalgia OR *spin* pain OR backache OR lumbago) AND (pilates OR pilates method)	Title, Abstract or Keyword
Physiotherapy Evidence Database	1928–2014	low back pain AND pilates	Title and Abstract
Proquest (Dissertations and Theses, Medical and Health Complete, Nursing and Allied Health Source)	1928–2014	(low back pain OR dorsalgia OR *spin* pain OR backache OR lumbago) AND (pilates OR pilates method)	Title, Abstract, or Subject Heading
Scopus	1960–2014	(low back pain AND pilates) OR (dorsalgia AND pilates) OR (*spin* pain AND pilates) OR (backache AND pilates) OR (lumbago AND pilates)	Title, Abstract, or Keyword
Sport Discus	1975–2014	(low back pain OR dorsalgia OR *spin* pain OR backache OR lumbago) AND (pilates OR pilates method)	Title, Abstract, or Keyword
Web of Science	1977–2014	(low back pain OR dorsalgia OR *spin* pain OR backache OR lumbago) AND (pilates OR pilates method)	Topic or Title

meet the criteria, they received a score of "zero". Individual item scores were then summated to provide a total score of methodological quality out of 16, with higher scores reflecting greater methodological quality. Once quality scores were calculated, these were divided into five qualitative categories of poor (score = 0–8), fair (score = 9–10), good (score = 11–12), very good (score = 13–14) and excellent (score = 15–16) methodological quality, as defined in previous research [38].

Data Extraction and Syntheses

The number of included RCTs and their methodological quality were summarised using descriptive statistics. The author(s), year of publication, and details regarding participants, interventions, comparison treatments, outcome measures, were extracted from RCTs by the primary author (CW), and tabulated. To determine whether a meta-analysis of study findings could be performed, the clinical and statistical heterogeneity of RCTs was assessed [15,40–41].

Clinical heterogeneity of RCTs was assessed by comparing differences in the population, intervention, comparison treatments,

Table 2. Modified Guidelines for use of the McMasters Critical Appraisal Form for Quantitative Studies[34].

Item	Essential Criteria
1. Purpose	Do the authors clearly state that the aim of the study, which is to evaluate the effect of Pilates exercise in individuals diagnosed with chronic low back pain (CLBP)?
2. Literature review	Do the authors justify, by identifying gaps in the literature, the need to undertake further research into the effectiveness of Pilates exercise for individuals diagnosed with CLBP?
3. Study design	Have the authors used a randomised controlled trial to answer study aims, that is, to evaluate the effectiveness of Pilates exercise in people with CLBP?
4. Blinding	Have the authors used assessor blinding to minimise bias?
5. Sample description	Have the authors described the sample in terms of age, gender, and at least one measure of disability due to CLBP?
6. Sample size	Have the authors justified their sample size through a power calculation or post hoc analysis (and recruited sufficient numbers)?
7. Ethics and consent	Have the authors documented ethical approval for the research and gained informed consent by participants?
8. Validity of outcomes	Did the authors use outcome measures that are valid for use in people with CLBP to assess all outcome variables?
9. Reliability of outcomes	Did the authors use outcome measures that are reliable for use in people with CLBP to assess all outcome variables?
10. Intervention description	Did the authors provide sufficient information to enable reproduction of the intervention?
11. Statistical significance	Did the authors report the results for at least one outcome measure in line with study aim and in terms of statistical significance?
12. Statistical analysis	Did the authors use appropriate statistical analyses in evaluating results according to their aim?
13. Clinical importance	Did the authors reflect on the clinical importance of results for people diagnosed with CLBP?
14. Conclusions	Did the authors provide appropriate conclusions considering the study method and results?
15. Clinical implications	Did the authors discuss clinical implications of the results in terms of treatment of CLBP and in directing further research?
16. Study limitations	Did the authors identify limitations of the study methodology and results?

outcome measures, and timing of reassessment of individual studies [15]. Statistical heterogeneity was assessed by calculation of an i^2 statistic of studies with similar comparison treatment groups using the Cochrane Review Manager (version 5.2) software [41–43]. If i^2 was greater than 75%, studies were considered to have substantial heterogeneity [41]. If substantial clinical and statistical heterogeneity were present, pooling results in a meta-analysis was deemed inappropriate.

Key findings of RCTs were expressed in terms of between-group mean differences and 95% confidence intervals. If between-group mean differences and 95% confidence intervals were not provided by RCTs, these were calculated from post-treatment mean values and standard deviations using the Physiotherapy Evidence Database calculator [44]. For the randomised cross-over trial, the between-group mean difference and 95% confidence interval was calculated from the first comparison time period between the Pilates exercise and control group, as the carryover effect in relation to time of treatment and pain intensity was statistically significant [21].

Results for each outcome measures were considered to be statistically significant if the 95% confidence interval of the between group difference did not cross "zero" [45]. If a 95% confidence interval was unable to be calculated from results given, a p value less than 0.05 for the between group comparison was considered to indicate statistical significance [45]. Results were considered to be clinically significant in this review if the mean between-group difference was greater than the minimal clinically important difference reported in the literature [46,47].

Results

Search Results

A total of 267 "hits" were obtained with database searching, and an additional RCT was identified when reviewing reference lists of previous systematic reviews (Figure 1) [48]. The majority of studies identified by this search strategy were excluded due to being duplicates (n = 115) or not being an RCT (n = 95). Other studies were excluded as they were not published in the English language (n = 16), did not assess the effectiveness of Pilates exercise in people with CLBP compared to other treatment (n = 17), were published in an abstract format (n = 8).

There was 100% agreement between the 2 reviewers regarding the 14 RCTs included in this review (Figure 1) [21,23–26,48–56]. Four RCTs were described in academic theses [48,49,51,53] and 10 were published in academic journals [21,23–26,50,52,54–56]. It should be noted that 2 RCTs were reported across 2 papers but only 1 paper was included in this review to avoid duplication of findings [22,23,55,57]. For one RCT, the paper that was published in a peer-reviewed journal was selected over the thesis to extract results [55,57]. For the other RCT, the paper reporting on changes in pain and functional ability in the short and long term was included [23], rather than the paper reporting on outcomes only in the short term [22].

Methodological Quality

There was 95% agreement between the two reviewers regarding item scores of the McMaster Critical Review Form for Quantitative Studies. This represents "almost perfect" inter-rater reliability (kappa score = 0.88, p = 0.00) [39]. Discussion with the third reviewer was required to reach consensus regarding the adequacy of the description of Pilates exercise [27], presence of assessor bias [21], documentation of informed consent and ethical approval [51], use of valid and reliable outcome measures [51], and discussion of the statistical significance and clinical importance

of results [48,49]. One of the RCTs was published by an author of this review (PM) [23]. To avoid bias, this author was not involved in the stages of review of this RCT [23].

The methodological quality of studies ranged from 4 to 16, representing "poor" to "excellent" methodological quality (Table 3). RCTs published in the past 2 years were generally of higher quality, as were those published in journals compared to academic theses. According to the McMaster Quantitative Review Form, strengths in the methodological quality of most RCTs related to the provision of a clear purpose (Item 1), description of participants (Item 5), and documentation of ethic approval and consent (Item 7) [34]. The majority of RCTs also provided results in terms of statistical significance (Item 11) and conducted appropriate statistical analyses (Item 12) [34].

Several RCTs, however, did not ensure assessor blinding (item 4), recruit an adequate sample size (Item 6), or document the validity and/or reliability of outcome measures (Item 8, 9) [34]. Other RCTs did not provide adequate detail of Pilates exercise programs for replication (Item 10), or discuss the clinical importance of results (Item 14) (Table 3) [34].

Description of Included Studies

A summary of the population, intervention, comparison, and outcome measures for each RCT is provided in Table 4 and 5. The number of participants per RCT ranged from 12 to 83, while the mean age of participants across RCTs ranged between 21 to 49 years of age. The ratio of female to male participants ranged from 5:1 through to 1:1, except in one study where only females were recruited [54].

In terms of the Pilates interventions, most RCTs described supervised exercise programs delivered in 30 to 60-minute sessions, 1–3 times per week, for 4–15 weeks (Table 4, 5). Home exercises were incorporated in 6 RCTs as part of the Pilates exercise intervention [25,26,48,52,54,55]. The supervision ratios of clients per therapist for supervised sessions ranged from 11:1 to 1:1, although not all RCTs provided this information. Use of specialised Pilates exercise equipment, such as a Reformer, was reported in 5 RCTs [21,23,26,49,55].

Pilates exercise was compared to usual care and physical activity in 9 RCTs, massage therapy in 1 RCT, and other forms of exercise in 4 RCTs (Table 4, 5). Usual care and physical activity could involve unknown other treatments [53,56], no treatment [25,50,52], education [24], medications [24,48,55], or consultations with health professionals, such as physiotherapists [48,55]. Other forms of exercise ranged from cycling [23], McKenzie exercise [54], traditional lumbar stabilisation exercise [51], and a mixed form of exercise including stretching, strengthening and stabilisation [26].

Variable outcome measures were used to investigate the effectiveness of Pilates exercise in reducing pain and improving functional ability in people with CLBP (Table 4, 5). These included the Visual Analog Scale and Numerical Rating Scale (11 and 101 point scales) for pain, and the Roland Morris Disability Questionnaire, Oswestry Disability Questions, Quebec Score, and the Miami Back Index for functional ability [33,47]. Treatment outcomes were measured at different time periods, ranging from 4 to 24 weeks.

Heterogeneity of Included Studies

Significant clinical heterogeneity was noted across RCTs in terms of the study population, intervention, and outcome assessment (Table 4, 5). Though all RCTs studied people with CLBP, some included people with acute and subacute symptoms, or other diagnoses [21,49,55]. Pilates exercise interventions also

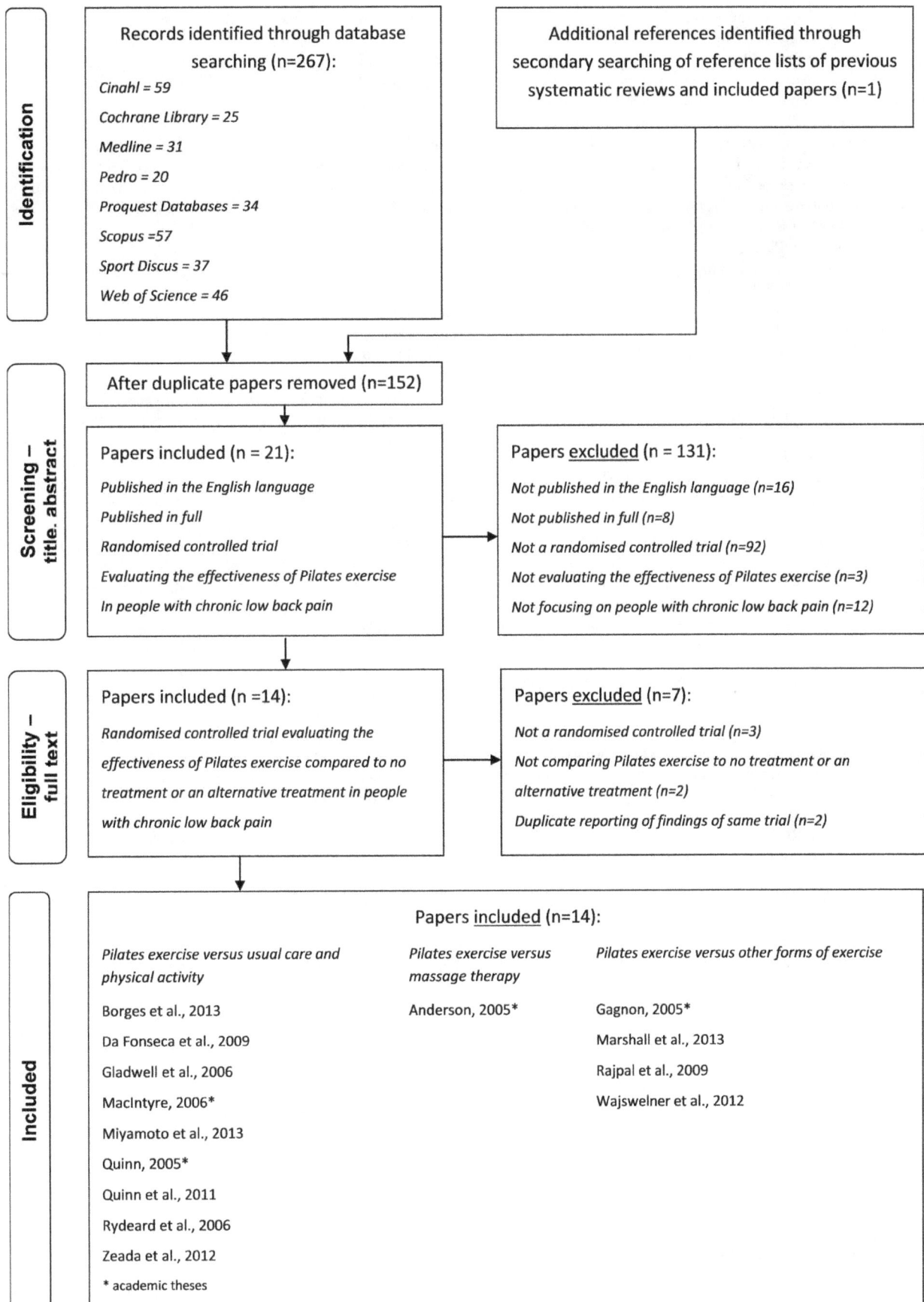

Identification

Records identified through database searching (n=267):

Cinahl = 59

Cochrane Library = 25

Medline = 31

Pedro = 20

Proquest Databases = 34

Scopus =57

Sport Discus = 37

Web of Science = 46

Additional references identified through secondary searching of reference lists of previous systematic reviews and included papers (n=1)

After duplicate papers removed (n=152)

Screening – title. abstract

Papers included (n = 21):

Published in the English language

Published in full

Randomised controlled trial

Evaluating the effectiveness of Pilates exercise

In people with chronic low back pain

Papers excluded (n = 131):

Not published in the English language (n=16)

Not published in full (n=8)

Not a randomised controlled trial (n=92)

Not evaluating the effectiveness of Pilates exercise (n=3)

Not focusing on people with chronic low back pain (n=12)

Eligibility – full text

Papers included (n =14):

Randomised controlled trial evaluating the effectiveness of Pilates exercise compared to no treatment or an alternative treatment in people with chronic low back pain

Papers excluded (n=7):

Not a randomised controlled trial (n=3)

Not comparing Pilates exercise to no treatment or an alternative treatment (n=2)

Duplicate reporting of findings of same trial (n=2)

Included

Papers included (n=14):

Pilates exercise versus usual care and physical activity

Borges et al., 2013

Da Fonseca et al., 2009

Gladwell et al., 2006

MacIntyre, 2006*

Miyamoto et al., 2013

Quinn, 2005*

Quinn et al., 2011

Rydeard et al., 2006

Zeada et al., 2012

* academic theses

Pilates exercise versus massage therapy

Anderson, 2005*

Pilates exercise versus other forms of exercise

Gagnon, 2005*

Marshall et al., 2013

Rajpal et al., 2009

Wajswelner et al., 2012

Figure 1. Results of Literature Search.

varied in terms of the duration of the intervention, level of supervision, incorporation of home exercises, education, and use of specialised equipment. Outcomes were also measured with different outcome measures at different time periods.

Comparison treatments also varied considerably across RCTs (Table 4, 5). When Pilates exercise was compared to usual care and physical activity, participants could access variable therapies depending on the RCT [24,48,55]. Usual physical activity also varied with some studies focusing on participants who were highly active [55,56], while the others did not. When Pilates exercise was compared to other forms of exercise, comparison exercise regimes were either similar to Pilates exercise [26,51], or quite distinct [23]. Also, in some studies, participants could access other interventions as well [26,51].

Significant statistical heterogeneity was also observed when comparing outcomes achieved with Pilates exercise versus usual care and physical activity for pain ($i^2 = 90\%$, p<0.001), and functional ability ($i^2 = 87\%$, p<0.00001) between 4 and 12 weeks. Similarly, significant statistical heterogeneity was noted when comparing pain relief achieved with Pilates exercise versus other forms of exercise ($i^2 = 83\%$, p = 0.0006) between 4 and 8 weeks. Pooling individual study findings in a meta-analysis, then, was deemed inappropriate for these variables in the short term, given the clinical and statistical heterogeneity of RCTs [40,41].

Moderate statistical heterogeneity was noted when comparing improvements in functional ability with Pilates exercise and other forms of exercise in the short term (4–8 weeks) ($i^2 = 44\%$, p = 0.17). At 24 weeks, mild statistical heterogeneity was evident when Pilates exercise was compared with other forms of exercise across the 2 RCTs for pain ($i^2 = 25\%$, p = 0.25) and functional ability ($i^2 = 9\%$, p = 0.29) [23,26]. Nevertheless, the clinical heterogeneity of RCTs comparing Pilates exercise to other forms of exercise suggested a meta-analysis would be of limited benefit [40,41].

Findings of Included Studies

Pilates exercise versus usual care and physical activity. Four high quality RCTs reported a statistically significant difference in pain relief with Pilates exercise in the short term (4–15 weeks) [21,24,25,55]. Two high quality RCTs, and one poor quality RCT, however, disagreed with these findings [48,50,52]. At 24 weeks, no statistically significance difference in pain relief with Pilates exercise and education versus education alone was reported (Table 6) [24].

The statistically significant improvements in pain reported in the short term were clinically significant in 3 out of 4 RCTs [21,24,25]. This is because mean difference scores exceeded the minimal clinically important difference for their respective outcome measures. For example, Borges et al. (2013) and Quinn, Barry, and Barry (2011) described a mean reduction (and 95% confidence interval) on the Visual Analog Scale of 4.1 (1.8 to 6.3) and 1.5 (0.9 to 2.1) points respectively [21,25]. The minimal clinically important difference for the Visual Analog Scale in people with CLBP has been reported in the literature as between 1.5 to 2 points [46,47].

Similarly, Miyamoto, Costa, Glavanin, and Cabral (2013) reported a mean reduction (and 95% confidence interval) of pain on the 11 point Numerical Rating Scale of 2.2 (1.1 to 3.2) points where the minimal clinically important difference was 2 points [47]. Meanwhile, Rydeard, Leger, and Smith (2006) did not report a clinically significant improvement in pain, that is a mean reduction (and 95% confidence interval) of 15.6 (13.4 to 17.8) points on the 101 point Numerical Rating Scale [55]. This is lower than the estimated minimal clinically important difference of 20 points [46].

With regards to functional ability, 3 high quality RCTs reported statistically significant improvements with Pilates exercise in the short term (4–12 weeks) [24,48,55]. In contrast, 2 high quality RCTs and 3 poor quality RCTs did not [25,50,52,53,56]. Meanwhile, at 24 weeks, no statistically significance difference in improvement in functional ability with Pilates exercise with education versus education alone was reported (Table 7) [24].

Statistically significant short-term improvements in functional ability with Pilates exercise were not clinically significant. For example, MacIntyre (2005) and Miyamoto et al. (2013) reported a mean improvement (and 95% confidence interval) of 2.6 (1.5 to 5.2) and 2.7 (1.0 to 4.4) on the Roland Morris Disability Questionnaire respectively. These changes were less than the minimal clinically important distance of 3.5 to 5 points [46,47]. Similarly, Rydeard et al. (2006) reported a mean change (and 95% confidence interval) of 1.2 (1.1 to 1.4) points on the Oswestry Disability Questionnaire which is below the minimal clinically important difference of 10 points [46,47].

Pilates exercise versus massage therapy. Only one RCT of fair quality compared the effectiveness of Pilates exercise to massage therapy [49]. This RCT did not report any statistically significant differences in pain or functional ability between groups at 6 weeks (Table 8, 9). As a consequence, there were no clinically significant differences noted between Pilates exercise and massage therapy.

Pilates exercise versus other forms of exercise. When Pilates exercise was compared to other forms of exercise, conflicting results in terms of pain relief were reported in the short term (4–8 weeks) [23,26,51,54]. One high quality and low quality RCT reported statistically significant improvements [23,54], while another high quality and low quality RCT did not [26,51]. At 24 weeks, though, there was agreement in 2 high quality RCTs that Pilates exercise resulted in equivalent improvements in pain as other forms of exercise (Table 8) [23,26].

The improvement in pain suggested in one high quality and low quality RCT in the short term was not clinically significant [23,54]. For example, Marshall, Kennedy, Brooks, and Lonsdale (2013) reported a mean decrease (and 95% confidence interval) of 1.1 (0.1 to 2.1) points on the Visual Analog Scale, and Rajpal, Arora, and Chauhan (2009) reported a mean decrease (and 95% confidence interval) of 1.4 (0.7 to 2.1) points on the Visual Analog Scale [23,54]. These scores were less than the minimal clinically important difference of 1.5–2 points on the Visual Analog Scale [46,47].

With regards to functional ability, one high quality RCT reported a statistically significant improvement with Pilates exercise over other forms of exercise in the short term [23]. In contrast, another high quality and low quality RCT did not report a statistically significant difference in improvement [26,51]. At 24 weeks, however, 2 high quality RCTs agreed that Pilates exercise offered similar improvements in functional ability as other forms of exercise (Table 9) [23,26].

The statistically significant improvement in functional ability reported by Marshall et al. (2013) in the short term was not clinically significant [23]. This is because the mean improvement (and 95% confidence interval) in functional ability was 6.5 (1.1 to 11.8) points on the Oswestry Disability Index which is less than the minimal clinically important difference of 10 points [23,46,47].

Discussion

This systematic review provides an update on the effectiveness of Pilates exercise in reducing pain and improving functional ability in people with CLBP based on current evidence. It provides

Table 3. Methodological Quality of Included Studies - McMaster Critical Review Form for Quantitative Studies [34].

Study	Individual Item																Total (/16)	Qualitative Descriptor [38]
	1	2	3	4	5	6	7	8	9	10	11	12	13	14	15	16		
Pilates exercise versus usual care and physical activity																		
1. Borges et al., 2013 [21]	1	1	1	1	1	1	1	0	0	1	1	1	0	1	1	1	13	Very good
2. da Fonseca et al., 2009 [50]	1	1	0	0	0	1	0	0	0	0	1	0	0	0	0	0	4	Poor
3. Gladwell et al., 2006 [52]	1	0	1	1	1	0	1	1	1	1	1	0	1	1	1	1	13	Very Good
4. MacIntyre, 2006 [48]	1	1	1	1	1	1	1	1	1	1	1	0	1	1	1	1	15	Excellent
5. Miyamoto et al., 2013 [24]	1	1	1	1	1	1	1	1	1	1	1	1	1	1	1	1	16	Excellent
6. Quinn, 2005 [53]	1	1	1	0	0	0	0	0	0	0	1	0	0	0	0	0	6	Poor
7. Quinn et al., 2011 [25]	1	1	1	1	1	0	1	0	1	1	1	1	1	1	1	0	13	Very good
8. Rydeard et al., 2006 [55]	1	1	1	1	0	1	1	1	0	1	1	1	1	1	1	1	14	Very good
9. Zeada et al., 2012 [56]	1	0	0	0	1	0	0	0	1	0	0	0	0	0	0	0	4	Poor
Pilates exercise versus massage or other forms of exercise																		
10. Anderson, 2005 [49]	1	1	1	1	1	0	0	0	0	1	0	1	0	1	1	1	10	Fair
11. Gagnon, 2005 [51]	1	1	1	0	1	0	1	0	0	0	1	1	0	1	1	1	10	Fair
12. Marshall et al., 2013 [23]	1	1	1	1	1	1	1	1	0	1	1	1	1	1	1	1	15	Excellent
13. Rajpal et al., 2009 [54]	0	0	0	0	0	0	0	0	1	1	1	0	0	0	0	1	5	Poor
14. Wajswelner et al., 2012 [26]	1	1	1	1	1	1	1	1	1	1	1	1	1	1	1	1	16	Excellent

Table 4. Description of Included Studies- Pilates exercise versus usual care and physical activity.

Study	Population	Intervention and Comparison	Outcome Measures [Timing]
1. Borges et al., 2013 [21]	22 participants with chronic low back pain (CLBP) and Human T-Lymphotrophic Virus	Pilates: 2 X 60 minute supervised sessions per week for 15 weeks; Equipment = Mat, Cadillac, Reformer; Supervision Ratio = ?11 clients: 1 therapist; Standardised protocol	Short Form – 36 - Pain
	Gender (Female: Male) = 2.7: 1.0	No Pilates: no change in daily activities for 15 weeks	Visual Analog Scale - Pain
	Age$^\&$ (years) = 48.3 (10.0)		[0, 15 weeks]
	Baseline Pain Intensity$^\&$ (/10)^a = Pilates 7.2 (2.4); Comparison 6.9 (2.5)		
2. da Fonseca et al., 2009 [50]	17 people with CLBP	Pilates: 2 sessions per week for 15 sessions; Equipment = Mat	Visual Analog Scale – Pain
	Gender (Female: Male) = 2.4: 1.0	No Pilates: continue usual physical activity but no treatment apart from medications	[0, 7–8 weeks]
	Age$^\&$ (years) = 33.1(11.6)		
	Baseline Pain Intensity$^\&$ (/10)^a = Pilates 5.9 (2.0); Comparison 6.1 (1.8)		
3. Gladwell et al., 2006 [52]	34 people with non-specific CLBP	Pilates: 60 minutes, 1 X per week for 6 weeks (as well as home exercises); Equipment: Mat	Oswestry Disability Questionnaire
	Gender (Female: Male) = 4:1	No Pilates: usual physical activity, no treatment apart from medication	Visual Analog Scale – Pain
	Age$^\&$(years) = 40.6(9.7)		[0, 6 weeks]
	Baseline Pain Duration$^\&$ (years) = 10.4 (10.1)		
4. MacIntyre, 2006 [48]	32 participants with CLBP	Pilates: 1 X 60 minute supervised mat session per week and 3 X 10 minute home exercises sessions per week for 12 weeks; General protocol	Roland Morris Disability Questionnaire
	Gender (Female: Male) Pilates = 3.0: 1.0; Comparison = 4.3: 1.0	No Pilates	Visual Analog Scale – Pain
	Age$^\&$ (years) Pilates = 33.2 (7.7); Comparison = 46.7 (14.4)	(Both groups could undertake physiotherapy and exercise as required)	[0, 3, 12 weeks]
	Baseline Pain Intensity$^\&$ (/10)^a = Pilates 5.1 (2.0); Comparison 4.8 (1.7)		
	Baseline Disability$^\&$ (/24)^t = Pilates 7.0 (3.1); Comparison 7.4 (3.4)		
5. Miyamoto et al., 2013 [24]	86 participants with non-specific CLBP	Pilates: 2 X 60 minute supervised mat sessions per week for 6 weeks with education; Supervision ratio = 1:1; General protocol but graded to individual ability	Numeric Rating Scale (11 point) - Pain
	Gender (Female: Male) = Pilates 5.0: 1.0; Comparison 3.8: 1.0	No Pilates: Education booklet and physiotherapy advice 2X per week for 6 weeks (Both groups could take medication as required)	Roland Morris Disability Questionnaire
	Age$^\&$ (years) = Pilates 40.7 (11.8); Comparison 38.3 (11.4)		[0, 6, 24 weeks]
	Baseline Pain Intensity$^\&$ (/10)$^+$ = Pilates 6.6 (1.5); Comparison 6.5 (1.7)		
	Baseline Disability$^\&$ (/24)^t = Pilates 9.7 (4.5); Comparison 10.5 (5.4)		
6. Quinn, 2005 [53]	22 participants with CLBP	Pilates: 2 X 45–60 minute supervised mat sessions per week for 12 weeks; Standardised protocol	Oswestry Disability Questionnaire
	Age$^\&$ (years) = Pilates 46.3 (6.7) years; Comparison 34.7 (7.3)	No Pilates: usual daily activities for 12 weeks, and no new exercise program	[0, 12 weeks]
	Baseline Disability$^\&$ (/100)^s = Pilates 25.9 (10.7); Comparison 22.0 (8.7)		
7. Quinn et al., 2011 [25]	29 participants with CLBP who had undergone physiotherapy treatment but had poor core stability and residual pain	Pilates: 1 X 60 minute supervised mat sessions and 5 X 15 minute home exercises per week for 8 weeks; Supervision ratio = 3–6:1; Standardised protocol but modified as required	Roland Morris Disability Questionnaire
	Age$^\&$ (years) = Pilates 41.8 (13.8); Comparison 44.1 (12.5)	No Pilates: (or further treatment) for 8 weeks	Visual Analog Scale– Pain
	Baseline Pain Intensity$^\&$ (/100)$^\wedge$ = Pilates 40.4 (14.6); Comparison 39.9 (19.9)		[0, 8 weeks]

Table 4. Cont.

Study	Population	Intervention and Comparison	Outcome Measures [Timing]
	Baseline Disability$^{\&}$ (/24) ^{t} = Pilates 6.9 (4.6); Comparison 7.7 (5.0)		
8. Rydeard et al., 2006 [55]	39 physically active participants with subacute, recurrent, or chronic low back pain	Pilates: 3 X 60 minute supervised sessions and 6 X 15 minute home exercises per week for 4 weeks; Equipment: Mat, Reformer; Standardised protocol	Numerical Rating Scale (101 point) – Pain
	Gender (Female: Male) = Pilates 2.0: 1.0; Comparison 1.6: 1.0	No Pilates: continued regular activity and consultation with medical and health care professionals	Roland Morris Disability Questionnaire - Hong Kong
	Age$^{\&}$ (years) = Pilates 37.0 (9.0); Comparison 34.0 (8.0)		[0, 4 weeks]
	Baseline Pain Intensity$^{\&}$ (/100)^b = Pilates 23.0 (17.7); Comparison 30.4 (17.6)		
	Baseline Disability$^{\&}$ (/24)^t = Pilates 3.1(2.5); Comparison 4.2 (3.6)		
9. Zeada, 2012 [56]	20 athletes with chronic low back pain	Pilates: 4 sessions per week for 8 weeks; Equipment: Mat; Standardised protocol	Roland Morris Disability Questionnaire
	Age$^{\&}$ (years) = Pilates 23.5 (2.4); Comparison 26.2(3.6)	No Pilates: 8 weeks	[0, 8 weeks]
	Baseline Disability$^{\&}$ (/24)^t = Pilates 7.4(1.2); Comparison 6.5 (0.9)		

$^{\&}$values represent Mean [Standard Deviation];
^{a}as measured by Visual Analog Scale (11 point);
^{t}as measured by Roland Morris Disability Questionnaire;
$^+$as measured by Numerical Rating Scale (11 point);
$^\$$as measured by Oswestry Disability Index;
$^\wedge$as measured by Visual Analog Scale in mm;
^{b}as measured by the Numerical Rating Scale (101 point).

a meta-synthesis of findings from 14 RCTs, including recently published RCTs that have not been included in other reviews [21,23–26,48–56]. A meta-analyses was not conducted due to the heterogeneity of RCTs [40,41].

Pilates exercise versus usual care and physical activity

Pilates exercise results in statistically significant improvements in pain and functional ability in the short term in people with CLBP. This conclusion is based on the balance of evidence, where more high quality RCTs have reported these findings [21,24,25,55]. In addition, short term improvements in pain may be clinically significant, but not improvements in functional ability [45–47].

Another conclusion of this review is that superior improvements with Pilates exercise compared to usual care and physical activity is unlikely at 24 weeks. This is based on research evidence of one high quality RCT that has investigated the longer term effect of Pilates exercise [24]. In this RCT, though, participants had ceased Pilates exercises at 6 weeks, and it is not known if a longer lasting effect may have been present if the intervention was continued for more than 6 weeks, as is recommended in the literature [13].

These systematic review findings are similar to those of another review in that a statistically significant reduction in pain with Pilates exercise was achieved when compared to no Pilates exercise [17]. This current review clarifies, though, that this improvement may only be in the short term, and that this change may be clinically significant. In relation to functional ability, these review findings contrast with other systematic reviews as a statistically significant improvement in functional ability in the short term was identified [6,7,17]. This difference may be due to inappropriate

meta-analyses in some reviews and variable grouping of comparison treatments [13]. The size of functional improvements in RCTs in this review, however, do not appear to be clinically significant [46,47].

It should be acknowledged that not all RCTs in this review agreed regarding the effectiveness of Pilates exercise compared to usual care and physical activity [48,50,52,53]. Different results may be explained by the variable methodological quality of RCTs. For example, the majority of high quality RCTs reported statistically significant findings (4/6), while lower quality RCTs did not (2/2) [50,53].

Different results may also be due to small sample sizes or co-interventions within RCTs. Three of the 4 RCTs that did not find statistically significant findings were under-powered with small sample sizes, meaning that treatment changes may have been less easily detected [50,52,53]. The other RCT had a large sample size, but allowed the comparison group to access other interventions, such as physiotherapy and medications [48]. This may have led to the effectiveness of Pilates exercise being under estimated as the between group difference in outcome may have been reduced.

In addition, different RCT outcomes may have related to variable Pilates exercise regimes. For example, RCTs with statistically significant results prescribed supervised exercise sessions more than once a week, often with the use of specialised equipment [21,24,25,55]. It is therefore recommended that clinicians replicate Pilates exercise programs contained within RCTs with statistically significant results to maximise treatment outcomes.

Table 5. Description of Included Studies- Pilates exercise versus massage or other forms of exercise.

Study	Population	Intervention and Comparison	Outcome Measures [Timing]
1. Anderson, 2005 [49]	21 people with chronic or recurrent low back pain	Pilates: 2 X 50 minute supervised sessions per week for 6 weeks; Equipment = Reformer; Standardised protocol	Miami Back Index – Pain and Disability
	Gender (Female: Male) = 0.9: 1.0	Massage: 2 X 30 minute sessions per week for 6 weeks	Oswestry Disability Questionnaire
	Age[&] (years) = Pilates 42.4 (12.0); Comparison 44.0 (13.7)		[0, 6 weeks]
	Baseline Pain Intensity[&] (/10)[#] = Pilates 6.4 (2.5); Comparison 7.3 (1.7)		
	Baseline Disability[&] (/100)[$] = Pilates 18.6 (5.9); Comparison 16.7 (4.2)		
2. Marshall et al., 2013 [23]	64 participants with CLBP	Pilates: 3 X 50–60 minute supervised sessions per week for 8 weeks; Equipment = Mat, Reformer; Supervision Ratio = 10 clients: 1 therapist; Standardised protocol	Oswestry Disability Questionnaire
	Gender (Female: Male) = 1.7: 1.0	Cycling: 3 X 50–60 minutes supervised indoor stationary cycle training for 8 weeks	Visual Analog Scale – Pain
	Age[&] (years) 36.2(6.2)		[0, 8, 24 weeks]
	Baseline Pain Intensity[&] (/10)[a] = Pilates 3.6 (2.1); Comparison 4.5 (2.5)		
	Baseline Disability[&](/100)[$] = Pilates 25.4 (11.2); Comparison 24.0 (11.9)		
3. Gagnon, 2005 [51]	12 participants with acute and chronic low back pain	Pilates: 1–2 X 30–45 minute supervised mat sessions per week for 6–7 weeks; Standardised protocol	Revised Oswestry Disability Index
	Gender (Female: Male) = Pilates 5.0: 1.0; Comparison 2.0: 1.0	Traditional lumbar stabilisation exercise: 1–2 X 30–45 minute supervised mat sessions per week for 6–7 weeks	Visual Analog Scale – Pain
	Age[&] (years) = Pilates 36.0 (11.4); Comparison 30.3 (12.4)	(Both groups could continue physiotherapy treatment and home exercises as indicated)	[0, 4, 6–7 weeks]
	Baseline Pain Intensity[&] (/10)[a] = Pilates 3.9 (2.5); Comparison 2.1 (1.7)		
	Baseline Disability[&] (/100)[$] = Pilates 17.2 (6.1); Exercise 15.8 (3.7)		
4. Rajpal et al., 2009 [59]	40 females 20–30 years old with postural CLBP	Pilates exercise: Daily home exercise (10 repetitions with 10 second hold) over 4 weeks – progressed from crook lying, 4 point kneeling and knee extension on fit ball	Visual Analog Scale – Pain
	Age (years): Mean = 21.8	McKenzie exercise: Daily postural correction exercises (15–20 repetitions, 3 X per day) in sitting and standing	[0, 4 weeks]
5. Wajswelner et al., 2012 [26]	83 participants with CLBP or stiffness	Pilates: 2 X 60 minute supervised sessions per week, and daily home exercises for 6 weeks; Equipment: Mat, Reformer, Trapeze Table; Supervision Ratio: 4 clients: 1 therapist; Individualised, based on directional preferences	Numerical Rating Scale (11 point) - Pain
	Gender (Female: Male) = Pilates 1.3: 1.0; Comparison 1.2: 1.0	General exercise: 2 X 60 minute supervised sessions per week (including aerobic, stretching, strengthening, and stabilisation exercise) and daily home exercises for 6 weeks; Supervision Ratio: 4 clients: 1 therapist	Quebec Scale - Pain and Disability
	Age[&] (years) = Pilates 49.3 (14.1); Comparison 48.9(16.4)	(Both groups could utilise analgesic medication as required but no other form of treatment)	[0, 6, 12, 24 weeks]
	Baseline Pain Intensity[&] (/10)[+] = Pilates 4.9 (1.6); Comparison 4.6 (1.8)		
	Baseline Disability[&] (/100)[t] = Pilates 28.1 (11.4); Comparison 23.9 (14.0)		

[&]values represent Mean [Standard Deviation];
[#]as per Miami Back Index;
[$]as measured by Oswestry Disability Index;
[a]as measured by Visual Analog Scale (11 point);
[+]as measured by Numerical Rating Scale (11 point);
[t]as measured by Roland Morris Disability Questionnaire.

Pilates exercise versus massage therapy

Only one RCT compared Pilates exercise to massage therapy [49]. No statistically significant difference in improvements in pain or functional ability was noted at 6 weeks. More high quality RCTs, though, are required to confirm these findings due to the "fair" methodological quality of this RCT [34,38].

Table 6. Effectivenessof Pilates exercise versus usual care and physical activity in reducing pain in people with chronic low back pain.

Study	Methodological Quality [Score]	Population [Sample size]	Intervention and Comparison	Outcome Measure(s)	Assessment Timing	Mean Difference [95% confidence interval]
1. Borges et al., 2013 [21]	Very good [13/16]	Chronic low back pain [n = 64]	Pilates exercise versus no change in physical activity	Visual Analog Scale	15 weeks	−4.1 [−6.3 to −1.8][a]
2. da Fonseca et al., 2009 [50]	Poor [4/16]	Chronic low back pain [n = 17]	Pilates exercise versus no Pilates exercise	Visual Analog Scale	7–8 weeks	−1.9 [−5.0 to 1.2]
3. Gladwell et al., 2006 [52]	Very good [13/16]	Chronic low back pain [n = 34]	Pilates exercise versus usual care and physical activity	Visual Analog Scale – Present Pain	6 weeks	−0.2 [−0.8 to 0.4]
				Visual Analog Scale - Pain Diary	6 weeks	−0.3 [−0.9 to 0.3][+]
4. MacIntyre, 2006 [48]	Excellent [15/16]	Non-specific chronic low back pain [n = 86]	Pilates exercise versus no change in physical activity[s]	Visual Analog Scale	3 weeks	−0.4 [−1.7 to 0.9]
					12 weeks	−1.6 [−3.2 to 0.0]
5. Miyamoto et al., 2013 [24]	Excellent [16/16]	Chronic low back pain for more than 6 months [n = 22]	Pilates exercise and education versus education alone	Numerical Rating Scale (11 point)	6 weeks	−2.2 [−3.2 to −1.1][a]
					24 weeks	−0.9 [−1.9 to 0.1]
6. Quinn et al., 2011 [25]	Very good [14/16]	Chronic low back pain after physiotherapy [n = 29]	Pilates exercise versus no Pilates exercise	Visual Analog Scale	8 weeks	−1.5 [−2.1 to −0.9][a]
7. Rydeard et al., 2006 [55]	Very good [14/16]	Subacute, chronic, or recurrent low back pain, physically active [n = 39]	Pilates exercise versus no change in physical activity[s]	Numerical Rating Scale (101 point)	4 weeks	−15.6 [−17.8 to −13.4][a]

[a]statistically significant between group difference;
[+]reported as statistically significant in study, but not calculated in this review;
[s]with or without usual care.

Table 7. Effectiveness of Pilates exercise compared to usual care and physical activity in improving functional ability in people with chronic low back pain.

Study	Methodological Quality [Score]	Population [Sample size]	Intervention and Comparison	Outcome Measure(s)	Assessment Timing	Mean Difference [95% confidence interval]
1. Gladwell et al., 2006 [52]	Very good [13/16]	Chronic low back pain [n = 34]	Pilates exercise versus usual care and physical activity	Oswestry Disability Questionnaire	6 weeks	0.0 [−8.5 to 8.5]
2. MacIntyre, 2006 [48]	Excellent [15/16]	Non-specific chronic low back pain [n = 86]	Pilates exercise versus no change in physical activity[s]	Roland Morris Disability Questionnaire	3 weeks	−0.6 [−2.6 to 1.5]
					12 weeks	−2.6 [−5.2 to −0.1][a]
3. Miyamoto et al., 2013 [24]	Excellent [16/16]	Chronic low back pain for greater than 6 months [n = 22]	Pilates exercise and education versus education alone	Roland Morris Disability Questionnaire	6 weeks	−2.7 [−4.4 to −1.0][a]
					24 weeks	−1.4 [−3.1 to 0.0]
4. Quinn, 2005 [53]	Poor [6/16]	Chronic low back pain [n = 22]	Pilates exercise versus usual physical activity	Oswestry Disability Questionnaire	12 weeks	−7.1 [−17.6 to 3.4]
5. Quinn et al., 2011 [25]	Very good [14/16]	Chronic low back pain after physiotherapy [n = 29]	Pilates exercise versus no Pilates exercise	Oswestry Disability Questionnaire	8 weeks	1.3 [not given but p> 0.05]
6. Rydeard et al., 2006 [55]	Very good [14/16]	Subacute, chronic, or recurrent low back pain, physically active [n = 39]	Pilates exercise versus no change in physical activity[s]	Oswestry Disability Questionnaire	4 weeks	−1.2 [−1.4 to −1.0][a]
7. Zeada et al., 2012 [56]	Poor [4/16]	Athletes with chronic low back pain [n = 20]	Pilates exercise versus no Pilates exercise	Roland Morris Disability Questionnaire	8 weeks	1.7 [−0.4 to 3.8][+]

[s]with or without usual care;
[a]statistically significant between group difference;
[+]reported as statistically significant in the study.

Table 8. Effectiveness of Pilates exercise versus massage or other forms of exercise in reducing pain in people with chronic low back pain.

Study	Methodological Quality [Score]	Population [Sample size]	Intervention and Comparison	Outcome Measure(s)	Assessment Timing	Mean Difference [95% confidence interval]
1. Anderson, 2005 [49]	Fair [10/16]	Chronic or recurrent low back pain [n = 21]	Pilates exercise versus massage	Miami Back Index (Pain)	6 weeks	−10.8 [−25.9 to 4.3]
2. Marshall et al., 2013[23]	Excellent [15/16]	Chronic low back pain [n = 64]	Pilates exercise versus stationary cycling	Visual Analog Scale (Current pain)	8 weeks	−1.1 [−2.1 to −0.1][a]
					24 weeks	−1.4 [−2.6 to −0.2]
				Visual Analog Scale (Worst pain)	8 weeks	−0.4 [−1.4 to 0.6]
3. Gagnon, 2005 [51]	Fair [10/16]	Acute and chronic low back pain [n = 12]	Pilates exercise versus lumbar stabilisation	Visual Analog Scale	4 weeks	0.8 [−1.3 to 2.9]
					6–7 weeks	0.6 [−1.7 to 2.8]
4. Rajpal et al., 2009 [54]	Poor [5/16]	Females with chronic low back pain [n = 40]	Pilates exercise versus McKenzie exercise	Visual Analog Scale	4 weeks	−1.4 [−2.1 to −0.7][a, $]
5. Wajswelner et al., 2012 [26]	Excellent [16/16]	Chronic low back pain [n = 83]	Pilates exercise versus general exercise (mixed)	Numerical Rating Scale (11 point)	6 weeks	−0.5 [−1.3 to 0.3]
					12 weeks	−0.6 [−1.5 to 0.3]
					24 weeks	0.3 [−0.7 to 1.2]

[a]statistically significant between group difference;
[$]based on comparison of pre and post treatment scores.

Pilates exercise versus other forms of exercise

Based on current evidence, it is difficult to conclude on the short-term effectiveness of Pilates exercise in people with CLBP compared to other forms of exercise. Statistically significant improvements in pain and functional ability have been reported in one high quality RCT [23], but not in other high quality RCTs [26]. The clinical significance of reported statistically significant improvements is also unlikely [23,46,47]. There is consensus across high quality RCTs, though, that people with CLBP will experience equivalent improvements in pain and functional ability

with Pilates exercise or alternative forms of exercise at 24 weeks [23,26].

Authors of this review therefore suggest that Pilates exercise is unlikely to provide superior improvements in pain and functional ability compared to other forms of exercise, at least in the long term. Findings of this review are similar to those of previous systematic reviews in that improvements in pain and functional ability with Pilates exercise compared to other forms of exercise have not been reported as statistically significant [6,7,17]. This

Table 9. Effectiveness of Pilates exercise versus massage or other forms of exercise in improving functional ability in people with chronic low back pain.

Study	Methodological Quality [Score]	Population [Sample size]	Intervention and Comparison	Outcome Measure(s)	Assessment Timing	Mean Difference [95% confidence interval]
1. Anderson, 2005 [49]	Fair [10/16]	Chronic or recurrent low back pain [n = 21]	Pilates exercise versus massage therapy	Miami Back Index (Disability)	6 weeks	−7.9 [−1.4 to 0.3]
				Oswestry Disability Questionnaire	6 weeks	−4.0 [−10.0 to 2.0]
2. Marshall et al., 2013 [23]	Excellent [15/16]	Acute and chronic low back pain [n = 12]	Pilates exercise versus stationary cycling	Oswestry Disability Index	8 weeks	−6.5 [−11.8 to −1.1][a]
					24 weeks	4.4 [−0.7 to 9.5]
3. Gagnon, 2005 [51]	Fair [10/16]	Chronic low back pain [n = 32]	Pilates exercise versus lumbar stabilisation	Oswestry Disability Index	4 weeks	−3.0 [−11.1 to 5.1]
					6–7 weeks	−2.2 [−10.9 to 6.5]
4. Wajswelner et al., 2012 [26]	Excellent [16/16]	Chronic low back pain [n = 83]	Pilates exercise versus general exercise	Quebec Score	6 weeks	1.8 [−3.1 to 6.7]
					12 weeks	−0.8 [−6.4 to 4.8]
					24 weeks	−1.1 [−5.8 to 3.6]

[a]statistically significant between group difference.

review is different, however, in that it acknowledges that there could be differences in the short term.

There are two reasons why authors of this review have not ruled out the possibility of Pilates exercise offering superior short-term benefit over other forms of exercise. First, one of the two RCTs that reported no difference in the short term was of "fair" methodological quality [34,38]. This meant that findings were likely to be more biased than that of higher quality RCTs [38]. Second, comparison exercise treatments were variable and it could be possible that Pilates exercise is more effective than some types of exercise, but not others. When Pilates exercise was compared to a distinctly different form of exercise, cycling, there was a statistically significant difference in outcome [23]. When compared to exercises involving lumbar stabilisation, however, no difference was noted [26,51]. Future research should investigate the relative effectiveness of Pilates exercise to different forms of exercise.

Limitations

Limitations of this systematic review relate to the inclusion of only RCTs published in the English language and consequent language bias. Of the 16 studies excluded based on their language, however, only 2 appeared to be potentially relevant RCTs when reviewing titles and abstracts translated into the English language [58,59]. Another limitation was the focus of this review on outcomes of pain and functional ability in people with CLBP. Other outcomes may have also been clinically important, such as quality of life [33,60]. In addition, the methodological quality of RCTs was summarised by a total score out of 16 using the McMaster Quantitative Review Form criteria [34]. This approach can lead to oversimplification of methodological quality as all items of the scale are weighted evenly [61].

The strength of the review findings was also influenced by the availability and diversity of primary evidence. The limited number of RCTs that had compared Pilates exercise to massage therapy and other forms of exercise lessened the certainty of results [15]. The small sample sizes and short term follow up of many RCTs also affected the precision of findings [62]. Moreover, the heterogeneity of study populations, interventions, comparison treatments, outcome measures, and timing of reassessment prevented conduction of meaningful meta-analyses of RCTs [40,41].

Conclusion

According to this systematic review, Pilates exercise results in statistically significant improvements in pain and functional ability in the short term compared to usual care and physical activity in people with CLBP [21,24,25,55]. Changes in pain are more likely to be clinically significant than improvements in functional ability. At 24 weeks, though, improvements with Pilates exercise and education may be equivalent to those achieved with education alone [24]. When Pilates exercise is compared to massage therapy or other forms of exercise, equivalent improvements in pain and functional ability have been reported in people with CLBP [23,26,49].

Implications

This systematic review provides an update on the effectiveness of Pilates exercise in people with CLBP that may be used to assist clinical decision-making. Future research should investigate optimal Pilates exercise regimes for people with CLBP, including appropriate frequencies and length of programs, supervision ratios, use of home exercises, and specialised equipment [13]. Future RCTs should also investigate the long term efficacy of Pilates exercise to other treatments, such as massage, and confirm if there is any difference in effectiveness between Pilates exercise and various forms of exercise, such as aerobic exercise versus lumbar stabilisation [15]. Research into whether some people with CLBP may benefit from Pilates exercise more than others may also assist in clinical decision-making on whether Pilates exercise is suitable for individual clients [63,64].

Author Contributions

Analyzed the data: CW BH. Wrote the paper: CW. Reviewed manuscript: CW BH AB GK PM.

References

1. Charlton JE (2005) Core Curriculum for Professional Education in Pain, 3rd ed. Seattle: International Association of the Study of Pain Press.
2. Dagenais S, Caro J, Haldeman S (2008) A systematic review of low back pain cost of illness studies in the United States and internationally. Spine J 8: 8–20.
3. Hoy D, March L, Brooks P, Woolf A, Blyth F, et al. (2010) Measuring the global burden of low back pain. Best Pract Res Clin Rheumatol 24: 155–165.
4. Woolf AD, Pfleger B (2003) Burden of major musculoskeletal conditions. Bull World Health Organ 81: 646–656.
5. Brennan S, French H (2008) A questionnaire survey of the knowledge and use of Pilates based exercise for chronic low back pain amongst Irish physiotherapists. Phys Ther Rev 13: 212–213.
6. Aladro-Gonzalvo AR, Araya-Vargas GA, Machado-Diaz M, Salazar-Rojas W (2013) Pilates-based exercise for persistent, non-specific low back pain and associated functional disability: A meta-analysis with meta-regression. J Bodyw Mov Ther 17: 125–136.
7. Pereira LM, Obara K, Dias JM, Menacho MO, Guariglia DA, et al. (2012) Comparing the Pilates method with no exercise or lumbar stabilization for pain and functionality in patients with chronic low back pain: Systematic review and meta-analysis. Clin Rehabil 26: 10–20.
8. Latey P (2001) The Pilates method: History and philosophy. J Bodyw Mov Ther 5: 275–282.
9. Wells C, Kolt GS, Bialocerkowski A (2012) Defining Pilates exercise: A systematic review. Complement Ther Med 20: 253–262.
10. Hayden JA, van Tulder MW, Tomlinson G (2005) Systematic review: Strategies for using exercise therapy to improve outcomes in chronic low back pain. Ann Intern Med 142: 776–785.
11. Macedo LG, Maher CG, Latimer J, McAuley JH (2009) Motor control exercise for persistent, nonspecific low back pain: A systematic review. Phys Ther 89: 9–25.
12. Pillastrini P, Gardenghi I, Bonetti F, Capra F, Guccione A, et al. (2012) An updated overview of clinical guidelines for chronic low back pain management in primary care. Joint Bone Spine 79: 176–185.
13. Wells C, Kolt GS, Marshall P, Bialocerkowski A (2014) The definition and application of Pilates exercise to treat people with chronic low back pain: A Delphi survey of Australian physical therapists. Phys Ther 94, doi:10.2522/ptj.20130030
14. Da Luz MA, Costa LOP, Fuhro FF, Manzoni ACT, Oliveira NTB, et al. (2014) Effectiveness of mat Pilates or equipment-based Pialtes exercises in patiences with chronic nonspecific low back pain: A randomised controlled trial. Phys Ther 94: 623–631, doi 10.2522/ptj.20130277.
15. Wells C, Kolt GS, Marshall P, Hill B, Bialocerkowski A (2013) Effectiveness of Pilates exercise in treating people with chronic low back pain: A systematic review of systematic reviews. BMC Medical Research Methodology 13: 7. Available: http://www.biomedcentral.com/1471-2288/13/7. Accessed 4 February 2014.
16. La Touche R, Escalante K, Linares MT (2008) Treating non-specific chronic low back pain through the Pilates Method. J Bodyw Mov Ther 12: 364–370.
17. Lim ECW, Poh RLC, Low AY, Wong WP (2011) Effects of Pilates-based exercises on pain and disability in individuals with persistent non-specific low back pain: A systematic review with meta-analysis. J Orthop Sports Phys Ther 41:70–80.
18. Miyamoto GC, Costa LO, Cabral CM (2013) Efficacy of the Pilates method for pain and disability in patients with chronic nonspecific low back pain: A

systematic review with meta-analysis. Braz J Phys Ther 17:517–532, doi 10.1590/S1413-35552012005000127.

19. Posadzki P, Lizis P, Hagner-Derengowska M (2011) Pilates for low back pain: A systematic review. Complement Ther Clin Pract 17: 85–89.

20. Costa LOP, Hancock M, Maher C, Ostelo RWJG, Cabral CMN, et al. (2012) Pilates for low back pain (Protocol). Cochrane Database of Systematic Reviews 12:CD010265, doi: 10.1002/14651858.CD010265.

21. Borges J, Baptista AF, Santana N, Souza I, Kruschewsky RA, et al. (2014) Pilates exercises improve low back pain and quality of life in patients with HTLV-1 virus: A randomised crossover clinical trial. J Bodywork and Movt Ther 18: 68–74.

22. Brooks C, Kennedy S, Marshall PW (2012) Specific trunk and general exercise elicit similar changes in anticipatory postural adjustments in patients with chronic low back pain: A randomized controlled trial. Spine 37: E1543–E1550.

23. Marshall PW, Kennedy S, Brooks C, Lonsdale C (2013) Pilates exercise or stationary cycling for chronic nonspecific low back pain: Does it matter? A randomised controlled trial with 6 month follow-up. Spine 38: E952–959.

24. Miyamoto GC, Costa LOP, Glavanin T, Cabral CMN (2013) Efficacy of the addition of modified Pilates exercises to minimal intervention in patients with chronic low back pain: A randomised controlled trial. Phys Ther 93: 310–320. doi 10.2522/ptj.20120190.

25. Quinn K, Barry S, Barry L (2011) Do patients with chronic low back pain benefit from attending Pilates classes after completing conventional physiotherapy treatment? Physiotherapy Ireland 32:5–12.

26. Wajswelner H, Metcalf B, Bennell K (2012) Clinical pilates versus general exercise for chronic low back pain: Randomized trial. Med Sci Sports Exerc 44: 1197–1205.

27. Kunz R, Vist GE, Oxman AD (2007) Randomisation to protect against selection bias in healthcare trials. Cochrane Database Syst Rev 2: Article Number MR000012Article Number MR000012.

28. National Health and Medical Research Council (NHMRC) (2009) NHMRC additional levels of evidence and grades for recommendations for developers of guidelines. Canberra: National Health and Medical Research Council.

29. Collins J, Fauser B, Bart CJM (20050 Balancing the strengths of systematic and narrative reviews. Hum Reprod Update 11:103–104.

30. Cook D, Mulrow C, Haynes R (1997) Systematic reviews: Synthesis of best evidence for clinical decisions. Ann Intern Med 126: 376–380.

31. Hopewell S, Clarke M, Moher D, Wager E, Middleton P, et al. (2008) CONSORT for reporting randomised trials in journal and conference abstracts. Lancet 371:281–283.

32. Hayden JA, van Tulder MW, Malmivaara A, Koes BW (2005) Exercise therapy for treatment of non-specific low back pain. Cochrane Database Syst Rev 3: Article Number CD000335.

33. Chapman JR, Norvell DC, Hermsmeyer JT, Bransford RJ, DeVine J, et al. (2011) Evaluating common outcomes for measuring treatment success for chronic low back pain. Spine 36: S54–68.

34. Law M, MacDermid J (1998) Evidence-based rehabilitation (2nd Ed.). Thorofare, New Jersey: Slack.

35. Katrack P, Bialocerkowski AE, Massy-Westropp N, Kumar VSS, Grimmer KA (2004) A systematic review of the content of critical appraisal tools. BMC Med Res Methodol 4:22. Available: http://www.biomedcentral.com/1471-2288/4/22. Accessed 4 February 2014.

36. Lekkas P, Larson T, Kumar S, Grimmer K, Nyland L, et al. (2007) No model of clinical education for physiotherapy students is superior to another: A systematic review. Aust J Physiother 53: 19–28.

37. Schabrun SM, Hillier S (2009) Evidence for the retraining of sensation after stroke: A systematic review. Clin Rehabil 23: 27–39.

38. Daly A, Bialocerkowski A (2009) Does evidence support physiotherapy management of adult complex regional pain syndrome type one: A systematic review. Eur J Pain 13: 339–353.

39. Viera AJ, Garrett JM (2005) Understanding inter-observer agreement: The kappa statistic. Family Medicine 37: 360–363.

40. Fletcher J (2007) What is heterogeneity and is it important? BMJ 334:94–96.

41. Higgins JPT, Thompson SG, Deeks JJ, Altman DG (2003) Measuring inconsistency in meta-analyses. BMJ 327: 557–560. Available: http://www.bmj.com/content/327/7414/557. Accessed 7 May 2014.

42. Riley RD, Higgins JPT, Deeks J (2011) Interpretation of random effects meta-analyses. BMJ 342: d549. Available: http://www.bmj.com/content/342/bmj.d549. Accessed 7 May 2014.

43. The Cochrane Collaboration (2012) Review Manager (RevMan) [Computer program]. Version 5.2 Copenhagen: The Nordic Cochrane Centre.

44. Herbert R (2013) Confidence Interval Calculator. Available: http://www.pedro.org.au/english/downloads/confidence-interval-calculator/. Accessed 7 May 2014.

45. Van Tulder M, Malmivaara A, Hayden J, Koes B (2007) Statistical significance versus clinical importance: Trials on exercise therapy for chronic low back pain as example. Spine 32:1785–1790.

46. Ostelo RW, de Vet HC (2005) Clinically important outcomes in low back pain. Best Pract Res Clin Rheumatol 19: 593–607.

47. Ostelo RW, Deyo RA, Stratford P, Waddell G, Croft P, et al. (2008) Interpreting change scores for pain and functional status in low back pain: Towards international consensus regarding minimal importance change. Spine 33: 90–94.

48. MacIntyre L (2006) The effect of Pilates on patients' chronic low back pain: A pilot study [dissertation]. Johannesburg: University of the Witwatersrand.

49. Anderson B (2005). Randomised clinical trial comparing active versus passive approaches to the treatment of recurrent and chronic low back pain [dissertation]. Miami, Florida: University of Miami.

50. da Fonseca JL, Magini M, de Freitas TH (2009) Laboratory gait analysis in patients with low back pain before and after a Pilates intervention. J Sport Rehabil 18:269–282.

51. Gagnon LH (2005) Efficacy of Pilates exercises as therapeutic intervention in treating patients with low back pain [dissertation]. Knoxville: University of Tennessee.

52. Gladwell V, Head S, Haggar M, Beneke R (2006) Does a program of Pilates improve chronic nonspecific low back pain? J Sport Rehabil 15:338–350.

53. Quinn J (2005) Influence of Pilates-based mat exercise on chronic lower back pain [dissertation]. Boca Raton, FL: Florida Atlantic University.

54. Rajpal N, Arora M, Chauhan V (2008) The study on efficacy of Pilates and McKenzie exercise in postural low back pain – A rehabilitative protocol. Physiotherapy and Occupational Therapy Journal 1:33–56.

55. Rydeard R, Leger A, Smith D (2006) Pilates-based therapeutic exercise: Effect on subjects with nonspecific chronic low back pain and functional disability: A randomized controlled trial. J Orthop Sports Phys Ther 36: 472–484.

56. Zeada MA (2011) Ffects of Pilates on low back pain and urine catecholamine. Ovidius University Annals, Series Physiotherapy Education and Sport 12:41–47.

57. Rydeard RA (2001) Evaluation of a targeted exercise rehabilitation approach and its effectiveness in the treatment of pain, functional disability and muscle function in a population with longstanding unresolved low back pain [dissertation]. Kingston, Canada: Queens University.

58. Kawanishi CY, de Oliveira MR, Coelho VS, Parreira RB, de Oliveira RF, et al. (2011) Effect of Pilates exercise on trunk function and pain in patients with low back pain [Portuguese]. Revista Terapia Manual 9:410–417.

59. Montero-Camra J, Sierra-Silvestre E, Monteagudo-Saiz AM, Lepez-Fernandez J, Lopez-Lopez A, et al. (2013) Active eccentric stretch against passive analytical hamstring stretch in subacute or chronic non-specific low back pain: A pilot trial [Spanish]. Fisioterapia 35: 206–213, doi 19.1016/j.ft.2012.10.004.

60. Dworkin RH, Turk DC, Farrar JT, Haythornthwaite JA, Jensen MP, et al. (2005) Core outcome measures for chronic pain clinical trials: IMMPACT recommendations. Pain 113: 9–119.

61. Colle F, Rannou F, Revel M, Fermanian J, Poiraudeau S (2002) Impact of quality scales on levels of evidence inferred from a systematic review of exercise therapy and low back pain. Arch Phys Med Rehabil 83: 1745–1752.

62. Noordzij M, Tripepi Giovanni, Dekker FW, Zoccali C, et al. (2010) Sample size calculations: Basic principles and common pitfalls. Nephrol Dial Transplant 25: 1388–1393.

63. Stolze LR, Allison SC, Childs JD (2012) Derivation of a preliminary clinical prediction rule for identifying a subgroup of patients with low back pain likely to benefit from Pilates-based exercise. J Orthop Sports Phys Ther 42: 425–436.

64. Wells C, Kolt GS, Marshall P, Bialocerkowski A (2014) Indications, benefits, and risks of Pilates exercise for people with chronic low back pain: A Delphi survey of Pilates trained physical therapists. Phys Ther, doi 10.2522/ptj20130568.

2

The Association between the History of Cardiovascular Diseases and Chronic Low Back Pain in South Koreans

In-Hyuk Ha[1,2]*, Jinho Lee[1,3], Me-riong Kim[1], Hyejin Kim[1], Joon-Shik Shin[1]

1 Jaseng Medical Foundation, Jaseng Hospital of Korean Medicine, Seoul, Republic of Korea, 2 Graduate School of Public Health & Institute of Health and Environment, Seoul National University, Gwanak-ro, Gwanak-gu, Seoul, Korea, 3 Department of Herbology, Graduate School of Korean Medicine, Kyung Hee University, Seoul, Republic of Korea

Abstract

Background: Cardiovascular disease and related risk factors have been suggested as a mechanism leading to atherosclerosis of the lumbar vessels and consequent lumbar pain or sciatica. But there is continued controversy concerning its generalization. This study examined whether cardiovascular disease or its risk factors were associated with chronic low back pain (cLBP) in Koreans.

Methods: Health surveys and examinations were conducted on a nationally representative sample (n = 23,632) of Koreans. A total of 13,841 eligible participants (aged 20 to 89 years) were examined to determine the association between cardiovascular disease, the Framingham risk score, major cardiovascular risk factors (blood pressure, diabetes, cholesterol, and smoking habits) and chronic LBP.

Results: The total prevalence of cLBP was 16.6% (men: 10.8%, women: 21.1%) and that in patients with a history of cardiovascular diseases was 36.6% (men: 26.5%, women: 47.1%). The results showed that patients' medical history of cardiovascular disease was significantly associated with cLBP in both men and women when adjusted for covariates (men: OR 2.16; 95%CI 1.34~3.49; women: OR 2.26; 95%CI 1.51~3.38). No association was observed between cLBP and the Framingham risk score, medication for hyperlipemia, hypertension, diabetes, and major cardiovascular risk factors (systolic blood pressure, total cholesterol, high density lipoprotein cholesterol, triglycerides, glucose and smoking habits) in either men or women.

Conclusions: The prevalence of cLBP is correlated to a history of cardiovascular disease, but not to the major cardiovascular risk factors from the Framingham study. Further studies on whether these results were affected by psychological factors in patients with a history of cardiovascular diseases or whether new potential risk factors from the artery atherosclerosis hypothesis applying to Koreans exist are needed.

Editor: Yiru Guo, University of Louisville, United States of America

Funding: The authors have no support or funding to report.

Competing Interests: The authors have declared that no competing interests exist.

* E-mail: hanihata@gmail.com

Introduction

Low back pain (LBP) is a common disorder which negatively impacts both individual and society. 70 to 80% of adults suffer from low back pain at some point in their lives [1]. Approximately 6 to 10% patients who initially suffer from acute LBP develop chronic LBP or experience repeated fluctuating pain episodes, and health care services are needed to counteract symptoms which in turn incur substantial social costs [2]. LBP is the fifth most frequent reason for clinic visits in the United States [3]. In addition, indirect costs related to work loss are also substantial with many patients reporting dysfunction and disruption of daily activities and work due to pain, and 2% of the U.S. work-force are compensated for back injuries each year [4]. Therefore, a more accurate and efficient screening system for risk factors of chronic LBP seems important for better understanding and prevention of the transition to chronic pain and disability.

There have been many studies aiming to determine the cause of LBP, and it has usually been accepted that biomechanical loading of the spine [5], smoking [6], psychosocial influences [7], obesity [8], and BMI [9,10] are causes of low back pain. Studies on whether cardiovascular disease and its risk factors could be a cause of low back pain initially began with the evaluation of 56 postmortem lumbar aortograms. Eighty-eight percent of subjects with back pain history had one or more missing lumbar arteries which was high when compared with the 59% of age-matched controls [11]. Atherosclerosis of the lumbar arteries has received continued attention as a possible underlying factor for back disorders as ischemia of the lumbar spine can cause damage or degeneration of the main structure causing pain [12]. Studies have also been conducted not only on atherosclerosis, but also on the association of serum lipids and blood pressure, which can be the cause of atherosclerosis and perhaps back pain [1].

The Framingham Heart Study introduced the concept of risk factors in cardiovascular diseases by identifying common factors that contribute to cardiovascular disease by following its development over 50 years [13]. The Framingham risk score estimates the 10 year risk of cardiovascular disease by assessing the following factors which affect cardiovascular disease – gender, age, systolic blood pressure (SBP), use of hypertension treatment, smoking habits, diabetes mellitus, total cholesterol, and high density lipoprotein(HDL) cholesterol [14]. Therefore, the Framingham risk score could be useful in examining the association between cardiovascular risk factors and chronic LBP.

The present study aimed to find out whether the Framingham risk score and main risk factors of cardiovascular diseases such as blood pressure, diabetes, cholesterol and smoking habits, as determined by the Framingham study were associated with chronic LBP. The possible confounding effects of socioeconomic status (education, income and occupation), lifestyle risk factors (alcohol drinking and exercise habits) and BMI, which is closely related to serum lipid, were considered in the analysis. The study sample was representative of the Korean adult population.

Methods

2.1. Study Population and Sampling

This study was based on data obtained from the Korean National Health and Nutritional Examination Survey (KNHANES) IV (2007–2009), which used a rolling sampling design that involved a complex, stratified, multistage, probability-cluster survey of a representative sample of the non-institutionalized civilian population of South Korea. The survey was performed by the Korean Ministry of Health and Welfare and had three components: the health survey, health examination, and nutrition survey. Further information can be found in "The 4th (2007–2009) KNHANES Sample Design" and the 1st~3rd Sample Design reports, which are available on the KNHANES website [15]. The data from KHANES is available on request by email if the applicant logs onto the 'Korea National Health and Nutrition Examination Survey' website and specifies which annual reports he or she needs. The KNHANES IV (2007–2009) examination and health survey was completed by 23,632 subjects (74.5% of the total target population of 31,705). The present analysis was confined to 13,841 respondents aged 20 to 89 years who answered the back pain examination survey and had no missing values of covariance or cardiovascular risk factors.

2.2. Chronic Low Back Pain

Chronic LBP patients were defined as individuals who reported episodes of back pain lasting three months or longer during the previous year in the health survey.

2.3. Cardiovascular Disease Patients, Cerebrovascular Disease Patients

Cardiovascular disease patients were defined as individuals who reported having suffered from cardiac infarction or angina. Cerebrovascular disease patients were defined as individuals who reported having experienced ischemic stroke(s).

2.4. The Framingham Risk Score

Of the 13,841 total target population, individuals with cardiovascular or cerebrovascular disease history were excluded, and 13,299 patients were assessed for the association between Framingham risk scores, hyperlipemia, hypertension, and diabetes medication, and chronic LBP. The Framingham risk score was calculated through an algorithm using the serum total cholesterol(TChol) level. This algorithm divided the subjects in 9 groups by age and further divided them into 5 subgroups within 4 categories(total cholesterol level, high-density lipoprotein cholesterol level, systolic blood pressure, diastolic blood pressure). We assigned risk values to each group according to their gender. The subjects were categorized into subgroups by whether or not they currently smoked or had diabetes, and again assigned risk values according to their gender. The Framingham risk score was calculated as the sum of the values resulting from these 6 steps. Conclusively, the possibility of risk factors with regard to the calculator prepared by R.B. D'Agostino et al. [16] was obtained and the outcomes were classified into five groups according to risk. The group with the highest risk factor was compared to the other groups.

2.5. Hyperlipemia, Hypertension and Diabetes

In the Seventh Joint National Committee on the Prevention, Detection, Evaluation, and Treatment of High Blood Pressure (JNC 7), prehypertension was defined to be systolic blood pressure (SBP) in the range of 120 mmgHg to 139 mmgHg, or diastolic blood pressure (DBP) from 80 mmHg to 89 mmHg. Hypertension was defined when SBP was above 140 mmHg, DBP was above 90 mmHg or when taking medication for blood pressure control. Following National Cholesterol Education Program Adults Treatment Panel III(NCEP ATPIII) [17], hypercholesterolemia was defined when TChol was above 240 mg/dl or when patients were already on medication for control of hypercholesterolemia. Triglycerides(TG) above 200 mg/dl was defined as hyperlipidemia and HDL below 40 mg/dl was defined as low HDL cholestrolemia. According to the American Diabetes Association, impaired fasting glucose was defined as a fasting glucose level between 110 mg/dL to 125 mg/dL. Fasting glucose level above 126 mg/dl or those on insulin medication treatment were defined as diabetes.

2.6. Cardiovascular Risk Factors

We investigated the cardiovascular risk factors of 10,592 people who had no history of cardio-cerebrovascular disease and no history of medication taken for hyperlipemia, hypertension, or diabetes. Smoking status was divided into three categories; current smokers, past smokers and nonsmokers. Systolic and diastolic pressure are presented as the mean value of the second and third blood pressure measurements out of three independent measurements. Serum concentrations of TChol, HDL cholesterol, TG, and glucose after a minimum 8 hour fast were analyzed. For BP analyses, the upper half of the group(>148 mmHg) with systolic blood pressure above 140 mmHg was compared to the prehypertension(120–138 mmHg) and normal blood pressure groups(≤119 mmHg), and the upper half of the group(> 95 mmHg) with diastolic blood pressure above 90 mmHg was compared to the prehypertension(80–89 mmHg) and normal groups(≤79 mmHg). In analyzing total cholesterol and TG, the upper half of the groups with values above normal range(cholesterol≥255 mg/dl, triglycerides≥255 mg/dl) were compared to the upper(cholesterol 183–239 mg/dl, triglycerides≥255 mg/dl) and lower halves of the normal range groups(cholesterol≤182, triglycerides≤102). The lower half(≤35 mg/dl) of patients in the hypoalphalipoproteinemia group was compared to the upper(≥ 51 mg/dl) and lower halves(40–50 mg/dl) of the normal range group(≥40 mg/dl). For glucose, the diabetic group(≥126 mg/dl), impaired fast glucose group(110–125 mg/dl) and normal group(≤ 109 mg/dl) were compared.

Table 1. Associations by cardiovascular and cerebrovascular disease with chronic low back pain in Koreans aged 20 to 89 years.

		n (cases)	Adjusted for age OR	95% CI	Fully adjusted[a] OR	95% CI
Cardiovascular diseases						
Men	No	5925(618)	1.00		1.00	
	Yes	147(39)	2.09	1.32–3.30	2.16	1.34–3.49
Women	No	7629(1571)	1.00		1.00	
	Yes	140(66)	2.43	1.64–3.60	2.26	1.51–3.38
Cerebrovascular diseases						
Men	No	5934(622)	1.00		1.00	
	Yes	138(35)	1.74	1.02–2.97	1.53	0.91–2.58
Women	No	7631(1566)	1.00		1.00	
	Yes	138(71)	2.14	1.41–3.24	1.95	1.28–2.97

Logistic regression analysis. Odds ratios (OR) and 95% confidence intervals (CI).
[a]Adjusted for age, education, household income, occupation, BMI, alcohol drinking and exercise habits.

All blood analyses were carried out by Seoul Institution of Medicine and Science and Neodin Medical Institute (NMI) which are both institutions certified by the Korean Ministry of Health and Welfare.

2.7. Covariates

The gender, age, socioeconomic status, and lifestyle of subjects were analyzed. Education was classified as ≤6, 7–9, 10–12 or >13 years of formal education. Households were broken into income quartiles by gender and age according to the average monthly household income adjusted for family size using the equivalence scale (monthly household income/number of household members). Occupation classification was further divided from the Korean Standard Classification of Occupation, 6th revision into 7 groups; (a) administrator, manager, or professional practitioner, (b) office worker, (c) service or retail industry worker, (d) agriculture or fishery industry worker, (e) equipment mechanic or machinery operator, (f) manual worker, and (g) unemployed. BMI (kg/m^2) was categorized into 3 brackets according to physical measurements (<18.5, 18.5–24.9, 25≤). Alcohol consumption was divided into two categories; nondrinkers (those with no alcohol consumption during the past year or whose frequency of alcohol intake was less than once a month) and drinkers (those with alcohol consumption at least once a month). Regular exercise patterns were sorted according to whether subjects did heavy exercise (running, climbing, fast biking, etc.) at least 20 minutes/session, 3 times/week, light exercise (swimming, tennis doubles, volleyball, etc.) at least 30 minutes/session, 5 times/week, or walked at least 30 minutes/session, 5 times/week during the past week.

2.8. Statistical Analysis

Logistic regression analysis was used to estimate associations between cardiovascular diseases, the Framingham risk score, hypertension, hypercholesterolemia, hypertriglyceridemia, hypoalphalipoproteinemia, diabetes, medication, serum lipid levels, blood glucose levels, blood pressure, smoking and low back pain with adjustments made for covariates. The statistical packages for Social Science for Windows, version 11.0 (SPSS Inc., Chicago, IL, U.S.A.) were used. Population weights were applied to the analyses to correct the distributions of the cluster sample regarding Primary Sampling Unit, covariance, and significance to correspond with those of the Korean population.

2.9. Ethics Statement

The interviewer was not given any prior information about a participant before he/she performed the interview, and all participants provided written consent to participate in the survey. The study protocol was approved by the Institutional Review Board of Jaseng Hospital of Korean Medicine in Seoul, Korea.

Results

The total prevalence of chronic LBP was 16.6% (10.8% in men and 21.1% in women) and that of chronic LBP in patients who suffered from cardiovascular diseases was 36.6% (26.5% in men and 47.1% in women). In both men and women, the prevalence of chronic LBP was higher in subjects with a history of cardiovascular diseases than those with no history of cardiovascular diseases(Fully adjusted OR was 2.16 in men and 2.26 in women) (Table 1). The average and standard deviation of age, blood pressure, total cholesterol, HDL, TG, glucose levels and Framingham risk scores in patients who had no history of cerebro-cardiovascular diseases are listed by gender in Table 2. The covariates used were education, household income, occupation, BMI, alcohol drinking and exercise habits. Table 3 shows the age-adjusted relationships of covariates with chronic LBP.

There were no statistically significant differences between the groups in the Framingham risk scores. In addition, there was no significant association between hyperlipidemia, hypertriglyceridemia, hypoalphalipoproteinemia, and diabetes with chronic LBP. The prevalence of chronic LBP was significantly lower in men who had hypertension compared to those who didn't, but no associations were seen among women (Table 4).

Diastolic pressure was associated with chronic LBP in both men and women, and glucose was found to be associated in women (Table 5).

The subjects with normal systolic blood pressure(≤79) had a higher incidence of cLBP than those in the upper half of the group(>95 mmHg) with diastolic blood pressure above 90 mmHg(the age adjusted OR was 2.12 in men and 1.61 in women). The estimates were little affected by the addition of covariates in the model. There was no relationship between

Table 2. Descriptive statistics of cardiovascular risk factors [a].

	Men	Women
	mean(S.D.)	mean(S.D.)
Age(years)	47.8 (15.4)	48.3 (16.0)
Systolic blood pressure(mmHg)	120.7 (15.9)	115.5 (18.0)
Diastolic blood pressure(mmHg)	79.6 (10.6)	74.1 (10.5)
Total cholesterol(mg/dl)	187.0 (34.7)	187.5 (35.7)
HDL- cholesterol(mg/dl)	47.9 (12.0)	53.3 (12.7)
Triglycerides(mg/dl)	156.7 (126.2)	114.1 (79.4)
Glucose(mg/dl)	99.1 (24.0)	96.1 (22.9)
Framingham risk score(%)	12.8 (12.9)	10.8 (13.0)
Medication of hypertension[b]	14.1%	16.3%
Medication of hyperlipemia[b]	2.1%	3.5%
Medication of diabetes[b]	5.3%	5.1%

[a]Subjects with no history of cardiovascular disease or cerebrovascular disease.
[b]Percentage of patients on medication for hypertension, hyperlipidemia or diabetes in total subjects.

systolic blood pressure, total cholesterol, TG, HDL, or smoking with chronic LBP in either men or women. For a more contrastive comparison, we divided the abnormal value group into 2 groups and compared the most extreme measurement group with normal ranges.

Discussion

Our study found that the risk of chronic LBP increased in both men and women who had a history of cardiovascular diseases. But the Framingham risk score which predicts the danger of cardiovascular disease and almost all major cardiovascular risk factors were not associated with chronic LBP. The study sample was representative of Korean men and women aged 20 to 89 years. Our results are consistent with previous studies that reported cardiovascular diseases are associated with chronic LBP. Several studies have reported that, similar to our study results, cardiovascular diseases are related to LBP [11,18] and lumbar disc degeneration[19–23] using the atherosclerosis hypothesis.

It cannot be stated that cardiovascular disease risk factors are associated with chronic LBP just on the basis that cardiovascular diseases and vessel abnormality are related with chronic LBP. In our study results, although there was a strong connection between chronic LBP and cardiovascular diseases, no consistent associations were found between chronic LBP and the major or "traditional" risk factors, especially the major Independent Risk Factors for CHD [14], which include serum total cholesterol, HDL cholesterol, triglycerides, diabetes mellitus and smoking. The association of these risk factors with chronic LBP has been a matter of controversy in many studies. High cholesterol [24,25], high LDL cholesterol [24,25], low HDL cholesterol [26], high triglycerides [24,25,27], diabetes [28] and hypertension [28,29] have been found to be significantly and independently associated with LBP.

A systematic review by Shiri et al. [1] on cardiovascular and lifestyle risk factors and the relationship with lumbar radicular pain (sciatica) found obesity, a long smoking history, and serum C-reactive protein to be associated with sciatica, whereas no consistent associations between sciatica and serum lipid levels or

high blood pressure were found. Another study reported that there was no association between diabetes and LBP [30].

Contrary to our assumption that hypertension patients would have a higher incidence of LBP, diastolic blood pressure was shown to have a negative correlation with LBP in both men and women. These results may result from lower susceptibility to musculoskeletal pain (ex. LBP) in people with high blood pressure [31]. Adverse to our initial prediction, the diabetic group presented a lower prevalence rate of low back pain when compared to the normal group. This may possibly be an error due to the small diabetic group.

Some major strengths of our study are that the sample group is a large-scale, nationally representative sample of Koreans, and the health examination and questionnaire surveys were conducted by trained interviewers in a standardized manner. Moreover, we analyzed not only the association between each major risk factor of cardiovascular disease and chronic LBP, but also whether cardiovascular risk factors could successfully predict chronic LBP using the Framingham risk score, and in this analyses, we were able to control for a number of potential confounders of chronic LBP, such as age, gender, BMI, household income, occupation, education, exercise, and alcohol drinking habits.

Two nationally representative sample studies on the relationship between LBP and cardiovascular disease risk factors have been published recently, and they are each based on the Finnish [32] and Norwegian population [27]. Leino-Arjas et al. reported that serum total cholesterol, LDL cholesterol and triglyceride levels had a significant association with sciatica in the Finnish population, and Heuch et al. reported that HDL cholesterol and triglycerides were related to LBP in the Norwegian population, which are not consistent with our results. This contrast between nationalities may result from the difference in dependent variables (sciatica vs. chronic LBP) or possibly the ethnic and cultural environmental diversities between Caucasians and Asians. A vast body of studies show across various ethnicities and cultures that relatively high risk factors of associated diseases are not necessarily reflected in the incidence rate [33,34] and that occurrence rates within similar disease groups demonstrate racial differences [35].

Also, our study revealed that Koreans are relatively healthy. The incidence rate of chronic LBP of ≥3 months was 10.8% in

Table 3. Associations by background factors with age-adjusted odds ratios (OR) and 95% confidence intervals (CI) for chronic low back pain among Koreans aged 20 to 89 years[a].

	Men			Women		
	n(case)	OR	95% CI	n(case)	OR	95% CI
Household income						
Low	972(168)	1.00		1583(541)	1.00	
Fairly low	1416(150)	0.88	0.66–1.17	1880(371)	0.78	0.64–0.94
Fairly high	1653(148)	0.84	0.61–1.16	1999(311)	0.75	0.61–0.92
High	1757(123)	0.69	0.50–0.95	2039(281)	0.69	0.55–0.86
Education(years)						
≤6	1060(212)	1.00		2442(541)	1.00	
7–9	712(104)	0.95	0.70–1.28	788(371)	0.71	0.56–0.90
10–12	2124(174)	0.72	0.53–0.99	2524(311)	0.58	0.45–0.74
>13	1902(99)	0.52	0.37–0.74	1747(281)	0.49	0.37–0.65
Occupation						
Administrator, manager, or professional practitioner	946(52)	1.00		748(61)	1.00	
Office worker	599(23)	0.58	0.33–1.02	493(31)	0.66	0.40–1.09
Service or retail industry worker	723(34)	0.75	0.46–1.22	1073(155)	1.23	0.87–1.74
Agriculture or fishery industry worker	707(163)	2.76	1.77–4.32	701(296)	3.07	2.01–4.67
Equipment mechanic or machinery operator	1181(101)	1.25	0.86–1.81	207(33)	1.63	0.87–3.06
Manual worker	492(54)	1.25	0.78–2.01	766(149)	1.17	0.80–1.72
Unemployed(student, housewife, etc.)	1150(162)	1.78	1.18–2.67	3513(779)	1.41	1.00–1.99
Regular exercise						
No	2346(213)	1.00		3402(623)	1.00	
Yes	3452(376)	1.07	0.84–1.35	4099(881)	1.28	1.11–1.48
Alcohol drinking						
No	1471(201)	1.00		4532(1071)	1.00	
At least once a month	4327(388)	0.85	0.67–1.07	2969(433)	0.88	0.75–1.04
BMI(kg/m²)						
<18.5,	205(30)	1.00		403(50)	1.00	
18.5–24.9	3558(379)	0.78	0.46–1.32	4965(929)	1.15	0.80–1.65
25≤	2035(180)	0.75	0.43–1.29	2133(525)	1.26	0.86–1.84

Logistic regression analysis.
[a]Subjects with no history of cardiovascular disease or cerebrovascular disease.

Korean men and 21.1% in women, whereas it was 21% in Norwegian men and 26% in women. Koreans showed better health statistics in the anthropometric risk factor indices than Finnish and Norwegian populations too and this may have partially caused the racial differences in the association with cardiovascular risk factors. The fact that other studies did not consider cerebrovascular diseases occurring in relation with atherosclerosis may have relatively influenced the results as well.

Furthermore, 8-hour fasting prior to laboratory examination was conducted in our study to achieve higher accuracy in the cholesterol and triglyceride measures. However, the Finnish population underwent 4-hour fasting, and the Norwegian population were not regulated for the amount of fasting, but were adjusted for covariates statistically instead.

The limitations of the present study are as follows; first, the cross-sectional design of this study does not allow for definite conclusions be drawn about the causal relationship; second, the hypothesis that atherosclerosis of lumbar arteries may lead to disc degeneration, which may, in turn, cause chronic LBP or sciatica in

people with cardiovascular disease or its risk factors is a weak point in that the low back region is infamous for its asymptomatic abnormalities [36].

Accordingly, even if the lumbar intervertebral disc or surrounding structures happen to be damaged or altered by atherosclerosis, there may be an absence of chronic LBP symptoms, rendering it difficult to affirm their correlation.

Also, we did not recognize the possibility of a direct correlation between cardiovascular disease and LBP, and this may be at variance with the atherosclerosis hypothesis proposed in this study. Additional limitations are that a major risk factor of cardiovascular disease – LDL cholesterol – was not included as a variable in our study, and that a minimum 8 hour fast may not have been enough to achieve completely reliable blood results regarding TG.

The reason why almost all major cardiovascular risk factors were not associated with chronic LBP in our study could be because of low statistical power due to the limited number of cases in the data or other potential biases due to the cross-sectional design nature of the study. These possibilities set aside, the results

Table 4. Associations by Framingham risk score and cardiovascular risk factors with chronic low back pain in Koreans aged 20 to 89 years[a].

	Men					Women				
	n(case)	Adjusted for age		Fully adjusted[c]		n(case)	Adjusted for age		Fully adjusted[c]	
		OR	95% CI	OR	95% CI		OR	95% CI	OR	95% CI
Framingham risk score[b]										
High	1159(219)	1.00		1.00		1500(603)	1.00		1.00	
Middle	2320(235)	0.77	0.56–1.05	0.89	0.65–1.21	3001(607)	0.84	0.68–1.03	0.89	0.72–1.09
Low	2319(135)	0.93	0.57–1.51	1.11	0.65–1.91	3000(294)	1.00	0.71–1.42	1.25	0.86–1.82
Hypertension										
Normal	2152(224)	1.00		1.00		4122(607)	1.00		1.00	
Prehypertension	1820(169)	0.89	0.68–1.16	0.90	0.68–1.18	1489(305)	0.93	0.78–1.13	0.89	0.73–1.08
Hypertension	1826(196)	0.63	0.48–0.83	0.63	0.47–0.85	1890(592)	0.97	0.80–1.17	0.92	0.75–1.11
Hypercholesterolemia										
No	5272(538)	1.00		1.00		6643(1273)	1.00		1.00	
Yes	526(51)	0.77	0.53–1.12	0.80	0.55–1.18	858(231)	0.91	0.74–1.12	0.92	0.74–1.13
Hypertriglyceridemia										
No	4490(469)	1.00		1.00		6722(1277)	1.00		1.00	
Yes	1308(120)	0.88	0.69–1.12	0.90	0.70–1.16	779(227)	1.15	0.94–1.41	1.10	0.90–1.35
Hypoalphalipoproteinemia										
No	3822(382)	1.00		1.00		6040(1121)	1.00		1.00	
Yes	1976(207)	0.97	0.78–1.20	0.98	0.78–1.24	1461(383)	1.13	0.96–1.32	1.07	0.91–1.25
Diabetes										
Normal	3891(373)	1.00		1.00		5723(1048)	1.00		1.00	
Impaired Fasting Glucose	1340(138)	0.87	0.69–1.10	0.90	0.71–1.15	1179(278)	0.89	0.74–1.07	0.87	0.72–1.05
Diabetes	567(78)	0.94	0.68–1.29	0.94	0.67–1.30	599(178)	0.86	0.68–1.08	0.82	0.65–1.03

Logistic regression analysis. Odds ratios (OR) and 95% confidence intervals (CI).
[a]Indicates subjects with no history of cardiovascular or cerebrovascular diseases. Diagnosis was made when patients met international standards or were already on medications for associated diseases.
[b]High indicates the uppermost quintile of the highest, middle 2nd and 3rd quintiles and lowest two quintiles.
[c]Adjusted for age, education, household income, occupation, BMI, alcohol drinking and exercise habits.

Table 5. Associations by cardiovascular risk factors with chronic low back pain among Koreans aged 20 to 89 years[a].

	Men	Adjusted for age		Fully adjusted[c]		Women	Adjusted for age		Fully adjusted[c]	
	n(case)	OR	95% CI	OR	95% CI	n(case)	OR	95% CI	OR	95% CI
Systolic blood pressure(mmHg)[b]										
Hypertension (≥148)	224(32)	1.00		1.00		203(49)	1.00		1.00	
Hypertention((140–148)	218(22)	0.86	0.43–1.69	0.85	0.42–1.71	209(62)	1.39	0.82–2.35	1.33	0.78–2.26
Pre-hypertension (120–139)	1585(156)	1.22	0.74–2.02	1.29	0.78–2.13	1153(267)	1.54	0.99–2.39	1.46	0.94–2.28
Normal (≤119)	2767(250)	1.30	0.81–2.08	1.44	0.90–2.31	4462(628)	1.40	0.90–2.17	1.43	0.92–2.22
Diastolic blood pressure(mmHg)[b]										
Hypertension (≥95)	360(22)	1.00		1.00		200(35)	1.00		1.00	
Hypertension(90–95)	466(37)	1.48	0.81–2.69	1.54	0.84–2.80	220(45)	1.43	0.79–2.57	1.48	0.81–2.68
Prehypertension (80–89)	1514(122)	1.68	0.95–2.97	1.76	0.99–3.12	1092(217)	1.47	0.94–2.31	1.56	1.00–2.44
Normal (≤79)	2454(279)	2.12	1.23–3.63	2.15	1.24–3.75	4515(709)	1.61	1.06–2.45	1.71	1.12–2.62
Total cholesterol(mg/dl)[b]										
Hypercholesterolemia (≥255)	169(15)	1.00		1.00		212(43)	1.00		1.00	
Hypercholesterolemia(240–255)	185(16)	1.13	0.49–2.61	1.23	0.53–2.86	213(40)	0.95	0.54–1.67	0.92	0.51–1.66
Upper normal (183–239)	2207(204)	1.37	0.72–2.61	1.47	0.77–2.81	2813(538)	1.27	0.85–1.90	1.22	0.81–1.84
Lower normal (≤182)	2233(225)	1.57	0.83–2.96	1.64	0.87–3.10	2789(385)	1.31	0.88–1.97	1.29	0.85–1.96
Triglycerides(mg/dl)[b]										
Hypertriglyceridemia (≥268)	511(49)	1.00		1.00		225(47)	1.00		1.00	
Hypertriglyceridemia(200–268)	518(42)	0.79	0.47–1.34	0.81	0.47–1.40	223(49)	0.93	0.54–1.61	1.01	0.58–1.77
Upper normal (103–199)	1884(182)	0.93	0.64–1.36	0.99	0.65–1.52	2760(498)	0.99	0.67–1.45	1.07	0.72–1.58
Lower normal (≤102)	1881(187)	0.99	0.67–1.46	0.96	0.65–1.44	2819(412)	1.13	0.76–1.67	1.24	0.83–1.86
HDL- cholesterol(mg/dl)[b]										
Upper normal (≥51)	1803(186)	1.36	0.92–2.00	1.32	0.87–1.99	2713(400)	1.10	0.76–1.57	1.17	0.81–1.68
Lower normal (40–50)	1837(185)	1.49	1.01–2.20	1.43	0.96–2.13	2653(490)	1.19	0.84–1.69	1.23	0.86–1.76
Hypoalphalipoproteinemia(35–40)	522(39)	0.78	0.46–1.31	0.75	0.44–1.27	356(53)	0.77	0.48–1.26	0.76	0.47–1.25
Hypoalphalipoproteinemia (≤35)	632(50)	1.00		1.00		305(63)	1.00		1.00	
Glucose(mg/dl)										
Diabetes (≥126)	167(16)	1.00		1.00		86(13)	1.00		1.00	
Impaired fast glucose (110–125)	296(25)	0.64	0.28–1.45	0.63	0.27–1.46	191(40)	1.65	0.75–3.64	1.78	0.80–3.98
Normal (≤109)	4331(419)	1.21	0.61–2.39	1.22	0.61–2.43	5750(953)	2.05	1.02–4.14	2.24	1.10–4.55
Smoking										
Smoker	2291(189)	1.00		1.00		375(910)	1.00		1.00	
Past history of smoking	1618(192)	1.02	0.79–1.32	1.08	0.83–1.41	329(47)	0.92	1.60	0.95	0.55–1.64
Non-smoker	885(79)	1.15	0.82–1.61	1.16	0.82–1.64	5323(910)	0.98	0.64–1.50	1.00	0.65–1.53

Logistic regression analysis. Odds ratios (OR) and 95% confidence intervals (CI).
[a]Subjects with no history of cardiovascular disease, cerebrovascular disease or intake of medication for hyperlipemia, hypertension or diabetes.
[b]Following international standards, comparison between the upper half of the high risk group and the upper and lower halves of the normal group.
[c]Adjusted for age, education, household income, occupation, BMI, alcohol drinking and exercise habits.

of our study can be largely interpreted from two different standpoints. Firstly, cLBP may be associated with psychological and/or sensitivity factors of cardiovascular disease patients unrelated to the atherosclerosis hypothesis. Individuals who reported having suffered from cardiac infarction or angina may be more sensitive and susceptible to pain in general. Although recent studies using national data from Finnish [32] and Norwegian populations [27] also did not consider psychological factors, as cLBP is closely related with psychological conditions, the potential relationship should be given due consideration.

Secondly, risk factors that are not necessarily "traditional" risk factors but related to the atherosclerosis hypothesis may be associated with chronic LBP in Koreans. For many years, serum cholesterol level has been viewed to be the single most significant biochemical marker in predicting the risk of cardiovascular disease, but it has since showed limitations as a preventive measure; i.e., failing to prevent cardiovascular disease even after successful "primary prevention" through reduction of risk factors [37]. Therefore more studies are focusing on novel serum markers, including C-reactive protein and homocysteine [38], as cardiovascular disease also occurs in many people with normal lipidemia levels and traditional risk factors were unable to predict the occurrence of cardiovascular disease in these patients. Also, Briggs et al. reported in a recent study that within abnormal BMI groups(BMI>30), patients with elevated C-reactive protein had a higher LBP occurrence rate with a higher OR of 2.87(95% CI

1.18–6.96) [26,38]. Along these lines, perhaps a more significant connection may be drawn between chronic LBP in Koreans and a new cardiovascular risk factor.

In conclusion, our study indicates a strong relationship between chronic LBP and cardiovascular diseases. However, we were unable to confirm the cause of this relationship. Therefore, further large-scale studies on the association between various cardiovas-

cular risk factors (such as high-sensitivity C-reactive protein) and chronic LBP considering psychological factors are called for.

Author Contributions

Conceived and designed the experiments: IHH JSS. Performed the experiments: MRK. Analyzed the data: HJK. Wrote the paper: IHH JHL.

References

1. Shiri R, Karppinen J, Leino-Arjas P, Solovieva S, Varonen H, et al. (2007) Cardiovascular and lifestyle risk factors in lumbar radicular pain or clinically defined sciatica: A systematic review. Eur Spine J 16: 2043–2054.
2. Andersson GB (1999) Epidemiological features of chronic low-back pain. Lancet 354: 581–585.
3. Deyo RA, Mirza SK, Martin BI (2006) Back pain prevalence and visit rates: Estimates from U.S. national surveys, 2002. Spine (Phila Pa 1976) 31: 2724–2727.
4. Frymoyer JW, Cats-Baril WL (1991) An overview of the incidences and costs of low back pain. Orthop Clin North Am 22: 263–271.
5. Keyserling WM (2000) Workplace risk factors and occupational musculoskeletal disorders, part 1: A review of biomechanical and psychophysical research on risk factors associated with low-back pain. AIHAJ 61: 39–50.
6. Goldberg MS, Scott SC, Mayo NE (2000) A review of the association between cigarette smoking and the development of nonspecific back pain and related outcomes. Spine (Phila Pa 1976) 25: 995–1014.
7. Hoogendoorn WE, van Poppel MN, Bongers PM, Koes BW, Bouter LM (2000) Systematic review of psychosocial factors at work and private life as risk factors for back pain. Spine (Phila Pa 1976) 25: 2114–2125.
8. Leboeuf-Yde C (2000) Body weight and low back pain. A systematic literature review of 56 journal articles reporting on 65 epidemiologic studies. Spine (Phila Pa 1976) 25: 226–237.
9. Shiri R, Karppinen J, Leino-Arjas P, Solovieva S, Viikari-Juntura E (2010) The association between obesity and low back pain: A meta-analysis. Am J Epidemiol 171: 135–154.
10. Heuch I, Heuch I, Hagen K, Zwart JA (2013) Body mass index as a risk factor for developing chronic low back pain: A follow-up in The Nord-Trondelag Health Study. Spine (Phila Pa 1976) 38: 133–139.
11. Kauppila LI, Tallroth K (1993) Postmortem angiographic findings for arteries supplying the lumbar spine: Their relationship to low-back symptoms. J Spinal Disord 6: 124–129.
12. Kauppila LI (2009) Atherosclerosis and disc degeneration/low-back pain–a systematic review. Eur J Vasc Endovasc Surg 37: 661–670.
13. Dawber TR, Kannel WB (1966) The Framingham study. an epidemiological approach to coronary heart disease. Circulation 34: 553–555.
14. Wilson PW, D'Agostino RB, Levy D, Belanger AM, Silbershatz H, et al. (1998) Prediction of coronary heart disease using risk factor categories. Circulation 97: 1837–1847.
15. Ministry of Health and Welfare, Korea Centers for Disease Control and Prevention (2013) Ministry of health and welfare, available on:https://knhanes.cdc.go.kr/knhanes/index.do. 2013.
16. D'Agostino RB S, Vasan RS, Pencina MJ, Wolf PA, Cobain M, et al. (2008) General cardiovascular risk profile for use in primary care: The Framingham heart study. Circulation 117: 743–753.
17. National Cholesterol Education Program (NCEP) Expert Panel on Detection, Evaluation, and Treatment of High Blood Cholesterol in Adults (Adult Treatment Panel III) (2002) Third report of the national cholesterol education program (NCEP) expert panel on detection, evaluation, and treatment of high blood cholesterol in adults (adult treatment panel III) final report. Circulation 106: 3143–3421.
18. Svensson HO, Vedin A, Wilhelmsson C, Andersson GB (1983) Low-back pain in relation to other diseases and cardiovascular risk factors. Spine (Phila Pa 1976) 8: 277–285.
19. Kurunlahti M, Kerttula L, Jauhiainen J, Karppinen J, Tervonen O (2001) Correlation of diffusion in lumbar intervertebral disks with occlusion of lumbar arteries: A study in adult volunteers. Radiology 221: 779–786.
20. Kauppila LI, Mikkonen R, Mankinen P, Pelto-Vasenius K, Maenpaa I (2004) MR aortography and serum cholesterol levels in patients with long-term nonspecific lower back pain. Spine (Phila Pa 1976) 29: 2147–2152.
21. Takeyachi Y, Yabuki S, Arai I, Midorikawa H, Hoshino S, et al. (2006) Changes of low back pain after vascular reconstruction for abdominal aortic aneurysm and high aortic occlusion: A retrospective study. Surg Neurol 66: 172–6; discussion 177.
22. Tokuda O, Okada M, Fujita T, Matsunaga N (2007) Correlation between diffusion in lumbar intervertebral disks and lumbar artery status: Evaluation with fresh blood imaging technique. J Magn Reson Imaging 25: 185–191.
23. Turgut AT, Sonmez I, Cakit BD, Kosar P, Kosar U (2008) Pineal gland calcification, lumbar intervertebral disc degeneration and abdominal aorta calcifying atherosclerosis correlate in low back pain subjects: A cross-sectional observational CT study. Pathophysiology 15: 31–39.
24. Leino-Arjas P, Kaila-Kangas L, Solovieva S, Riihimaki H, Kirjonen J, et al. (2006) Serum lipids and low back pain: An association? A follow-up study of a working population sample. Spine (Phila Pa 1976) 31: 1032–1037.
25. Leino-Arjas P, Solovieva S, Kirjonen J, Reunanen A, Riihimaki H (2006) Cardiovascular risk factors and low-back pain in a long-term follow-up of industrial employees. Scand J Work Environ Health 32: 12–19.
26. Briggs MS, Givens DL, Schmitt LC, Taylor CA (2013) Relations of C-reactive protein and obesity to the prevalence and the odds of reporting low back pain. Arch Phys Med Rehabil 94: 745–752.
27. Heuch I, Heuch I, Hagen K, Zwart JA (2010) Associations between serum lipid levels and chronic low back pain. Epidemiology 21: 837–841.
28. Jhawar BS, Fuchs CS, Colditz GA, Stampfer MJ (2006) Cardiovascular risk factors for physician-diagnosed lumbar disc herniation. Spine J 6: 684–691.
29. Hemingway H, Shipley M, Stansfeld S, Shannon H, Frank J, et al. (1999) Are risk factors for atherothrombotic disease associated with back pain sickness absence? the whitehall II study. J Epidemiol Community Health 53: 197–203.
30. Hestbaek L, Leboeuf-Yde C, Manniche C (2003) Is low back pain part of a general health pattern or is it a separate and distinctive entity? A critical literature review of comorbidity with low back pain. J Manipulative Physiol Ther 26: 243–252.
31. Hagen K, Zwart JA, Holmen J, Svebak S, Bovim G, et al. (2005) Does hypertension protect against chronic musculoskeletal complaints? The Nord-Trondelag Health Study. Arch Intern Med 165: 916–922.
32. Leino-Arjas P, Kauppila L, Kaila-Kangas L, Shiri R, Heistaro S, et al. (2008) Serum lipids in relation to sciatica among finns. Atherosclerosis 197: 43–49.
33. Ford ES, Giles WH, Dietz WH (2002) Prevalence of the metabolic syndrome among US adults: Findings from the third national health and nutrition examination survey. JAMA 287: 356–359.
34. Sumner AE, Cowie CC (2008) Ethnic differences in the ability of triglyceride levels to identify insulin resistance. Atherosclerosis 196: 696–703.
35. Sumner AE (2009) Ethnic differences in triglyceride levels and high-density lipoprotein lead to underdiagnosis of the metabolic syndrome in black children and adults. J Pediatr 155: S7.e7–11.
36. Jensen MC, Brant-Zawadzki MN, Obuchowski N, Modic MT, Malkasian D, et al. (1994) Magnetic resonance imaging of the lumbar spine in people without back pain. N Engl J Med 331: 69–73.
37. Pearson TA (2002) New tools for coronary risk assessment: What are their advantages and limitations? Circulation 105: 886–892.
38. Ridker PM (2001) High-sensitivity C-reactive protein: Potential adjunct for global risk assessment in the primary prevention of cardiovascular disease. Circulation 103: 1813–1818.

3

Return to Work Coordination Programmes for Work Disability: A Meta-Analysis of Randomised Controlled Trials

Stefan Schandelmaier[1]*, Shanil Ebrahim[2], Susan C. A. Burkhardt[1], Wout E. L. de Boer[1], Thomas Zumbrunn[3], Gordon H. Guyatt[2], Jason W. Busse[2,4], Regina Kunz[1]

1 Academy of Swiss Insurance Medicine, University Hospital Basel, Basel, Switzerland, 2 Department of Clinical Epidemiology and Biostatistics, McMaster University, Hamilton, Ontario, Canada, 3 Clinical Trial Unit, University Hospital Basel, Basel, Switzerland, 4 Department of Anesthesia, McMaster University, Hamilton, Ontario, Canada

Abstract

Background: The dramatic rise in chronically ill patients on permanent disability benefits threatens the sustainability of social security in high-income countries. Social insurance organizations have started to invest in promising, but costly return to work (RTW) coordination programmes. The benefit, however, remains uncertain. We conducted a systematic review to determine the long-term effectiveness of RTW coordination compared to usual practice in patients at risk for long-term disability.

Methods and Findings: Eligible trials enrolled employees on work absence for at least 4 weeks and randomly assigned them to RTW coordination or to usual practice. We searched 5 databases (to April 2, 2012). Two investigators performed standardised eligibility assessment, study appraisal and data extraction independently and in duplicate. The GRADE framework guided our assessment of confidence in the meta-analytic estimates. We identified 9 trials from 7 countries, 8 focusing on musculoskeletal, and 1 on mental complaints. Most trials followed participants for 12 months or less. No trial assessed permanent disability. Moderate quality evidence suggests a benefit of RTW coordination on proportion at work at end of follow-up (risk ratio = 1.08, 95% CI = 1.03 to 1.13; absolute effect = 5 in 100 additional individuals returning to work, 95% CI = 2 to 8), overall function (mean difference [MD] on a 0 to 100 scale = 5.2, 95% CI = 2.4 to 8.0; minimal important difference [MID] = 10), physical function (MD = 5.3, 95% CI = 1.4 to 9.1; MID = 8.4), mental function (MD = 3.1, 95% CI = 0.7 to 5.6; MID = 7.3) and pain (MD = 6.1, 95% CI = 3.1 to 9.2; MID = 10).

Conclusions: Moderate quality evidence suggests that RTW coordination results in small relative, but likely important absolute benefits in the likelihood of disabled or sick-listed patients returning to work, and associated small improvements in function and pain. Future research should explore whether the limited effects persist, and whether the programmes are cost effective in the long term.

Editor: Michael Fehlings, University of Toronto, Canada

Funding: No funding was received for this study. The authors were salaried by their institutions. SE is a recipient of the Canadian Institutes of Health Research doctoral award. JB is supported by a New Investigator Award from the Canadian Institutes of Health Research and the Canadian Chiropractic Research Foundation.

Competing Interests: All authors have completed the Unified Competing Interest form at www.icmje.org/coi_disclosure.pdf (available on request from the corresponding author) and declare: no support from any organisation for the submitted work; asim, the Department of Insurance Medicine at the University Hospital in Basel, is funded in part by donations from public insurance companies and a consortium of private insurance companies (affiliated Authors: SS, SB, WdB, RK); JWB acts as a consultant to Prisma Health Canada, which is a private incorporated company funded by employers and insurers that consults on and manages long-term disability claims; no other relationships or activities that could appear to have influenced the submitted work. There are no patents, products in development or marketed products to declare.

* E-mail: sschandelmaier@uhbs.ch

Introduction

Long-term sickness absence secondary to illness or injury is associated with reduced quality of life [1,2], and considerable socioeconomic costs [3–9]. Both patients who are unable to work and the society benefit from return to work (RTW) [2]. However, RTW often requires overcoming challenges, including coping with on-going health problems, re-establishing work functioning, and finding suitable alternative work if a previous job is no longer available [10]. Lack of cooperation between patients, employers, healthcare providers, and insurers may also complicate RTW

[1,10]. The Organisation for Economic Co-operation and Development (OECD) postulated in 2010 that "more people with disability could work if they were helped with the right supports at the right time" through better "cross-agency co-operation" and "systematic and tailored engagement with clients" [1].

Following this intuitively appealing approach, social and private insurers have increasingly implemented RTW coordination services for people receiving wage replacement benefits [11]. RTW coordination, however, demands considerable effort from the affected individual, health professionals, and employers, often without compensation, and is associated with substantial direct costs for insurers. Involved parties thus require reliable information about the effectiveness of RTW coordination to gauge whether RTW coordination is warranted [1].

Existing systematic reviews of RTW interventions have not focused on RTW coordination [12–22]. Therefore, we conducted a systematic review and meta-analysis of randomised controlled trials (RCTs) addressing the effectiveness of RTW coordination compared to usual practice on disability, RTW, function, quality of life and satisfaction in employees receiving wage replacements benefits.

Methods

Document S1 shows the protocol of the review.

Eligibility Criteria

Eligible studies met the following criteria: (1) random allocation of adult participants to RTW coordination or usual care, (2) inclusion of participants of whom at least 80% were continuously off work (full or part time sick leave or on disability benefit) for at least four weeks and employed at the time of sick listing, and (3) report of disability status or RTW as an outcome. We defined RTW coordination as involving a direct assessment leading to an individually tailored RTW plan implemented by a RTW-coordinator or team who coordinates services and communication among involved stakeholders.

We excluded employer initiated RTW coordination programmes because they typically focus on prevention of sick leave, and encounter fewer barriers in implementing workplace-directed interventions than insurance or third party RTW coordinators.

Identification of Studies and Data Collection

We carried out a systematic search of MEDLINE, EMBASE, CINAHL, PsycINFO, and the Cochrane Central Register of Controlled Trials from inception to April 2, 2012. Our search strategy combined possible synonyms of RTW coordination (e.g. case management or multidisciplinary rehabilitation), sick leave and disability with a filter for RCTs (see Document S2). We screened reference lists of relevant articles to identify additional eligible trials. Two reviewers independently and in duplicate screened titles and abstracts in any language, reviewed articles in full text, and extracted data from eligible trials. They resolved discrepancies by discussion to achieve consensus. We contacted study authors if information about eligibility criteria, methodological components, or outcome data was incomplete or conflicting.

Assessment of Risk of Bias

Two reviewers independently assessed randomisation sequence generation, concealment of allocation, blinding of participants, RTW coordinators, and outcome assessors, completeness of data, whether participants were analysed in the group to which they were initially randomised, and whether selective outcome reporting occurred. Cluster RCTs were assessed for recruitment bias [23], and appropriate statistical analysis [23]. We assessed blinding of outcome assessment and completeness of data separately for RTW outcomes and patient reported outcomes (PROs). We used a modified Cochrane risk of bias instrument [23], with response options of "definitely yes", "probably yes", "probably no", and "definitely no" with definitely and probably yes ultimately assigned high risk of bias and probably and definitely no assigned low risk of bias [24]. Because of the small number of studies for each outcome, we were unable to address publication bias or explore explanations for variability in results [23].

Data Analysis

We conducted random effects meta-analyses (MAs) using RevMan 5.1 [25] and R 2.15.0 [26]. If available, we used baseline-adjusted effect estimates. In case of missing values, we analysed the available data without imputations to prevent biased weighting of studies [23]. We used I^2 to estimate heterogeneity [23].

We expressed pooled effects of dichotomous outcomes as risk ratios and calculated illustrative absolute risk differences by using the median baseline risk. We pooled effects of continuous outcomes as differences between group means (mean differences).

We felt the most important outcome was RTW that persisted over the long term; if we found varying measures of RTW, we therefore focused on the one that best reflected long-term outcome. If studies with time to event outcomes failed to report hazard ratios (HR), we extracted individual patient data from survival curves, verified the extraction by re-plotting, and then calculated the HR and associated 95% confidence interval (CI). If data extraction was not possible, we calculated HRs and 95% CIs based on log-rank-tests [27].

Five reviewers independently grouped all PROs by consensus into 9 categories: Overall function, physical function, social function, mental function, general health, pain, depression, anxiety, and patient satisfaction. We preferred change scores to end scores in order to correct for possible baseline differences, but we pooled both types of scores as change scores were not available for all trials. We transformed PROs expressed in different units to units on the scale of the most familiar instrument before we pooled mean differences [28]. This allowed us to enhance the interpretation of the summary effect by considering an anchor based minimal important difference (MID) on that instrument. Specifically, we rescaled *overall function* into the 0 to 100 scale of the Oswestry Disability Index (MID = 10 [29–34]), *physical, mental and social function* into the 0 to 100 scale of the SF-36 (MIDs = 8.4, 7.3, and 11.7 [35], respectively) and *pain* into a 0 to 100 visual analogue scale (MID = 10 [36]). In a second step, we used the rescaled outcomes to calculate the proportion of participants who improved by at least one MID in each group of each trial which allowed us to calculate and pool risk differences (RD) [28].

We conducted sensitivity analysis if a study reported several definitions of a RTW-outcome, e.g. full-time and part-time RTW versus full-time only (specified in footnotes of table 3). If more than one study reported several definitions, we conducted meta-analyses of all possible combinations, that is six for *proportion at work at end of study* and six for *proportion ever returned to work*.

Reporting and Rating Quality of Evidence

The PRISMA statement [37] guided our reporting and the GRADE framework [38] guided our assessment of confidence in the meta-analytic estimates.

Results

Identification of Eligible Trials and Data Collection

Of 2459 citations, 15 articles [39–55] describing 9 RCTs proved eligible (figure 1). We approached 12 authors of whom 10 replied and 7 provided additional information about 7 studies [39–44,46] (footnotes in tables 1, 2, 3, 4).

Characteristics of Included Trials

Table 1 shows characteristics of studies and populations. Participants were consenting volunteers in all but one study in which participants received no official information about the intervention [46]. Table 2 shows characteristics of interventions

2269 unique articles identified by search of titles and abstracts
Source: MEDLINE (n=1648), Embase (n=344), CINAHL (n=908), PsycINFO (n=82), Cochrane Central Register of Controlled Trials (n=327), and reference lists of relevant articles

143 full text articles assessed for eligibility

128 articles rejected
Reasons: Study protocol, no randomised controlled trial, > 20% of participants unemployed at time of sick listing or less than 4 weeks on sick leave, no face-to-face contact between RTW-coordinator and participant, no individualised RTW-plan, no RTW-outcome, control group not usual practice

9 randomised controlled trials (15 articles) included in systematic review and meta-analysis

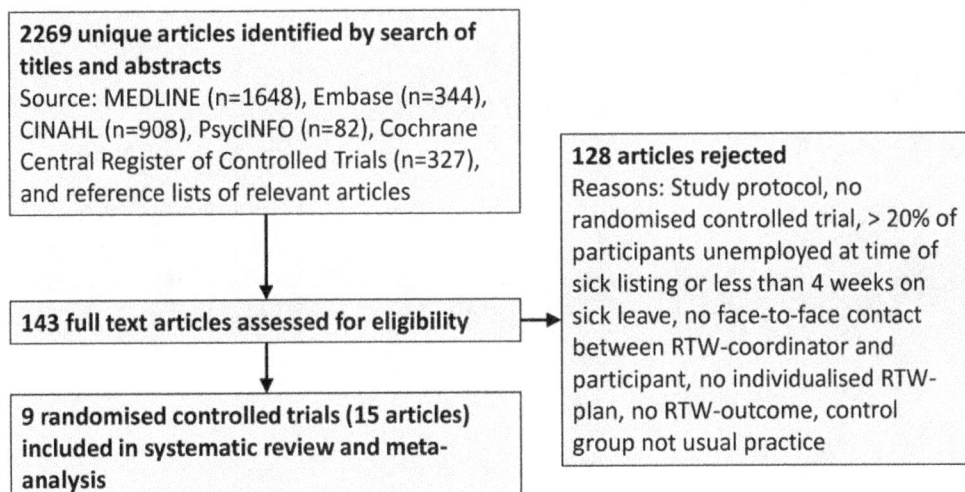

Figure 1. Study selection. Last update of electronic search to April 2, 2012.

and comparisons. No study specified the financial resources available to the RTW coordinators for patient support. In five studies [39,40,43,45,46], some participants assigned to practice as usual may have received RTW coordination.

Table 3 shows details of the reported outcome measures. The outcome *proportion at work at end of study* best reflected long-term in contrast to *time until stable RTW* and *proportion ever returned to work* that provided information regarding the first episode of RTW or the first episode of RTW of a specific duration, and *sickness absence days* that expressed the duration of all episodes of sickness absence.

Risk of Bias

Table 4 presents our assessment of risk of bias. See footnotes of table 4 for unclear or incomplete reporting of outcomes that we could not clarify with authors. Most studies concealed allocation and conducted an analysis-as-randomised. Blinding of personnel, participants and assessors of patient reported outcomes (self-administered questionnaires) was impossible. Loss to follow-up was substantial in most studies.

Effects and Confidence in Estimates

Table 5 shows the evidence profile of the meta-analytic estimates of important outcomes and Table S1 the summary of findings table for all outcomes. The heterogeneity was low across all outcomes but risk of bias (high attrition or selective reporting), imprecision and indirectness limited our confidence in the estimates.

All pooled effects of RTW outcomes significantly favoured RTW coordination (figure 2). The *proportion at work at end of study* increased by a factor of 1.08 (95% confidence interval (CI) 1.03 to 1.13, moderate confidence). This corresponds to an absolute effect of 5 in 100 more individuals returning to work (95% CI 2 more to 8 more). The pooled hazard ratio of *time until stable RTW* was 1.34 (95% CI 1.12 to 1.36, moderate confidence). The *proportion of ever returning to work* increased by a factor of 1.07 (95% CI 1.00 to 1.13, low confidence), corresponding to 4 more per 100 (95% CI, 0 more to 8 more). Total *sickness absence days* decreased by 36 workdays per year (95% CI, 17 to 56, moderate confidence). Sensitivity analysis did not reveal any substantial differences in our pooled estimates or heterogeneity.

Figure 3 shows meta-analyses of PROs. Expressed on a 0 to 100 scale, RTW coordination improved *mean overall function* by 5.2 (95% CI 2.4 to 8.0; MID = 10, moderate confidence), *physical function* by 5.3 (95% CI 1.4 to 9.1; MID = 8.4, moderate confidence), *pain* by 6.1 (95% CI 3.1 to 9.2; MID = 10, moderate confidence), *mental function* by 3.1 (95% CI 0.7 to 5.6; MID = 7.3, moderate confidence) and *social function* by 3.1 (95% CI –0.6 to 6.8; MID = 11.7, low confidence). When we used the MIDs to calculate risk differences, RTW coordination increased the proportion of participants who improved considerably in *overall function* by 9% (95% CI 4 to 15%), *physical function* by 8% (95% CI 2 to 14%), *pain* by 8% (95% CI 2 to 13%), *mental function* by 6% (95% CI 0 to 11%), and *social function* by 4% (95% CI –2 to 10%).

Figure S1 shows the output of the RevMan software including the raw data.

Discussion

We found moderate quality evidence that RTW coordination interventions result in small relative increases in RTW. Assuming a typical risk of 43 in 100 individuals not returning to work, this small relative effect implies an absolute effect of 5 in 100 more returning to work. If maintained over the long term, many would consider this an important benefit. We also found moderate quality evidence that the intervention results in small improvements in function and pain. We found no evidence that one type of RTW coordination programme was superior to another.

Our findings gain credence from the rigor of the review. We performed a comprehensive search, adjudicated eligibility and extracted data independently and in duplicate, obtained additional information from 7 authors, performed appropriate primary and sensitivity analyses and evaluated confidence in estimates of effect using the GRADE approach [38].

Our review has limitations. First, given the small number of studies for each outcome, we were unable to address publication bias. Second, we pooled change and end scores for the PROs. In theory, standard deviations of the two scores might differ substantially, leading to different weighting of individual studies in the meta-analysis [23]. However, there is evidence that SDs of change scores often do not appreciably differ from end scores [56]. Third, results from two cluster RCTs uncorrected for intra-cluster

Table 1. Characteristics of studies and populations (at time of randomisation).

Trial (country)	Sample size	Year(s), method of recruitment	Health condition	mean age (SD) [years]	% men	type of claim	length of work absence [months]
Bültmann 2009 (Denmark)	119	2004/2005, consecutive cases of sick leave registers of 4 municipalities	Musculoskeletal, not mental disorder	43.7 (11.3)	45	Full sick leave, not permanent disability	1 to 3
Davey 1994 (United Kingdom)	50	1990/1991, review of personal injury claim files of four participating personal injury insurances	Injuries likely to result in absences from work of six months or more	39.4 (11.5)	75	Full sick-leave, not permanent disability	median 20 (range 3 to 55)
Donceel 1999 (Belgium)	710 in 60 clusters	1997/1997, consecutive cases of insurance offices (= clusters)	Surgery for disc herniation	39.2 (n.r.)	65	Full sick leave	2 to 2.5
Feuerstein 2003 (Unites States of America)	205	1999/2000, claim database of the Department of Labour's Office of Workers' Compensation Programs	Work related upper extremity disorder	46.0 (8.6)[1]	22[1]	Full or part-time sick-leave	1 to 6[2]
Lambeek 2010 (Netherlands)	134	2005-2007, visitors of 4 outpatient clinics	Non-specific chronic low back pain, not mental disorder	46.2 (9.1)	58	Full or part-time sick leave, not permanent disability	3 or more
Lindh 1998 (Sweden)	611	1995/1996, consecutive cases of 7 social insurance offices	Non-specific chronic musculoskeletal pain	39.5 (n.r.)	38	Full sick-leave	3 or more
Purdon 2006 (United Kingdom)	1423	2003/2004, attracted by marketing of RTW-coordination-providers	Any condition likely to result in a <50% chance to return to work without intervention, 1/3 mental and 1/3 musculoskeletal disorders	44 (n.r.)	43	Full sick leave, not permanent disability	1,5 to 6
Rossignol 2000 (Canada)	110	1995/1996, consecutive cases of regional office of the Quebec Workers' Compensation Board	Any work-related injury to the middle or lower vertebral column, not surgery or multiple injuries	37.6 (10.1)	72	Full sick-leave, not permanent disability	1 to 2
Van der Feltz-Cornelis 2010 (Netherlands)	60 in 24 clusters	2007, review of medical files and prospective selection by occupational physicians (= clusters)	Anxiety, depression, somatoform disorder	42, range 24-59 (n.r.)	42	Full sick leave, not permanent disability	mean 4.7, range 0.25 to 10.6

RTW = return to work, n.r. = not reported.
[1] As inferred from a subsample of 131 participants.
[2] From personal correspondence.

Table 2. Characteristics of interventions and comparisons.

Study: intervention title	Provider(s) of RTW-coordination:	Affiliation of RTW-coordinator(s)	Process of RTW-coordination	Duration	Consumption of health care and other services	Adherence of RTW-coordinators and participants	Usual practice
Bültmann 2009: "Coordinated and Tailored Work rehabilitation"	1 rehab. team: OP, occupational PT, chiropractor, psychologist, social worker, experience and training n.r.	N.r.	Standardised assessment of disability and functioning, identification of barriers for RTW; individually tailored RTW-plan, actions directed at worker, workplace, and environment. Social worker coordinates with workplace and municipality case manager	Maximal 3 month	Increase	all patients received RTW-plan	Optional case management from municipal case managers
Davey 1994: "Rehabilitation co-ordinator service"	1 coordinator: PT, experience in care coordination, no specific training	Academic rehab. unit	Assessment at the participant's home, RTW-plan with focus on involving each claimant to the fullest possible extent, coordinator discussed plan with a psychologist and a physician, monitoring, making changes as appropriate	6 month	Increase	N.r.	No restriction
Donceel 1999: "New guideline for medical advisers"	30 medical advisers: social insurance physicians, experience and training n.r.	One private insurer	Monthly follow-up: Clinical and functional assessment, exploration of barriers for RTW, advice on legal criteria, gradual RTW, exercise, and normal course of work incapacity, encouragement of rehab., communication with treating physicians; case discussion with colleagues; referral to rehab. if no RTW after 3-4 months[3]	As long as participant on disability benefit	N.r.	no drop-outs[3]	30 medical advisers, focus on corporal damage, little rehab. efforts
Feuerstein 2003: "Integrated case management"	32 nurse case managers: 2 day training in ergonomic assessment and workplace accommodations, problem solving approach, experience in coordination of medical care	US Department of Labour	Semi structured interview, ergonomic worksite assessment, case management plan with workplace accommodation, applying problem solving process, monitoring, coordination of medical care (detailed list of workplace accommodations reported[2])	4 month, variable	N.r.	N.r.	33 Nurse case managers, focus on medical care, no training in a structured protocol
Lambeek 2010: "Integrated care"	2 case managers: OPs, 2-day training program	University hospital	Individualised RTW-plan, coordination of care, communication with occupational therapists (mandatory workplace intervention based on participatory ergonomics) and physical therapists (mandatory graded activity program using cognitive behavioural principles). Conference calls every three weeks, strict timing.	67 (SD 32) calendar days	Decrease	N.r.	Guidance from OPs, GPs and other health professionals. averagely 0.2 visits to case managers
Lindh 1998: "Multidisciplinary rehabilitation programme"	1 rehab. team: rehab. physician, nurse, physical therapist, psychotherapist, psychologist, occupational therapist, social worker, vocational counsellor, experience and training n.r.	Outpatient rehab. clinic	Medical, functional, psychological and social assessment, RTW-plan, weekly team conferences, regular meetings with participant and spouse	Individually regulated	N.r.	N.r.	Physical therapy and other rehab. measures
Purdon 2006[1]: "Job Retention and Rehabilitation"	Case managers, experience and training n.r.	4 third-party case management providers	Point of contact for clients, giving advice, gate keeping to other services, sometimes providing services, coordination of medical care, rehab, employer, ergonomic workplace assessment, occupational therapy, advising on welfare rights, career, CV preparation, and job search.	20 to 36 weeks	No change	88% received RTW-plan, 72% of those followed the plan	No systematic aid; low levels of work support
Rossignol 2000: "Program for coordination of primary health care"	1 team: 2 primary care physicians, 1 nurse, experience and training n.r.	N.r.	Standardised medical assessment, RTW-plan according to clinical guideline for back pain. Assisting the treating physicians in finding and scheduling diagnostic and therapeutic procedures, cooperation with Worker's Compensation, standardised weekly telephone talk	Until RTW	No change	N.r.	Instruction to continue with treating physician

28

Back Pain: Assessment and Treatment

Table 2. Cont.

Study: intervention title	Provider(s) of RTW-coordination:	Affiliation of RTW-coordinator(s)	Process of RTW-coordination	Duration	Consumption of health care and other services	Adherence of RTW-coordinators and participants	Usual practice
Van der Feltz-Cornelis 2010: "psychiatric consultation model"	12 OPs, training in diagnosis and treatment of mental disorders. consulted by 2 psychiatrist trained in improvement of work functioning	Company of participant	Psychiatric assessment, collaborative RTW-plan, coordination of plan and monitoring by OP	Until RTW	N.r.	N.r.	Care from OP[2] and mental health care professionals

RTW = return to work, n.r. = not reported, OP = occupational physician, PT = physical therapist, GP = general practitioner, rehab. = rehabilitation.
[1]The trial compared three intervention arms with usual practice. We considered only the arm "combined intervention" because the other arms were restricted to either workplace or health care interventions.
[2]In the Dutch system, each company is obliged to have company insurance for sick leave and to offer their employees access to occupational health care. Occupational physicians provide social-medical guidance for sick listed employees with the aim to return to work (RTW) as quickly as possible. Usually, occupational physicians are organised as third party service providers.
[3]From personal correspondence.

dependency may have spuriously increased precision, thus overweighting these studies in the meta-analysis.

Comparison with Other Systematic Reviews

Our study selection partly overlaps with related systematic reviews that defined RTW interventions from different points of view. They compared usual practice to RTW interventions that either included a specific workplace component [12–15], applied RTW-interventions to a population with a specific health condition [16–19], or explored them within a specific country only [20–22]. Two of these systematic reviews (with 3/42 [17] or 0/10 [13] studies overlapping) addressed RTW coordination in a subgroup analysis (RTW coordination as a subgroup of RTW-interventions). Both suggested that RTW coordination improved RTW [13,17] whereas effects on PROs remained unclear [13]. However, much like other related reviews, they did not perform a meta-analysis. Reasons included poor study quality [15] or high heterogeneity in the RTW interventions [15,17,18]. Only one systematic review (1/6 studies overlapping) conducted a meta-analysis, concluding with low confidence that RTW interventions with an active workplace involvement improve RTW outcomes [12].

Other reviews also noted limitations in the evidence that we identified. Evidence regarding the effectiveness of RTW interventions suffers from poor descriptions of interventions and controls [12,13], insufficient information beyond one year follow-up [13,18], and paucity of studies on participants with mental health problems [12,13]. Further, a systematic review of 34 RCTs (3 overlapping) and 8 cohort studies found evidence of possible publication bias [17].

Applicability of Findings

Applicability of the results is enhanced by recruitment through insurance registers that ensured a representative selection of claimants. The prompt initiation of interventions after work absence and the high intensity of support are consistent with the OECD recommendations that social insurances or corresponding benefit authorities should apply RTW coordination at an early stage and resources should shift from passive benefits towards RTW programmes [1].

Diversity and limitations in the description of both RTW coordination interventions, and the nature of usual practice, advise on cautious interpretation and application of our results. Most studies focused on organisational features, such as composition of the team, distribution of roles, and standardisation of initial assessment. Interventions differed in degree of standardisation, and in the roles and backgrounds of intervention providers. Information regarding training and experience of RTW coordinators, resources available, and adherence of coordinators and participants were typically lacking. Descriptions of the usual practice controls were even more limited.

The striking consistency of results from study to study in virtually all outcomes ameliorated the unease about variability in interventions and controls. If variability were very important, one would not expect to see such consistency.

All but 2 studies [42,45] (85% of participants in the review) focused on claimants with musculoskeletal complaints. Recent statistics from high-income countries show that new disability claimants with psychiatric disorders (30 to 40%) have outnumbered those with musculoskeletal complaints [1]. Although the results from the two studies that did enrol a substantial proportion [42] or an exclusive sample [45] of claimants with psychiatric complaints showed similar results to other studies, generalizing results to these populations is questionable.

Table 3. Characteristics of outcomes.

Study	Follow-up	Return to work outcomes (definition); patient reported outcomes (assigned outcome group)
Bültmann 2009	12 months	**RTW[1]:** proportion at work at end of study[16], sickness absence (mean number of work days off including all episodes of sick leave); **PROs[17,18]:** pain during last month (pain), Oswestry Low Back Pain Disability Questionnaire (general function); **Not analysed:** pain during last week (n.r.)
Davey 1994	6 months	**RTW[2]:** proportion at work (full or part time), proportion ever returned to work (full or part time); **PROs[17]:** Hospital Anxiety and Depression Scale[5] (depression), Nottingham Health Profile (physical and social function)[5]; **Not analysed:** self-rated anxiety
Donceel 1999	12 months	**RTW[4]:** proportion at work at end of study (full time) = proportion ever returned to work, time until RTW[6] (full-time, "stable" at end of follow up)
Feuerstein 2003	16 months	**RTW[1]:** time until RTW[7,8,9,10,11] (full time), proportion ever returned to work (full time)[8,10,11]; **PROs[17]:** Patient satisfaction, Upper extremity function scale[7] (pain), SF-12[7] (physical and mental function); **Not analysed:** Levine symptom scale (overlap with other functional scales)
Lambeek 2010	12 months	**RTW[3]:** time until RTW (full-time, for at least 4 weeks), proportion ever returned to work[8], sickness absence (mean number of work days off including all episodes of sick leave); **PROs:** Roland disability questionnaire (physical function)[18], visual analogue scale (pain)[18], EQ5D (general function)[7,17]
Lindh 1998	60 months[12]	**RTW[1]:** proportion at work at end of study[8,10,12,13] (full or part time), proportion ever returned to work[8,10,12,13] (full or part time)
Purdon 2006	20 to 36 weeks	**RTW[2]:** proportion at work at end of study, proportion ever returned to work (full-time, for at least 2 weeks[14]); **PROs[17]:** SF-36 (physical, mental and social function, pain, general health); **Not analysed:** Hospital Anxiety and Depression Scale[15], cumulative sickness absence[15], cumulative Incidence of RTW for a spell of 13 weeks[14]; SF-36 (physical role, emotional role, energy/fatigue), self-assessed general health, health improvement
Rossignol 2000	6 months	**RTW[1]:** time until RTW (full or part time, for at least 2 days)[11]; **PROs[18]:** visual analogue scale (pain), Quebec Back Pain Disability Scale (physical function), Oswestry low back pain disability questionnaire (overall function); **Not analysed:** Dallas pain questionnaire (overlap with other functional scales), Health care satisfaction (n.r.)
Van der Feltz-Cornelis 2010	6 months	**RTW[3]:** time until RTW (full-time, for at least 4 weeks, all who returned stayed at work)[8,10,13], proportion at work at end of study[10,13] = proportion ever returned to work[10,13]; **PROs[18]:** PHQ9 (depression); **Not analysed:** PHQ15, SCL-90 (no subscales reported), EQ5D (reported in Quality Adjusted Life Years)

RTW = return to work, PROs = patient reported outcomes, n.r. = not reported.

Data source: [1] administrative data,

[2] diary, interview, or survey, [3] combination of diary or interview and administrative data,

[4] not reported.

[5] SD not reported. We imputed missing standard deviations (SDs) with the weighted average of the SDs of the remaining trials.

[6] Hazard ratio estimated from log-rank test.

[7] From personal correspondence.

[8] Data extracted from graph.

[9] Time between a claimant's initial evaluation by a case manager (not randomization) and RTW.

[10] Missing or unclear number of participants.

[11] Cessation of disability benefits as surrogate for RTW (Rossignol, Feuerstein).

[12] Data presented for two subgroups (immigrant and swedes) which we recombined. Only the number of patients who started the intervention reported. To prevent attrition bias at 60 month, we used 18 month data (ensuring a slightly longer follow up than other studies) and conducted sensitivity analysis using 15 or 12 months.

[13] Data in graph conflicting with text or table.

[14] RTW for at least 2, 6 or 13 weeks reported. We disregarded the 13 weeks outcome which most participants could not achieve due to short follow-up. To ensure longest follow-up, we used 2 weeks and conducted sensitivity analysis using 6 weeks.

[15] Data presented in groups, variance not estimable.

[16] Full-time and part-time RTW reported separately. We used full time RTW and conducted sensitivity analyses using part-time combined with full-time.

[17] End scores.

[18] Change scores.

Table 4. Methodological components.

Study	Random sequence adequately generated?	Allocation concealed?	Participants and RTW-coordinators blinded?	RTW-outcome assessor blinded?	PRO- outcome assessor blinded?	Loss to follow-up of RTW-outcomes [%]	Loss to follow-up of PROs [%]	Intention to treat analysis[1]	Selective reporting[2]	Other
Bültmann 2009	Y	Y[3]	N	Y	N	5	34	Y	?	
Davey 1994	Y	Y	N	N	N	0	0	Y	?	
Donceel 1999	Y	Y	N[4]	N	n.a.	0	n.a.	(Y)	?	9
Feuerstein 2003	Y	N[3]	N	(N)	N	40[3]	36–61	(N)	Y[5,8]	
Lambeek 2010	Y	Y	N	Y	N	7	13	Y	N	
Lindh 1998	(N)	(N)	N	Y	n.a.	?	n.a.	Y	Y[6,8]	
Purdon 2006	Y	Y[3]	N	N	N	28	29	Y	?	
Rossignol 2000	Y	Y	N	Y	N	0	18	Y	?	
V. d. Feltz-Cornelis 2010	Y	Y	N	Y	N	18	27	Y	Y[7,8]	9

RTW = return to work, PRO = patient reported outcomes, Y = yes, (Y) = probably Yes, N = No, (N) = probably no, ? = unclear, n.a. = not applicable.
[1] Participants analysed in the group to which they were initially assigned.
[2] "No" if protocol published and all outcomes correctly reported; "?" if no protocol published and selective reporting not obvious.
[3] From personal correspondence.
[4] Participants were probably not aware of the intervention.
[5] RTW-outcomes not published, incomplete outcome information (see table 3).
[6] Results presented in subgroups, incomplete outcome information (see table 3).
[7] Primary outcome not mentioned in protocol.
[8] Incomplete outcome information (see table 3).
[9] Cluster randomised trials: No risk of recruitment bias. Baseline information of individual clusters not reported. Effects of RTW-outcomes not corrected for possible design effects (risk of inflated precision).

Table 5. Evidence Profile, relevant outcomes.

Quality assessment						No of participants		Effect		Confidence in estimate	Importance
No of studies	Design	Risk of bias	Inconsistency	Indirectness	Imprecision	RTW-coordination	Usual care	Relative (95% CI)	Absolute		
Proportion at work et end of study											
6	randomised trials	serious[1,2]	no serious inconsistency	no serious indirectness	no serious imprecision	794/1279 (62.1%)	656/1138 (57.6%)	RR 1.08 (1.03 to 1.13)	5 more per 100 (from 2 more to 7 more)	⊕⊕⊕ MODERATE	CRITICAL
Overall function (range of scores: 0-100; Better indicated by higher values)											
4	randomised trials	serious[1]	no serious inconsistency	no serious indirectness	no serious imprecision	716	558	–	MD 5.2 higher (2.4 to 8.0 higher)	⊕⊕⊕ MODERATE	IMPORTANT
Physical function (range of scores: 0-100; Better indicated by higher values)											
5	randomised trials	serious[1]	no serious inconsistency	no serious indirectness	no serious imprecision	729	619	–	MD 5.3 higher (1.4 to 9.1 higher)	⊕⊕⊕ MODERATE	IMPORTANT
Pain (range of scores: 0-100; Better indicated by lower values)											
6	randomised trials	serious[1,4]	no serious inconsistency	no serious indirectness	no serious imprecision	784	646	–	MD 6.1 lower (3.1 to 9.2 lower)	⊕⊕⊕ MODERATE	IMPORTANT
Social function (range of scores: 0-100; Better indicated by higher values)											
2	randomised trials	serious[1]	no serious inconsistency	no serious indirectness	serious[5]	589	470	–	MD 3.1 higher (0.6 lower to 6.8 higher)	⊕⊕ LOW	IMPORTANT
Mental function (range of scores: 0-100; Better indicated by higher values)											
2	randomised trials	serious[1,2]	no serious inconsistency	no serious indirectness	no serious imprecision	599	512	–	MD 3.1 higher (0.7 to 5.6 higher)	⊕⊕⊕ MODERATE	IMPORTANT

[1]Risk of attrition bias.
[2]Risk of reporting bias.
[3]Total population size less than 400.
[4]Use of unvalidated instruments.
[5]Confidence interval encloses no effect and meaningful difference.

Study	RTW coord. (Events) Patients	Usual practice (Events) Patients	Weight (%)	Effect (95% CI)	Favours usual practice ↔ Favours RTW coord.
Proportion at work at end of study				Relative risk	
Davey	(3) 33	(2) 17	0.1	0.77 (0.14 to 4.19)	
Lindh	(114) 238	(116) 226	7.0	0.93 (0.78 to 1.12)	
Van der Feltz–Cornelis	(22) 26	(21) 25	4.2	1.01 (0.79 to 1.28)	
Purdon	(326) 571	(244) 458	19.1	1.07 (0.96 to 1.20)	
Donceel	(310) 345	(299) 365	66.1	1.10 (1.03 to 1.16)	
Bültmann	(51) 66	(29) 47	3.5	1.25 (0.97 to 1.62)	
Total (I² = 0.0%)	(826) 1279	(711) 1138	100.0	1.08 (1.03 to 1.13)	
Time until return to work				Hazard ratio	
Feuerstein	59	64	14.7	1.11 (0.75 to 1.62)	
Rossignol	54	56	12.0	1.16 (0.76 to 1.79)	
Donceel	345	365	54.7	1.31 (1.11 to 1.53)	
Van der Feltz–Cornelis	25	24	6.4	1.70 (0.93 to 3.11)	
Lambeek	63	61	12.3	1.90 (1.24 to 2.90)	
Total (I² = 13.6%)	546	570	100.0	1.34 (1.14 to 1.56)	
Proportion ever returned to work				Relative risk	
Davey	(3) 33	(2) 17	0.1	0.77 (0.14 to 4.19)	
Lindh	(147) 238	(154) 226	15.5	0.91 (0.79 to 1.04)	
Van der Feltz–Cornelis	(22) 26	(21) 25	5.9	1.01 (0.79 to 1.28)	
Rossignol	(42) 54	(41) 56	7.1	1.06 (0.86 to 1.31)	
Purdon	(355) 545	(272) 458	24.0	1.10 (0.99 to 1.21)	
Donceel	(310) 345	(299) 365	39.5	1.10 (1.03 to 1.16)	
Lambeek	(50) 65	(44) 69	6.6	1.21 (0.97 to 1.51)	
Feuerstein	(20) 59	(17) 64	1.2	1.28 (0.74 to 2.19)	
Total (I² = 20.5%)	(949) 1365	(850) 1280	100.0	1.07 (1.00 to 1.13)	
Sickness absence days				Mean difference	
Lambeek	63	61	61.8	29.9 (5.0 to 54.9)	
Bültmann	66	47	38.2	46.0 (14.3 to 77.8)	
Total (I² = 0.0%)	129	108	100.0	36.1 (16.5 to 55.7)	

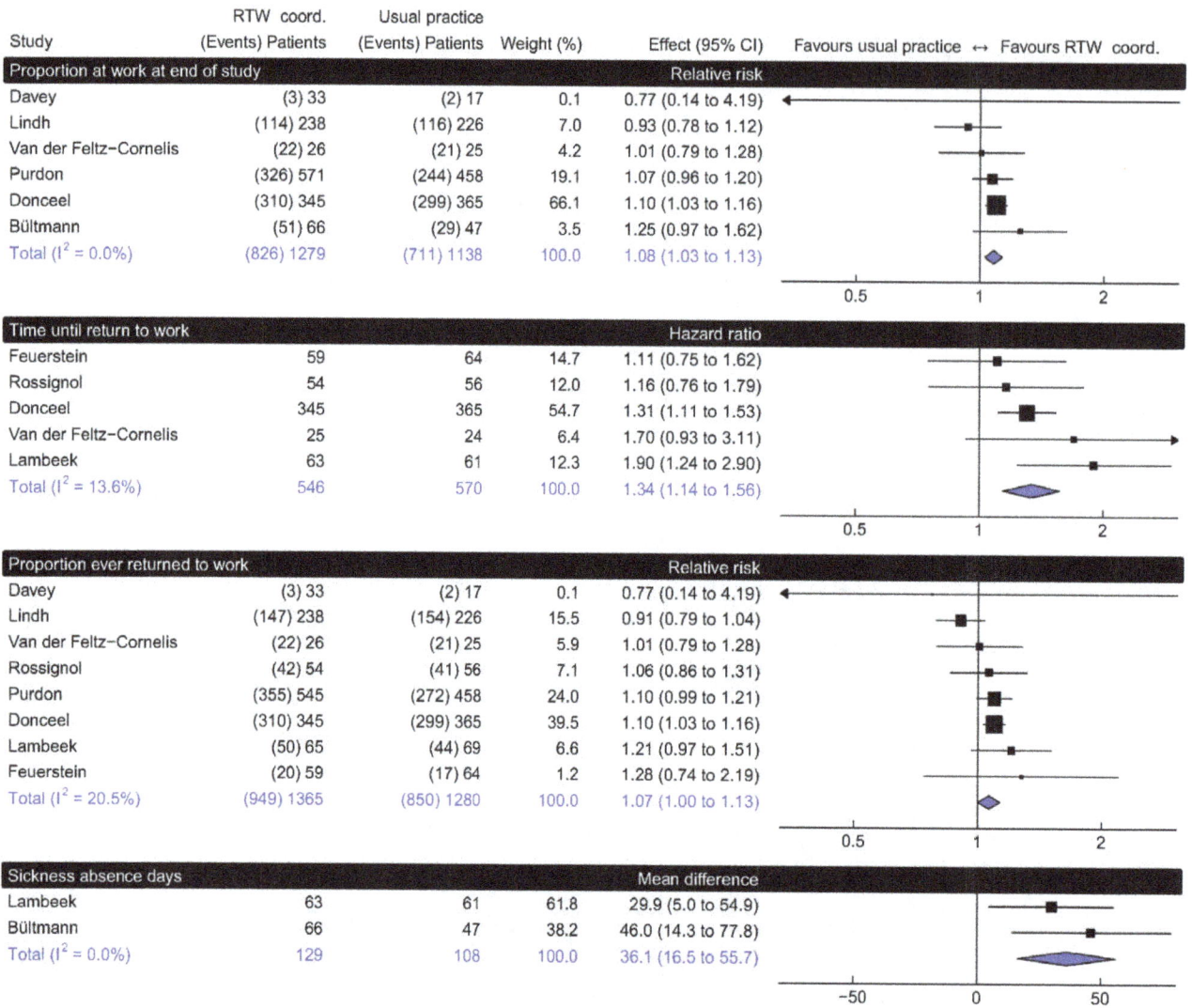

Figure 2. RTW-outcomes. RTW coord. = return to work coordination.

Judging the importance of our measured relative effect size is challenging. An absolute difference in the proportion at work at end of study - of the order of 5% suggested by the results of this review - could be important if maintained over the long term. Indeed, many are likely to agree that an absolute reduction in the proportion on long-term disability would be important. However, follow-up was generally too short to inform results over the long-term. Only one study assessed work stability after initial work resumption but reported the results incompletely [47].

Two studies conducted an economic analyses based on the outcome *cumulative sickness absence* [39,50] one year after randomisation. They both concluded that RTW coordination compared to usual practice was cost effective from a societal perspective, that is by considering the cost of the intervention, health care utilisation, and loss of productivity. The societal perspective leaves out the cost of wage replacement, which is considered a redistribution of wealth, and, therefore, does not inform about the impact of RTW coordination on social security savings. In contrast, an economic analysis from an insurance perspective would integrate this information. Cost effectiveness from an insurance perspective may occur only in the long-term and depend mainly on savings related to fewer disability pensions [57].

Implications for Research

Results to date suggest small but possibly important benefits of RTW coordination. Determining the long-term benefits and the cost effectiveness of the programmes will require trials with low risk of bias (concealment, blinding of outcome assessors and statisticians, minimal missing data), measuring long-term outcomes of work force retention and long-term disability (including pensions). This would also enable extending the research on comparing different definitions of RTW outcomes [58]. We require studies in specific populations that represent the majority of disabled individuals, including both musculoskeletal and psychiatric problems. We strongly encourage researchers of RTW interventions to describe interventions, comparisons, and settings more systematically to enable comparability of studies and facilitate transfer into practice.

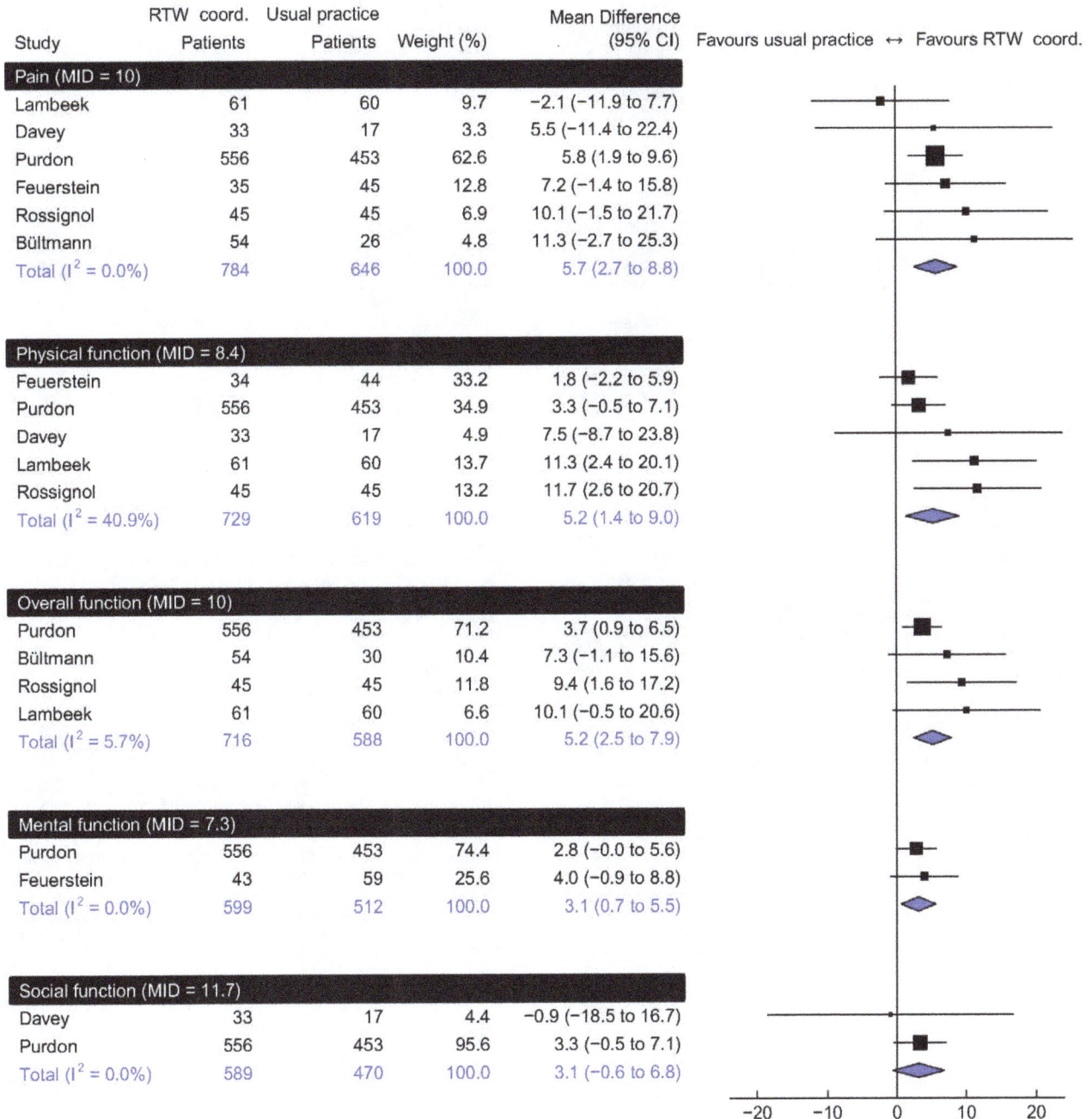

Figure 3. Patient reported outcomes. Individual trials' outcomes expressed on a 0 to 100 scale. RTW coord. = return to work coordination. MID = minimal important difference.

Supporting Information

Figure S1   RevMan output for all outcomes including raw data.

Table S1   Summary of findings for all outcomes.

Document S1   Protocol.

Document S2   PubMed search strategy.

Acknowledgments

We thank the study authors Johannes Anema, Judith Bosmans, Ute Bültmann, Peter Donceel, Susan Purdon, Michel Rossignol, and William Shaw for their unhesitant cooperation and for providing data; Urs Brügger, Julian Higgins and Stephen Walter for valuable advice.

Author Contributions

Conceived and designed the experiments: RK SS SB JB GG. Performed the experiments: SS RK SB WdB SE JB. Analyzed the data: TZ SS RK GG. Wrote the paper: SS SE SB WdB TZ JB GG RK. Developed the search strategy: SS RK. Performed the study selection: SS SB RK WdB.

Appraised study quality: RK SS. Extracted study characteristics and outcome data: SE RK SS TZ. Performed consensus exercises: SE JWB SS

RK WdB. Contributed to the interpretation and discussion of the results: SS SE SB WdB TZ JB GG RK.

References

1. OECD (2010) Sickness, Disability and Work: Breaking the Barriers. A Synthesis of Findings across OECD Countries. Paris: OECD Publishing. p.
2. Gordon Waddell, Burton KA (2006) Is Work Good for Your Health and Well-Being? London: The Stationery Office. p.
3. Frymoyer JW, Cats-Baril WL (1991) An overview of the incidences and costs of low back pain. Orthop Clin North Am 22: 263–271.
4. Nachemson A (1994) Chronic pain - the end of the welfare state? Qual Life Res 3 Suppl 1: S11–17.
5. Abenhaim L, Suissa S (1987) Importance and economic burden of occupational back pain: a study of 2,500 cases representative of Quebec. J Occup Med 29: 670–674.
6. Labriola M, Lund T (2007) Self-reported sickness absence as a risk marker of future disability pension. Prospective findings from the DWECS/DREAM study 1990–2004. Int J Med Sci 4: 153–158.
7. Lund T, Kivimäki M, Labriola M, Villadsen E, Christensen KB (2008) Using administrative sickness absence data as a marker of future disability pension: the prospective DREAM study of Danish private sector employees. Occup Environ Med 65: 28–31. doi:10.1136/oem.2006.031393.
8. Kivimäki M, Forma P, Wikström J, Halmeenmäki T, Pentti J, et al. (2004) Sickness absence as a risk marker of future disability pension: the 10-town study. J Epidemiol Community Health 58: 710–711. doi:10.1136/jech.2003.015842.
9. Gjesdal S, Bratberg E (2003) Diagnosis and duration of sickness absence as predictors for disability pension: Results from a three-year, multi-register based and prospective study. Scand J Public Health 31: 246–254. doi:10.1080/14034940210165154.
10. Young AE, Roessler RT, Wasiak R, McPherson KM, van Poppel MNM, et al. (2005) A developmental conceptualization of return to work. J Occup Rehabil 15: 557–568. doi:10.1007/s10926-005-8034-z.
11. Young AE, Wasiak R, Roessler RT, McPherson KM, Anema JR, et al. (2005) Return-to-work outcomes following work disability: stakeholder motivations, interests and concerns. J Occup Rehabil 15: 543–556. doi:10.1007/s10926-005-8033-0.
12. van Oostrom SH, Driessen MT, de Vet HC, Franche R-L, Schonstein E, et al. (2009) Workplace interventions for preventing work disability. Cochrane Database Syst Rev. doi:10.1002/14651858.CD006955.pub2.
13. Franche R-L, Cullen K, Clarke J, Irvin E, Sinclair S, et al. (2005) Workplace-based return-to-work interventions: a systematic review of the quantitative literature. J Occup Rehabil 15: 607–631. doi:10.1007/s10926-005-8038-8.
14. Kuoppala J, Lamminpää A (2008) Rehabilitation and work ability: a systematic literature review. J Rehabil Med 40: 796–804. doi:10.2340/16501977-0270.
15. Carroll C, Rick J, Pilgrim H, Cameron J, Hillage J (2010) Workplace involvement improves return to work rates among employees with back pain on long-term sick leave: a systematic review of the effectiveness and cost-effectiveness of interventions. Disabil Rehabil 32: 607–621. doi:10.3109/09638280903186301.
16. Meijer EM, Sluiter JK, Frings-Dresen MHW (2005) Evaluation of effective return-to-work treatment programs for sick-listed patients with non-specific musculoskeletal complaints: a systematic review. Int Arch Occup Environ Health 78: 523–532. doi:10.1007/s00420-005-0622-x.
17. Palmer KT, Harris EC, Linaker C, Barker M, Lawrence W, et al. (2011) Effectiveness of community- and workplace-based interventions to manage musculoskeletal-related sickness absence and job loss: a systematic review. Rheumatology (Oxford, England): 1–13. doi:10.1093/rheumatology/ker086.
18. Hlobil H, Staal JB, Spoelstra M, Ariëns GAM, Smid T, et al. (2005) Effectiveness of a return-to-work intervention for subacute low-back pain. Scand J Work Environ Health 31: 249–257.
19. Elders LA, van der Beek AJ, Burdorf A (2000) Return to work after sickness absence due to back disorders–a systematic review on intervention strategies. Int Arch Occup Environ Health 73: 339–348.
20. Clayton S, Bambra C, Gosling R, Povall S, Misso K, et al. (2011) Assembling the evidence jigsaw: insights from a systematic review of UK studies of individual-focused return to work initiatives for disabled and long-term ill people. BMC Public Health 11: 170. doi:10.1186/1471-2458-11-170.
21. Bambra C, Whitehead M, Hamilton V (2005) Does "welfare-to-work" work? A systematic review of the effectiveness of the UK's welfare-to-work programmes for people with a disability or chronic illness. Soc Sci Med 60: 1905–1918. doi:10.1016/j.socscimed.2004.09.002.
22. Hayday S, Rick J, Carroll C, Jagger N, Hillage J (2008) Review of the Effectiveness and Cost Effectiveness of Interventions, Strategies, Programmes and Policies to Help Recipients of Incapacity Benefits Return to Employment (Paid and Unpaid). Brighton: Institute for Employment Studies. p.
23. Higgins JPT, Green S (2011) Cochrane Handbook for Systematic Reviews of Interventions Version 5.1.0 [updated March 2011]. Higgins JPT, Green S, editors The Cochrane Collaboration. p. Available:www.cochrane-handbook.org.
24. Akl EA, Sun X, Busse JW, Johnston BC, Briel M, et al. (2012) Specific instructions for estimating unclearly reported blinding status in randomized trials

25. were reliable and valid. J Clin Epidemiol 65: 262–267. doi:10.1016/j.jclinepi.2011.04.015.
25. The Nordic Cochrane Centre, The Cochrane Collaboration (2011) Review Manager (RevMan). Copenhagen. p.
26. R Development Core Team (2011) (n.d.) R: A language and environment for statistical computing. Vienna, Austria: R Foundation for Statistical Computing. p. Available:http://www.R-project.org/.
27. Parmar MK, Torri V, Stewart L (1998) Extracting summary statistics to perform meta-analyses of the published literature for survival endpoints. Stat Med 17: 2815–2834.
28. Thorlund K, Walter SD, Johnston BC, Furukawa TA, Guyatt GH (2011) Pooling health-related quality of life outcomes in meta-analysis - a tutorial and review of methods for enhancing interpretability. Research Synthesis Methods 2: 188–203. doi:10.1002/jrsm.46.
29. Lauridsen H, Hartvigsen J, Manniche C, Korsholm L, Grunnet-Nilsson N (2006) Responsiveness and minimal clinically important difference for pain and disability instruments in low back pain patients. BMC Musculoskeletal Disorders 7: 82.
30. Copay AG, Glassman SD, Subach BR, Berven S, Schuler TC, et al. (2008) Minimum clinically important difference in lumbar spine surgery patients: a choice of methods using the Oswestry Disability Index, Medical Outcomes Study questionnaire Short Form 36, and pain scales. Spine J 8: 968–974.
31. Ostelo RWJG, De Vet HCW (2005) Clinically important outcomes in low back pain. Best Pract Res Clin Rheumatol 19: 593–607.
32. Fisher K (2008) Assessing clinically meaningful change following a programme for managing chronic pain. Clin Rehabil 22: 252–259. doi:10.1177/0269215507081928.
33. Hägg O, Fritzell P, Nordwall A (2003) The clinical importance of changes in outcome scores after treatment for chronic low back pain. Eur Spine J 12: 12–20.
34. Ostelo RWJG, Deyo RA, Stratford P, Waddell G, Croft P, et al. (2008) Interpreting change scores for pain and functional status in low back pain: towards international consensus regarding minimal important change. Spine 33: 90–94. doi:10.1097/BRS.0b013e31815e3a10.
35. Kosinski M, Zhao SZ, Dedhiya S, Osterhaus JT, Ware JE Jr (2000) AID-ANR1O>3.0.CO;2-M.
36. Dworkin RH, Turk DC, McDermott MP, Peirce-Sandner S, Burke LB, et al. (2009) Interpreting the clinical importance of group differences in chronic pain clinical trials: IMMPACT recommendations. Pain 146: 238–244. doi:10.1016/j.pain.2009.08.019.
37. Moher D, Liberati A, Tetzlaff J, Altman DG (2009) Preferred Reporting Items for Systematic Reviews and Meta-Analyses: The PRISMA Statement. J Clin Epidemiol 62: 1006–1012. doi:10.1016/j.jclinepi.2009.06.005.
38. Guyatt GH, Oxman AD, Vist GE, Kunz R, Falck-Ytter Y, et al. (2008) GRADE: an emerging consensus on rating quality of evidence and strength of recommendations. BMJ 336: 924–926. doi:10.1136/bmj.39489.470347.AD.
39. Bültmann U, Sherson D, Olsen J, Hansen CL, Lund T, et al. (2009) Coordinated and tailored work rehabilitation: a randomized controlled trial with economic evaluation undertaken with workers on sick leave due to musculoskeletal disorders. J Occup Rehabil 19: 81–93. doi:10.1007/s10926-009-9162-7.
40. Lambeek LC, van Mechelen W, Knol DL, Loisel P, Anema JR (2010) Randomised controlled trial of integrated care to reduce disability from chronic low back pain in working and private life. BMJ 340: c1035. doi:10.1136/bmj.c1035.
41. Rossignol M, Abenhaim L, Séguin P, Neveu a, Collet JP, et al. (2000) Coordination of primary health care for back pain. A randomized controlled trial. Spine 25: 251–258.
42. Purdon S, Stratford N, Taylor R, Natarajan L, Bell S (2006) Impacts of the Job Retention and Rehabilitation Pilot. Changes.
43. Feuerstein M, Huang GD, Ortiz JM, Shaw WS, Miller VI, et al. (2003) Integrated case management for work-related upper-extremity disorders: impact of patient satisfaction on health and work status. J Occup Environ Med 45: 803–812. doi:10.1097/01.jom.0000079091.95532.92.
44. Davey C (1994) The implementation and evaluation of a rehabilitation co-ordinator service for personal injury claimants.
45. van der Feltz-Cornelis CM, Hoedeman R, de Jong FJ, Meeuwissen JA, Drewes HW, et al. (2010) Faster return to work after psychiatric consultation for sicklisted employees with common mental disorders compared to care as usual. A randomized clinical trial. Neuropsychiatr Dis Treat 6: 375–385.
46. Donceel P, Du Bois M, Lahaye D (1999) Return to work after surgery for lumbar disc herniation. A rehabilitation-oriented approach in insurance medicine. Spine 24: 872–876.
47. Lindh M (1997) A randomized prospective study of vocational outcome in rehabilitation of patients with non-specific musculoskeletal pain: A multidisciplinary approach to patients identified after 90 days of sick-leave. Scan J Rehab Med 29: 103–112.

48. Davey C (1993) Evaluating a rehabilitation co-ordinator service for personal injury claimants. International journal of rehabilitation research 16: 49–53.

49. Farrell C, Nice K, Lewis J, Sainsbury R (2006) Experiences of the Job Retention and Rehabilitation Pilot. Pensions.

50. Lambeek LC, Bosmans JE, Van Royen BJ, Van Tulder MW, Van Mechelen W, et al. (2010) Effect of integrated care for sick listed patients with chronic low back pain: economic evaluation alongside a randomised controlled trial. BMJ 341: c6414. doi:10.1136/bmj.c6414.

51. Lambeek LC, Anema JR, van Royen BJ, Buijs PC, Wuisman PI, et al. (2007) Multidisciplinary outpatient care program for patients with chronic low back pain: design of a randomized controlled trial and cost-effectiveness study. BMC public health 7: 254. doi:10.1186/1471-2458-7-254.

52. Lambeek LC, van Mechelen W, Buijs PC, Loisel P, Anema JR (2009) An integrated care program to prevent work disability due to chronic low back pain: a process evaluation within a randomized controlled trial. BMC musculoskeletal disorders 10: 147. doi:10.1186/1471-2474-10-147.

53. Lincoln AE, Feuerstein M, Shaw WS, Miller VI (2002) Impact of Case Manager Training on Worksite Accommodations in Workers' Compensation Claimants With Upper Extremity Disorders. Journal of Occupational and Environmental Medicine 44: 237–245. doi:10.1097/00043764-200203000-00011.

54. Shaw WS, Feuerstein M, Lincoln AE, Miller VI, Wood PM (2001) Case management services for work related upper extremity disorders. Integrating workplace accommodation and problem solving. AAOHN J 49: 378–389.

55. van der Feltz-Cornelis CM, Meeuwissen J a C, de Jong FJ, Hoedeman R, Elfeddali I (2007) Randomised controlled trial of a psychiatric consultation model for treatment of common mental disorder in the occupational health setting. BMC health services research 7: 29. doi:10.1186/1472-6963-7-29.

56. Busse JW, Montori VM, Krasnik C, Patelis-Siotis I, Guyatt GH (2009) Psychological Intervention for Premenstrual Syndrome: A Meta-Analysis of Randomized Controlled Trials. Psychother Psychosom 78: 6–15. doi:10.1159/000162296.

57. Busch H, Bodin L, Bergström G, Jensen IB (2011) Patterns of sickness absence a decade after pain-related multidisciplinary rehabilitation. Pain 152: 1727–1733. doi:10.1016/j.pain.2011.02.004.

58. Steenstra IA, Lee H, de Vroome EMM, Busse JW, Hogg-Johnson SJ (2012) Comparing Current Definitions of Return to Work: A Measurement Approach. J Occup Rehabil [Epub ahead of print]. doi:10.1007/s10926-011-9349-6.

4

Diaphragm Postural Function Analysis Using Magnetic Resonance Imaging

Pavel Vostatek[1]*, Daniel Novák[1], Tomas Rychnovský[2], Šarka Rychnovská[2]

1 Department of Cybernetics, Czech Technical University in Prague, Prague, Czech Republic, **2** AVETE OMNE Physiotherapy Center, Filmarska 19, Prague, Czech Republic

Abstract

We present a postural analysis of diaphragm function using magnetic resonance imaging (MRI). The main aim of the study was to identify changes in diaphragm motion and shape when postural demands on the body were increased (loading applied to a distal part of the extended lower extremities against the flexion of the hips was used). Sixteen healthy subjects were compared with 17 subjects suffering from chronic low back pain and in whom structural spine disorders had been identified. Two sets of features were calculated from MRI recordings: dynamic parameters reflecting diaphragm action, and static parameters reflecting diaphragm anatomic characteristics. A statistical analysis showed that the diaphragm respiratory and postural changes were significantly slower, bigger in size and better balanced in the control group. When a load was applied to the lower limbs, the pathological subjects were mostly not able to maintain the respiratory diaphragm function, which was lowered significantly. Subjects from the control group showed more stable parameters of both respiratory and postural function. Our findings consistently affirmed worse muscle cooperation in the low back pain population subgroup. A clear relation with spinal findings and with low back pain remains undecided, but various findings in the literature were confirmed. The most important finding is the need to further address various mechanisms used by patients to compensate deep muscle insufficiency.

Editor: Junming Yue, The University of Tennessee Health Science Center, United States of America

Funding: This work has been supported by the research program CVUT SGS.SGS10/279/OHK3/3T/13 and by Ministry of Education, Youth and Sport of the Czech Republic with the grant number MSM6840770012 entitled "Transdisciplinary Research in Biomedical Engineering II". The funders had no role in study design, data collection and analysis, decision to publish, or preparation of the manuscript.

Competing Interests: Tomas and Sarka Rychnovska are employees of Avete omne company. They have no financial interest in the research. The authors declare no other potential conflicts of interest with respect to the authorship and/or publication of this article.

* E-mail: vostapav@fel.cvut.cz

Introduction

The diaphragm and deep stabilization muscles of the body have been described as an important functional unit for dynamic spinal stabilization [1,2]. The diaphragm precedes any movement of the body by lowering and subsequently establishing abdominal pressure which helps to stabilize the lumbar part of the spine. Proper activation of the diaphragm within the stabilization mechanism requires the lower ribs to be in an expiratory (low) position. During the breathing cycle, the lower ribs have to stay in the expiratory position and only expand to the sides. This is an important assumption for the straight and stabilized spine. Under these conditions, the motion of the diaphragm during respiration is smooth, and properly helps to maintain abdominal pressure.

Dysfunction of the cooperation among diaphragm, abdominal muscles, pelvic floor muscles and the deep back muscles is the main cause of vertebrogenic diseases and structural spine findings such as hernia, spondylosis and spondylarthrosis [3,4]. Diaphragm function control is a broad and important issue for a number of fields of investigation, including pulmonology [5], chest surgery [6], rehabilitation [7] and gastroenterology [8]. However, studies dealing with the lumbar stabilization system mostly do not include diaphragm activity monitoring [9]. A traditional objective of studies dealing with diaphragm function is the diaphragm respiratory function [10]; studies focused on postural function are rare.

Studies focused on diaphragm activation with the aim of posture stabilization include Hodges [11–14], who concluded phase modulation corresponding to the movement of the upper limbs in diaphragm electromyography records. Some works deal with various modes of diaphragm functions in various respiration types [15,16] or in situations not directly related to respiration, e.g. activation during breath holding [17]. These studies have always concentrated on healthy subjects who did not exhibit symptoms of respiratory disease or vertebrogenic problems.

The use of magnetic resonance imaging for diaphragm assessment

Studies dealing with diaphragm motion using MRI are taken as a valid method for intrathoracic movement investigations [18]. Gierada [19] assessed MRI artifacts and concluded that MRI is a valid method for diaphragm image processing. Gierada [20] also used MRI for observing the anteroposterior size of the thorax, the height of the diaphragm during inspiration and expiration, and also the ventral and dorsal costophrenic angle during maximal breathe in and out. Kotani [21] and Chu [22] assessed chest and diaphragm movements for scoliosis patients. Suga [23] compared healthy subjects and subjects with chronic obstructive pulmonary disease (COPD), measuring the height, excursions and anteroposterior (AP) size of the diaphragm with the zone of apposition. Paradox diaphragm movements for subjects with COPD were investigated by Iwasawa [10]. Iwasawa used deep breath sequences while comparing diaphragm height and costophrenic angles. The study consisted of healthy subjects and subjects with scoliosis. Kotani [21] concluded that there was ordinary diaphragm motion with limited rib cage motion in the scoliosis group. The position of the diaphragm was measured relative to the apex of the lungs to the highest point of the diaphragm. Chu [22] compared healthy subjects against subjects with scoliosis, finding the same amount of diaphragm movement for both groups. The scoliosis group had the diaphragm significantly lower in the trunk and relatively smaller lung volumes. The distance between the apex of the lungs and the diaphragm ligaments was measured by Kondo [24], comparing young and old subjects. The effect of intraabdominal pressure on the lumbar part of the spine was observed by MRI and pressure measurement by Daggfeldt and Thorstensson [25]. Differences in diaphragm movement while performing thoracic or pulmonary breathing with the same spirometric parameters were tested by Plathow [26]. Plathow also examined the vital capacity of the lungs compared with 2D and 3D views in [27]. He concluded that there was a better correlation between the lung capacity and the 3D scans. In another study, Plathow focused on dynamic MRI. He proved significant correlations among diaphragm length and spirometric values vital capacity (VC), forced expiratory volume (FEV1) and other lung parameters [28].

Relation of structural spine findings and LBP

The causes of LBP and their relations to spinal findings have been the subject of several studies, and continue to be a significant study topic. Harris [29] examined intervertebral discs from 123 subjects concluding comprehensiveness of the objective. Jensen [30] assessed low back magnetic resonance imaging (MRI) with the goal of finding structural changes related to LBP. Jensen found no direct connection between certain types of structural changes and LBP. The only structural change related to pain was disk protrusion. Carragee [31] studied MRI findings of 200 subjects after a period of low LBP, and found no direct significant MRI finding related to low back pain.

The way in which the diaphragm is used for non-breathing purposes is affected by it's recruitment for respiration [32]. There is evidence that the presence of respiratory disease is a stronger predictor for low back pain than other established factors [33]. However, the relationship between the respiratory function and the postural function is widely disregarded [34]. Body muscles coordination for posture stabilization is a complex issue, and the role of the diaphragm in this cooperation has not been intensively studied [35].

In this paper we presents an assessment of a non-respiratory diaphragm function via visual monitoring provided by magnetic resonance imaging (MRI). The main goal is to separate respiratory diaphragm movements from non-respiratory diaphragm movements, and then to evaluate their role in body stabilization. The subjects included in the study consisted of a group of healthy volunteers and a group of volunteers in whom structural spine disorders had been identified, and who suffered from chronic low back pain (lasting for one year at least). To the best of our knowledge, there has been no similar work dedicated to the postural function of the diaphragm in pathological cases.

We investigated diaphragm reactability and movement during tidal breathing and breathing while a load was applied to the lower limbs. We used diaphragm movement harmonicity, frequency and range for both respiratory and postural movements as assessed

parameters. Another part of the parameters was acquired from static measurements, where we assessed diaphragm inclination, height and position in the trunk. Differences between healthy and pathological subjects were evaluated statistically. The results of our work should help in understanding the diaphragm function in the posture stabilization system, with possible implications for physiological practice.

Materials and Methods

1.1 Subjects groups

Two groups of volunteers were selected:

- C_1 — without a pathological condition (n = 16, 11 women, 5 men, control group), id numbers 1–16.
- C_2 — with a structural pathological condition of the spine localized in the lumbar spine area (n = 17, 8 women, 9 men, pathological group), id numbers 17–33.

Neither the healthy subjects nor the pathological subjects had any pulmonary disease. The average age of the control group was 35 years (in the 23–56 age span). The average age in the pathological subjects was 42 years (in the 23–65 age span). Detailed characteristics of the two groups are summarized in Table 1.

Structural findings in the pathological subjects were confirmed by the previous MRI in the lumbar spine area. The study excluded patients with an inborn defect of the spine or a defect acquired traumatically. All pathological subjects had suffered from low back pain of various intensity and frequency for at least one year (classifying the LBP as chronic). Types of the spinal pathologies are presented in Tab 2. The intensity of the LBP was determined using the visual analog pain scale (VAS) with a range of 0–10. The subjects indicated their current pain on the day of imaging and their overall pain in the course of one month before imaging. Length and frequency of the pain symptoms are shown in Table 2. The resulting scores are shown in Table 2. The VAS values for the control group C_1 were zeros for all subjects.

Acute pain was not the criteria for selection of the pathological group. The main criteria was the spinal findings, which is documented in Table 3.

Due to a distinct inter-group difference in age, a paired t-test was performed to confirm no statistical significance among the groups. The resulting p-value (p = 0.08) showed no statistical difference at the 5% significance level. Normality of the age distribution within the groups by the Kolmogorov-Smirnov test ($p_{C1} = 0.89, p_{C2} = 0.55$) confirmed normal distribution of the data. No differences in the mean for all other parameters in Table 1 were confirmed with great significance ($p > 0.2$).

Table 1. Details of the study groups (mean ± standard deviation).

	C_1	C_2
Age	35 ± 11	42 ± 11
Weight (kg)	71 ± 15	78 ± 16
Height (cm)	172 ± 10	174 ± 6
Sternum height (cm)	20.9 ± 1.61	21.4 ± 1.77
Thorax height (cm)	30 ± 2.1	30.2 ± 1.7

C_1 is the control group, C_2 is the pathological group.

Table 2. Pathological subjects' low back pain intensity, pain location and duration.

Subject id	VAS_a	VAS_m	Pain frequency	Pain loc.	LBP duration (years)
17	1.1	6.2	twice a week	Cp, Lp	4
18	5.9	6.6	continuous	Cp, Lp	3
18	0	0	once or twice a year	Lp	20
20	0	2.4	twice a week	Lp	1
21	7.1	1.9	continuous	Lp	10
22	0.9	0.9	once or twice a mont	Lp	27
23	0.5	0.1	once or twice a year	Lp	2
24	5.1	3.1	continuous	Lp, Thp	4
25	6.3	7.1	continuous	Cp, Lp	22
26	5.3	5.3	continuous	Lp	1
27	0.2	6.4	once or twice a month	Cp,Lp	5
28	6.2	2.8	once or twice a year	Lp	16
29	2.2	4.9	once a month	Cp, Lp	9
30	6.6	8.9	once or twice a year	Lp	7
31	0	5.4	four times a month	Cp,Lp	1
32	2	3.7	continuous	Lp	5
33	0	7.7	continuous	Cp,Lp	30

Low back pain intensity values of the pathological subjects determined by visual analog scale (VAS for group C_1 was all zeros). VAS_a represents the actual pain felt on the day when the subject was measured. VAS_m represents the pain felt in a period of one month before the measurements. All subjects exhibited different frequency of pain occurence and duration of the symptoms.

1.2 Study settings

Diaphragm activity was monitored under two different situations:

- S_1 — subjects lie supine on their backs during tidal breathing.
- S_2 — subjects lie supine on their backs during tidal breathing while loading is applied to the distal part of their extended lower extremities against the flexion of the hips. The applied pressure was of the 4th grade according to Janda's muscle test [36]. The subjects ensured that no additional pain was induced by the maneuver.

1.3 Ethics Statement

All patients provided written, informed consent for participation in the study and the study was approved by the Ethics Committee of the Motol University Hospital in Prague, Czech Republic.

1.4 Data Acquisition

The healthy group was examined in an open Siemens MRI apparatus, with a 0.23 T magnet and the NUMARIS/4 syngo MRI 2004A software load version. The length of each recorded sequence was 18 s. During this time, 77 images were recorded at regular intervals. The subject was in a supine position, using a size large body coil. The projection plane was placed sagittally in the axial topogram directed paravertebrally on the right side, midway through the center of the vertebral body and the edge of the thoracic wall. The width of each layer was 33 mm. The true FISP dynamic sequence was used, configured as follows: 1 NSA, matrix 240×256 pixels, TR 4.48 ms, TE 2.24 ms, FA 90, TSE1, FOV 328 mm.

The pathological study group was scanned by General Electric SIGNA HDx MRI, with a 1.5 T magnet and the 14-M5A software load version. The length of each recorded sequence was 22.2 s, resulting in the acquisition of 60 images. The projection plane was placed sagittally in the axial topogram directed paravertebrally on the right side, midway through the center of the vertebral body and the edge of the thoracic wall. The width of each layer was 15 mm. The GE FIESTA Cine dynamic sequence was used, configured as follows: 1 NSA, matrix 256×256 pixels, TR 3.1 ms, TE 1.3 ms, FA 55, FOV 420 mm.

The proposed processing methodology is indifferent to distinct images resolution, e.g. the resolution of the control group: 1.37 mm/pixel, pathological group: 1.64 mm/pixel. Three markers, 20-ml syringes filled with water, were placed on the skin surface of each subject on his right side. They are shown as hyper signal marks on the body surface (see for example Figure 1). The first marker was placed in the mid-clavicular line at the level of the jugular notch, and the second marker was placed at the level of the inferior 10-rib costal margin. The last marker was placed on the back of the subject at the level of the thoracolumbar junction.

The spatial resolution of our images was sufficient for proper diaphragm contour recognition on each sequence. In addition, the temporal resolution was sufficient, with a maximum recorded breathing frequency of 0.54 Hz. The diaphragm contour areas were not affected by artifacts. Image brightness was the only varying parameter, and there was no significant effect on the resulting differential curves.

1.5 MRI Processing

In order to assess diaphragm activity, the **differential curve** (dif-curve) was calculated across all MR images. Firstly, let us define the **differential area** (a_t) as the area bordered by the diaphragm in the lowest position from the sequence and the diaphragm in current (t-th) image — see Figure 1. The image containing the lowest placed diaphragm is called the background

Table 3. Pathological subjects' spine findings.

Subject id	Spine pathology
17	canal stenosis
18	disc protrusion
18	disc prolapse
20	disc degeneration
21	spondylolysis L5/S1, disc protrusion L5/S1
22	disc protrusion L1/L2, L2/L3
23	disc degeneration L4/L5
24	canal stenosis
25	canal stenosis
26	disc degeneration L4/L5 a L5/S1
27	disc degeneration L4/L5, end plates degeneration Th11/12
28	canal stenosis, end plates degeneration Th11/12 a Th12/L1
29	spinal canal stenosis, disc degeneration L4/L5 and L5/S1
30	spine stenosis, disc degeneration L4/L5 with protrusion
31	disc degeneration L4/L5 a L5/S1 with protrusion
32	disc protrusion L1/L2, L2/L3, canal stenosis, lig. flava hypertrophy
33	disc prolapse C5/C6

Pathological spinal condition observed during MRI spinal examination.

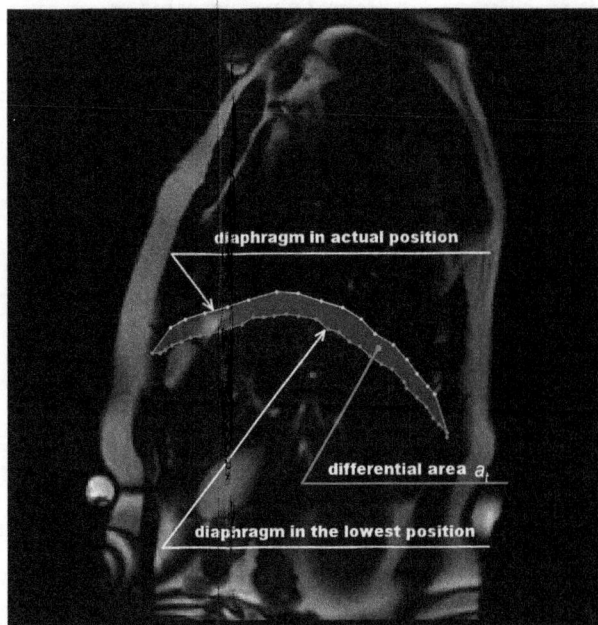

Figure 1. Differential area definition. Figure shows t-th image from a sequence with corrensponding diaphragm contour. The t-th diaphragm contour together with the lowest placed diaphragm contour in the sequence form the diferential area a_t.

picture. Secondly, the dif-curve is defined as the time series of a_t, measured in mm^2. Hence, the dif-curve is an integral quantity which characterizes the diaphragm motion in the same manner as spirometry, but it consists strictly of diaphragm movement. The algorithm for a_t calculation is shown in Figure 2A–C. Typical dif-curves are shown in Figures 3, 4.

1.6 Extraction of respiratory and postural movements from the dif-curve

Each digitally sampled signal can be expressed as the sum of a finite number of harmonic waves of different amplitudes and phases. Decomposition of the signal into harmonic components is traditionally represented by the harmonic spectrum of the signal. The spectrum denotes the relation between the amplitudes and the frequencies of the harmonic waves. Typical dif-curves spectra are shown in Figure 3. Each peak in the spectrum stands for one harmonic component. If the diaphragm worked only for respiration with stable depth of the motion it would lead to a simple spectrum with a single peak corresponding to the breathing frequency. This motion would be fully described by a single sine wave. Diaphragm motion is more complex, and often involves other non-respiratory movements. However, due to the harmonic properties of respiration, the harmonic spectrum is useful for dif-curve processing.

We chose to model diaphragm motion by two sine waves corresponding to respiratory and non-respiratory movements. These waves are extracted from the dif-curve spectrum by the inverse Fourier transform. The two models are shown in Figure 3A,B. The original dif-curve is plotted by a solid line. The respiratory model is called a **respiratory curve (res-curve)**. The non-respiratory model is called a **postural curve (pos-curve)**. The res-curve fully characterizes the respiratory movement by frequency and amplitude. The pos-curve provides a model of a postural global range by a pos-curve amplitude. If there were several peaks that together compose the final respiratory or

postural part of the signal, we chose by visual inspection the peak that best described the values of the original signal (peaks and subsequent pos-curves are marked in Figure 3 by a green square).

The relation between breath regularity and the spectrum complexity of the corresponding dif-curves is summarized in Fig. 3. Fig. 3A,C provides an example of a dif-curve with the corresponding spectrum for a person whose respiratory movements are widely regular. In the corresponding spectrum there is one significant peak, which represents the subject's respiration marked by a red dot. The diaphragm respiratory movement is also modulated by other movements. This causes the occurrence of smaller peaks besides the respiratory peak. These peaks capture smaller parts of the diaphragm movement. Fig. 3B,D shows a more complex dif-curve with less regular respiration. The spectrum (Fig. 3D) has a clearly visible peak, which corresponds to the respiration (marked by a red dot) and, again at lower frequencies, there are peaks which modulate the respiratory movement. This time, however, the peaks capture a much bigger part of the diaphragm movement.

Three typical dif-curves with corresponding respiratory and postural models for both situations, S_1 and S_2, are shown in Figure 4. There is a clearly visible respiratory function (A) with a big postural movement in situation S_2 (B) for subject 11. Subject 25 (in E, F) did not respire for the first six seconds of the imaging in situation S_2, and then the respiration became regular. The subject 24 (C, D) exhibited almost no respiration during situation S_2. Dif-curves including no respiration led to exclusion of the subject from further statistical data processing.

1.7 MR Parameters Extraction

Two sets of parameters were extracted on the basis of diaphragm MRI activity: **Dynamic parameters** are based on dif-curve processing. The main aim of introducing dynamic parameters was to assess which part of diaphragm motion is

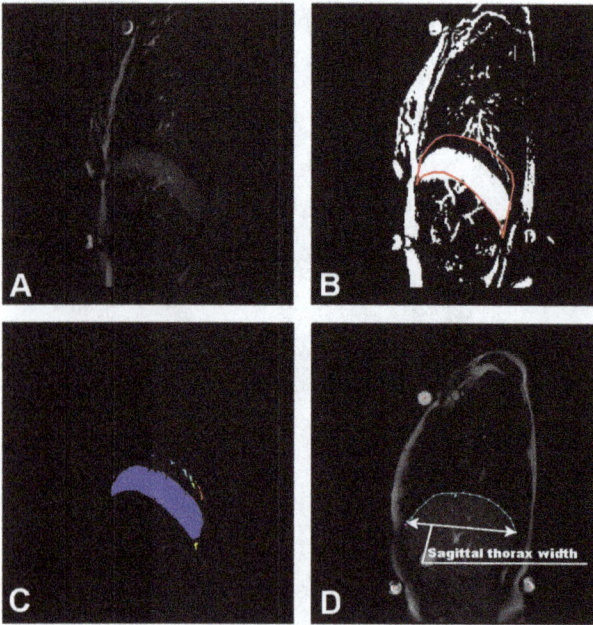

Figure 2. Differential area calculation. Image on t-th position in a sequence is subtracted from the background image (the image with the lowest placed diaphragm) (A). Subtracted image is thresholded, providing a binary image with a clearly visible crescent corresponding to movement of the diaphragm (B). The red-bordered part, surrounding the highest and the lowest diaphragm position from the whole sequence reducing the space for crescent location. Continuous image parts inside the border are labeled and the part corresponding to diaphragm movement is than processed (C). Some of the extracted parameters were normalized using the thorax width measure shown here (D).

related to respiration, and how significant non-respiratory movements are.

- Frequency and amplitude of res-curve: f_r, respectively a_r.

- Amplitude of pos-curve: a_p.
- Amplitudes ratio of res-curve and pos-curve: $r_{pr} = \frac{a_p}{a_r}$.
- Range of diaphragm motion measured in 3 different points placed on diaphragm surface rg_i, $i \in 1,2,3$. See Figure 5. Measured in mm.
- The percentage of energy yielded by the three biggest spectrum lines: p_3.
- Standard deviation, skewness and kurtosis of the dif-curve: $\sigma_{DC}, \gamma_{DC}, \beta_{DC}$.

Static parameters assess diaphragm shape and position. For the static parameters, the following features were extracted in order to analyze the anatomic characteristics of the diaphragm:

- Diaphragm inclination in the sagittal plane in caudal position: dec_a. Angle measured as shown in Figure 6.
- Height of a strip overlapping the diaphragm contour parallel diaphragm inclination: h_d — see Figure 7.
- Vertical distance from anterior point used for rg_3 and back marker (syringe): d_p. This parameter corresponds to the diaphragm height in the thorax. See Figure 8.

1.8 Statistical Analysis

A paired t-test was used to identify differences between the control and the pathological group. The significance of the statistical test is marked by symbol *, or by symbol ** if level of significance was below $p < 0.05$, respectively $p < 0.001$, as indicated in Tables 4, 5, 6 in Section 2. A Kolmogorov-Smirnov (KS) analysis was performed, to assess the normality of the data.

The correlation (by Pearson's correlation coefficient) between all parameters and the subjects body mass index (BMI) was assessed in order to eliminate an effect on the results. The parameters affected by BMI dependence were in situation $S_1 : p_3, h_d$ and in situation $S_2 : a_r, \beta_{DC}, \gamma_{DC}, d_p$. A possible way to suppress the correlation with BMI was to normalize the parameters by the width of the subject's thorax (Figure 2E, the width was determined during the lowest position of the diaphragm). However, no influence on the statistical results was observed after normaliza-

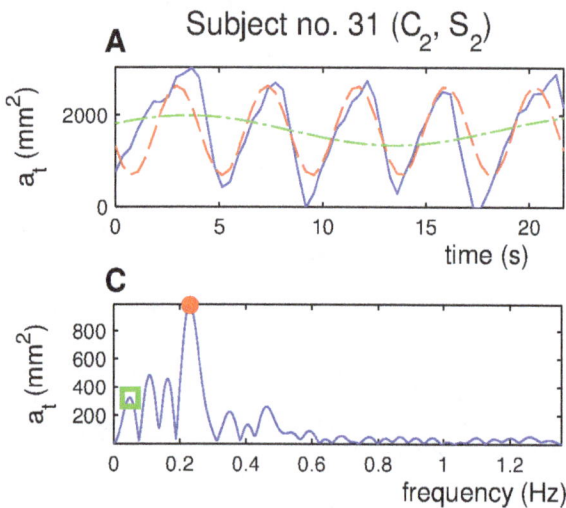

Figure 3. Dif-curves (A, B, solid line) and appropriate spectra (C, D, solid line). Extracted res-curves (red dashed line, A, B) and pos-curves (green dotted line, A, B) with corresponding spectral peaks (C, D) marked in the spectra with a red dot (respiratory peak) and a green square (postural peak).

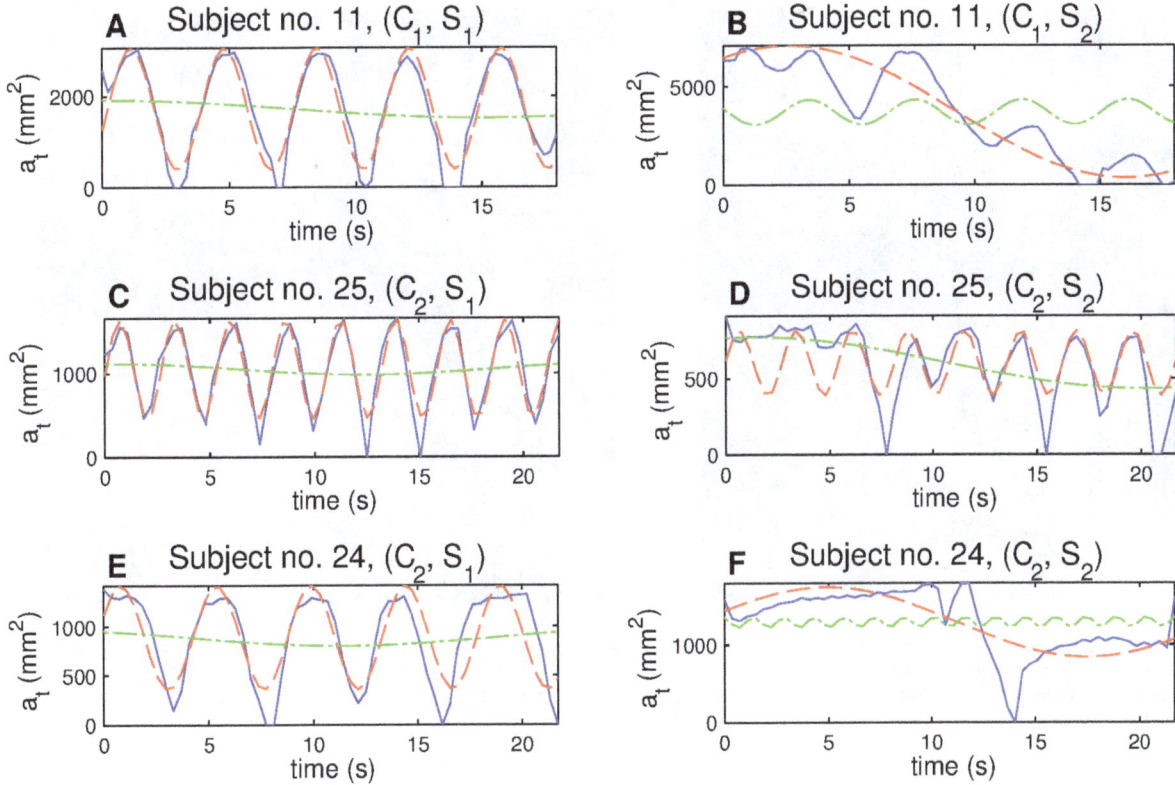

Figure 4. Dif-curves (solid line) and extracted res-curves (red dashed line) and pos-curves (green dotted line). Example of harmonic breathing (A), breath with a strong postural part after the load occurred (B), harmonic breath which became partly non-harmonic after the load occurred (C, D), and breath which almost lost its ability of respiration movement ability after the load occurred (E, F).

tion, except for parameter h_d, which t-test results changed by two orders of magnitude (though there was no change in significance). In order to keep results clear, all were kept in the original units, with the exception of h_d, which is in normalized form.

All extracted features were treated for outlier values. Outlier values were determined as follows:

$$\text{proper data range} = \langle P_{25} - w \cdot (P_{75} - P_{25}), P_{75} + w \cdot (P_{75} - P_{25}) \rangle \quad (1)$$

P_k stands for k-th percentile, w is a constant set by default to 1.5. This value ensures approximately 99.3 percent coverage of the data, when the data is normally distributed. Data outside this range is likely to consist of error values or marginal data that distorts the statistics.

Secondly, as stated in the methodology section (Sec. 1.6), patients were present in our datasets whose respiration did not exhibit proper respiration movement. These subjects were also excluded from the statistical evaluation — four subjects, all from the pathological group C_2 (id numbers: 19, 24, 27, 29).

Results

The results are presented in Tables 4, 5, 6.

2.1 Dynamic parameters

2.1.1 Respiratory and postural curves. We concluded significantly faster respiration in pathological group in both observed situations S_1, S_2, with $p < 0.05$. Respiratory frequency

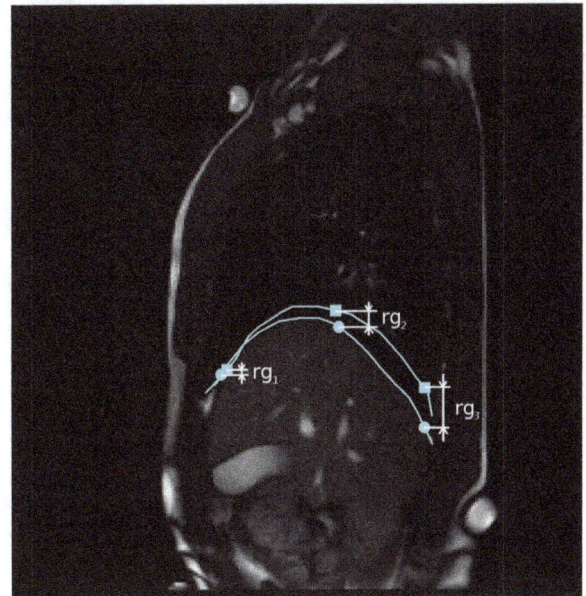

Figure 5. Parameters rg_i. Parameters rg_i are computed as vertical subtraction of caudal from cranial diaphragm position. The three parameters correspond to the anterior (rg_1), middle (rg_2) and posterior (rg_3) diaphragm part. Points were spread evenly on the diaphragm contour with small constant drift of rg_1 and rg_3 from the contour margins.

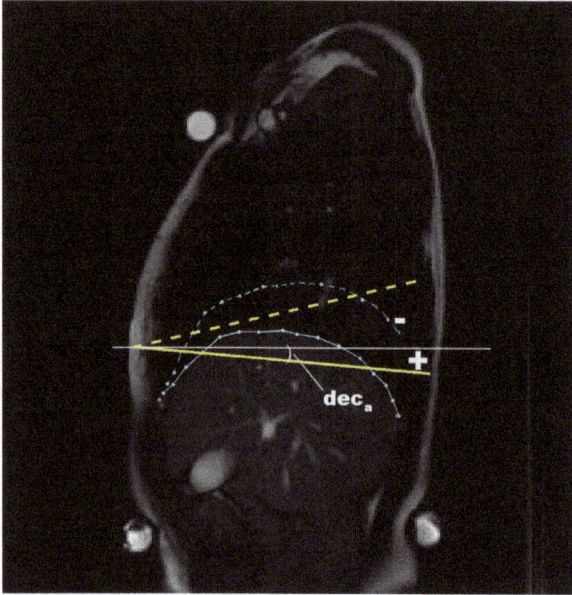

Figure 6. Measurement of the diaphragm inclination. Inclination of the diaphragm was measured by angle between the line fitted to the diaphragm contour and horizontal axis. The inclination was measured during the caudal diaphragm position.

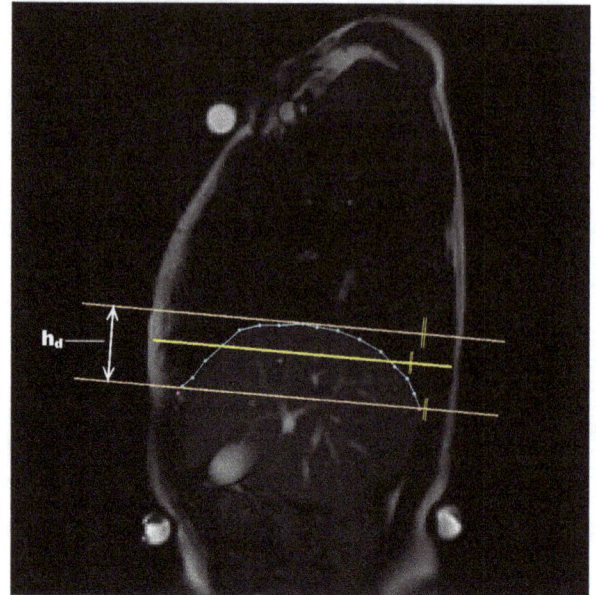

Figure 7. Measurement of the diaphragm height h_d**.** Measurement was done during the diaphragm caudal position. The middle line is the line fitted to the diaphragm contour by least squares method.

did not change much for the control group after a load was applied to the lower limbs ($0.21 Hz$ in S_1, $0.22 Hz$ in S_2). By contrast, the frequency of the pathological group rose significantly ($p=0.01$). The height of the diaphragm respiratory movements reflected by the respiratory curve amplitude (a_r) resulted in very significant difference among the groups, with $p<0.001$ in both situations S_1,S_2. As in the case of respiratory frequency, there was no change in respiratory curve amplitude in the control group when a load was applied to the lower limbs ($1823\ mm^2\ S_1$, $1928\ mm^2\ S_2$). By contrast, the pathological group showed lowered excursions when load was applied ($870\ mm^2\ S_1$, $540\ mm^2\ S_2$). The inter-situational difference was significantly different amongst the groups with $p=0.004$. In comparison with the pathological group, the control group had 3 times bigger excursions in situation S_1, and 6.5 times bigger excursions in the situation S_2.

In order to compare diaphragm excursions in mm, rg_i parameters were introduced. The diaphragms excursions was measured in three points laid on the diaphragm contour — anterior, central and posterior part (see Figure 5). The control group exhibited a significantly bigger motion range than the pathological group in both situations ($p<0.001$). In addition, the measurements showed great motion of the posterior diaphragm part than of the anterior part. In S_1, the antero-posterior ratio was 2.2 within the control group and 4.2 within the pathological group. In S_2, the control group raised the range of the posterior part to 56.5 mm, resulting in an antero-posterior ratio of 2.5. The pathological group, by contrast, raised the range in the anterior area and reduced the range in posterior area, resulting in an antero-posterior ratio of 2.3.

The range of postural movements (the amplitude of the postural curve a_p) was great in the control group (C_1: $380\ mm^2\ S_1$, $660\ mm^2\ S_2$, C_2: $260\ mm^2\ S_1$, $570\ mm^2\ S_2$), with the only statistically significant difference in situation S_1 ($p=0.04$). For both groups, the amplitude of the postural curve rose when a load was applied to the lower limbs, while the rises in C_1 and C_2 did not

differ significantly ($p=0.27$). The amplitude ratio of the res-curve and the pos-curve r_{pr} shows which type of diaphragm motion dominates in the overall motion. When this parameter is greater than 1, it means that postural moves of the diaphragm are bigger than the respiratory moves, and vice versa. Moreover, in situation S_2 the range of motion in the pathological group was equally distributed between respiratory and postural movement ranges (r_{pr} 0.95, meaning 50% of the total motion range by postural motion

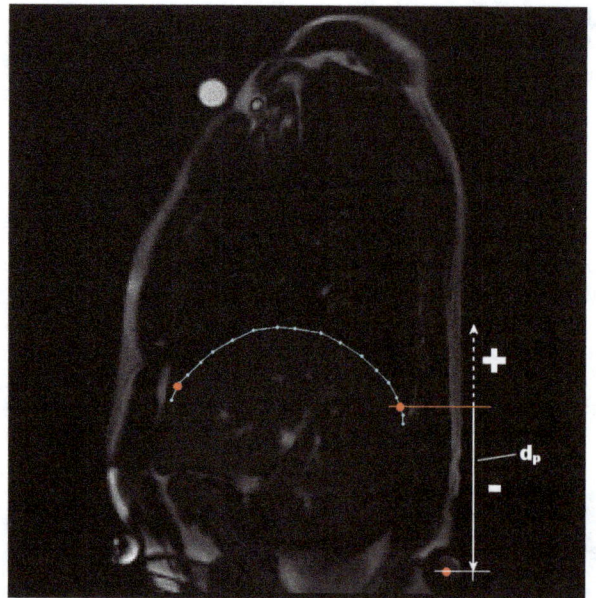

Figure 8. Measurement of the diaphragm height in the trunk. The figure indicates when the height is negative (the diaphragm higher than the back marker) and when the height is positive (the diaphragm placed under the back marker).

Table 4. Dynamic parameters results, first part.

		f_r (Hz)	a_r (mm²)	r_{pr} (−)	a_p (mm²)	p_3 (%)
S_1	C_1	0.21 ± 0.06	1823 ± 873	0.3 ± 0.2	378 ± 163	46.7 ± 7.8
	C_2	0.26 ± 0.06	870 ± 297	0.31 ± 0.21	258 ± 152	29.7 ± 6.3
	p	*	**	−	*	**
S_2	C_1	0.22 ± 0.08	1928 ± 864	0.30 ± 0.12	659 ± 353	45.9 ± 5.3
	C_2	0.34 ± 0.1	540 ± 314	0.95 ± 0.61	574 ± 402	24.5 ± 5.8
	p	*	**	*	−	**
$S_2 - S_1$	C_1	0.006 ± 0.07	300 ± 740	-0.02 ± 0.25	160 ± 470	-1.6 ± 6.6
	C_2	0.083 ± 0.08	-360 ± 190	0.7 ± 0.55	320 ± 310	-9.2 ± 3.8
	p	*	*	**	−	*

$S_{1,2}$ stands for the monitoring situations, $C_{1,2}$ stands for the subjects groups, p stands for p-value of the student's t-test among the groups. $S_2 - S_1$ stands for subtraction of parameter — assess change of the parameter after a load was applied to the lower limbs. The parameters are: frequency (f_r) and amplitude (a_r) of res-curve. Amplitude of pos-curve (a_p). Amplitudes ratio of res-curve and pos-curve (r_{pr}). The percentage of energy yielded by the three biggest spectrum lines (p_3).

and 50% by respiratory motion), while both in situation S_1 and in situation S_2 the control group had the same ratio of postural and respiratory movements of 0.3 (23% of the total motion range for postural motion and 77% for respiratory motion).

2.1.2 Diaphragm motion harmonicity and central moments. The most important dif-curve shape parameter is its harmonicity, reflected by parameter p_3. When the patient loses control over the diaphragm motion, the dif-curve loses its typical harmonic shape and the three biggest spectral lines carry less of the signal energy (see Section 1.6). The control group was able to keep the harmonicity almost at the same level in both situations (S_1 46.7%, S_2 46%), while the pathological group achieved a significantly (p-values $< 10^{-7}$) lower percentage (S_1 29.7%, S_2 25.5%). For the pathological group, the decrease in the p_3 value was significantly bigger (p-value 0.002) bigger than decrease for the control group.

The third central statistical moment, skewness (γ_{DC}), elegantly characterizes the centering of the dif-curve around it's mean value. This parameter can be used to indicate whether the patient kept the diaphragm longer in inspiratory position or in expiratory position. Naturally, harmonic breath would lead to zero skewness. If the diaphragm is kept longer in inspiratory (caudal) position there is positive skewness, and if the diaphragm is kept in longer in

respiratory (cranial) position there is negative skewness. In S_1, both the control and the pathological group had negative skewness (C_1: -0.11, C_2: -0.65). However, the control group exhibited big variance (positive skewness in a case of 6 subjects). For the pathological group, all values were negative except in the case of one subject. The difference is significant ($p < 0.001$), despite big variance in the control group. In S_2, the mean skewness values were C_1: -0.13, C_2: -0.57. The control group became more consistent, while the pathological group exhibited great variance for this parameter. This is due to an increase in the influence of the postural part of the diaphragm movement. The difference between groups C_1, C_2 was significant, with $p = 0.02$. There was no significant change, either in the control or in pathological group, when a load was applied to the lower limbs ($p = 0.87$).

The fourth central statistical moment kurtosis can be used to study control over the diaphragm movement. Harmonic motion shows lower kurtosis than more random, worse controlled motion. In situation S_1, the control group had a lower kurtosis parameter (1.92) than pathological group (2.23), with a significant difference, $p = 0.03$. In situation S_2, the kurtosis parameter for the control group fell to 1.67, and for the pathological rose to 2.89, which raised the significance of the inter-group difference (p-value $= 3 \cdot 10^{-6}$).

Table 5. Dynamic parameters results, second part.

		σ_{DC}	γ_{DC}	β_{DC}	rg_1 (mm)	rg_2 (mm)	rg_3 (mm)
S_1	C_1	1416 ± 607	-0.11 ± 0.46	1.92 ± 0.39	21.1 ± 10.1	40.7 ± 13.4	47.1 ± 12.3
	C_2	786 ± 218	-0.65 ± 0.20	2.23 ± 0.33	7 ± 7.7	21.7 ± 5.7	29.8 ± 6.6
	p	**	**	*	**	**	**
S_2	C_1	1711 ± 624	-0.13 ± 0.29	1.67 ± 0.10	22.1 ± 10.8	46.1 ± 14.3	56.5 ± 17.7
	C_2	670 ± 290	-0.57 ± 0.66	2.89 ± 0.68	10.1 ± 6.1	20.6 ± 8.6	23.7 ± 8.1
	p	**	*	**	**	**	**
$S_2 - S_1$	C_1	300 ± 650	0.084 ± 0.37	-0.14 ± 0.51	0.95 ± 11	5.4 ± 15	6.5 ± 19
	C_2	-96 ± 210	0.11 ± 0.66	0.49 ± 0.79	4.6 ± 6.2	-0.36 ± 7	-5.4 ± 8.8
	p	*	−	*	−	−	*

$S_{1,2}$ stands for the monitoring situations, $C_{1,2}$ stands for the subjects groups, p stands for p-value of the student's t-test among the groups. $S_2 - S_1$ stands for subtraction of parameter — assess change of the parameter after a load was applied to the lower limbs. The parameters are: standard deviation (σ_{DC}), skewness (γ_{DC}) and kurtosis (β_{DC}) of the dif-curve. Range of diaphragm motion measured in 3 different points placed on diaphragm surface $rg_i, i \in 1,2,3$.

2.2 Static parameters

The diaphragm height, described by the h_d parameter (higher h_d means a more bulging diaphragm), differs significantly between the groups, both in situation S_1 (p-value = 0.001) and in situation S_2 (p-value = 0.003). The parameter was independent of postural load, and has a very similar value for both situation S_1 and situation S_2: 0.25 for the control group, and 0.32 for the pathological group. The parameter was normalized by the anteroposterior size of the thorax. In addition, the dependency of the parameter on the patient's pain intensity was revealed (see Section 2.4).

The inclination of the diaphragm in caudal position (dec_a) differs significantly between the groups in the two observed situations (S_1, $p = 0.0005$, S_2, $p = 0.02$). The difference between situation S_1 and situation S_2 was not great (within the standard deviation range), and was statistically the same for both groups ($p = 0.27$). The mean inclination in situation S_1 was 23.8° in the control group and 15° for the pathological group, i.e. the control group kept the diaphragm in a more vertical position.

The diaphragm height in the thorax (d_p) differs considerably between the groups ($p < 10^{-10}$). The control group kept the diaphragm below the back marker in both situations. In situation S_1 the value was 2.9 cm, and in situation S_2 the value was 3.5 cm. The diaphragm was lowered by 0.6 cm on an average, which is a small value in comparison with the standard deviation of the values. In situation S_1 the pathological group had the diaphragm in a position 6.4 cm above the back marker, on an average, and 5.1 cm above the marker in situation S_2. The average difference is 1.3 cm. No statistically significant difference (p-value 0.15) was found among the diaphragm shifts after a load was applied to the lower limbs.

2.3 Summary

We concluded that there was slower and deeper respiratory motion (parameters f_r, a_r) for both observed situations. In addition, after the postural demands rose in situation S_2, the breathing speed increased significantly ($p = 0.01$) in the pathological group. In the same manner the breath depth (a_r) lessened significantly ($p = 0.004$) in the pathological group. There were bigger postural moves in the control group, and they remained bigger in both

situations, rising equally for each group. The res/pos ratio r_{pr} shows great domination of postural moves in the pathological group. As the respiratory moves lowered when there was a load, the ratio rose greatly in the pathological group, and the difference between the groups became significant. A very significant difference in harmonicity emerged, which is denoted by the p_3, β_{DC} parameters. These parameters indicates a much more harmonic diaphragm movement in the control group, with or without a load. In addition, β_{DC} increased significantly ($p = 0.02$) in both situations in the pathological group. The diaphragm motion in the thorax was symmetrical for the control group.

The results for the static parameters revealed that the diaphragm of the control group was flatter (parameter h_d) in both situations. The inclination of the diaphragm was greater (i.e. it was more verticalized) in the control group. The pathological group had the diaphragm placed significantly higher in the trunk, as indicated by the d_p parameter.

2.4 Correlation between pain intensity (VAS), pain duration and the measured parameters

A correlation analysis between VAS of the subjects' LBP intensity and the measured parameters revealed that the only correlated parameter was h_d ($p = 0.045$). A significant correlation emerged only in situation S_2 (Figure 9). The only significant correlation was detected for VAS summarized for the month before imaging. There was no significant correlation between diaphragm motion harmonicity or range and the intensity of the subjects' LBP. No correlation was detected between the parameters and pain duration either.

Discussion

Studies of diaphragm motion using MRI are taken as a valid method for intrathoracic movement investigations [18–20]. Plathow [18] assessed diaphragm length using dynamic MRI in the mid-coronal plane by 1.5 T magnetic resonance, and concluded that the spatial and time resolution is sufficient for acquiring the breathing sequences. Gierada [20] also used a 1.5 T MRI device for measuring the height of the excursions of the diaphragm at three different points in several sagittal planes. Gierada [19] assessed MRI artifacts and concluded that MRI is a valid method for diaphragm image processing along the diaphragm contour. Suga [23] used breathing MRI (BMRI) for comparing healthy subjects and subjects with chronic obstructive pulmonary disease (COPD), measuring excursions and the length of the apposition of the diaphragm in supine position. Suga concluded that BMRI is a useful non-invasive method with good spatial and temporal resolution.

The extracted parameters were selected in a way that allows a wide spectrum of diaphragm properties to be assessed. A novel method involves evaluating harmonicity using statistical methods (kurtosis) or harmonic spectrum processing. Some similar parameters to ours can be found in the literature — measurements of cranio-caudal excursions of the diaphragm [23,26,37–39] and the anteroposterior and lateral proportion of the diaphragm [21,22]. Plathow [40] measured shortening of the diaphragm contour in the sagittal and frontal plane. The height and anteroposterior proportion of the diaphragm were assessed in [10,20,24]. Miyamoto [41] assessed the curvature of the diaphragm. Differences between the diaphragm in inspiratory and expiratory positions, measured by Gierada [20] and Takazakura [42], were used to determine the height of the diaphragm motion. Gierada [19] compared the movement of the ventral and dorsal part of the

Table 6. Static parameters results.

		h_d (–)	dec_a (°)	d_p (mm)
S_1	C_1	0.25 ± 0.06	23.8 ± 7.1	29 ± 28
	C_2	0.32 ± 0.05	15 ± 5.6	−64 ± 18
	p	*	**	**
S_2	C_1	0.25 ± 0.05	24.8 ± 9.6	35 ± 20
	C_2	0.31 ± 0.06	17.8 ± 5.8	−51 ± 17
	p	*	*	**
$S_2 - S_1$	C_1	0.0009 ± 0.04	1.7 ± 6	6.6 ± 20.7
	C_2	−0.02 ± 0.03	3.6 ± 3.1	15.8 ± 14.1
	p	–	–	–

$S_{1,2}$ stands for the monitoring situations, $C_{1,2}$ stands for the subjects groups, p stands for p-value of the student's t-test among the groups. $S_2 - S_1$ stands for subtraction of parameter — assess change of the parameter after a load was applied to the lower limbs. The parameters are: diaphragm inclination in the sagittal plane in caudal position (dec_a). Height of a strip overlapping the diaphragm contour (h_d). The diaphragm height in the thorax (d_p).

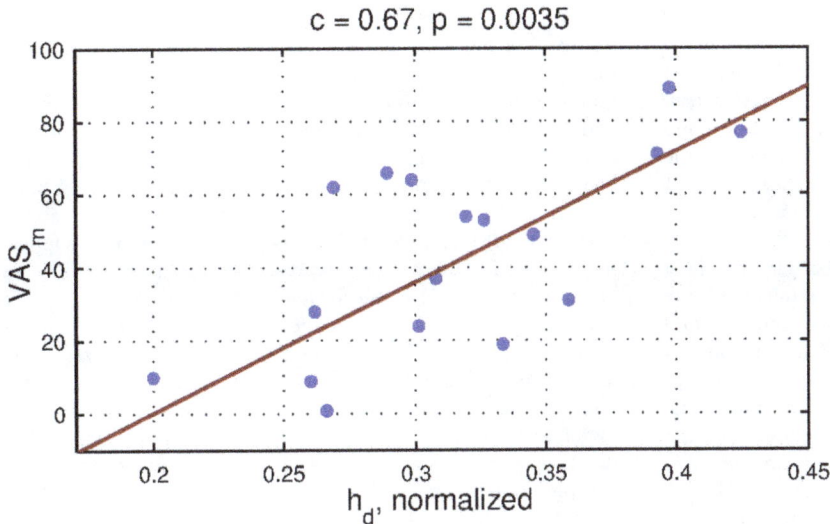

Figure 9. Correlation between VAS_m **parameter and** h_d **parameter in situation** S_2. Diaphragm height were the only diaphragm parameter which was statistically significantly correlated (p = 0.0035) with the subjects' low back pain indicated during the month before imaging. Pearson correlation coefficient was 0.67.

diaphragm using MRI. Kolar [17] used measurements of the differential area.

In the results section, we concluded that there is a statistically significant difference in the range of motion (ROM) of the diaphragm. A two and three times greater ROM was noted in the control group, than in the pathological group in situations S_1 and S_2. In addition, the average diaphragm excursions rg_2 (central part) in situation S_1 were 40 mm in the control group and 22 mm in the pathological group. In situation S_2, rg_2 was 46 mm in the control group and 21 mm in the pathological group. The diaphragm excursions rose from the ventral part to the dorsal part. Gierada [20] also concluded that there was a bigger motion range in the ventral diaphragm of the diaphragm than in the dorsal part. Kondo, who studied the correlation between lung volume and diaphragm motion, came to the same conclusion in [17]. Kolar [39] observed diaphragm excursions 27.3 ± 10.2 mm in the apex and 39 ± 17.6 mm in the dorsal part during tidal breathing. Takazakura [42] showed a difference of 20 mm within the highest point of the diaphragm motion when sitting and when supine. Taking into account the large range of diaphragm motions reported in the literature [43], our measurements prove to be consistent.

When considering changes in the range of diaphragm motion after pressure was applied to the lower limbs, the ROM values for the control group rose on an average, but there was great variance in the group, and the rise was bigger in the posterior part than in the anterior part. The ROM values for the pathological group rose in the anterior part of the diaphragm, and lessened in the posterior diaphragm part. In contrast to our measurements, Kolar [44] observed an opposite change in the same situations. In Kolar's case, the range of motions was the same during tidal breathing, but the group with LBP had lower excursions of the anterior part of the diaphragm. The subjects in Kolar's study had the diaphragm at the same height in the trunk, despite the symptoms. We observed that the diaphragm was significantly higher for the pathological group. This may be a mechanism by which the pathological group was able to keep the diaphragm excursions more evenly spread after the postural demands increased.

We also observed that the diaphragm was more contracted in the posterior part for the control group. Diaphragm inclination measurements showed significant lowering of the posterior part of the diaphragm relative to the anterior part of the diaphragm for the control group. The pathological group kept the diaphragm in a more horizontal position. The average changes in inclination after a rise in postural demands were only small in comparison with variance of the inclination. The height of the diaphragm contour (h_d) above the zone of apposition was also measured as a significant parameter between the groups of subjects. Suwatana-pongched [43] concluded that there was flattening of the diaphragm in the older population in his study. Our results did not show any significant age-related correlation of diaphragm flatness. Instead, the only significant correlation that we observed was between diaphragm height and the LBP intensity of the pathological group during the month before the measurements were made. The correlation was significant in situation S_2. We assume that this diaphragm bulging is due to worse ability to contract the diaphragm properly. To the best of our knowledge, there are no results in the literature for measurements of diaphragm flatness in subjects suffering from LBP. Worse ability to contract the diaphragm in the pathological group is also supported by the significantly higher position in the trunk.

Other questions which emerge in relation to LBP intensity are the effects of acute pain. These would bias our findings, as the study focused on long time changes in the motion patterns of the diaphragm. The first factor is the pain induced by the applied load. This was controlled by our methodology, and the subjects ensured that no additional pain was induced by postural load. The second factor concerns differences in pain intensity perceived on the day of measurement, and the influence of the pain on the results. An important consideration is that the pain was chronic, and so we assume a tendency of the muscles to overload the spine, and some influence of the observed structural degenerative spinal findings. The range of pain intensity on the day of measurement of the patients is wide, from 0 to 8.9 (refer to Table 2). This wide range of pain intensity is useful for revealing a possible dependency of the parameters on acute perception of the pain. The best practice would be to classify the subjects into groups according to pain, and to treat the groups statistically. However, the kind of evaluation was not possible, because we would have needed many more study subjects. A second option was to examine the correlation between pain intensity and the measured parameters. No correlation was concluded between measured parameters and pain intensity except for bulging (i.e. long term pain) of the diaphragm, as was discussed above. The results indicate that, as the pain is long term, the patients do not change their respiratory patterns according to fluctuations in the chronic LBP.

It was concluded that a useful method for comparing the ratio of actual respiratory-related motions with other motions of the diaphragm is to separate the differential curve into respiratory and non-respiratory movements of the diaphragm. This division was inspired by various works. In [45–47] the postural and respiratory functions of the diaphragm were assessed using invasive EMG. Hodges [3,46,48] described tonic and respiratory activation during the breathing cycle and superimposition of the electromyographic signals phasically related to harmonic limb movement. Hodges also used the harmonic spectrum in his investigation of muscle cooperation for compensating breathing movements in body posture. Our study showed a non-negligible proportion of non-respiratory diaphragmatic motion, referred to as postural movements. These movements formed one third of the diaphragm motion range, on an average, in tidal breathing. The rise in the range of postural motions when there is an increase in postural demands on the body confirms the participation of the diaphragm in postural mechanisms. Separating the respiratory signal from the postural signal was important in cases when postural movements start to form a large proportion of the diaphragm motion, as in situation S_2 for the pathological group. A simple investigation of the differential curve does not show significant lowering of the respiratory motion range, but after the signals are separated significant changes are revealed in both the postural and the respiratory parts of the movement.

The significant differences in the harmonicity of the diaphragm motion observed in this study indicate changes in the central nervous system related to diaphragm function in subjects with pathological spinal findings suffering from various intensities of chronic low back pain. Low back pain is a wide-spread and widely studied phenomenon. Alternating respiratory patterns and ana-tomical changes in the diaphragm have been assessed in LBP subjects. Studies concluding increased susceptibility to pain and injury [1,13,49] identified differences in muscle recruitment in people suffering from LBP. Janssens [50] used fatigue of inspiratory muscles, and observed altered postural stabilizing strategy in healthy subjects. Jenssens also observed non-worsening stabilization with an already altered stabilizing strategy in subjects suffering from LBP. Grimstone [51] measured respiration-related body imbalance in subjects suffering from LBP, observing worse stability in subjects with LBP. Kolar [44] investigated differences in diaphragm contractions between healthy subjects and LBP subjects. He observed lesser contractions in the posterior part of the diaphragm while the postural demands on the lower limbs increased, and he suspected that intra-abdominal pressure lowering might be the underlying mechanism of LBP. Roussel [34] assessed the altered breathing patterns of LBP subjects during lumbopelvic motor control tests, concluding that some subjects used an altered breathing pattern to provide stronger support for spinal stability.

In our measurements, we did not observe the same diaphragm excursions in the posterior part of the diaphragm for healthy subjects and for subjects suffering from LBP as were observed by [44]. The excursions were reduced in the pathological group. In contrast with Kolar's findings [44], we concluded that there was

also lowering of the diaphragm inspiratory position in the pathological group in situation S_2. Our measurements support the hypothesis of less diaphragm contraction in the pathological group, with a significant correlation between diaphragm bulging and the intensity of the patient's low back pain. We did not conclude that any other parameters than diaphragm flatness were dependent on the intensity of the subjects' back pain. A high position in the trunk also supports the hypothesis of worse ability to contract the diaphragm in LBP subjects. These findings support the hypothesis that changed diaphragm recruitment would be an important underlying factor for low back pain [33].

In the pathological group, the abdominal muscles lack the ability to hold the ribs in lower position. For this reason, the insertion parts of the diaphragm are not fixed and the diaphragm muscle changes its activation. The diaphragm is disharmonic in its motion, which causes problems with providing respiration and at the same time retaining abdominal pressure. The muscle principle for spine stabilization is therefore violated, and is replaced by a substitute model, which tends more easily toward the emergence of low back pain, spine degeneration or disc hernia.

Reversed causation is always a possibility, i.e. it is possible that the diaphragm behavior is changed in order to stabilize the spine after the deep intrinsic spinal muscles fail. During these changes, breathing patterns may occur, e.g. breath holding and decreased diaphragm excursions. Both of these phenomena were observed in the pathological group in our study. Roussel [34] identified various spinal stability enhancement mechanisms, concluding that a further sub-classification would be needed for the group of LBP patients, according to the variety of spinal supportive mechanisms that they use. Few investigations have been made of diaphragm and breathing patterns, and further research is of basic importance [35].

Some limitations of the the harmonic model of respiratory and postural movements need to be addressed. The modeled breath has to be periodic and preferably harmonious. The breath frequency has to be stable within the observed sequence. If these conditions are not fulfilled the results will be biased. Our measurements were suitable for using the sine model. All subjects displayed stable frequency of breathing. However it is desirable to extend the model to observe the time dependence of the parameters. The sine wave model of diaphragm postural function works well for assessing the range of postural motion. A more complex model needs to be created for a more detailed inspection of the postural function. Magnetic resonance imaging is a reliable method for making detailed observations and assessments of the diaphragm. A restriction of dynamic assessment is the frequency of the movement. This is limited by the sampling (imaging) frequency, which is currently quite low. Thus the diaphragm can be recruited in stabilizing compensation only in static loadings.

3.1 Conclusions and future works

Our study shows a way to compare the diaphragm motion within the group of controls without spinal findings and those who have a structural spinal finding, e.g. a hernia, etc., not caused by an injury. In this way, we confirm our experience of the influence of the diaphragm on spinal stability and respiration. The control group show a bigger range of diaphragm motion with lower breathing frequency. The diaphragm also performs better harmonicity (coordination) within its movement. The postural and breathing components are better balanced. This fact is very important for maintaining the intraabdominal pressure, which helps to support the spine from the front. For this reason, it plays a key role in treating back pain, hernias, etc. In the group of controls we also found a lower position of the diaphragm while it was in inspiration position in tidal breathing and also while being loaded. These facts also support the ability of the diaphragm to play a key role in maintaining the good stability of the trunk. It is also important that we are able to separate the phases of diaphragm movement. This supports both the postural function and the breathing function of this muscle due to MR imaging.

Our findings consistently affirmed worse muscle cooperation in the low back pain population subgroup. A clear relation to spinal disorders and low back pain remains inconclusive, but various findings in the literature have been confirmed. Probably the most important conclusion is that there is a need to further address various mechanisms used by patients to compensate deep muscle insufficiency. We have proposed a technique for assessing respiration properties, and have also separated the diaphragm movement that is not linked with respiration.

This study supports our clinical experience, which is based on observations of the difference in motor control of the respiratory and stabilization muscles in patients with and without low back pain. Our clinical experience has indicated that the function is different. This motor control ability to use trunk stabilization muscles needs to be learned by patients with back pain. We believe that diaphragm movements imaging could be a tool for diagnostic support for muscle imbalance in this area. Postural motions of the diaphragm could predict dispositions to vertebrogenic problems or could help when seeking to correct these problems. To verify this suggestion, it is necessary to broaden the group of subjects and to establish a norm for the healthy population.

Author Contributions

Conceived and designed the experiments: TR SR PV DN. Performed the experiments: TR SR. Analyzed the data: PV DN. Wrote the paper: PV DN.

References

1. Lewit K (1980) Relation of faulty respiration to posture and with clinical implications. The Journal of the American Osteopathic Association : 525–529.
2. Barr KP, Griggs M, Cadby T (2005) Lumbar stabilization: Core concepts and current literature, part 1. American journal of physical medicine and rehabilitation : 473–480.
3. Hodges PW, Richardson CA (1999) Altered trunk muscle recruitment in people with low back pain with upper limb movement at different speeds. Archives of physical medicine and rehabilitation : 1005–1012.
4. Cholewicki J, Ivancic PC, Radebold A (2002) Can increased intra-abdominal pressure in humans be decoupled from trunk muscle co-contraction during steady state isometric exertions? European journal of applied physiology : 127–133.
5. Cohen E, Mier A, Heywood P, Murphy K, Boultbee J, et al. (1994) Excursion-volume realtion of the right hemidiaphragm measured by ultrasonography and respiratory airow measurement. Thorax : 885–889.
6. Smolkov L, Mek M (2006) Fyzioterapie a pohybov lba u chronickch plicnch onemocnn. Blue Wings, Praha.
7. Kapandji IA (1998) The physiology of the joints. Volume 3. The trunk and the vertebral column. Churchill Livingstone, London.
8. Troyer AD, Estenne M (1981) Limitations of measurement of transdiaphragmatic pressure in de-tecting diaphragmatic weakness. Thorax : 169–174.
9. Cholewicki J, McGill SM (1996) Mechanical stability of the in viva lumbar spine: implications for injury and chronic low back pain. Clinical biomechanics (Bristol, Avon) : 1–15.
10. Iwasawa T, Kagei S, Gotoh T, Yoshiike Y, Matsushita K, et al. (2002) Magnetic resonance analysis of abnormal diaphragmatic motion in patients with emphysema. European Respiratory Journal : 225–231.
11. Hodges PW, Butler JE, McKenzie DK, Gandevia SC (1997) Contraction of the human diaphragm during rapid postural adjustments. Journal of Physiology : 539–548.
12. Hodges PW, Richardson CA, et al. (1997) Relationship between limb movement speed and associ- ated contraction of the trunk muscles. Ergonomics : 539–548.
13. Hodges PW, Gandevia SC, Richardson CA (1997) Contractions of specific abdominal muscles in postural tasks are affected by respiratory maneuvers. Journal of Applied Physiology : 753–760.
14. Hodges PW (2001) Changes in motor planning of feedforward postural responses of the trunk muscles in low back pain. Experimental brain research : 261–266.
15. Sharp JT, Goldberg NB, Druz WS, Fishman HC, Danon J (1977) Thoracoabdominal motion in chronic obstructive pulmonary disease. The American review of respiratory disease : 47–56.
16. Troyer AD (1997) Effect of hyperination on the diaphragm. The European respiratory journal : official journal of the European Society for Clinical Respiratory Physiology : 708–713.
17. Kolar P, Neurwith J, Sanda J, Suchanek V, Svata Z, et al. (2009) Analysis of diaphragm movement during tidal breathing and during its activation while breath holding using mri synchronized with spirometry. Physiol Res : 383–392.
18. Plathow C, Ley S, Zaporozhan J, Schöbinger M, Gruenig E, et al. (2006) Assessment of reproducibility and stability of different breath-hold maneuvres by dynamic mri: comparison between healthy adults and patients with pulmonary hypertension. Eur Radiol : 173–179.
19. Gierada DS, Curtin JJ, Erickson SJ, Prost RW, Strandt JA, et al. (1997) Fast gradient echo magnetic resonance imaging of the normal diaphragm. Journal of Thoracic Imaging : 70–74.
20. Gierada D, Curtin J, Erickson S, Prost R, Strandt J, et al. (1995) Diaphragmatic motion: Fast gradient-recalled-echo mr imaging in healthy subjects. Radiology : 879–884.
21. Kotani T, Minami S, Takahashi K, Isobe K, Nakata Y, et al. (2004) An analysis of chest wall and diaphragm motions in patients with idiopathic scoliosis using dynamic breathing mri. Spine : 298–302.
22. Chu WC, Li AM (2006). Spine : 2243–2249.
23. Suga K, Tsukuda T, Awaya H (1999) Impaired respiratory mechanics in pulmonary emphysema: evaluation with dynamic breathing mri. J Magn Reson Imaging : 510–520.
24. Kondo T, Kobayashi I, Taguchi Y, Hayama N, Tajiri S, et al. (2005) An analysis of the chest wall motions using the dynamic mri in healthy elder subjects. Tokai Journal Experimental and Clinical Medicine : 15–20.
25. Daggfeldt K, Thorstensson A (2003) The mechanics of back-extensor torque production about the lumbar spine. Journal of Biomechanics : 815–825.
26. Plathow C, Zimmermann H, Fink C, Umathum R, Schöbinger M, et al. (2005) Inuence of different breathing maneuvers on internal and external organ motion: use of fiducial markers in dynamic mri. International journal of radiation oncology, biology, physics : 238–245.
27. Plathow C, Schoebinger M, Fink C, Ley S (2005) Evaluation of lung volumetry using dynamic three-dimensional magnetic resonance imaging. investigative radiology. Investigative Radiology : 173–179.
28. Plathow C, Fink C, Sander A, Ley S, Puderbach M, et al. (2005) Comparison of relative forced expiratory volume of one second with dynamic magnetic resonance imaging parameters in healthy subjects and patients with lung cancer. Journal of magnetic resonance imaging : 212–218.
29. Harris RI, Macnab I (1954) Structural changes in the lumbar intervertebral discs; their relationship to low back pain and sciatica. J Bone Joint Surg Br : 304–322.
30. Jensen MC, Brant-Zawadzki MN, Obuchowski N, Modic MT, Malkasian D, et al. (1994) Magnetic resonance imaging of the lumbar spine in people without back pain. The New England journal of medicine : 69–73.
31. Carragee E, Alamin T, Cheng I, van den Haak TFE, Hurwitz E (2006) Are first-time episodes of serious lbp associated with new mri findings? Spine J : 624–635.
32. McGill SM, Sharratt MT, Seguin JP (1995) Loads on spinal tissues during simultaneous lifting and ventilatory challenge. Ergonimics : 1772–1792.
33. Smith MD, Russell A, Hodges PW (2005) Disorders of breathing and continence have a stronger associ-ation with back pain than obesity and physical activity. The Australian journal of physiotherapy: 11–16.
34. Roussel N, Nijs J, Truijen S, Vervecken L, Mottram S, et al. (2009) Altered breathing patterns during lumbopelvic motor control tests in chronic low back pain: a casecontrol study. European Spine Journal : 1066–1073.
35. Courtney R (2009) The function of breathing and its dysfunctions and their relationship to breath-ing therapy. International Journal of Osteopathic Medicine : 78–85.
36. Janda V (1996) Funkcni svalovy test [in czech]. Grada Publishing, Praha.
37. Edlik O, Sakarya ME, Uzun K, Harman M, Temizoz O, et al. (2004) Demonstrating the effect of theophylline treatment on diaphragmatic movement in chronic obstructive pulmonary disease patients by mruoroscopy. Eur J Radiol : 150–154.
38. Unal O, Arslan H, Uzun K, Ozbay B, Sakarya ME (2000) Evaluation of diaphragmatic movement with mr fluoroscopy in chronic obstructive pulmonary disease. Clin Imaging : 347–350.
39. Kondo T, Kobayashi I, Taguchi Y, Ohta Y, Yanagimachi N (2000) A dynamic analysis of chest wall motions with mri in healthy young subjects. Respirology : 19–25.
40. Plathow C, Fink C, Ley S (2004) Measurement of diaphragmatic length during the breathing cycle by dynamic mri: comparison between healthy adults and patients with an intrathoracic tumor. european radiology. Eur Radiol : 1392–1399.

41. Miyamoto K, Katsuji S, Kazuaki M (2002) Fast mri used to evaluate the effect of abdominal belts during contraction of trunk muscles. Spine : 1749–1754.
42. Takazakura R, Takahashi M, Nitta N, Murata K (2004) Diaphragmatic motion in the sitting and supine positions: Healthy subject study using a vertically open magnetic resonance system. J Magn Reson Imaging : 605–609.
43. Suwatanapongched T, Gierada DS, Slone RM, Pilgram TK, Tuteur PG (2003) Variation in di-aphragm position and shape in adults with normal pulmonary function. Chest : 2019–2027.
44. Kolar P, Sulc J, Kyncl M, Sanda J, Cakrt O, et al. (2012) Postural function of the diaphragm in persons with and without chronic low back pain. The Journal of orthopaedic and sports physical therapy : 352–362.
45. Skladal J, Ruth C (1978) Some remarks concerning the postural activity of the diaphragm in man. Agressologie : 45–46.
46. Hodges PW, Gandevia SC (2000) Activation of the human diaphragm during a repetitive postural task. The Journal of physiology : 165–175.

47. Butler JE, McKenzie DK, Gandevia SC (2001) Discharge frequencies of single motor units in human diaphragm and parasternal muscles in lying and standing. J Appl Physiol : 147–154.
48. Hodges PW, Gurfinkel VS, Brumagne S, Smith TC, Cordo PC (2002) Coexistence of stability and mobility in postural control: evidence from postural compensation for respiration. Experimental Brain Research : 293–302.
49. Hungerford B, Gilleard W, Hodges PW (2003) Evidence of altered lumbopelvic muscle recruitment in the presence of sacroiliac joint pain. Spine : 1593–1600.
50. Janssens L, Brumagne S, Polspoel K, Troosters T, McConnell A (2010) The effect of inspiratory muscles fatigue on postural control in people with and without recurrent low back pain. Spine : 1088–1094.
51. Grimstone SK, Hodges PW (2003) Impaired postural compensation for respiration in people with recur-rent low back pain. Experimental brain research : 218–224.

5

Ultrasonographic Assessment of Enthesitis in HLA-B27 Positive Patients with Rheumatoid Arthritis, a Matched Case-Only Study

Antonio Mera-Varela[1,2], Aida Ferreiro-Iglesias[1], Eva Perez-Pampin[1], Marisol Porto-Silva[1], Juan J. Gómez-Reino[1,2], Antonio Gonzalez[1]*

1 Research Laboratory 10 and Rheumatology Unit, Instituto de Investigacion Sanitaria – Hospital Clinico Universitario de Santiago, Santiago de Compostela, Spain, **2** Department of Medicine, University of Santiago de Compostela, Santiago de Compostela, Spain

Abstract

Introduction: HLA-B27 has a modifier effect on the phenotype of multiple diseases, both associated and non-associated with it. Among these effects, an increased frequency of clinical enthesitis in patients with Rheumatoid Arthritis (RA) has been reported but never explored again. We aimed to replicate this study with a sensitive and quantitative assessment of enthesitis by using standardized ultrasonography (US).

Methods: The Madrid Sonography Enthesitis Index (MASEI) was applied to the US assessment of 41 HLA-B27 positive and 41 matched HLA-B27 negative patients with longstanding RA. Clinical characteristics including explorations aimed to evaluate spondyloarthrtitis and laboratory tests were also done.

Results: A significant degree of abnormalities in the entheses of the patients with RA were found, but the MASEI values, and each of its components including the Doppler signal, were similar in HLA-B27 positive and negative patients. An increase of the MASEI scores with age was identified. Differences in two clinical features were found: a lower prevalence of rheumatoid factor and a more common story of low back pain in the HLA-B27 positive patients than in the negative. The latter was accompanied by radiographic sacroiliitis in two HLA-B27 positive patients. No other differences were detected.

Conclusion: We have found that HLA-B27 positive patients with RA do not have more enthesitis as assessed with US than the patients lacking this HLA allele. However, HLA-B27 could be shaping the RA phenotype towards RF seronegativity and axial involvement.

Editor: Chi Zhang, University of Texas Southwestern Medical Center, United States of America

Funding: The study was supported by grants 10CSA918040PR from the Xunta de Galicia (http://www.sergas.e/MostrarContidos_N3_T01.aspx?IdPaxina = 10142) and PI08/0744 of the Instituto de Salud Carlos III (http://www.isciii.es/) that are partially financed by the European Regional Development Fund of the European Union. The funders had no role in study design, data collection and analysis, decision to publish, or preparation of the manuscript.

Competing Interests: The authors have declared that no competing interests exist.

* E-mail: antonio.gonzalez.martinez-pedrayo@sergas.es

Introduction

Research in the genetic component of RA etiology has experienced a marked progress in recent years with the identification of a large number of susceptibility loci [1,2]. However, there are still many unsolved questions. Among them the relative to genotype-phenotype relationships are very prominent. It is expected that genotypes will have an important role in shaping the RA phenotype and that identification of these relationships will help manage patients in a personalized manner. The most established relationship has been the observed between a large number of RA susceptibility factors and the production of anti-citrullinated protein antibodies (ACPA). The earlier discovered association of the shared epitope (SE) with severe RA, including progression of erosive arthritis, seems to be explained by SE association with ACPA production. Other lines of active research in this field include the search for genetic factors modifying progression of erosions [3,4], or response to treatment

[5,6] and of loci associated with ACPA negative patients [7,8]. Some of these studies are focused in RA susceptibility loci [4,6,8], which are good candidates because of their involvement in the disease mechanisms. Additional candidates are the genetic factors associated with related diseases. These loci are also of known functional relevance and they have the potential of being involved in subgroups of RA patients sharing clinical characteristics with the disease where the loci were identified.

One of these candidates is HLA-B27 [9,10,11,12,13]. It is strongly associated with ankylosing spondylitis (AS) and with other spondyloarthritis (SpA), but not with RA [14,15]. HLA-B27 has also modifier effects on the phenotype that have been observed in its associated diseases and in some non-HLA-B27 associated diseases. Among the HLA-B27 associated diseases, there are multiple reports showing earlier disease onset, more involvement of sacroiliac and spine joints, a higher tendency to chronicity and more prevalence of back pain in HLA-B27 positive than in negative patients [16,17,18,19,20,21]. In addition, non-HLA-B27 associated diseases can be modified to show higher prevalence of archetypical AS clinical features. For example, HLA-B27 positive patients with inflammatory bowel disease show an increased prevalence of sacroiliitis, spondylitis and enthesitis [22,23]. HLA-B27 also increases the prevalence of sacroiliitis in patients with familial Mediterranean fever [24]; and of sacroiliitis, inflammatory back pain and enthesitis in children with Juvenile Idiopathic Arthritis [25,26]. Therefore, it is not surprising that some researchers have thought the presence of HLA-B27 could modify the phenotypes of patients with RA towards resembling SpA. There have been some reports in this direction [9,10,11,12,13], but all these studies were done more than a decade ago and none of their findings have become established. One of these studies reported an increased prevalence of clinical enthesitis in patients with early arthritis fulfilling RA criteria [9].

Enthesitis, the inflammation of the entheses, is very prevalent and relatively specific of all forms of SpA motivating its inclusion as part of the disease classification criteria [15,27]. Enthesitis is present in early SpA and, occasionally, it is the unique disease manifestation for some time. This has lead some authors to consider enthesitis the primary lesion in this group of diseases [28]. Now we have the possibility to identify early enthesitis when it is not yet clinically apparent either to patients or to physical exploration thanks to magnetic resonance imaging and ultrasonography (US) [29,30,31,32,33]. This property of US has been applied to a variety of clinical situations demanding sensitive evaluation. Examples include SpA with subclinical enthesopathy [34], recurrent acute anterior uveitis without SpA [35], long term dialysis [36], and patients with psoriasis without psoriatic arthritis [36,37], showing in all these cases an increased frequency of abnormalities. US evaluation has also shown an increased frequency of abnormalities in patients with RA relative to healthy controls in spite of the complete absence of clinical enthesitis [38,39]. Only one of these studies assessed HLA-B27, concerning recurrent anterior uveitis, and it found that enthesitis was associated with this HLA allele [35].

Therefore, we have now the opportunity to analyze the prevalence of enthesitis in RA patients stratified for HLA-B27 status with the sensitivity and accuracy allowed by US. With this aim, we have selected all available RA patients positive for HLA-B27 in our hospital and matched RA patients negative for HLA-B27. The two groups were compared with the Madrid Sonography Enthesitis Index (MASEI) [31], focused anamnesis and physical exploration. No differences in the MASEI or any of its components were detected. This result excludes a role of HLA-B27 in the enthesal abnormalities of these patients. However, a modifier effect of HLA-B27 on the phenotype of the patients with RA was suggested by its association with RF negative status and a more frequent story of low back pain.

Materials and Methods

Ethics statement

All patients gave their written informed consent to participate. Sample collection and the study protocol were approved by the Comite de Investigacion Clinica de Galicia (Spain).

Selection of patients

DNA and serum samples from patients with RA according to ACR classification criteria were used [40]. All patients were of Spanish ancestry and were attending the Rheumatology Unit of the Hospital Clinico Universitario de Santiago. HLA-B27 positive patients were selected. Gender, age at disease onset and current

age of these patients was used to select matched HLA-B27 negative patients at a 1:1 ratio. Patients were invited to participate in the study and they gave their written informed consent. The rheumatologist and the nurse involved in recruitment and evaluation of the patients were blind to their HLA-B27 status.

Laboratory studies

Two complementary genotyping reactions were used to determine the HLA-B27 status (available from the authors upon request). The first PCR was based on the method of Bon et al. [41]. It amplifies HLA-B*2701-*2706 alleles, which are the most common in the Caucasian population and the most associated with AS. The second PCR used a combination of 3 primers described by Faner et al. [42]. It amplifies a larger number of alleles than the first, from HLA-B*2701 to *2724 except for HLA-B*2718 and HLA-B*2723. PCR amplification was done with a multiplex PCR system (KAPA2G fast HotStart, Kapa Biosystems, Woburn, MA). Detection of the PCR products was performed with single-base extension (SNaPshot Multiplex Kit from Applied Biosystems, Foster City, CA) using probes targeting a non polymorphic base. In this way, the most frequents alleles of HLA-B27 were covered by two PCR. Four samples were positive only in the second amplification, which is consistent with the low frequency of the rare alleles in Spain [43].They were excluded from analysis because of their more uncertain status.

HLA-DBR1 alleles were determined by a sequencing based typing method (SBT) using the AlleleSEQR HLA-DRB1 Typing kit (Abbott Diagnostics, Abbott Park, Germany), which includes bidirectional sequencing of the second exon of DRB1. Ambiguous samples were additionally sequenced with group-specific primers (AlleleSEQR HLA-DRB1 GSSP, Abbott). The anti-CCP status of the patients was determined using the EDIA ACPA Kit (Euro-Diagnostica, Arnhem, The Netherlands). Quantification and setting of the cut-off level at 5 units/ml were done according to the manufacturer's instructions. RF status was determined by rate nephelometry with the IMMAGE Immunochemistry Systems (Beckman Coulter, Ireland), which covers all Ig isotypes.

Clinical and Ultrasound evaluation

Patient history was reviewed and a specific anamnesis of symptoms and signs characteristic of HLA-B27 associated diseases was conducted. Physical exploration was done looking for signs of axial involvement with instruments developed for SpA as the Schober test, BASDAI and BASFI scores and assessment of the lateral trunk flexion. A modified Schober test according with Moll and Wright was used[44]. Inflammatory back pain was defined as lumbar pain at night or with morning stiffness that does not improve with rest or that improves with exercise and that persists for more than a month. Plain antero-posterior pelvic radiographs were evaluated for the presence of sacroiliitis. This assessment was independently done by two rheumatologists in a blind form.

In addition, the presence of enthesitis was evaluated by a rheumatologist experienced in US focused on articular and periarticular locations and blind to the HLA-B27 status of patients. A General Electric LogiqQ7 US machine with a 10–14 MHz linear array transducer was used. The power Doppler setting was standardized with a pulse repetition frequency (PRF) of 500 Hz with a low wall filter and 35–40 dB of gain. The Madrid Sonography Enthesitis Index (MASEI) was used for quantitative and standardized assessment [31]. This index evaluates 6 features in 6 entheses. A value ≥ 18 has been defined as characteristic of SpA. The 6 features are enthesis thickness, structure, calcifications, erosions, bursae and power Doppler signal. The 6 bilaterally assessed locations are proximal plantar fascia, distal Achilles tendon, distal and proximal patellar tendon insertion, distal quadriceps tendon and brachial triceps tendon.

Statistical analysis

HLA-B27 positive patients with RA were considered cases and the matched HLA-B27 negative patients were controls. Demographic, clinical, laboratory, radiographic and ultrasound characteristics were compared between the two groups using Student T test or the Fisher exact test for contingency tables depending on the quantitative or qualitative nature of the variables, respectively. Detailed US results were compared with the Man-Whitney U test and non-parametric statistics because they showed many zero values. All analyses were done with Statistica 7.0 (StatSoft, Tulsa, OK). Differences with P<0.05 were considered statistically significant.

Results

Analysis of 672 patients with RA identified 65 that were HLA-B27+, the remaining 607 were HLA-B27- (11 additional patients showed an uncertain HLA-B27 status and were not included). The HLA-B27 positive subgroup of patients showed less RF positive subjects, 50.0 %, than the HLA-B27 negative subgroup 64.6 % (P = 0.025). Also the ACPA status showed a trend to decreased prevalence in this subgroup (Table 1). However, there were not more patients with low titers of ACPA (between 5 and 45 units) in the HLA-B27 positive (33.3 %) than in the HLA-B27 negative subgroup (32.8 %). The other characteristics, gender, age at disease onset, erosive arthritis and carrier status of the SE, were similar in the two subgroups of patients (Table 1).

A total of 41 HLA-B27 positive patients were available and willing to participate in the study. One HLA-B27- patient was selected for each HLA-B27+ patient trying to match them for gender, age at disease onset and current age. The resulting groups were very similar not only in the selected variables but also in other characteristics as height, weight, serology and SE status (Table 2). During the visit for evaluation one of the patients in the HLA-B27 positive subgroup was found to have SpA in spite of his previous classification as RA and was excluded from further analysis. Specific anamnesis and physical evaluation of the patients were done blind to their HLA-B27 status. They disclosed a higher prevalence of low back pain, mechanical or inflammatory, in the

HLA-B27 positive subgroup, 27.5 %, than in the HLA-B27 negative subgroup, 7.5 %, P = 0.037. This difference was similarly distributed between inflammatory and mechanical pain (Table 3). No other symptom or evaluation showed differences between the two patient groups. Specifically there were not differences in modified Schober's test, BASDAI or BASFI scores or in the lateral flexion of the spine (Table 3). A few patients reported a story of past skin lesions that could correspond to psoriasis but without differences between the two subgroups.

Two rheumatologists that were blind to the HLA-B27 status of the patients evaluated plain pelvic radiographs for the presence of sacroiliitis. Their assessment was fully concordant identifying 2 patients with sacroiliitis. The two were positive for HLA-B27. This was not significantly different from the result in the HLA-B27 negative subgroup, but we investigated it further. A review of the two patients with sacroiliitis did not challenge their classification as RA: the two showed erosive RA and one of them was positive for ACPA and homozygous for the SE. The two patients had a story of inflammatory low back pain.

Systematic evaluation of the entheses following the MASEI procedure (representative images in Figure 1) yielded no differences between the two subgroups of patients (Table 4). Mean MASEI values were even nominally lower in the HLA-B27 positive subgroup. Also, the threshold score of 18 proposed as specific of AS [31], was not discriminating between the two subgroups: there were 13 patients above this value in the HLA-B27 positive subgroup and 10 in the HLA-B27 negative subgroup. In addition, no difference was detected with any of the components of the index (Table 4). This is specially relevant for the power Doppler signal (Figure 2) because it has been differentially associated with SpA relative to other diseases including RA [39]. But no difference was detected comparing the whole distribution of values (Table 4), or the percentage of

Table 1. Characteristics of the patients with RA in function of the HLA-B27 subgroup.

	HLA-B27-	HLA-B27+	P value
Women %	77.6 (471/607)[a]	72.3 (47/65)	0.3
Age of disease onset, mean (SD)	46.3 (14.8)	44.9 (16.7)	0.5
Rheumatoid Factor % [b]	64.6 (369/571)	50.0 (30/60)	0.025
Anti-CCP %	63.0 (376/597)	50.8 (33/65)	0.05
Anti-CCP median (IQR) [c]	93.3 (32.8–198.0)	67.4 (18.7–141.3)	0.3
Carrier SE %	53.3 (286/537)	56.4 (31/55)	0.7
Erosive arthritis %	65.8 (369/561)	61.7 (37/60)	0.5

[a]Number with the feature/total number of patients with available information.
[b]Median and IQR were 122 (61–445) in the HLA-B27- subgroup and 235 (128–366) in the HLA-B27+ subgroup (P = 0.8). This information was available only for 127 RF+ patients.
[c]Median and interquartile range of the anti-CCP positive patients.

Table 2. Characteristics of the patients recruited for detailed analysis in function of the HLA-B27 subgroup.

	HLA-B27-	HLA-B27+	P value
Women %	73.2 (30/41)[a]	80.5 (33/41)	0.6
Age of disease onset, mean (SD)	41.9 (15.7)	43.9 (17.3)	0.6
Current age, mean (SD)	64.8 (15.2)	64.4 (14.7)	0.9
Weight, mean (SD)	68.8 (12.2)	68.3 (13.7)	0.8
Height, mean (SD)	159.5 (7.8)	158.3 (8.7)	0.5
Ever smoking %	24.4 (10/41)	24.4 (10/41)	1
Rheumatoid factor %	55.0 (22/40)	50.0 (20/40)	0.8
Anti-CCP %	40.0 (16/40)	51.2 (21/41)	0.4
Carrier of SE %	55.0 (22/40)	57.9 (22/38)	0.8
Erosive arthritis %	65.0 (26/40)	53.9 (21/39)	0.4
Biologics %	50.0 (20/40)	60.0 (24/40)	0.5
Anti-TNF [b]	60.0 (12/20)	45.8 (11/24)	0.4
Rituximab	15.0 (3/20)	16.7 (4/24)	1.0
Abatacept	10.0 (2/20)	20.8 (5/24)	0.4
Tocilizumab	15.0 (3/20)	16.7 (4/24)	1.0
Methotrexate	65.0 (13/20)	83.3 (20/24)	0.2
Leflunomide	20.0 (4/20)	0.0 (0/24)	0.04

[a]Number with the feature/total number of patients with available information.
[b]Including Etanercept, Adalimumab and Infliximab.

Table 3. Results of the anamnesis and exploration of recruited patients in function of the HLA-B27 subgroup.

	HLA-B27-	HLA-B27+	P value
Back pain %	7.5 (3/40)	27.5 (11/40)	0.037
Inflammatory back pain %	2.5 (1/40)	12.5 (5/40)	0.2
Non-inflammatory back pain %	5.0 (2/40)	15.5(6/40)	0. 3
Story of 'psoriatic' lesions %	7.3 (3/40)	5.0 (2/40)	1.0
Schober's test, mean (SD)	3.7 (1.0)	3.8 (1.0)	0.9
Right lateral flexion, mean (SD)	13.2 (4.0)	12.7 (4.4)	0.6
Left lateral flexion, mean (SD)	13.4 (4.3)	11.8 (3.6)	0.1
BASDAI, mean (SD)	4.3 (2.5)	4.6 (2.4)	0.6
BASFI, mean (SD)	2.9 (2.4)	3.4 (2.2)	0.4
Sacroiliitis Rx %	0.0 (0/34)[a]	5.7 (2/35)	0.3

[a]Number with the feature/total number of patients with available information.

positive signals (9/40 in HLA-B-27 positive patients *vs.* 13/41 in HLA-B27 negative patients) or the mean values in the patients showing Doppler signals (4.7 *vs.* 4.6, in the HLA-B27 positive and negative patients, respectively). The only associations we identified were unrelated with the HLA-B27 status: a significant increase of the MASEI value in men relative to women (not shown), and an increase of the score with age due to calcifications (not shown). The two patients with sacroiliitis lacked signs of enthesitis (MASEI values of 4 and 8).

Discussion

Our analyses have not shown any specific enthesal abnormality in the HLA-B27 positive patients with RA. The sensitive and quantitative evaluation allows us to exclude a significant HLA-B27 modifier effect towards enthesitis in the RA patients. However, an excess of patients in the HLA-B27 positive group referred a story of low back pain that in two of the patients was associated with radiographic sacroiliitis. These findings together with a lower prevalence of RF keep open the possibility of a modifier effect of the HLA-B27 allele on the phenotype of RA patients, but excluding the presence of enthesis.

Our primary aim was to compare the frequency of enthesitis between HLA-B27 positive and negative patients with RA using systematic US examination. This imaging technology has shown sensitivity for detecting a high percentage of SpA patients with subclinical enthesitis [15,29,30,31,32,33,34,39]. It is applied with

scoring protocols that help differentiate SpA patients from controls, from subjects that have suffered mechanical injury and from other forms of inflammatory arthritis [31,32,33]. Specifically, the MASEI protocol used here has shown high sensitivity and specificity and it is very comprehensive because it includes assessment of 6 features in 6 enthesal sites and both grey scales and power Doppler [31,33]. The assessment of power Doppler is a distinct advantage of this method over the most commonly used GUESS procedure for our study because the Doppler signal is the most specific feature distinguishing SpA from mechanical and RA enthesal abnormalities [39].

We have found significant abnormalities in the entheses of patients with RA confirming findings of previous US studies [38,39,45]. However, no differences were found between HLA-B27 positive and negative patients, even for components of the index that are more specific for SpA like the Doppler signal. Therefore, it is clear that the presence of HLA-B27 does not induce enthesal pathology in RA patients and that all the abnormalities found in these patients are produced with independence of this genetic factor.

Other interesting aspect of our MASEI results is that only patients older than 50 years of age showed values over the threshold identifying patients with AS or SpA [31,33]. Therefore, our results do not question the specificity of this threshold for early SpA, which starts most often below this age. An increase of enthesal abnormalities with age was already shown more than a decade ago [46]. It was described as independent of the underlying disease and, as in our study, to be mostly due to calcification.

Two of the other clinical features we have analyzed were different between HLA-B27 positive and negative patients with RA. The first was the prevalence of RF, which was less common in HLA-B27 positive patients. It was accompanied by a trend to lower prevalence of ACPA. This result could imply either association of HLA-B27 with RF seronegative RA or misclassification of patients. The latter possibility can be reasonably excluded because we only found a patient with SpA among the 41 that were specifically revised. In addition, the HLA-B27+ RF- patients were not different in any respect from the HLA-B27- RF- subgroup. For example, the HLA-B27+RF- and B27-RF- patients were comparable at percentage of ACPA+, 26.7 % vs. 25.6 %, erosive arthritis, 51.7 % vs. 45.7 %, or percentage of carriers of SE, 44.4 % vs. 43.1 %, respectively. This leaves us with the possibility that HLA-B27 could be a susceptibility factor for RF seronegative RA. Only studies in additional sample collections will be needed to clarify this matter.

An increased prevalence of low back pain was also associated with HLA-B27 in the patients with RA. This outcome from the anamnesis was combined with the identification of two patients

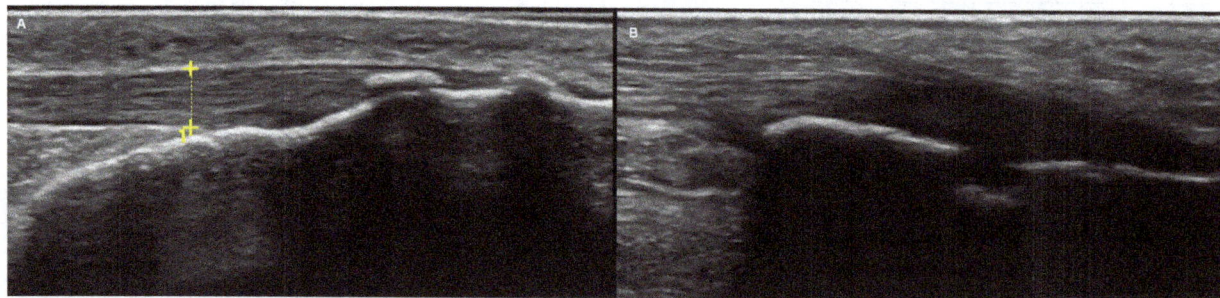

Figure 1. Representative images of features detected with US exploration. A) Example of analysis of the Achilles tendon thickness measured between the two yellow crosses in one patient, and B) Erosion detected in the superior pole of the calcaneous in a different patient.

Table 4. Ultrasonographic evaluation of the entheses following the MASEI procedure.

	HLA-B27-	HLA-B27+	P value
MASEI, mean (SD)	14.2 (9.3)	13.6 (8.8)	0.7
MASEI, median $(_{10-90}R)$*	11.0 (5−24)	11.5 (4−27)	0.7
MASEI >18, %	24.4 (10/41)	32.5 (13/40)	0.5
- structure, median $(_{10-90}R)$	0 (0−1)	0 (0−1.5)	0.8
- thickness, median $(_{10-90}R)$	2 (0−5)	2 (0−5)	0.08
- erosion, median $(_{10-90}R)$	3 (0−6)	0 (0−10.5)	0.8
- calcification, median $(_{10-90}R)$	7 (2−13)	5 (2.5−14)	0.7
- Doppler, median $(_{10-90}R)$	0 (0−6)	0 (0−3)	0.3
- bursitis, median $(_{10-90}R)$	0 (0−1)	0 (0−1)	0.8

*The range between percentiles 10 and 90.

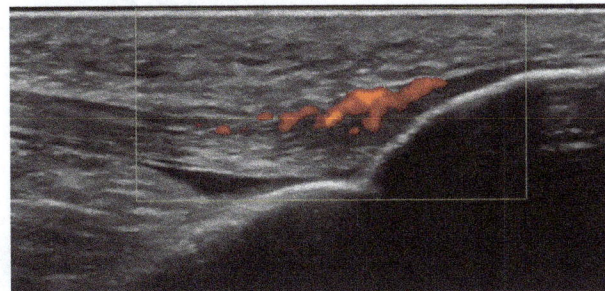

Figure 2. Positive power Doppler signal identifying tibial tuberosity enthesitis. The signal (in red) is detected in the tibial insertion of the patellar ligament in one of the studied patients.

with radiographic sacroiliitis among the patients with inflammatory low back pain. The two results are in agreement with the idea that HLA-B27 could modify RA towards the axial joints. This idea is supported by previous studies showing association between sacroiliitis and HLA-B27, both in HLA-27-associated diseases [17,19,20,21], and in some non-associated diseases [22,23,24,26] including RA [10,12,13]. In fact, this is the unique association with HLA-B27 that has been replicated in different RA studies. However, two previous studies did not found differences in the sacroiliac joints between HLA-B27 positive and negative patients with RA [47,48]. These findings should motivate new studies directed to the analysis of low back pain and to the identification of sacroiliitis. MRI will be the technology of choice for these studies because it is very sensitive for incipient changes in the sacroiliac joints [29], and it could provide more definitive results than radiography given the small size of the HLA-B27 positive subgroup.

In relation with the low back pain association, it could be argued that its presence questions the classification of the patients as RA. However, this type of reasoning is incompatible with the aim of our study. When the aim is to identify patients with RA

showing phenotypes resembling SpA, we need to consider classification of RA before doing any extra analysis and keep this classification constant along the study.

Conclusions

We have found that HLA-B27 positive patients with RA do not have more enthesitis as assessed with US than those lacking this allele. However, these patients referred a more prevalent story of low back pain and were more often seronegative for RF than the HLA-B27 negative patients indicating that HLA-B27 could be shaping the RA phenotype in other directions deserving further and more focused analysis.

Acknowledgments

Authors acknowledge the patients with RA participating in this study by their availability and generosity. AF-I has a pre-doctoral bursary from the Instituto de Salud Carlos III (Spain).

Author Contributions

Conceived and designed the experiments: AM-V AG. Performed the experiments: AM-V AF-I EP-P MP-S JJG-R. Analyzed the data: AM-V AF-I AG. Wrote the paper: AM-V AF-I AG.

References

1. Gregersen PK (2010) Susceptibility genes for rheumatoid arthritis - a rapidly expanding harvest. Bull NYU Hosp Jt Dis 68: 179–182.
2. Plenge RM, Raychaudhuri S (2010) Leveraging human genetics to develop future therapeutic strategies in rheumatoid arthritis. Rheum Dis Clin North Am 36: 259–270.
3. Knevel R, Krabben A, Brouwer E, Posthumus MD, Wilson AG, et al. (2012) Genetic variants in IL15 associate with progression of joint destruction in rheumatoid arthritis: a multicohort study. Ann Rheum Dis.
4. van der Linden MP, Feitsma AL, le Cessie S, Kern M, Olsson LM, et al. (2009) Association of a single-nucleotide polymorphism in CD40 with the rate of joint destruction in rheumatoid arthritis. Arthritis Rheum 60: 2242–2247.
5. Plant D, Bowes J, Potter C, Hyrich KL, Morgan AW, et al. (2011) Genome-wide association study of genetic predictors of anti-tumor necrosis factor treatment efficacy in rheumatoid arthritis identifies associations with polymorphisms at seven loci. Arthritis Rheum 63: 645–653.
6. Cui J, Saevarsdottir S, Thomson B, Padyukov L, van der Helm-van Mil AH, et al. (2010) Rheumatoid arthritis risk allele PTPRC is also associated with response to anti-tumor necrosis factor alpha therapy. Arthritis Rheum 62: 1849–1861.
7. Padyukov L, Seielstad M, Ong RT, Ding B, Ronnelid J, et al. (2011) A genome-wide association study suggests contrasting associations in ACPA-positive versus ACPA-negative rheumatoid arthritis. Ann Rheum Dis 70: 259–265.
8. Seddighzadeh M, Gonzalez A, Ding B, Ferreiro-Iglesias A, Gomez-Reino JJ, et al. (2012) Variants Within STAT Genes Reveal Association with Anticitrullinated Protein Antibody-negative Rheumatoid Arthritis in 2 European Populations. J Rheumatol 39: 1509–1516.

9. El-Gabalawy HS, Goldbach-Mansky R, Smith D, 2nd, Arayssi T, Bale S, et al. (1999) Association of HLA alleles and clinical features in patients with synovitis of recent onset. Arthritis Rheum 42: 1696–1705.
10. Jajic Z, Jajic I (1991) HLA-B27 antigen and rheumatoid arthritis. Acta Med Iugosl 45: 195–202.
11. Jaraquemada D, Ollier W, Awad J, Young A, Silman A, et al. (1986) HLA and rheumatoid arthritis: a combined analysis of 440 British patients. Ann Rheum Dis 45: 627–636.
12. Rantapaa Dahlqvist S, Nordmark LG, Bjelle A (1984) HLA-B27 and involvement of sacroiliac joints in rheumatoid arthritis. J Rheumatol 11: 27–32.
13. Rundback JH, Rosenberg ZS, Solomon G (1993) The radiographic features of rheumatoid arthritis in HLA-B27-positive patients. Skeletal Radiol 22: 263–267.
14. Reveille JD, Maganti RM (2009) Subtypes of HLA-B27: history and implications in the pathogenesis of ankylosing spondylitis. Adv Exp Med Biol 649: 159–176.
15. Dougados M, Baeten D (2011) Spondyloarthritis. Lancet 377: 2127–2137.
16. Feldtkeller E, Khan MA, van der Heijde D, van der Linden S, Braun J (2003) Age at disease onset and diagnosis delay in HLA-B27 negative vs. positive patients with ankylosing spondylitis. Rheumatol Int 23: 61–66.
17. Skare TL, Leite N, Bortoluzzo AB, Goncalves CR, Da Silva JA, et al. (2012) Effect of age at disease onset in the clinical profile of spondyloarthritis: a study of 1424 Brazilian patients. Clin Exp Rheumatol 30: 351–357.
18. Queiro R, Torre JC, Gonzalez S, Lopez-Larrea C, Tinture T, et al. (2003) HLA antigens may influence the age of onset of psoriasis and psoriatic arthritis. J Rheumatol 30: 505–507.
19. Chung HY, Machado P, van der Heijde D, D'Agostino MA, Dougados M (2011) HLA-B27 positive patients differ from HLA-B27 negative patients in

clinical presentation and imaging: results from the DESIR cohort of patients with recent onset axial spondyloarthritis. Ann Rheum Dis 70: 1930–1936.

20. Kaarela K, Jantti JK, Kotaniemi KM (2009) Similarity between chronic reactive arthritis and ankylosing spondylitis.A 32-35-year follow-up study. Clin Exp Rheumatol 27: 325–328.

21. Queiro R, Sarasqueta C, Belzunegui J, Gonzalez C, Figueroa M, et al. (2002) Psoriatic spondyloarthropathy: a comparative study between HLA-B27 positive and HLA-B27 negative disease. Semin Arthritis Rheum 31: 413–418.

22. Rodriguez-Reyna TS, Martinez-Reyes C, Yamamoto-Furusho JK (2009) Rheumatic manifestations of inflammatory bowel disease. World J Gastroenterol 15: 5517–5524.

23. Orchard TR, Holt H, Bradbury L, Hammersma J, McNally E, et al. (2009) The prevalence, clinical features and association of HLA-B27 in sacroiliitis associated with established Crohn's disease. Aliment Pharmacol Ther 29: 193–197.

24. Kasifoglu T, Calisir C, Cansu DU, Korkmaz C (2009) The frequency of sacroiliitis in familial Mediterranean fever and the role of HLA-B27 and MEFV mutations in the development of sacroiliitis. Clin Rheumatol 28: 41–46.

25. Berntson L, Damgard M, Andersson-Gare B, Herlin T, Nielsen S, et al. (2008) HLA-B27 predicts a more extended disease with increasing age at onset in boys with juvenile idiopathic arthritis. J Rheumatol 35: 2055–2061.

26. Flato B, Smerdel A, Johnston V, Lien G, Dale K, et al. (2002) The influence of patient characteristics, disease variables, and HLA alleles on the development of radiographically evident sacroiliitis in juvenile idiopathic arthritis. Arthritis Rheum 46: 986–994.

27. Rudwaleit M, van der Heijde D, Landewe R, Akkoc N, Brandt J, et al. (2011) The Assessment of SpondyloArthritis International Society classification criteria for peripheral spondyloarthritis and for spondyloarthritis in general. Ann Rheum Dis 70: 25–31.

28. McGonagle D, Gibbon W, Emery P (1998) Classification of inflammatory arthritis by enthesitis. Lancet 352: 1137–1140.

29. Maksymowych WP (2009) Progress in spondylarthritis. Spondyloarthritis: lessons from imaging. Arthritis Res Ther 11: 222.

30. D'Agostino MA, Aegerter P, Bechara K, Salliot C, Judet O, et al. (2011) How to diagnose spondyloarthritis early? Accuracy of peripheral enthesitis detection by power Doppler ultrasonography. Ann Rheum Dis 70: 1433–1440.

31. de Miguel E, Cobo T, Munoz-Fernandez S, Naredo E, Uson J, et al. (2009) Validity of enthesis ultrasound assessment in spondyloarthropathy. Ann Rheum Dis 68: 169–174.

32. Balint PV, Kane D, Wilson H, McInnes IB, Sturrock RD (2002) Ultrasonography of entheseal insertions in the lower limb in spondyloarthropathy. Ann Rheum Dis 61: 905–910.

33. de Miguel E, Munoz-Fernandez S, Castillo C, Cobo-Ibanez T, Martin-Mola E (2011) Diagnostic accuracy of enthesis ultrasound in the diagnosis of early spondyloarthritis. Ann Rheum Dis 70: 434–439.

34. Ruta S, Gutierrez M, Pena C, Garcia M, Arturi A, et al. (2011) Prevalence of subclinical enthesopathy in patients with spondyloarthropathy: an ultrasound study. J Clin Rheumatol 17: 18–22.

35. Munoz-Fernandez S, de Miguel E, Cobo-Ibanez T, Madero R, Ferreira A, et al. (2009) Enthesis inflammation in recurrent acute anterior uveitis without spondylarthritis. Arthritis Rheum 60: 1985–1990.

36. Gutierrez M, Zeiler M, Filippucci E, Salaffi F, Becciolini A, et al. (2011) Sonographic subclinical entheseal involvement in dialysis patients. Clin Rheumatol 30: 907–913.

37. Naredo E, Moller I, de Miguel E, Batlle-Gualda E, Acebes C, et al. (2011) High prevalence of ultrasonographic synovitis and enthesopathy in patients with psoriasis without psoriatic arthritis: a prospective case-control study. Rheumatology (Oxford) 50: 1838–1848.

38. Genc H, Cakit BD, Tuncbilek I, Erdem HR (2005) Ultrasonographic evaluation of tendons and enthesal sites in rheumatoid arthritis: comparison with ankylosing spondylitis and healthy subjects. Clin Rheumatol 24: 272–277.

39. D'Agostino MA, Said-Nahal R, Hacquard-Bouder C, Brasseur JL, Dougados M, et al. (2003) Assessment of peripheral enthesitis in the spondylarthropathies by ultrasonography combined with power Doppler: a cross-sectional study. Arthritis Rheum 48: 523–533.

40. Arnett FC, Edworthy SM, Bloch DA, McShane DJ, Fries JF, et al. (1988) The American Rheumatism Association 1987 revised criteria for the classification of rheumatoid arthritis. Arthritis Rheum 31: 315–324.

41. Bon MA, van Oeveren-Dybicz A, van den Bergh FA (2000) Genotyping of HLA-B27 by real-time PCR without hybridization probes. Clin Chem 46: 1000–1002.

42. Faner R, Casamitjana N, Colobran R, Ribera A, Pujol-Borrell R, et al. (2004) HLA-B27 genotyping by fluorescent resonance emission transfer (FRET) probes in real-time PCR. Hum Immunol 65: 826–838.

43. Mathieu A, Paladini F, Vacca A, Cauli A, Fiorillo MT, et al. (2009) The interplay between the geographic distribution of HLA-B27 alleles and their role in infectious and autoimmune diseases: a unifying hypothesis. Autoimmun Rev 8: 420–425.

44. Moll JM, Wright V (1971) Normal range of spinal mobility. An objective clinical study. Ann Rheum Dis 30: 381–386.

45. Falsetti P, Frediani B, Fioravanti A, Acciai C, Baldi F, et al. (2003) Sonographic study of calcaneal entheses in erosive osteoarthritis, nodal osteoarthritis, rheumatoid arthritis and psoriatic arthritis. Scand J Rheumatol 32: 229–234.

46. Shaibani A, Workman R, Rothschild BM (1993) The significance of enthesopathy as a skeletal phenomenon. Clin Exp Rheumatol 11: 399–403.

47. Saraux A, Guedes C, Allain J, Valls I, Baron D, et al. (1997) HLA-B27 in French patients with rheumatoid arthritis. Scand J Rheumatol 26: 269–271.

48. Jurik AG, de Carvalho A, Graudal H (1987) Radiographic visualisation of seropositive rheumatoid arthritis in carriers of HLA-B27. RöFo - Fortschritte auf dem Gebiet der R 147: 14–20.

6

How Well Do Randomized Trials Inform Decision Making: Systematic Review Using Comparative Effectiveness Research Measures on Acupuncture for Back Pain

Claudia M. Witt[1,2]*, Eric Manheimer[1], Richard Hammerschlag[3], Rainer Lüdtke[4], Lixing Lao[1], Sean R. Tunis[5], Brian M. Berman[1]

1 University of Maryland School of Medicine, Center for Integrative Medicine, Baltimore, Maryland, United States of America, 2 Charité University Medical Center, Institute for Social Medicine, Epidemiology and Health Economics, Berlin, Germany, 3 Research Department, Oregon College of Oriental Medicine, Portland, Oregon, United States of America, 4 Carstens Foundation, Essen, Germany, 5 Center for Medical Technology Policy, Baltimore, Maryland, United States of America

Abstract

Background: For Comparative Effectiveness Research (CER) there is a need to develop scales for appraisal of available clinical research. Aims were to 1) test the feasibility of applying the pragmatic-explanatory continuum indicator summary tool and the six CER defining characteristics of the Institute of Medicine to RCTs of acupuncture for treatment of low back pain, and 2) evaluate the extent to which the evidence from these RCTs is relevant to clinical and health policy decision making.

Methods: We searched Medline, the AcuTrials™ Database to February 2011 and reference lists and included full-report randomized trials in English that compared needle acupuncture with a conventional treatment in adults with non-specific acute and/or chronic low back pain and restricted to those with ≥30 patients in the acupuncture group. Papers were evaluated by 5 raters.

Principal Findings: From 119 abstracts, 44 full-text publications were screened and 10 trials (4,901 patients) were evaluated. Due to missing information and initial difficulties in operationalizing the scoring items, the first scoring revealed inter-rater and inter-item variance (intraclass correlations 0.02–0.60), which improved after consensus discussions to 0.20–1.00. The 10 trials were found to cover the efficacy-effectiveness continuum; those with more flexible acupuncture and no placebo control scored closer to effectiveness.

Conclusion: Both instruments proved useful, but need further development. In addition, CONSORT guidelines for reporting pragmatic trials should be expanded. Most studies in this review already reflect the movement towards CER and similar approaches can be taken to evaluate comparative effectiveness relevance of RCTs for other treatments.

Editor: Laxmaiah Manchikanti, University of Louisville, United States of America

Funding: CMW received a travel grant by the Institute for Integrative Health a non-profit organization, Baltimore, United States of America. The funders had no role in study design, data collection and analysis, decision to publish, or preparation of the manuscript. No additional external funding received for this study.

Competing Interests: The authors have declared that no competing interests exist.

* E-mail: claudia.witt@charite.de

Introduction

Comparative Effectiveness Research (CER) has considerable potential to help health care providers as well as patients and clinicians to choose among currently available therapeutic options. Different definitions for CER have been published. In this paper we use the working definition as established by the Institute of Medicine (IOM) Committee, which defines CER as "the generation and synthesis of evidence that compares the benefits and harms of alternative methods to prevent, diagnose, treat, and monitor a clinical condition or to improve the delivery of care. The purpose of CER is to assist consumers, clinicians, purchasers, and policy makers to make informed decisions that will improve health care at both the individual and population levels" [1].

However, to date, the majority of clinical trials have assessed the efficacy of medical interventions rather than their effectiveness. To support more informed decision-making, there has been a call for more evidence on real world effectiveness from CER [2]. Available systematic reviews generally do not assess available evidence from a CER perspective – in other words, to examine the extent to which published trials are relevant to clinical and health policy decision making. On the contrary, appraisal of internal validity plays one of the most prominent roles in systematic reviews. For example, Cochrane reviews provide systematic information about possible bias within each study, but do not provide systematic information about the relevance of the study results for clinical and health policy decision-making.

For a better understanding of CER, it is essential to distinguish between 'efficacy' and 'effectiveness'. 'Efficacy' refers to "the extent to which a specific intervention is beneficial under ideal conditions" [3]. Many randomized controlled trials are efficacy trials, particularly those conducted for regulatory drug approval. They aim to produce the expected result for an intervention under carefully controlled conditions chosen to maximize the likelihood of observing an effect if it exists. The trial population and setting of efficacy trials can differ in important ways from the clinical settings in which the interventions are likely to be used [4]. By contrast, 'effectiveness' is a measure of the extent to which an intervention, when deployed in the field in routine circumstances, does what it is intended to do for a specific population [3], and therefore can often be more relevant to policy evaluation and the health care decisions of providers and patients.

For randomized trials, the distinction between explanatory and pragmatic randomized trials was introduced in the 1960 s by Schwarz and Lelloch [5] and is also used in the CONSORT extension [6], another milestone publication on practical trials [7] and the pragmatic-explanatory continuum indicator summary (PRECIS) [8]. However, the term 'explanatory' can be misleading since pragmatic trials can also use an explanatory (confirmatory) statistical approach. Because of this potential confusion, we will use the terms 'efficacy' and 'effectiveness' for labeling the ends of this continuum. It is important to note that there is no sharp distinction between efficacy and effectiveness trials. Rather these terms exist in a continuum and the site along this continuum may differ for different features of the trial design.

This is reflected in the PRECIS tool [8] that was primarily developed to guide the design of RCTs along 10 dimensions of the efficacy-effectiveness continuum. In addition, the IOM has described six characteristics of CER (see Table 1) [1]. Both sets of criteria share the intent of describing the features of research that help inform clinical and health policy decisions. Use of these tools to assess existing trials may offer insights about the specific ways in which existing research has fallen short, and provide specific ideas about how to improve the quality and relevance of future trials. It is of major interest whether the available research can inform stakeholders. Do the existing criteria that define 'pragmatism' and CER that were developed for planning trials that inform clinical decision could be applied to the published trials as a means of evaluating and strengthening the evidence base for CER? Licensing drug trials usually have their main focus on efficacy, using placebo controls and objective outcome measures whenever possible. Because of these regulatory aspects, non-pharmacological studies would serve as better examples to show the whole range of an existing efficacy-effectiveness continuum.

CER is especially valuable for those disorders that are the most common and most costly to society, have the highest morbidity rates, and a great degree of variation in their practice [9]. Low back pain has a high lifetime prevalence, is one of the most common reasons for visits to a physician [10] and results in high health care expenses [11]. An estimated 8 million Americans have used acupuncture as a treatment for persistent disabling pain conditions that include chronic low back pain [12], and clinical relevance of acupuncture for chronic low back pain in usual care is highlighted by a recent clinical expertise paper on acupuncture for chronic low back pain in the New England Journal of Medicine [13]. In this paper, we explore the efficacy/effectiveness continuum in the context of RCTs that assess the impact of acupuncture on low back pain.

This systematic review aims to 1) test the feasibility of applying the PRECIS tool and the IOM CER characteristics to RCTs of acupuncture for treatment of low back pain, and 2) evaluate the extent to which the evidence from these RCTs is relevant to clinical and health policy decision making.

Methods

Data sources and searches

We identified trials using the following search strategy:

- AcuTrials™ Database [14] Feb 10, 2011 searched for low back pain and a comparator group, which was standard care/usual care or no treatment. This database was created by the Research Department, Oregon College of Oriental Medicine, Portland, OR as a comprehensive database that includes all RCTs and systematic reviews on acupuncture published in English.
- Medline 1966 to Feb 17, 2011 searched for 'back pain and acupuncture' or 'back pain and Chinese Medicine' or 'back pain and Traditional Chinese Medicine' using the limits Clinical Trial, Meta-Analysis, Randomized Controlled Trial, English.
- Hand-searching for applicable trials, including the two most recent meta-analyses [15,16].

Study selection

Types of trials. We included controlled trials in which allocation to treatment was explicitly randomized. Trials were excluded that used an inappropriate method of randomization, e.g. open alternation or lottery.

Types of participants. Trials conducted among adult patients suffering from non-specific acute and/or chronic low back pain were included. Trials including patients with specific low back pain, e.g., sciatica or pelvic and lumbar pain during pregnancy, were excluded.

Types of interventions. The treatments considered had to at least involve needle insertion at acupuncture points, pain points or trigger points, and be described as acupuncture. The control interventions considered were conventional treatments (drugs, relaxation, physical therapies, self care etc.). Trials with additional acupuncture interventions based on usual care or other conventional interventions were included. Trials in which patients in the control group had no treatment or only rescue medication or TENS were excluded because they were not considered adequate conventional treatment interventions.

Types of publications. We included only English-language full papers that reported results of single trials. Follow-up publications, protocol publications, diagnostic trials, publications on intervention details, and publications that reported only economic results were excluded.

Sample size. Because we were mainly interested in the efficacy-effectiveness continuum and due to higher variance it is difficult to assess effectiveness with very small samples, we predefined arbitrary to include only those RCTs with ≥30 patients in the acupuncture group.

Data Extraction and Quality Assessment

Selection of trials and preliminary data extraction were performed by one rater (CMW). As a first step, references retrieved from Medline and the AcuTrials database were combined and duplicates were removed. All remaining abstracts were screened and trials that were clearly irrelevant were excluded (e.g., specific low back pain, only sham control or no control group, see Figure 1 for details). In addition, reference lists of recent systematic reviews [15,16] were checked, but did not reveal further unique trials. For the abstracts meeting inclusion criteria, the full papers were obtained and were formally re-checked to exclude ineligible papers. Information on methods, patients, interventions,

Table 1. Rating details using the PRECIS criteria and the IOM characteristics.

criteria	Rating# max. diff. points	Intraclass-correlation before/after	operationalization* good/moderate/difficult	comment	suggestions
PRECIS criteria					
1) eligibility criteria	1	−.12/.59	moderate	raters need good medical knowledge about the range of patients with this diagnosis in usual care	treatment guidelines could be used to aid decision making
2) treatment flexibility intervention group	0	.82/1.00	good	usual care situation differs in countries and even US States, number of treatment always limited in interventional trials	more details in CONSORT guidelines
3) practitioner expertise intervention group	1	.10/.69	moderate	expertise range differs between countries and even US States, often no data about usual care setting and limited information about selection procedure	more details in CONSORT guidelines
4) treatment flexibility control group	1	.58/.95	moderate	publications often don't provide enough information about co-interventions, number of treatment always limited in interventional trials	more details in CONSORT guidelines
5) practitioner expertise control group	1	.60/.92	moderate	publications don't provide enough information, expertise range differs between countries and even US States, often no data about usual care setting and limited information about selection procedure	more details in CONSORT guidelines
6) follow up intensity	1	.02/.36	difficult	trial situation always differs from usual care, influence of telephone interviews, or questionnaires is difficult to operationalize	clear operationalization needed
7) outcomes	1	−.20/−.20	difficult	raters need good knowledge about valid outcomes for the diagnosis, usual care situation on one end of the scale with no interference was difficult	more diagnoses specific standards e.g. in treatment guidelines needed
8) patients' compliance	2	.28/.62	difficult	publications don't provide enough information	could be included in CONSORT guidelines
9) practitioners' protocol adherence	1	.29/.68	difficult	publications don't provide enough information	could be included in CONSORT guidelines
10) primary analysis	1	−.12/.77	good	older publications do not provide this information systematic, most trials do ITT and the relevant topic of subgroup analyses is missing in PRECIS	aspect of subgroup analysis should be included (see IOM)
IOM criteria					
1) directly informing a specific clinical decision from the patient perspective or a health policy decision from the population perspective	3	−.17/.03	moderate	depends on health system, interpreted differently from different perspectives	
2) comparing at least two alternative interventions, each with the potential to be "best practice	2	−.09/.24	moderate	raters need good medical knowledge about treatments options and standards, treatment standards differ between countries, alternatives could be whole treatment packages and also usual care	treatment guidelines could be used to aid decision making
3) describing results at the population and subgroup levels	0	−.21/1.00	moderate	publications provide often none only partial results (e.g. p value for effect modification), items can be easily clearer operationalized	Data on effect modification, but also results for subgroups needed, should be included in CONSORT guidelines
4) measuring outcomes—both benefits and harms—that are important to patients	2	−.19/1.00	moderate	raters need good knowledge about valid outcomes for the diagnosis, difficult to decide which emphasis outcome and safety has in the rating	more diagnoses specific standards e.g. in treatment guideline needed that could linked

Table 1. Cont.

criteria	Rating# max. diff. points	Intraclass-correla-tion before/ after	operationa-lization* good/ moderate/ difficult	comment	suggestions
5) employing methods and data sources appropriate for the decision of interest	1	−.03/.03	moderate	publications don't provide enough information about the rational and setting for trial question	
6) conducted in settings that are similar to those in which the intervention will be used in practice.	2	.37/.69	moderate	publications don't provide enough information about usual setting for the intervention, setting differs between countries	more details in CONSORT guidelines

#after consensus max difference of points (scale 1–5, 1 = max. efficacy to 5 = max. effectiveness) for each of the trials for this criteria,
*qualitative result from the discussion within the consensus procedure.

outcomes and results was extracted from the included trials and entered into an Excel spreadsheet. Special attention was given to sample size, details and rationale of the intervention and comparator groups, the terminology used (efficacy or effectiveness), the test hypothesis (non-inferiority or superiority) and the effect size. If the effect size was not given in the original publications, it was extracted from published meta-analysis.

Data syntheses and analyses

The protocol of the systematic review was predefined. For all included trials, the efficacy-effectiveness continuum was assessed using both the ten PRECIS criteria [8] and the six Institute of Medicine (IOM) defining characteristics of CER [17] To allow a clearer approach, we converted the terminology from 'explanatory/pragmatic' to 'efficacy/effectiveness.' Assessment of trials (Table 2) was performed independently by 5 raters using an enhanced quantified version of the PRECIS and IOM characteristics with a scale of 1–5 for each criterion (1 = maximal efficacy to 5 = maximal effectiveness). This allowed calculation of inter-rater correlations and to present results in figures. The five raters came from different backgrounds (MD and PhD), each had more than 10 years of experience in clinical research, had worked on aspects of research methodology, and had experience in systematic reviews and acupuncture trials. Rating was done independently, results were sent from each rater to CMW, and RL performed the statistics. For the final results, each item was discussed in a conference call between all raters until a consensus was reached.

Agreements between raters (inter-rater reliability) were calculated separately for each item and each time point (before and after the consensus conference) by intraclass-correlations as defined by Shrout and Fleiss [18].

Results

Search Results

Altogether, 119 abstracts were identified: 115 from Medline and 4 additional from the AcuTrials™ database; no further unique abstracts were identified from the recent systematic reviews. Of these abstracts, 44 full papers were screened, and 10 trials, including 4901 total patients (2482 acupuncture and 2419 control) met the eligibility criteria and were subjected to data extraction (see Figure 1).

Included trials

One trial focused on acute low back pain [19], while all the others were on chronic pain low back pain. One trial included two

acupuncture groups: a standardized group and an individualized acupuncture group [20]. For this analysis, we used the individualized acupuncture group because we assumed this group to be closer to usual care. Within the 10 trials, four included a sham acupuncture group [21–24] and four included an economic analysis [22,25–27]. Only two trials used a complex intervention. In the trial by Cherkin [28], other Chinese medicine interventions such as cupping and moxibustion, were allowed. However, in the trial by Szczurko [29], acupuncture was delivered within a naturopathic treatment, which included exercise and dietary advice. All trials tested for superiority of acupuncture treatment. None of the trials aimed to evaluate the non-inferiority of acupuncture compared to conventional care. All ten trials were published in peer reviewed medical journals with relevant impact (Arch Int Med, BMJ, Am J Epi, Pain, PLOS One, Rheumatology, Spine).

Interrater Reliability of Ratings

Raters judged the general difficulty of applying the criteria on a scale from 0–10 (0 = very easy; 10 = very difficult) as 6 (median; range 2–7) for PRECIS and 8 (median; range 6–10) for the IOM criteria. The first independent ratings of the efficacy-effectiveness continuum were highly heterogeneous between trials and raters. This resulted in low inter-rater reliability estimates (Table 2). Missing information in the publications and difficulties in operationalizing the criteria were cited most frequently as the main reasons for the high rater variation in initial scoring of the trials (Table 1). Improved inter-rater reliability was found after the consensus discussion. The consensus process benefitted from each rater's experience in conducting and/or assessing trials on low back pain and acupuncture. Although there was still no full consensus between raters, the maximum difference was 2 points.

Mean Ratings of the Efficacy – Effectiveness Continuum

Details on the trials are presented in Table 2. The trials by Thomas et al [27] and Witt et al [26] that compared adjunctive acupuncture to usual care alone had high effectiveness scores on the efficacy-effectiveness continuum and could serve as examples for trials that aim to represent a usual care situation, whereas those trials which included an additional sham control arm [20,21,23,24] had higher efficacy scores representing a more experimental approach. This corresponded to the wording in the papers: Only those trials that included a sham control arm used the term 'efficacy;' all other trials used the term 'effectiveness'. Interestingly, most trials that scored higher on the efficacy side of the continuum were less standardized than usually observed in

PRISMA 2009 Flow Diagram

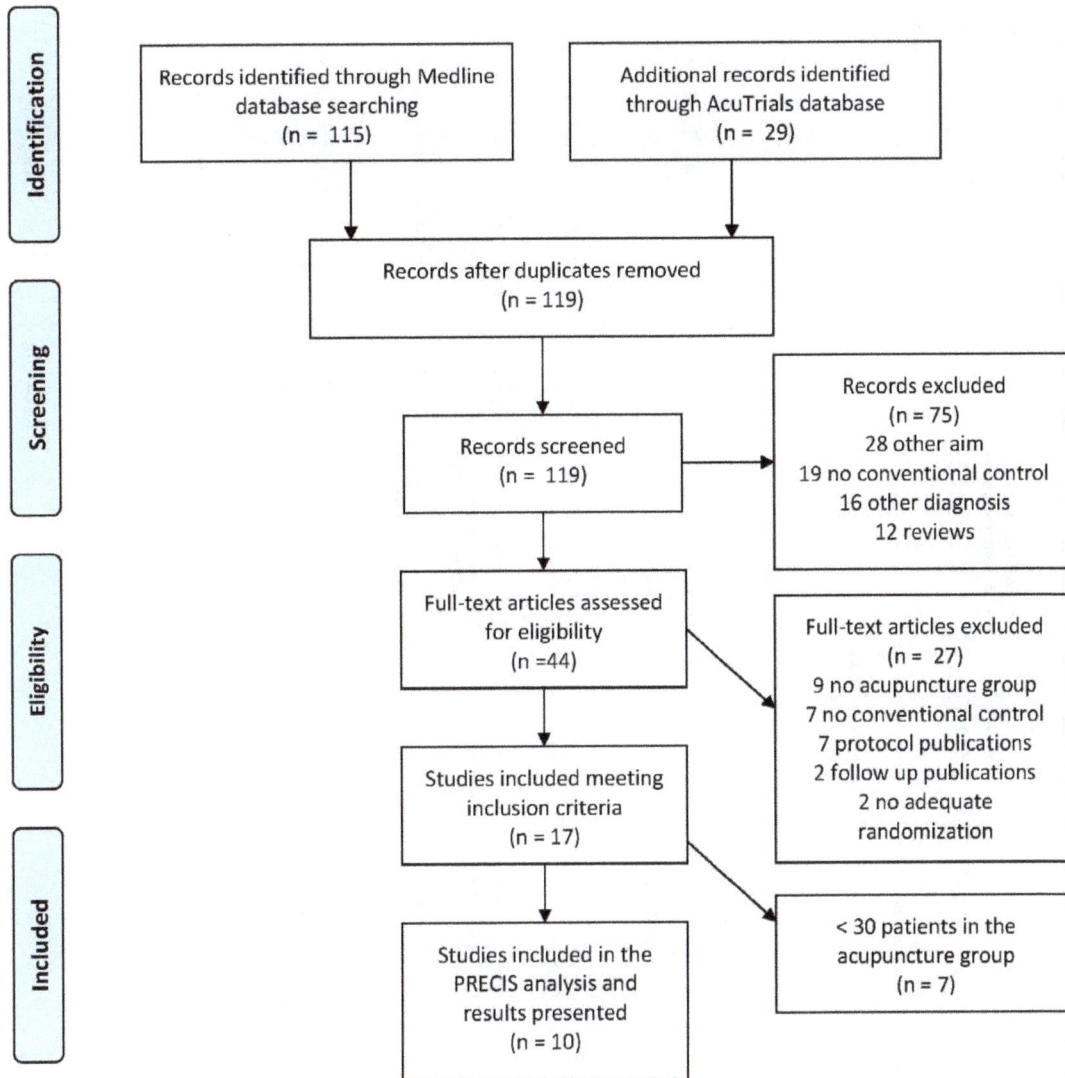

From: Moher D, Liberati A, Tetzlaff J, Altman DG, The PRISMA Group (2009). *Preferred Reporting Items for Systematic Reviews and Meta-Analyses: The PRISMA Statement. PLoS Med 6(6): e1000097. doi:10.1371/journal.pmed1000097*

For more information, visit www.prisma-statement.org.

Figure 1. Study selection.

drug research. The results showed that, for each trial, the placement along the efficacy-effectiveness continuum is multi-dimensional and varied for the different criteria within a given trial (Figure 2). Overall, when evaluating acupuncture as an adjunctive treatment that allowed more flexible treatment protocols, trials had higher effectiveness scores than trials that evaluated

acupuncture as a treatment alternative and used a more standardized treatment protocol (Figure 2).

An interesting exploratory observation is that those trials that reported more narrow eligibility criteria and a more standardized acupuncture intervention [23,24,30] resulted in larger effect sizes (≥0.5, Table 2) than trials that reported a more heterogeneous

Table 2. Trials on non specific low back pain with a conventional treatment comparator and >30 patients in the acupuncture group.

Author	N Acu/Con	Result SMD	Acupuncture #	Acu rational	Setting	Comparator details	Cointervention	Ad on comparator details presented	Rating PRECIS criteria (5=effectiveness/1=efficacy)										Rating IOM criteria (5–1)					
									1	2	3	4	5	6	7	8	9	10	1	2	3	4	5	6
Acute non specific low back pain																								
Eisenberg 2007 (19)	58/150	na	free, max 10 sessions	as usual	physicians, practitioners outpatient practices	treatment follows hospital guideline care (NSAID, muscle relaxants, education, activity alteration)	treatment follows hospital guideline care (NSAID, muscle relaxants, education, activity alteration)	yes number of visits	3.4	4.0	3.6	4.0	3.6	2.4	4.2	4.8	5.0	4.0	4.6	4.6	2.0	4.8	4.8	4.2
Chronic non specific low back pain																								
Witt 2006 (26)	1451/1390	0.43* (0.38;0.49)	needle, free, max 15 sessions	as usual	physicians outpatient practices	patients were free to seek care in the health insurance system	usual care	yes pain medication in both groups reported	4.4	5.0	4.0	5.0	5.0	3.6	4.4	4.4	5.0	4.0	4.6	4.0	2.8	4.6	4.8	4.0
Haake 2007 (21)	387/387	0.56* (0.43;0.70)	needle, semi-standard, 10 or 15 session	consen-sus	physicians outpatient practices	German guideline based treatment (physiotherapy, exercise, NSAID)	rescue medication	no conventional group type and frequency of treatment	3.0	2.0	3.0	4.0	3.8	2.8	4.4	4.2	3.2	4.0	4.4	4.6	1.0	4.2	4.8	4.0
Thomas 2006 (27)	160/81	0.34* (0.03;0.65)	needle, free, max 10 sessions	as usual	practitioners outpatient practices	treatment as provided by their GPs	treatment as provided by their GPs	yes both groups type of treatment	4.4	5.0	3.8	5.0	5.0	3.6	4.4	4.6	5.0	3.4	4.4	4.4	2.0	4.6	4.8	4.0
Cherkin 2009 (20)	157/161	na	needle, free, 10 sessions	by one diagnostician	2 research clinics, outpatients	treatment as provided by their physicians	self care book, usual care	yes % of patients with physician and practitioner visits	3.4	3.0	3.0	5.0	5.0	2.8	4.4	4.2	3.4	4.4	4.4	4.2	1.0	4.4	4.8	3.0
Cherkin 2001 (22)	94/90	0.24* (0.00;0.48)	needle +E-stim, max 10 sessions	consen-sus	practitioners outpatient practices	self care materials (book, videotapes)	usual care	yes treatments both groups; % patients with as non study visits	3.0	5.0	3.4	2.0	na	2.8	4.4	4.4	4.2	4.0	4.4	3.4	2.0	4.6	4.6	4.0
Molsberger 2002 (23)	65/60	0.62** (0.26;0.97)	needle, standard, 12 sessions	litera-ture	rehabi-litation clinic, inpatients	physiotherapy, exercise, education, mud packs, IR-heat, diclofenac (3×50 mg on demand)	physiotherapy, exercise, education, mud packs, IR-heat, diclofenac (3×50 mg on demand)	yes not presented	2.6	3.0	2.6	2.0	3.0	3.4	4.4	4.9	na	3.2	4.4	4.4	1.0	4.2	4.6	3.0
Leibing 2002 (24)	40/46	0.86** (0.42;1.31)	needle, standard, 20 sessions	litera-ture	university hospital outpatient clinic	physiotherapy	physiotherapy	yes not presented	3.4	1.0	2.0	2.4	2.2	3.2	4.4	4.8	na	3.2	4.0	4.4	1.0	4.2	4.8	2.8

Table 2. Cont.

Author	N Acu/ Con	Result SMD	Acupuncture #	Acu rational	Setting	Comparator details	Cointervention	Ad comparator on details presented	Rating PRECIS criteria (5-effectiveness/1-efficacy)										Rating IOM criteria (5-1)						
Szczurko 2007 (29)	39/30	na	needle, standard, 24 sessions	unclear	practitioners on site at a plant	self care booklet and physiotherapy advice and relaxation techniques		no percentage of patients compliant to dietry advice and to exercise	3.4	1.0	2.8	2.4	2.4	3.0	4.4	2.4	4.2		5.0	3.6	3.8	1.0	4.0	4.2	3.2
Meng 2003 (30)	31/24	0.50** (0.08;1.09)	needle, standard, 10 sessions	unclear	aneastesiologists at hospital, outpatients	treatment as before provided by their physicians (NSAID, aspirin, non narcotic analgesics)	treatment as before provided by their physicians (NSAID, aspirin, non narcotic analgesics)	yes patients with medication and use of other CAM treatments	2.6	2.0	2.8	3.4	5.0	3.0	4.6	3.8	na		3.0	4.0	4.6	3.0	4.2	4.6	3.2

Acu = acupuncture, Con = control, na = not available,
*primary endpoint from individual patient data meta-analysis (Vickers Trials 2010),
**short term effect on pain scales from recent meta-analysis (Yuan Spine 2008),
#standard = standardized treatment protocol, free = acupuncture as usual PRECIS: 1) Eligibility criteria, 2) Flexibility acu, 3) Practitioner expertise acu, 4) Flexibility control, 5) Practitioner Expertise control, 6) follow up, 7) Outcomes, 8)Patient compliance, 9) Practitioner adherence, 10) primary analysis IOM: 1) Informing decision making, 2) Comparing at least two alternatives, 3) Results for population and subgroups, 4) Patient relevant outcomes incl. safety, 5) Appropriate methods, 6) Setting close to reality.

patient sample and a flexible acupuncture treatment (effect size≤0.5, Table 2) [26,27].

Discussion

Using available criteria for planning CER to evaluate the efficacy-effectiveness continuum of published trials resulted in large heterogeneity between raters and items, which was partly solved by a consensus procedure. This was mainly due to information missing from the publications and to difficulties in operationalizing the criteria. Our focus on RCTs assessing acupuncture for low back pain allowed the inclusion of a number of high quality trials representing a broad spectrum of clinical research in the efficacy-effectiveness continuum. Trials that have a more flexible acupuncture treatment protocol and no further placebo control arm scored closer to effectiveness.

This is a systematic analysis that has tested the feasibility of appraising the efficacy-effectiveness continuum of randomized controlled trials. Advantages of the systematic review include its innovative scope on the process of appraisal, high quality studies covering the efficacy-effectiveness continuum, and that the scoring was done by 5 independent raters using two different sets of criteria. The review process benefitted from the experience of the selected raters in the design, performance and/or assessment of the field of research. Discussions between raters improved the inter-rater reliability significantly. This underlines the complex aspects of the efficacy-effectiveness continuum and the need for rater training. Limitations were that only one rater selected the papers, that secondary papers (e.g., on treatment details) were not included, and that randomized trials are only one part of CER and do not represent the whole spectrum of evidence. However, Cochrane reviews, which are often used to assist in decision-making, also focus on RCTs and primarily concentrate on the main paper presenting the results. Another limitation is that both criteria lists (PRECIS and IOM) were developed to guide new trials and not to assess published trials. However, the present study provides insights into the advantages and limitation of single items and indicates that, following the definition and main characteristics of CER, the ten PRECIS criteria and six IOM characteristics seem plausible candidates for the evaluation of existing research and could form a basis for a future evaluation instrument. That the items of the PRECIS tool have relevance for appraising published studies is supported by the very recent review by Koppenaal et al [31]. The authors used the PRECIS tool on two meta-analyses, scored the single items, and came to the conclusion that PRECIS can provide useful estimates on how single studies and the whole review are placed within the efficacy effectiveness continuum. Interestingly the authors used a similar scale from 1 to 5. However, they did either provide information on inter-rater variability nor details on advantages and limitations of single PRECIS items which can inform its further development.

The origin of some of the effect sizes presented in this review could be seen as a limitation. It was not the aim of this review to perform a meta-analysis and because of this effect sizes were taken from the literature and only used as an exploratory aspect for orientation.

The present findings reveal that the place of a trial in the efficacy-effectiveness continuum is multidimensional, indicating it is even more complicated to unambiguously label a trial as efficacy or effectiveness. From the scoring of the trials, it is clear that two of the RCTs [26,27] were designed mainly as effectiveness trials, whereas others were designed more as efficacy trials [23,24,29]. Interestingly, two of the trials [20,21], both including a sham control, standardized their acupuncture intervention much more

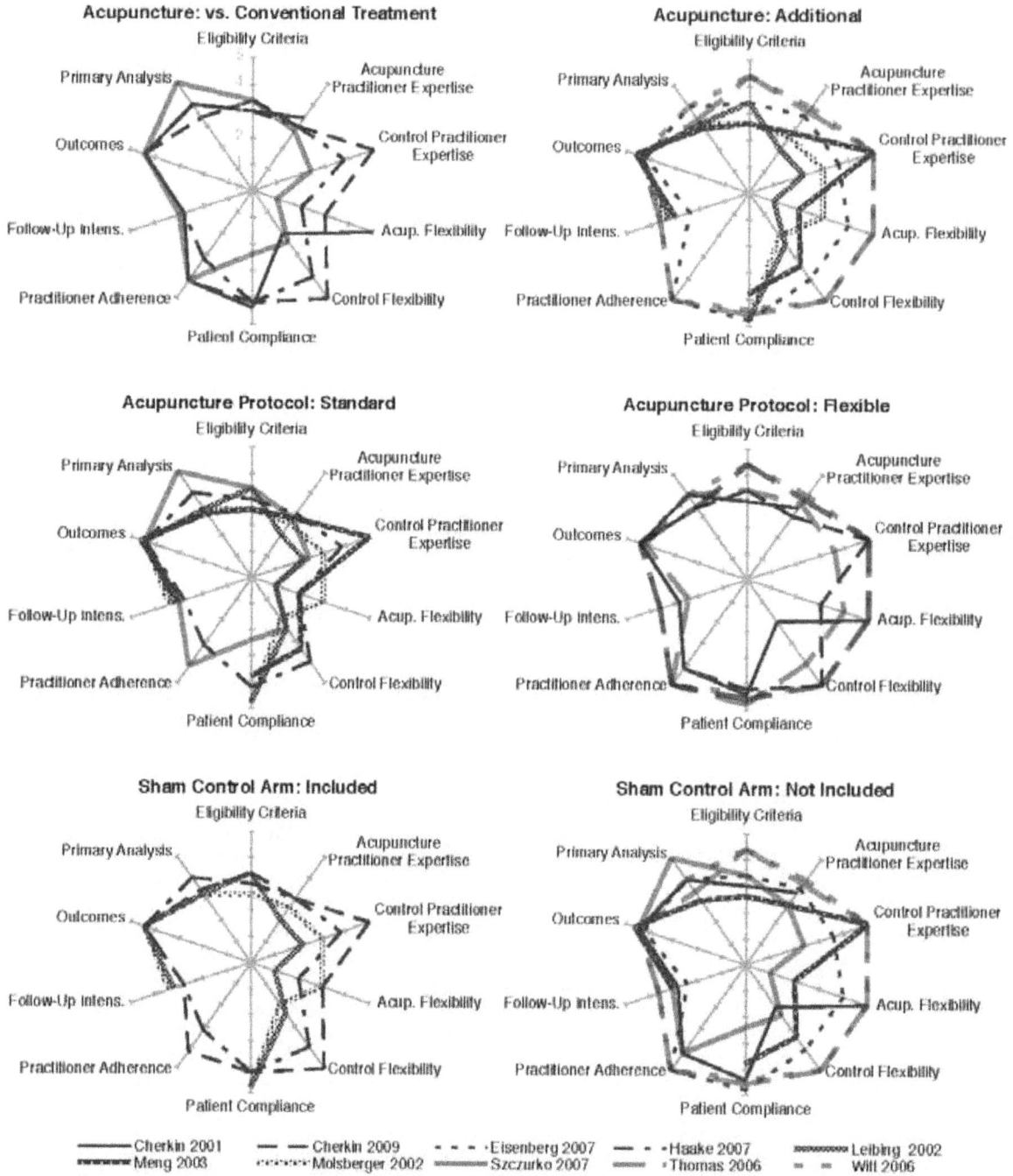

Figure 2. PRECIS scoring for the 10 included trials comparing different methodological aspects (second rating after consensus procedure), a larger rounder figure would correlate with a higher score on PRECIS representing more the effectiveness side.

than their conventional treatment control. None of the trials included all available patients, but eligibility criteria varied from relatively narrow to relatively wide.

In the early 1970's, when Asian medicine including acupuncture began its most recent migration to the West, researchers adopted the randomized controlled trial to investigate acupuncture without knowing Asian medicine had a long history [32]. Because of this evidence from those trials was often rejected as invalid and was therefore ignored. The discussion and demand for evidence that is generated in a way that satisfies decision-making

started early [33] and most studies in this review already reflect the movement toward an evidence base that can inform decisions makers. Acupuncture for low back pain can serve as a good example for different options of randomized studies within CER. On one hand, both large studies that evaluated acupuncture as adjunct to usual care represent a unique way that RCTs can more closely reflect the reality of a usual care setting [26,27]. On the other hand, those trials that had both a standard care/usual care control and a sham control arm, but still tried to keep their acupuncture intervention more flexible are good examples for a middle ground in the efficacy-effectiveness continuum [21]. Overall, the last decade of the acupuncture studies on low back pain provides useful information for the design of future randomized trials in other fields of non-pharmacological research.

In the scoring process of the trials appraising the eligibility criteria was not always easy. Therefore, it would be useful to analyze heterogeneity in addition to get better knowledge about the population in the studies [34]. It is important that trials with more heterogeneous populations result in higher outcome variances and smaller effect sizes, which must be taken into account when planning the sample sizes for future trials assessing CER.

Furthermore, CER is susceptible to systematic error [35]. The attempt to achieve methodological purity can result in clinically meaningless results, while attempting to achieve full generalizability can result in invalid and unreliable results. Achieving a creative tension between the two is crucial [36] and the relevance of the results has to be put into accordance with the rigor of the results. In CER, the evaluation of effect modifications and stratifications play a crucial role [37] to allow for conclusions on specific subgroups. This is one of the IOM criteria, but was not represented in the PRECIS score. Although the trials in our analysis were mainly published in high-ranking journals, none of the trials that scored more on the effectiveness side of the continuum gave detailed information about subgroups. For decision-making, this aspect should be strengthened in future trials and should be included in the criteria list for evaluation of the efficacy-effectiveness continuum.

One problem that came up during the rater consensus procedure was the information missing from the main publications. It is highly recommended to include in future review processes also all available secondary papers. However, in the case of the included studies information on selection procedure of

practitioners, as well as for patient compliance measures and practitioner adherence to protocol would not have been complete. In addition, it would be helpful to know more about the setting in which the treatment is typically carried out in each respective country and how much the trial setting differs from the clinical treatment setting. Although standards for reporting clinical trials (CONSORT [6], STRICTA [38]) mention the most relevant aspects, the above mentioned aspects, such as describing the usual setting for this treatment in detail and providing clear information on patients' compliance and practitioner adherence, are not adequately represented in the CONSORT guidelines and should be discussed in future revisions.

Conclusion

It is of high relevance for stakeholders to appraise the extent to which published trials are relevant to clinical and health policy decision-making. A systematic instrument, which can be also used in systematic reviews, needs further development. The available instruments for planning randomized studies for CER could provide a basis for this, but would need further development that includes more defined operational criteria and a rater's training manual. In addition, CONSORT guidelines for reporting RCTs should be more extended, fostering on reporting more details on CER relevant aspects. Most studies in this review already reflect the movement toward an evidence base that can inform both decision-makers and provide useful information for the design of randomized trials for other non-pharmacological treatments.

Author Contributions

Conceived and designed the experiments: CMW BB. Performed the experiments: RH EM RL LL CMW. Analyzed the data: CMW RL. Wrote the paper: CMW EM RH RL LL SRT BB.

References

1. Committee on Comparative Effectiveness Research Prioritization (2009) What is Comparative Effectiveness Research? In:, , Institute of Medicine (2009) Initial National Priorities for Comparative Effectiveness Research. Washington D.C.: The National Academies Press. 29 p.
2. Conway PH, Clancy C (2009) Comparative-Effectiveness Research – Implications of the Federal Coordinating Council's Report. N Engl J Med 361: 330.
3. Last J, Spasoff RA, Harris S (2001) A dictionary of epidemiology. Oxford: Oxford University Press.
4. Committee on Comparative Effectiveness Research Prioritization (2009) Optimizing Evidence. In: Institute of Medicine , ed. Initial National Priorities for Comparative Effectiveness Research. Washington D.C.: The National Academies Press. 31 p.
5. Schwarz D, Lelloch J (1967) Explanatory and pragmatic attitudes in therapeutical trials. J Chronic Dis 20: 637–647.
6. Zwarenstein M, Treweek S, Gagnier JJ, Altman DG, Tunis S, et al. (2008) Improving the reporting of pragmatic trials: an extension of the CONSORT statement. BMJ 337: a2390.
7. Tunis SR, Stryer DB, Clancy CM (2003) Practical clinical trials: increasing the value of clinical research for decision making in clinical and health policy. JAMA 290: 1624–1632.
8. Thorpe KE, Zwarenstein M, Oxman AD, Treweek S, Furberg CD, et al. (2009) A pragmatic-explanatory continuum indicator summary (PRECIS): a tool to help trial designers. CMAJ 180: E47–E57.
9. Fineberg H (2009) Foreword. In:, , Institute of Medicine (2009) Initial National Priorities for Comparative Effectiveness Research. Washington D.C.: The National Academies Press.
10. Deyo RA, Mirza SK, Martin BI (1976) Back pain prevalence and visit rates: estimates from U.S. national surveys, 2002. Spine 31: 2724–2727.
11. Luo X, Pietrobon R, Sun SX, Liu GG, Hey L (1976) Estimates and patterns of direct health care expenditures among individuals with back pain in the United States. Spine 29: 79–86.
12. Barnes PM, Powell-Griner E, McFann K, Nahin RL (2004) Complementary and alternative medicine use among adults: United States, 2002. Adv Data. pp 1–19.
13. Berman BM, Langevin HM, Witt CM, Dubner R (2010) Acupuncture for chronic low back pain. N Engl J Med 363: 454–461.

14. Oregon College of Oriental Medicine (2011) AcuTrials® Database. Available: http://acutrials.ocom.edu. Accessed 2011 Feb 10.
15. Yuan J, Purepong N, Kerr DP, Park J, Bradbury I, et al. (1976) Effectiveness of acupuncture for low back pain: a systematic review. Spine 33: E887–E900.
16. Rubinstein SM, van MM, Kuijpers T, Ostelo R, Verhagen AP, et al. (2010) A systematic review on the effectiveness of complementary and alternative medicine for chronic non-specific low-back pain. Eur Spine J 19: 1213–1228.
17. Committee on Comparative Effectiveness Research Prioritization (2009) Characteristics of CER. In: Institute of Medicine, ed. Initial National Priorities for Comparative Effectiveness Research. Washington D.C.: The National Academies Press. pp 37–39.
18. Shrout PE, Fleiss JL (1979) Interclass Correlations: Uses in Assessing Rater Reliability. Psychological Bulletin 86: 420–428.
19. Eisenberg DM, Post DE, Davis RB, Connelly MT, Legedza AT, et al. (2007) Addition of choice of complementary therapies to usual care for acute low back pain: a randomized controlled trial. Spine 32: 151–158.
20. Cherkin DC, Sherman KJ, Avins AL, Erro JH, Ichikawa L, et al. (2009) A randomized trial comparing acupuncture, simulated acupuncture, and usual care for chronic low back pain. Arch Intern Med 169: 858–866.
21. Haake M, Muller HH, Schade-Brittinger C, Basler HD, Schafer H, et al. (2007) German Acupuncture Trials (GERAC) for chronic low back pain: randomized, multicenter, blinded, parallel-group trial with 3 groups. Arch Intern Med 167: 1892–1898.
22. Cherkin DC, Eisenberg D, Sherman KJ, Barlow W, Kaptchuk TJ, et al. (2001) Randomized trial comparing traditional Chinese medical acupuncture, therapeutic massage, and self-care education for chronic low back pain. Arch Intern Med 161: 1081–1088.
23. Molsberger A, Diener HC, Krämer J, Michaelis J, Schäfer H, et al. (2002) GERAC-Akupunktur-Studien. Deutsches Ärzteblatt 99: B 1539–1541.
24. Leibing E, Leonhardt U, Koster G, Goerlitz A, Rosenfeldt JA, et al. (2002) Acupuncture treatment of chronic low-back pain – a randomized, blinded, placebo-controlled trial with 9-month follow-up. Pain 96: 189–196.
25. Eisenberg DM, Kessler RC, Van Rompay MI, Kaptchuk TJ, Wilkey SA, et al. (2001) Perceptions about complementary therapies relative to conventional therapies among adults who use both: results from a national survey. Ann Intern Med 135: 344–351.

26. Witt CM, Jena S, Selim D, Brinkhaus B, Reinhold T, et al. (2006) Pragmatic randomized trial of effectiveness and cost-effectiveness of acupuncture for chronic low back pain. American Journal of Epidemiology 164: 487–496.

27. Thomas KJ, MacPherson H, Thorpe L, Brazier J, Fitter M, et al. (2006) Randomised controlled trial of a short course of traditional acupuncture compared with usual care for persistent non-specific low back pain. BMJ 333: 623–626.

28. Cherkin DC, Deyo RA, Sherman KJ, Hart LG, Street JH, et al. (2002) Characteristics of visits to licensed acupuncturists, chiropractors, massage therapists, and naturopathic physicians. J Am Board Fam Pract 15: 463–472.

29. Szczurko O, Cooley K, Busse JW, Seely D, Bernhardt B, et al. (2007) Naturopathic care for chronic low back pain: a randomized trial. PLoS ONE 2: e919.

30. Meng CF, Wang D, Ngeow J, Lao L, Peterson M, et al. (2003) Acupuncture for chronic low back pain in older patients: a randomized, controlled trial. Rheumatology (Oxford) 42: 1–10.

31. Koppenaal T, Linmans J, Knottnerus JA, Spigt M (2011) Pragmatic vs. explanatory: An adaptation of the PRECIS tool helps to judge the applicability of systematic reviews for daily practice. J Clin Epidemiol.

32. Witt CM, MacPherson H, Kaptchuk TJ, Wahlberg A (2011) Efficacy, effectiveness and efficiency. In: Scheid V, MacPherson H, eds. Integrating East Asian Medicine into Contemporary Health Care. London: Churchill Livingstone.

33. Mason S, Tovey P, Long AF (2002) Evaluating complementary medicine: methodological challenges of randomised controlled trials. BMJ 325: 832–834.

34. Kent DM, Rothwell PM, Ioannidis JP, Altman DG, Hayward RA (2010) Assessing and reporting heterogeneity in treatment effects in clinical trials: a proposal. Trials 11: 85.

35. Strom BL (2007) Methodologic challenges to studying patient safety and comparative effectiveness. Med Care 45: S13–S15.

36. Godwin M, Ruhland L, Casson I, MacDonald S, Delva D, et al. (2003) Pragmatic controlled clinical trials in primary care: the struggle between external and internal validity. BMC Med Res Methodol 3: 28.

37. Witt CM, Schützler L, Lüdtke R, Wegscheider K, Willich SN (2011) Patient Characteristics and Variation in Treatment Outcomes: Which Patients Benefit Most From Acupuncture for Chronic Pain? Clin J Pain 27: 550–555.

38. MacPherson H, Altman DG, Hammerschlag R, Youping L, Taixiang W, et al. (2010) Revised STandards for Reporting Interventions in Clinical Trials of Acupuncture (STRICTA): extending the CONSORT statement. PLoS Med 7: e1000261.

Influence of Control Group on Effect Size in Trials of Acupuncture for Chronic Pain: A Secondary Analysis of an Individual Patient Data Meta-Analysis

Hugh MacPherson[1]*, Emily Vertosick[2], George Lewith[3], Klaus Linde[4], Karen J. Sherman[5], Claudia M. Witt[6,7], Andrew J. Vickers[2], on behalf of the Acupuncture Trialists' Collaboration[¶]

1 Department of Health Sciences, University of York, York, United Kingdom, 2 Memorial Sloan-Kettering Cancer Center, New York, New York, United States of America, 3 Faculty of Medicine, Primary Care and Population Sciences, University of Southampton, Southampton, United Kingdom, 4 Institute of General Practice, Technische Universität München, Munich, Germany, 5 Group Health Research Institute, Seattle, Washington, United States of America, 6 Center for Complementary and Integrative Medicine, University Hospital Zurich, Zurich, Switzerland, 7 Institute for Social Medicine, Epidemiology and Health Economics, Charité - Universitätsmedizin, Berlin, Germany

Abstract

Background: In a recent individual patient data meta-analysis, acupuncture was found to be superior to both sham and non-sham controls in patients with chronic pain. In this paper we identify variations in types of sham and non-sham controls used and analyze their impact on the effect size of acupuncture.

Methods: Based on literature searches of acupuncture trials involving patients with headache and migraine, osteoarthritis, and back, neck and shoulder pain, 29 trials met inclusion criteria, 20 involving sham controls (n = 5,230) and 18 non-sham controls (n = 14,597). For sham controls, we analysed non-needle sham, penetrating sham needles and non-penetrating sham needles. For non-sham controls, we analysed non-specified routine care and protocol-guided care. Using meta-regression we explored impact of choice of control on effect of acupuncture.

Findings: Acupuncture was significantly superior to all categories of control group. For trials that used penetrating needles for sham control, acupuncture had smaller effect sizes than for trials with non-penetrating sham or sham control without needles. The difference in effect size was −0.45 (95% C.I. −0.78, −0.12; p = 0.007), or −0.19 (95% C.I. −0.39, 0.01; p = 0.058) after exclusion of outlying studies showing very large effects of acupuncture. In trials with non-sham controls, larger effect sizes associated with acupuncture vs. non-specified routine care than vs. protocol-guided care. Although the difference in effect size was large (0.26), it was not significant with a wide confidence interval (95% C.I. −0.05, 0.57, p = 0.1).

Conclusion: Acupuncture is significantly superior to control irrespective of the subtype of control. While the choice of control should be driven by the study question, our findings can help inform study design in acupuncture, particularly with respect to sample size. Penetrating needles appear to have important physiologic activity. We recommend that this type of sham be avoided.

Editor: Yu-Kang Tu, National Taiwan University, Taiwan

Funding: The Acupuncture Trialists' Collaboration is funded by an R21 (AT004189I from the National Center for Complementary and Alternative Medicine (NCCAM) at the National Institutes of Health (NIH) to Dr Vickers) and by a grant from the Samueli Institute. Dr MacPherson's work on this project was funded in part by the National Institute for Health Research (NIHR) under its Programme Grants for Applied Research scheme (RP-PG-0707-10186). Dr. Witt's work has been supported by the Carstens Foundation within the grant for the Chair for Complementary Medicine Research. The views expressed in this publication are those of the author(s) and not necessarily those of the NCCAM, NHS, NIHR or the Department of Health in England. The funders had no role in study design, data collection and analysis, decision to publish, or preparation of the manuscript.

Competing Interests: The authors have declared that no competing interests exist.

* E-mail: hugh.macpherson@york.ac.uk

¶ Membership of the Acupuncture Trialists' Collaboration is provided in the Acknowledgments.

Introduction

One of the challenges of conducting a non-pharmacological clinical trial is choosing an appropriate control intervention. The simplest control arm is to offer patients routine clinical care without the experimental treatment. This controls for the expected course of the disease. However, the control arm can also be designed to control for other factors, for example, the non-specific effects associated with the time and attention that a patient receives from a clinician.

The choice of control is particularly problematic in acupuncture, which has seen a large increase in published trials in recent years [1]. In an individual patient data meta-analysis of high quality trials conducted by the Acupuncture Trialists' Collaboration [2], acupuncture reduced pain scores by 0.15 to 0.23 standard deviations in comparison to sham (placebo) acupuncture. When the control group did not involve sham, effect sizes ranged from 0.42 to 0.57 [2]. Yet within the general categories of control - those with sham and those without sham - there were marked differences in the exact nature of the intervention received in the control group. For example, trials with sham control included those with acupuncture needles inserted at points not thought to be active, needles that did not penetrate the skin, and non-needle approaches, such as detuned electrical devices. For trials without sham control, the control group in some were simply advised to "avoid acupuncture"; in other trials, both acupuncture and control groups were offered additional treatment, such as physical therapy for back pain.

In this paper, we aim to conduct an analysis of the Acupuncture Trialists' Collaboration dataset to determine how trial results vary by type of control. Specifically, we sought to determine the extent that effect sizes varied depending on whether needles were used for sham acupuncture, whether they penetrated the skin, and whether they were placed at or away from true acupuncture points. We also sought to determine whether there was variation in the effects of acupuncture associated with controls that did not involve sham, comparing "routine care", such as rescue medication made available to patients in both arms of the trial, with "protocolled care" where the control treatment was a standard care specified in the study protocol. Establishing effect sizes associated with commonly used types of controls will be of value in informing future clinical trial design for acupuncture, as well as helping the interpretation of published trial results.

Methods

Included Trials

Trials included in these analyses were identified through a systematic literature review that has been previously described [2]. The initial search was to November 2008, followed by a subsequent one conducted in December 2010. The searches included trials of acupuncture in four specified chronic pain conditions – non-specific musculoskeletal pain, shoulder pain, osteoarthritis, and chronic headache – where allocation concealment was determined unambiguously to be adequate. For trials of musculoskeletal pain, it was additionally specified that the current episode of pain must be of at least four weeks' duration. The search resulted in the identification of 31 trials.

Data Acquisition

Individual patient data were obtained from 29 trials. Data on the trial-level characteristics of the controls were obtained directly from trialists. Twenty trials with 5,230 patients had controls in the form of a sham acupuncture arm (Table 1), and 18 trials with 14,597 patients had non-sham controls (Table 2).

Outcome

The primary outcome used for this analysis was the primary pain endpoint as defined by the study authors. Where multiple criteria were considered in the primary outcome or if the primary outcome was inherently categorical, we used a continuous measure of pain intensity measured at the same time point as the original primary outcome. To make the various outcome measurements comparable between different trials, the primary endpoint of each was standardized by dividing by pooled standard deviation.

Types of Sham Acupuncture Controls

The characteristics we aimed to study in those trials with a sham acupuncture control group included whether or not a needle was used, whether a needle that penetrated the skin was used, whether

sham was performed on true acupuncture points or non-acupuncture points, and whether needle insertion was deep or superficial. Information on acupuncture characteristics was obtained from the trial manuscript supplemented by a questionnaire sent to trialists.

Trials were classified as "needle sham" if it was reported that either a penetrating or non-penetrating needle was used for sham acupuncture. A non-penetrating needle is a device specially developed for acupuncture research in which the needle retracts into the handle rather than penetrating the skin; however, the pressure of the needle against the skin is a very similar sensation to insertion. "Non-needle sham" included trials using non-needle methods of sham acupuncture, such as an inactivated laser or transcutaneous electric nerve stimulation (TENS) device. Needle sham trials were further classified as to whether or not the needle used in the sham acupuncture group penetrated the skin. Penetrating needles were almost always inserted at locations away from true acupuncture points (thereby investigating point location) while non-penetrating sham needles were either applied at the same points as in the true acupuncture group (testing exclusively skin penetration and not location) or at non-acupuncture points (investigating penetration and location simultaneously). For example, in the trial of Linde et al [3], needles were inserted superficially away from true acupuncture points; in contrast, the sham technique in the Kleinhenz et al [4] trial consisted of a special needle that retracted into the handle rather than penetrating through the skin at true acupuncture points.

We initially planned to investigate two other features of sham control: whether the depth of insertion for penetration was categorized by trialists as superficial or deep and whether sham was applied at or away from true acupuncture points. However, as shown in Table 1, only one trial reported using deep insertion in sham acupuncture [5]. For point location, there was strong collinearity with sham technique, with only techniques avoiding skin penetration using true acupuncture points.

As a sensitivity analysis, we re-analyzed the data excluding four trials which were determined by consensus among external reviewers as having an "intermediate likelihood of unblinding" [6][7][8][9]. However, after excluding these trials, only one remaining trial used non-needle sham acupuncture, limiting our ability to use meta-regression.

Types of Non-sham Controls

Trials that included controls without sham were categorized into two types: "routine care" and "protocolled care." Trials were identified as "routine care" if patients in both treatment and control groups had access to non-specified care as needed, such as rescue medications or other conventional care, but the use of such treatment was at the discretion of patients and doctors, with no specification in the protocol as to what treatments patients could receive. If protocols proscribed some treatments, such as surgery, but did not make specific recommendations as to allowable treatments, trials were defined as "routine care". Control groups where treatment consisted of information or education given to a patient ("attention control") were also considered to be routine care control groups. Trials were considered to be "protocolled care" if the care in the control group was specified in the study protocol. This was typically when the acupuncture group and the usual care control group both received an additional non-acupuncture treatment that was specifically indicated as part of the trial protocol. For example, trials that studied the effect of acupuncture and physical therapy compared to physical therapy alone were categorized as protocolled care.

Table 1. Sham Acupuncture-Controlled Trials, by Types of Sham Control.

Needle Used?	Penetrating?	True Acupuncture Points?	Depth of Insertion?	Trials
Yes	Yes	No	Superficial	Linde (2005) [3], Melchart (2005) [25], Diener (2006) [6], Scharf (2006) [26], Haake (2007) [11], Endres (2007) [27], Witt (2005) [28], Brinkhaus (2006) [29]
Yes	Yes	No	Deep	Berman (2004) [5] *
Yes	No	No	N/A	Vas (2008) [14]
Yes	No	Yes	N/A	Foster (2007) [24], Guerra (2004) [30], Kennedy (2008) [31], Kleinhenz (1999) [4], Vas (2004) [12], Vas (2006) [13]
No	No	No	N/A	Carlsson (2001) [9], Kerr (2003) [8]
No	No	Yes	N/A	Irnich (2001) [7], White (2004) [32]

*In this trial, penetrating needles were used on non-acupuncture points and non-penetrating needles were used on true acupuncture points. For the main analysis, we considered this trial as penetrating-needle sham used on non-acupuncture points.

In two trials there was a disagreement about whether the close specification of medication and other treatment in the control group constituted "protocolled care" or an active control group, which are excluded from analyses as per the review protocol [10]. The trial of acupuncture for migraine by Diener et al. [6] had a control group in which patients received standard pharmacological therapy for migraine prophylaxis. However, acupuncture and sham acupuncture groups did not receive prophylactic medication. The trial of acupuncture for lower back pain by Haake et al. [11] offered "routine management" up to and including physiotherapy, drugs and exercise to control group patients. Acupuncture and sham acupuncture patients had the same access to rescue medication as the "routine management" group, but did not have access to the same physiotherapy sessions or exercise consultations with physicians.

Statistical Methods

We used random-effects meta-regression to test the effect of each characteristic of sham acupuncture on the main effect estimate using the Stata command *metareg*. This command was also used to run a random-effects meta-regression to test the effect of routine versus protocolled care on the main effect estimate for usual care control groups. The main effect estimate of each trial was determined using linear regression, and the coefficient and standard error for each trial were entered as the dependent variable in the random-effects meta-regression.

A sensitivity analysis was performed excluding three trials by Vas et al. [12][13][14]. In our initial publication on effect size [2], we reported that these trials have very much larger effect sizes than average and that their exclusion resulted in heterogeneity becoming non-significant in the comparisons between acupuncture and sham. The trial of acupuncture for knee osteoarthritis by Berman et al. [5] used a combined insertion and non-insertion method for sham acupuncture. As a sensitivity analysis, we performed the analysis with this trial reclassified as using non-penetrating needles on true acupuncture points as well. We also excluded trials where the risk of bias from unblinding was not classed as being low. As a final sensitivity analysis of non-sham controlled trials, we excluded the trials by Haake et al. [11] and Diener et al. [6] for which there was disagreement as whether the control arm constituted active control, which is not eligible for analysis [10]. All analyses were conducted using Stata 12 (Stata Corp., College Station, TX).

Results

Sham acupuncture controls

Trial-level characteristics for sham-controlled trials are described in Table 3. The majority of sham-controlled trials (80%) used needle-based sham acupuncture. The number of trials using penetrating or non-penetrating needles was similar: seven trials used non-penetrating needles and nine trials used penetrating needles. All trials using penetrating needles placed these outside true acupuncture points, while only one of seven trials using non-penetrating needles did so.

Table 4 shows the effect sizes of sham-controlled acupuncture trials categorized by the type of sham. Acupuncture is significantly superior to sham irrespective of the type of sham control, both in the main analysis and in a sensitivity analysis excluding outlying studies. Table 4 also includes the results of the primary sensitivity analyses that excluded the Vas trials, which we had previously found to be outliers [2]. For example, not only was the effect size of the Vas trial for neck pain [13] about five times greater than the meta-analytic estimate, but between-trial heterogeneity was no longer statistically significant after excluding the Vas trials. Using the same rationale for exclusions, overall we found larger effect sizes were associated with acupuncture vs. non-penetrating sham needles (0.43; 95%CI: 0.01, 0.85) than vs. penetrating sham needles (0.17; 95%CI: 0.11, 0.23) although the difference between groups did not reach conventional levels of statistical significance.

Statistical comparisons between types of sham are given in Table 5, which shows the results of the random-effects meta-regression for sham-controlled trials. While trials that used needles as sham did not differ significantly from trials with non-needle sham (p≥0.2 for all comparisons), there is clear evidence of a greater effect size when acupuncture is compared against non-penetrating sham than when compared to penetrating sham. Trials using a penetrating needle had an effect size of −0.21 (95% C.I. −0.41, −0.01) standard deviations lower than trials that did not use a needle sham (p = 0.036). Trials that used penetrating needles for sham control had smaller effect sizes than those with non-penetrating sham or sham control without needles. The difference in effect size was −0.45 (95% C.I. −0.78, −0.12; p = 0.007). For the sensitivity analysis that excluded the Vas trials, this effect size reduced to −0.19 (95% C.I. −0.39, 0.01; p = 0.058). There were no significant differences between non-penetrating needles and sham techniques that did not involve needling.

In further sensitivity analyses, reclassification of the Berman trial had little effect on our results. For example, the comparison of

Table 2. Types of non-sham control group by trial: categorised as "protocolled care" or "routine care".

Trial	Control Group	Type of Control Group
Foster (2007) [24]	Advice and exercise: All three arms of the trial received advice and exercise. Patients received leaflet with information on knee osteoarthritis. Patients on NSAID therapy were allowed to continue with stable dose. Individualized exercises of progressive intensity for lower limb stretching, strengthening and balance (up to six 30-minute sessions over six weeks). Patients in the control arm did not receive verum or sham acupuncture.	Protocolled
Linde (2005) [3], Melchart (2005) [25]	Waiting list control: Control patients were not permitted to have prophylactic treatment for 12 weeks. All patients were allowed to treat acute headache as necessary (following current guidelines).	Routine
Thomas (2006) [33], Salter (2006) [34], Vickers (2004) [23]	General practitioner care: All patients received NHS treatment according to general practitioner's assessment and recommendation. Control patients did not receive acupuncture or any other specified interventions.	Routine
Berman (2004) [5]	Education-attention control: Patients in this arm attended six two-hour group sessions based for arthritis self-management, and received periodic educational materials by mail. Patients in the acupuncture and sham acupuncture arms did not participate in this intervention.	Routine
Cherkin (2001) [35]	Self-care education: Patients in this group received a book with information about back pain, treatment, improving quality of life and coping with emotional and interpersonal issues surrounding back pain. Patients also received two professionally-produced videos which addressed self-management of back pain and demonstrated exercises. Patients in the acupuncture and massage groups did not receive this educational material.	Routine
Scharf (2006) [26]	Conservative therapy: Patients in the conservative therapy group had 10 visits with physicians and received prescriptions for either diclofenac (up to 150 mg/day) or rofecoxib (25 mg/day) up to week 23. Patients in this group who had "partially successful" results were offered the choice of attending an additional five visits. Patients in the verum acupuncture and sham acupuncture groups were permitted to take up to 150 mg/day of diclofenac for the first two weeks and a total of 1 g of diclofenac during the rest of the study. Patients in both acupuncture groups and in the conservative management group received up to six sessions of physiotherapy. All patients were prohibited from taking any analgesics other than diclofenac and rofecoxib and any corticosteroids.	Protocolled
Diener (2006) [6]	Standard migraine treatment: Control group patients were treated according to the guidelines of the German Migraine and Headache Society. Patients had six to seven visits in which standard treatment was established. First choice of treatment was beta blockers, followed by flunarizine, and then valproic acid. Acute medication use was permitted in all groups.	Protocolled
Haake (2007) [11]	Conventional therapy: Patients in the conventional therapy group were treated according to German guidelines. Conventional therapy patients had 10 visits with physician or physiotherapist where physiotherapy, exercise and/or similar treatments were offered. Patients in all three arms were permitted to take NSAIDs up to the maximum daily dose.	Protocolled
Williamson (2007) [36]	Education and exercise: Patients in the control group were told they were in the "home exercise" group and received an exercise and advice leaflet.	Routine
Witt (2005) [28], Brinkhaus (2006) [29]	Waiting list control: Patients in the waiting list control group received no acupuncture treatment for eight weeks after randomization. All patients were allowed oral NSAIDs for pain as rescue medication. All patients were prohibited from taking corticosteroids or pain medication that acted on the central nervous system.	Routine
Witt (2006 – OA) [37], Witt (2006 – LBP) [38]	Conventional treatment: Patients in the control group were not allowed to use any kind of acupuncture during the first three months. All patients were allowed to use additional conventional treatments as needed.	Routine
Jena (2008) [39], Witt (2006 – Neck Pain) [40]	Conventional treatment: Patients in the control group were not allowed to use any kind of acupuncture during the first three months. All patients were allowed to use additional conventional treatments as needed.	Routine

penetrating needle vs. non-needle or non-penetrating needle gave a difference in effect size of 0.18 rather than 0.19 and a p value of 0.057 rather than 0.058. Excluding the four trials that were classified as "intermediate risk of unblinding" did not significantly change the effect sizes or p-values for most analyses. For example, the difference in effect size and 95% confidence interval when comparing penetrating needle sham to non-penetrating needle sham was -0.57 (-0.96, -0.18) in the main analysis, while the difference in effect size and 95% confidence for the same comparison was -0.57 (-0.98, -0.15) after excluding these four trials. However, the comparison with non-needle-based sham acupuncture included only one trial using non-needle sham. As a result, the standard error becomes much larger, and the p value

non-significant. Excluding the trials at intermediate risk of unblinding and the outlying Vas trials gave very similar results to the analyses excluding the outlying Vas trials alone. For example, the central estimate for the comparison of penetrating needle with non-needle sham changes from -0.21 to -0.18. Statistical significance was lost, presumably because of the limited number of trials remaining in the analysis (see Table S1, Supporting Information).

Non-sham controls

Trial-level characteristics for trials without sham controls are described in Table 2. The majority of these trials (72%) were

Table 3. Trial-level Characteristics for Trials with Sham Acupuncture Control Groups, N = 20.

Needle Used	
Yes	16 (80%)
No	4 (20%)
Penetrating Needle Used	
Yes	9 (45%)
No	7 (35%)
Non-needle	4 (20%)
True Acupuncture Points Used	
Yes	8 (40%)
No	12 (60%)
Superficial or Deep Sham	
Superficial	8 (40%)
Deep	1 (5%)
Non-penetrating sham	11 (55%)
Pain Type	
Low Back Pain	5 (25%)
Migraine	2 (10%)
Neck	3 (15%)
Osteoarthritis	5 (25%)
Shoulder	3 (15%)
Tension-type Headache	2 (10%)

Frequency (%).

Discussion

Principal findings

Acupuncture was significantly superior to sham irrespective of the type of sham control and superior to non-sham control irrespective of whether that constituted routine or protocolled care. That said, there were differences in effect sizes between trials with different control conditions. With regard to the types of sham control, we found that sham controls involving penetrating needles had smaller effect sizes than trials that did not use a needle control or where the needles in the control group did not penetrate the skin. An important implication is that the central estimates from our meta-analysis [2] may have underestimated the effects of acupuncture compared to sham. With regard to non-acupuncture controls, we found evidence that the effect size of acupuncture when compared to protocolled care is smaller than when compared to the less intensive routine care, although differences did not reach statistical significance.

There are two possible explanations for the differences in effect size by type of sham control: bias from unblinding and physiologic activity. It is plausible that penetrating needles are more credible to patients than non-penetrating approaches, such that patients are less likely to give biased responses on pain questionnaires. That said, there is no evidence in favor of such a hypothesis and considerable evidence against. In particular, the most common form of non-penetrating needle used was the "Streitberger" needle that has been carefully validated as a credible placebo in an empirical study. Indeed, study participants were unable to distinguish between the Streitberger needle and true acupuncture even when subject to both in crossover fashion [15]. The other explanation for our findings is that penetrating needles have important physiologic activity, that is, inserting an acupuncture needle superficially away from an acupuncture point may be less effective than deep insertion at a correct location, but nonetheless has some therapeutic activity against pain [16][17].

Relationship to the literature

There has been considerable interest in the literature regarding the appropriate choice of placebo controls for non-pharmacological therapies. One approach has been to investigate trials that included a placebo arm and a no-treatment arm, and then compare outcomes between these two, and in this way explore variations in the impact of the different types of placebo. An example of this is a Cochrane review of placebo controls covering a wide range of trials for different conditions, including some acupuncture trials [18]. In a sub-group analysis the authors found that trials using "physical placebos" (including sham acupuncture) were associated with greater placebo effects than trials with

classified as routine care. Table 6 provides further details of the control groups, separately by pain type.

The effect size for acupuncture in trials with routine care control (0.55, 95% CI 0.40, 0.70) was larger than when acupuncture was compared against protocolled care (0.29, 95% CI 0.01, 0.58). Although the difference in effect size was large, it was not significant (difference in effect size = 0.26, 95% CI −0.05, 0.57, p = 0.1). Removing the two studies [6] [11] in the sensitivity analysis had little effect on the effect size estimate (0.25, 95% CI −0.26, 0.76) for the comparison with protocolled care. The difference in effect size between trials utilizing protocolled vs. routine care was also similar (0.29, 95% CI −0.13, 0.72).

Table 4. Effect size of acupuncture compared to type of sham acupuncture control.

	Main Analysis		Excluding Vas et al. trials [12] [13] [14]	
	Number of Trials	Effect Size	Number of Trials	Effect Size
Needle sham	16	0.42 (0.19, 0.66)	13	0.22 (0.11, 0.33)
Non-needle sham	4	0.38 (0.19, 0.57)	4	0.38 (0.19, 0.57)
Non-penetrating needle	7	0.76 (0.31, 1.21)	4	0.43 (0.01, 0.85)
Penetrating needle	9	0.17 (0.11, 0.23)	9	0.17 (0.11, 0.23)
Non-needle and non-penetrating needle	11	0.63 (0.33, 0.94)	8	0.40 (0.18, 0.62)

Estimates obtained using meta-regression.

Table 5. Difference in effect sizes between types of sham control. Estimates obtained using meta-regression.

	Main Analysis			Excluding Vas et al. trials [12] [13] [14]		
	No. of Trials*	Change in Effect Size	p value	No. of Trials*	Change in Effect Size	p value
Needle vs. Non-needle sham	16 vs. 4	0.02 (−0.49, 0.53)	0.9	13 vs. 4	−0.17 (−0.43, 0.09)	0.2
Non-penetrating needle vs. Non-needle sham	7 vs. 4	0.35 (−0.28, 0.99)	0.3	4 vs. 4	0.01 (−0.45, 0.47)	1
Penetrating needle vs. Non-penetrating needle	9 vs. 7	−0.57 (−0.96, −0.18)	0.004	9 vs. 4	−0.19 (−0.47, 0.08)	0.2
Penetrating needle vs. Non-needle sham	9 vs. 4	−0.21 (−0.41, −0.01)	0.036	9 vs. 4	−0.21 (−0.41, −0.01)	0.036
Penetrating needle vs. Non-needle or Non-penetrating needle	9 vs. 11	−0.45 (−0.78, −0.12)	0.007	9 vs. 8	−0.19 (−0.39, 0.01)	0.058

*The number listed in the top row is the number of trials in the first comparison group. The number of trials listed in the bottom row is the number of trials in the second comparison group. For example, there were 16 needle sham-controlled trials and 4 non-needle sham-controlled in the main analysis.

pharmacological placebos [18]. This finding is consistent with the results of a trial that was specifically designed to compare a sham device (sham acupuncture) with an inert pill, the sham device being associated with a greater reduction of self-reported pain [19]. These results provide supportive evidence for our finding that different types of sham control lead to different estimates of treatment effects.

The data from the above Cochrane review of placebo controls were re-analysed by a different group of authors who observed that sham acupuncture interventions vs. no treatment have larger effects than other "physical placebos" vs. no treatment [20]. In a sub-analysis that is similar to what we report in this paper, they found that the standardised effect for acupuncture versus sham was similar for trials using penetrating sham needling (−0.43; 95%CI: −0.59, 0.28) compared to trials using non-penetrating sham (−0.37; 95%CI: −0.70, 0.04) [20]. By contrast, we found significantly smaller effect sizes when acupuncture was compared to sham acupuncture with penetrating needles (0.17; 95%CI: 0.11, 0.23) than when compared to non-penetrating needles (0.43; 95%CI: 0.01, 0.85). The differences might be explained by differences in the trials included - our data involved only chronic pain trials of methodologically high quality – and the greater precision afforded by individual patient data meta-analysis: note that the wide confidence intervals in the Cochrane data are consistent with the main estimates from the current analysis.

Table 6. Trial-level Characteristics for Trials with Non-sham Control Groups, N = 18.

Pain Type	Routine Care	Protocolled Care	Total
Headache	2	0	2
Migraine	1	1	2
Tension-Type Headache	1	0	1
Osteoarthritis	4	2	6
Lower Back Pain	3	2	5
Neck Pain	2	0	2
Total	13 (72%)	5 (28%)	18 (100%)

Frequency (%).

Study strengths and limitations

Combining patient data from 29 high-quality trials in a single database provides us for the first time with sufficient power to explore the role of controls in trials of acupuncture for chronic pain, because the power of meta-regression is strongly influenced by the number of trials and their variation. We were unable to address questions as to the depth and location of sham needle placement as only one trial used deep sham needle insertion and all sham-controlled trials that used true acupuncture points avoided penetrating needles. While the difference in effect size between routine and protocolled care is large and in the direction expected, it is associated with wide confidence intervals. Partially, this is due to the wide variety of non-sham controls, and the difficulty we had in categorizing them.

Even with this large dataset we do not have a full understanding of the different physiologic and psychologic effects of sham acupuncture. One limitation within the field generally is that the mechanisms for a persistent effect of acupuncture on chronic pain are incompletely understood and therefore we have no clear idea of whether a sham control inadvertently activates these mechanisms or not. This lack of understanding about the physiological mechanisms of acupuncture limits any firm conclusions we can draw regarding the extent that any of the sham controls discussed above can be considered as a true 'placebo'. Moreover when implementing sham acupuncture trials, the outcome may also be influenced by factors not included in our analysis, such as the believability of the control, prior knowledge of patients about acupuncture, whether the true acupuncture group was treated identically, the extent that practitioners were able to maintain equipoise, and practical implementation issues, such as how carefully the ring that comes with the Streitberger needle [15] was taped in place.

Implications for research

The research question remains the primary determinant on choice of control. In a strategy document developed with a range of collaborators using consensus methods, a useful distinction has been drawn between efficacy trials that seek to determine whether there are specific effects beyond the placebo in an ideal treatment environment, and effectiveness trials that seek to determine the overall impact of acupuncture in which specific and non-specific effects are combined [21]. Moreover research questions investigating the value of specific point location need to have sham needles located away from true acupuncture points while research questions testing skin penetration require non-penetrating sham needle controls applied at the same points as in the true acupuncture group.

The choice of a sham acupuncture control needs to be informed by consideration of the likely impact of the sham intervention. In the past, judgments on this have often used expert opinion on putative physiological activity of a sham control, even though we have yet to understand the mechanism(s) of the action of acupuncture [17]. A number of commentators have speculated that penetrating sham needling may be physiologically active and thus be an inappropriate sham control [16]. Our results provide support for this contention, suggesting that needle penetration should be avoided as a sham technique to control for non-specific effects associated with acupuncture in trials involving chronic pain patients. However sham acupuncture involving penetrating needles may well have a place when addressing questions of point specificity in explanatory trials. We are more cautious with regard to recommending the use of non-penetrating needles. Many forms of Japanese acupuncture use shallow insertion or non-insertion (the *toya hari* method) [22]. Using non-penetrating needles in controlled trials is not without its challenges: although apparently less active than other types of sham, we cannot assume that non-penetrating needles have complete physiologic inactivity; furthermore, there are practical questions regarding whether to enroll only acupuncture-naïve patients and whether practitioners can maintain equipoise in large trials over reasonable periods of time.

When sham acupuncture is not used, the choice of control is clearly driven by the research question. For instance, in the UK National Health Service (NHS) trial of acupuncture for chronic headache, the study question of Vickers et al was related to the effects of making acupuncture more widely available in primary care, a pragmatic comparison of "use acupuncture" and "avoid acupuncture" [23]. On the other hand, Foster et al. were interested in the impact of acupuncture when added to an existing rehabilitation program [24]. Yet our findings have clear implications for sample size calculations, with larger sample sizes needed in trials where care in the control arm is carefully specified.

Conclusion

From a large database of individual patient data from high-quality randomized trials, we found acupuncture to be significantly superior to control irrespective of the subtype of control. When compared against sham, trials with penetrating needles reported lower effect sizes for acupuncture than trials with non-penetrating needles or those that used non-needle sham. This suggests that penetrating needles have important physiologic activity, even when inserted superficially away from true acupuncture points. Accordingly, we recommend that this type of sham be avoided. In trials without sham control, we found that the effect size likely depends on the intensity of treatment in the control group, with smaller differences between acupuncture and protocol guided programs of treatment than between acupuncture and routine care. While the choice of control should be driven by the study question, these findings can help inform study design in acupuncture, particularly with respect to sample size.

Supporting Information

Table S1   Sensitivity analyses.

Acknowledgments

This is a study from the Acupuncture Trialists' Collaboration, which includes physicians, clinical trialists, biostatisticians, practicing acupuncturists and others. The collaborators within the Acupuncture Trialists' Collaboration are:

Claire Allen, BS, Cochrane Collaboration Secretariat, Oxford, England;

Mac Beckner, MIS, Information Technology and Data Management Center, Samueli Institute, Alexandria, Virginia;

Brian Berman, MD, University of Maryland School of Medicine and Center for Integrative Medicine, College Park; Maryland;

Benno Brinkhaus, MD, Institute for Social Medicine, Epidemiology and Health Economics, Charité University Medical Center, Berlin, Germany;

Remy Coeytaux, MD, PhD, Department of Community and Family Medicine, Duke University, Durham, North Carolina;

Angel M. Cronin, MS, Dana-Farber Cancer Institute, Boston, Massachusetts;

Hans-Christoph Diener, MD, PhD, Department of Neurology, University of Duisburg-Essen, Germany;

Heinz G. Endres, MD, Ruhr–University Bochum, Bochum, Germany;

Nadine Foster, DPhil, BSc(Hons), Arthritis Research UK Primary Care Centre, Keele University, Newcastle-under-Lyme, Staffordshire, England;

Juan Antonio Guerra de Hoyos, MD, Andalusian Integral Plan for Pain Management, and Andalusian Health Service Project for Improving Primary Care Research, Sevilla, Spain;

Michael Haake, MD, PhD, Department of Orthopedics and Traumatology, SLK Hospitals, Heilbronn, Germany;

Richard Hammerschlag, PhD, Oregon College of Oriental Medicine, Portland, Oregon;

Dominik Irnich, MD, Interdisciplinary Pain Centre, University of Munich, Munich, Germany;

Wayne B. Jonas, MD, Samueli Institute, Alexandria, Virginia;

Kai Kronfeld, PhD, Interdisciplinary Centre for Clinical Trials (IZKS Mainz), University Medical Centre Mainz, Mainz, Germany;

Lixing Lao, PhD, University of Maryland and Center for Integrative Medicine, College Park, Maryland;

George Lewith, MD, FRCP, Complementary and Integrated Medicine Research Unit, Southampton Medical School, Southampton, England;

Klaus Linde, MD, Institute of General Practice, Technische Universität München, Munich, Germany;

Hugh MacPherson, PhD, Complementary Medicine Evaluation Group, University of York, York, England;

Eric Manheimer, MS, Center for Integrative Medicine, University of Maryland School of Medicine, College Park, Maryland;

Alexandra Maschino, BS, Memorial Sloan-Kettering Cancer Center, New York, New York;

Dieter Melchart, MD, PhD, Centre for Complementary Medicine Research (Znf), Technische Universität München, Munich, Germany;

Albrecht Molsberger, MD, PhD, German Acupuncture Research Group, Duesseldorf, Germany;

Karen J. Sherman, PhD, MPH, Group Health Research Institute, Seattle, Washington;

Hans Trampisch, PhD, Department of Medical Statistics and Epidemiology, Ruhr–University Bochum, Germany;

Jorge Vas, MD, PhD, Pain Treatment Unit, Dos Hermanas Primary Care Health Center (Andalusia Public Health System), Dos Hermanas, Spain;

Andrew J. Vickers (collaboration chair), DPhil, Memorial Sloan-Kettering Cancer Center, New York, New York;

Norbert Victor, PhD (deceased), Institute of Medical Biometrics and Informatics, University of Heidelberg, Heidelberg, Germany;

Peter White, PhD, School of Health Sciences, University of Southampton, England;

Lyn Williamson, MD, MA (Oxon), MRCGP, FRCP, Great Western Hospital, Swindon, and Oxford University, Oxford, England;

Stefan N. Willich, MD, MPH, MBA, Institute for Social Medicine, Epidemiology, and Health Economics, Charité University Medical Center, Berlin, Germany;

Claudia M. Witt, MD, MBA, University Medical Center Charité and Institute for Social Medicine, Epidemiology and Health Economics, Berlin, Germany.

Data sharing policy:

The Acupuncture Trialists' Collaboration obtained some data that cannot be publicly deposited as this was a condition of us receiving the data from third parties. All summary data for the trial-level analyses will immediately be made available to investigators on request; requests for individual patient data will be considered on a case-by-case basis depending on the trials involved for the analysis concerned. Such data are fully de-identified.

Author Contributions

Analyzed the data: AV EV. Wrote the paper: HM AV EV. Co-ordinated the development and conduct of the study: HM. Designed the study: AV.

Gave input on the design of the study: HM CW GL KL KS. Wrote first draft of the Methods and Results sections: AV EV. Wrote first draft of the manuscript as a whole: HM. Gave comments on early drafts and approved the final version of the manuscript: HM EV GL KL KS CW AV. Had full access to all of the data in the study, takes responsibility for the integrity of the data and the accuracy of the data analysis: AV.

References

1. Han JS, Ho YS (2011) Global trends and performances of acupuncture research. Neurosci.Biobehav.Rev. 35(1873–7528):680–7.
2. Vickers AJ, Cronin AM, Maschino AC, Lewith G, MacPherson H, et al. (2012) Acupuncture for Chronic Pain: Individual Patient Data Meta-analysis.x Neurosci.Biobehav.Rev. 172(19):1444–53.
3. Linde K, Streng A, Jurgens S, Hoppe A, Brinkhaus B, et al. (2005) Acupuncture for patients with migraine: a randomized controlled trial. JAMA. 293:2118–25.
4. Kleinhenz J, Streitberger K, Windeler J, Gussbacher A, Mavridis G, et al. (1999) Randomised clinical trial comparing the effects of acupuncture and a newly designed placebo needle in rotator cuff tendinitis. Pain. 83:235–41.
5. BM, Lao L, Langenberg P, Lee WL, Gilpin AMK, et al. (2004) Effectiveness of acupuncture as adjunctive therapy in osteoarthritis of the knee: a randomized, controlled trial. Ann Intern Med. 141:901–10.
6. Diener HC, Kronfeld K, Boewing G, Lungenhausen M, Maier C, et al. (2006) Efficacy of acupuncture for the prophylaxis of migraine: a multicentre randomised controlled clinical trial. Lancet Neurol. 5:310–6.
7. D, Behrens N, Molzen H, Konig A, Gleditsch J, et al. (2001) Randomised trial of acupuncture compared with conventional massage and "sham" laser acupuncture for treatment of chronic neck pain. BMJ. 322(322(7302)):1574–8.
8. DP, Walsh DM, Baxter D (2003) Acupuncture in the management of chronic low back pain: a blinded randomized controlled trial. Clin J Pain. 19(6):364–70.
9. Carlsson CP, Sjölund BH (2001) Acupuncture for chronic low back pain: a randomized placebo-controlled study with long-term follow-up. Clin J Pain. 17(4):296–305.
10. Vickers AJ, Cronin AM, Maschino AC, Lewith G, MacPherson H, et al. (2010) Individual patient data meta-analysis of acupuncture for chronic pain: protocol of the Acupuncture Trialists' Collaboration. Trials. 11:90.
11. Haake M, Muller HH, Schade-Brittinger C, Basler HD, Schafer H, et al. (2007) German Acupuncture Trials (GERAC) for chronic low back pain: randomized, multicenter, blinded, parallel-group trial with 3 groups. Arch Intern Med. 167:1892–8.
12. Vas J, Mendez C, Perea-Milla E, Vega E, Panadero MD, et al. (2004) Acupuncture as a complementary therapy to the pharmacological treatment of osteoarthritis of the knee: randomised controlled trial. Br.Med.J. 329(1468-5833):1216.
13. Vas J, Perea-Milla E, Méndez C, Sánchez Navarro C, León Rubio JM, et al. (2006) Efficacy and safety of acupuncture for chronic uncomplicated neck pain: a randomised controlled study. Pain. 126(1–3):245–55.
14. Vas J, Ortega C, Olmo V, Perez-Fernandez F, Hernandez L, et al. (2008) Single-point acupuncture and physiotherapy for the treatment of painful shoulder: a multicentre randomized controlled trial. Rheumatology (Oxford). 47(6):887–93.
15. Streitberger K, Kleinhenz J (1998) Introducing a placebo needle into acupuncture research. Lancet. 352(0140–6736):364–5.
16. Lund I, Lundeberg T (2006) Are minimal, superficial or sham acupuncture procedures acceptable as inert placebo controls? Acupuncture in Medicine. 24(1):13–5.
17. Birch S (2006) A review and analysis of placebo treatments, placebo effects, and placebo controls in trials of medical procedures when sham is not inert. J Alternat Complement Med. 12:303–10.
18. Hróbjartsson A, Gøtzsche PC (2010) Placebo interventions for all clinical conditions. Cochrane Database Syst Rev. CD003974.
19. Kaptchuk TJ, Stason WB, Davis RB, Legedza ATR, Schnyer RN, et al. (2006) Sham device vs. inert pill: randomised controlled trial of two placebo treatments. BMJ. 332:391–7.
20. Linde K, Niemann K, Meissner K (2010) Are sham acupuncture interventions more effective than (other) placebos? A re-analysis of data from the Cochrane review on placebo effects. Forsch Komplementrmed. 17:259–64.
21. Witt CM, Aickin M, Baca T, Cherkin D, Haan MN, et al. (2012) Effectiveness guidance document (EGD) for acupuncture research - a consensus document for conducting trials. BMC Complementary and Alternative Medicine. 12(1):148.
22. Birch S, Felt R (1999) Understanding Acupuncture. Edinburgh: Churchill Livingstone.
23. Vickers AJ, Rees RW, Zollman CE, McCarney R, Smith CM, et al. (2004) Acupuncture for chronic headache in primary care: large, pragmatic, randomised trial. Br.Med.J. 328(1468–5833):744.
24. Foster NE, Thomas E, Barlas P, Hill JC, Young J, et al. (2007) Acupuncture as an adjunct to exercise based physiotherapy for osteoarthritis of the knee: randomised controlled trial. BMJ. 335:436.
25. Melchart D, Streng A, Hoppe A, Brinkhaus B, Witt C, et al. (2005) Acupuncture in patients with tension-type headache: randomised controlled trial. BMJ. 331:376–82.
26. Scharf H, Mansmann U, Streitberger K, Witte S, Kramer J, et al. (2006) Acupuncture and Knee Osteoarthritis: a three-armed randomized trial. Ann Intern Med. 145:12–20.
27. Endres HG, Böwing G, Diener H-C, Lange S, Maier C, et al. (2007) Acupuncture for tension-type headache: a multicentre, sham-controlled, patient- and observer-blinded, randomised trial. J Headache Pain. 8(5):306–14.
28. Witt C, Brinkhaus B, Jena S, Linde K, Streng A, et al. (2005) Acupuncture in patients with osteoarthritis of the knee: a randomised trial. Lancet. 366:136–43.
29. Brinkhaus B, Witt CM, Jena S, Linde K, Streng A, et al. (2006) Acupuncture in patients with chronic low back pain: a randomized controlled trial. Arch Intern Med.166:450–7.
30. Guerra de Hoyos JA, Andres Martin MdC, Bassas y Baena de Leon E, Vigára Lopez M, Molina López T, et al. (2004) Randomised trial of long term effect of acupuncture for shoulder pain. Pain. 112(3):289–98.
31. Kennedy S, Baxter GD, Kerr DP, Bradbury I, Park J, et al. (2008) Acupuncture for acute non-specific low back pain: a pilot randomised non-penetrating sham controlled trial. Complement Ther Med. 16(3):139–46.
32. White P, Lewith G, Prescott P, Conway J (2004) Acupuncture versus placebo for the treatment of chronic mechanical neck pain: a randomized, controlled trial. Ann.Intern.Med. 141(1539-3704):911–9.
33. Thomas KJ, MacPherson H, Thorpe L, Brazier J, Fitter M, et al. (2006) Randomised controlled trial of a short course of traditional acupuncture compared with usual care for persistent non-specific low back pain. BMJ. 333:623–6.
34. Salter GC, Roman M, Bland MJ, MacPherson H (2006) Acupuncture for chronic neck pain: a pilot for a randomised controlled trial. BMC Musculoskelet Disord. 7:99.
35. Cherkin DC, Eisenberg D, Sherman KJ, Barlow W, Kaptchuk TJ, et al. (2001) Randomized trial comparing traditional Chinese medical acupuncture, therapeutic massage, and self-care education for chronic low back pain. Arch. Intern. Med. 161(8):1081–8.
36. Williamson L, Wyatt MR, Yein K, Melton JT (2007) Severe knee osteoarthritis: a randomized controlled trial of acupuncture, physiotherapy (supervised exercise) and standard management for patients awaiting knee replacement. Rheumatology (Oxford). 46(9):1445–9.
37. Witt CM, Jena S, Brinkhaus B, Liecker B, Wegscheider K, et al. (2006) Acupuncture in patients with osteoarthritis of the knee or hip: a randomized, controlled trial with an additional nonrandomized arm. Arthritis Rheum. 54:3485–93.
38. Witt CM, Jena S, Selim D, Brinkhaus B, Reinhold T, et al. (2006) Pragmatic randomized trial evaluating the clinical and economic effectiveness of acupuncture for chronic low back pain. Am.J.Epidemiol. 164:487–96.
39. Jena S, Witt CM, Brinkhaus B, Wegscheider K, Willich SN (2008) Acupuncture in patients with headache. Cephalalgia. 28(9):969–79.
40. Witt CM, Jena S, Brinkhaus B, Liecker B, Wegscheider K, et al. (2006) Acupuncture for patients with chronic neck pain. Pain. 125:98–106.

Incomplete Reporting of Baseline Characteristics in Clinical Trials: An Analysis of Randomized Controlled Trials and Systematic Reviews Involving Patients with Chronic Low Back Pain

Maria M. Wertli[1]*, Manuela Schöb[1], Florian Brunner[2], Johann Steurer[1]

1 Horten Center for Patient Oriented Research and Knowledge Transfer, Department of Internal Medicine, University of Zurich, Zurich, Switzerland, **2** Department of Physical Medicine and Rheumatology, Balgrist University Hospital, Zurich, Switzerland

Abstract

Objective: The aim of this study was to evaluate the reporting of relevant prognostic information in a sample of randomized controlled trials (RCTs) that investigated treatments for patients with chronic low back pain (LBP). We also analysed how researchers conducting the meta-analyses and systematic reviews addressed the reporting of relevant prognostic information in RCTs.

Methods: We searched the Cochrane Database to identify systematic reviews that investigated non-surgical treatments for patients with chronic LBP. The reported prognostic information was then extracted from the RCTs included in the reviews. We used a purpose-defined score to assess the quantity of information reported in the RCTs. We also determined how the authors of systematic reviews addressed the question of comparability of patient populations between RCTs.

Results: Six systematic reviews met our inclusion criteria, and we analysed 84 RCTs. Based on the scores, the reporting of important prognostic variables was incomplete in almost half of the 84 RCTs. Information regarding patients' general health, social support, and work-related conditions was rarely reported. Almost half of the studies included in one of the meta-analyses provided insufficient information that did not allow us to determine whether patients in the primary trials were comparable.

Conclusions: Missing prognostic information potentially threatens the external validity (i.e. the generalizability or applicability) not only of primary studies but also of systematic reviews that investigate treatments for LBP. A detailed description of baseline patient characteristics that includes prognostic information is needed in all RCTs to ensure that clinicians can determine the applicability of the study or review results to their patients.

Editor: Laxmaiah Manchikanti, University of Louisville, United States of America

Funding: The authors have no support or funding to report.

Competing Interests: The authors have declared that no competing interests exist.

* E-mail: Maria.Wertli@usz.ch

Introduction

Assessing the external validity of randomized controlled trials (RCTs) is a key step in the critical appraisal of clinical studies. Many clinicians trust authors and journal editors to verify the high internal validity of the published studies (e.g., concealment of randomization list, information about drop-outs, intention to treat analysis), but physicians must decide for themselves whether the results apply to an individual patient. The information that is needed for this determination is reported in the Methods and Results sections of journal articles. The Methods section reports the eligibility criteria information, which states the patient qualifications for inclusion in the study. Patient characteristics are reported in the Results section; quite often, the article's Table 1 shows the distribution of characteristics of patients included in the study. Guidelines for reporting, e.g., the CONSORT Statement for randomized controlled trials [1], recommend not only a comprehensive description of eligibility criteria but also a list of baseline characteristics for important prognostic factors.

A complete description of relevant prognostic factors is particularly important in otherwise ill-defined diseases, such as chronic low back pain (CLBP). Several prognostic factors have been identified that can affect treatment effects in patients with CLBP, including age, duration of symptoms, first or recurrent episode, employment status, and comorbidities such as depression [2,3]. For example, a treatment is effective in patients without depression but be less effective or even ineffective in depressed patients [4].

Knowing the patients' baseline characteristics is important for interpreting study results, both for clinicians and for the researchers who conduct systematic reviews and meta-analyses. Pooling the results of primary studies with unknown or different distributions of relevant prognostic factors in the included

Table 1. Important prognostic risk factor domains and subdomains in patients with low back pain (modified from Hayden et al. [7]).

Domain	Subdomain	SQR Score*
General patient characteristics	Socio-demographic status Social support	Minimal requirement: ≥1 subdomain reported
Baseline health status	Overall health Overall psychological health Previous LBP	Minimal requirement: ≥1 subdomain reported
Work-related factors	Work: psychosocial demands Work: physical demands Work history Work place attributes	Minimal requirement: ≥1 subdomain reported
Current LBP	Clinical history Disability related to the complaint Changes related to complaint over time	Minimal requirement: ≥1 subdomain reported
Clinical examination findings	Physical examination findings Definition of NSLBP diagnosis[†] Changes found during the physical exam	Minimal requirement: ≥1 subdomain reported
Interactions with work/society	Compensation issues related to LBP	Minimal requirement: ≥1 subdomain reported

LBP: low back pain; NSLBP: nonspecific low back pain;
[†]To fulfil this subdomain, at least one more attribute (in addition to pain duration) had to be reported (e.g. disability, severity, pain referral) [30];
*SQR: Score for the quantity of reporting: Scoring SQR high: information reported in one or more subdomains for all six main domains; SQR moderate: information reported in one or more subdomains for five main domains; SQR low: information reported in one or more subdomains for four or fewer main domains.

population may lead to a biased result [5]. It is unclear whether authors report important prognostic information in sufficient detail in primary studies so as to be helpful in rational pooling of data in meta-analyses and systematic reviews.

The aim of the current study was to evaluate the reporting of relevant prognostic information in a selection of randomized controlled trials (RCTs) investigating treatment outcomes in patients with CLBP. We also determined whether the authors of systematic reviews addressed the question of comparability of patient populations between RCTs.

Methods

Study Design

Here we analysed primary studies included in CLBP-related systematic reviews in the Cochrane library. For the purpose of the current study, CLBP represents an ill-defined disease with high health care expenditure [6] for which important prognostic information is known to influence the course of the disease [3,7]. We aimed to include a complete set of trials for each treatment intervention; therefore, we analysed primary studies that were included in systematic reviews published in the Cochrane library. The Cochrane Collaboration Guideline [8,9,10] has published guidelines for the standardized assessment of baseline characteristics to facilitate comparison of systematic reviews. While this study is not a systematic review reporting will be based, if applicable, on the recommendations of the PRISMA statement [11].

Eligibility Criteria and Selection of Systematic Reviews

All systematic reviews that were published in the Cochrane library from its inception (1996) to December 2010 that investigated non-surgical treatments for CLBP were eligible for inclusion in our analysis. We searched the Cochrane library for the terms "chronic" and "non-specific low back pain" in the title, abstract, or keywords. Of the returned reviews, only RCTs published in English and German were eligible for further analysis due to the authors' lack of proficiency in other languages. Non-randomized trials and observational studies were excluded.

Two reviewers (MW and MS) independently screened the titles and abstracts of the identified systematic reviews to determine which ones met the pre-defined inclusion criteria. The full text of each RCT included in the systematic reviews were then

independently reviewed (MW and MS). Discrepancies between the two reviewers were discussed and resolved by consensus or by a third party (FB).

Data Extraction and Synthesis

One reviewer (MS) extracted data from the RCTs, including bibliographic data (authors, year of publication), eligibility criteria, and prognostic information. Prognostic information for LBP was defined a priori in collaboration with experienced clinicians (one internist, one rheumatologist, one general practitioner) and one methodologist in the field and by consulting the relevant literature [2,3].

We used the prognostic domains proposed by Hayden et al. [7] to categorize the information reported in the RCTs. These domains, which are considered to represent clinically meaningful groups, [2] have been used in previous research and are based on expert consensus [12]. The following six main domains were used: general patient characteristics, baseline health status, work-related factors, current low back pain (LBP), clinical examination findings, and interactions with work/society. Each main domain is divided into subdomains (e.g., current LBP is further divided according to the patient's clinical history, disability related to the complaint, and changes in the complaint over time). There were a total of 16 prognostic subdomains (Table 1). The six main domains represent a spectrum of important information that helps clinicians decide whether the study results are applicable to their patients.

One reviewer (MW) confirmed all of the extracted information and assigned the data to the appropriate subdomains. To quantify the amount of reported prognostic information for each RCT, we defined a Score for the Quantity of Reporting (SQR) for each one as follows: High SQR, information was reported for one or more subdomain in all six main domains; moderate SQR, information was reported for one or more subdomains in five of the six main domains; and low SQR, information was reported for one or more subdomains in four or fewer main domains (Table 1).

The SQR for each study was then compared to how the baseline characteristics were assessed in the systematic reviews. Assessment of the comparability of baseline characteristics in studies is defined in the Method guidelines for systematic reviews in the Cochrane Collaboration Back Review Group for Spinal Disorders [8] (first published in 1997). The relevant question is: "Are the baseline characteristics similar with regards to the most important prognostic factors?" The possible answers are "Yes/

Systematic reviews (SRs)
were identified by searching
the title, abstract and
keywords of papers included in
the Cochrane library:

N = 24

Number of SRs excluded after
screening the titles and abstracts:

n = 2 protocol
n = 15 not non-specific low back pain

Number of SRs meeting
eligibility criteria:

n = 7

Number of primary studies in
full-text articles assessed for
eligibility:

n = 100

Number of excluded full-text articles:

n = 1 French
n = 7 Japanese
n = 5 Chinese
n = 1 Polish
n = 1 Norwegian
n = 1 study included in two SR

n = 16

Number of studies included in
final analysis:

n = 84

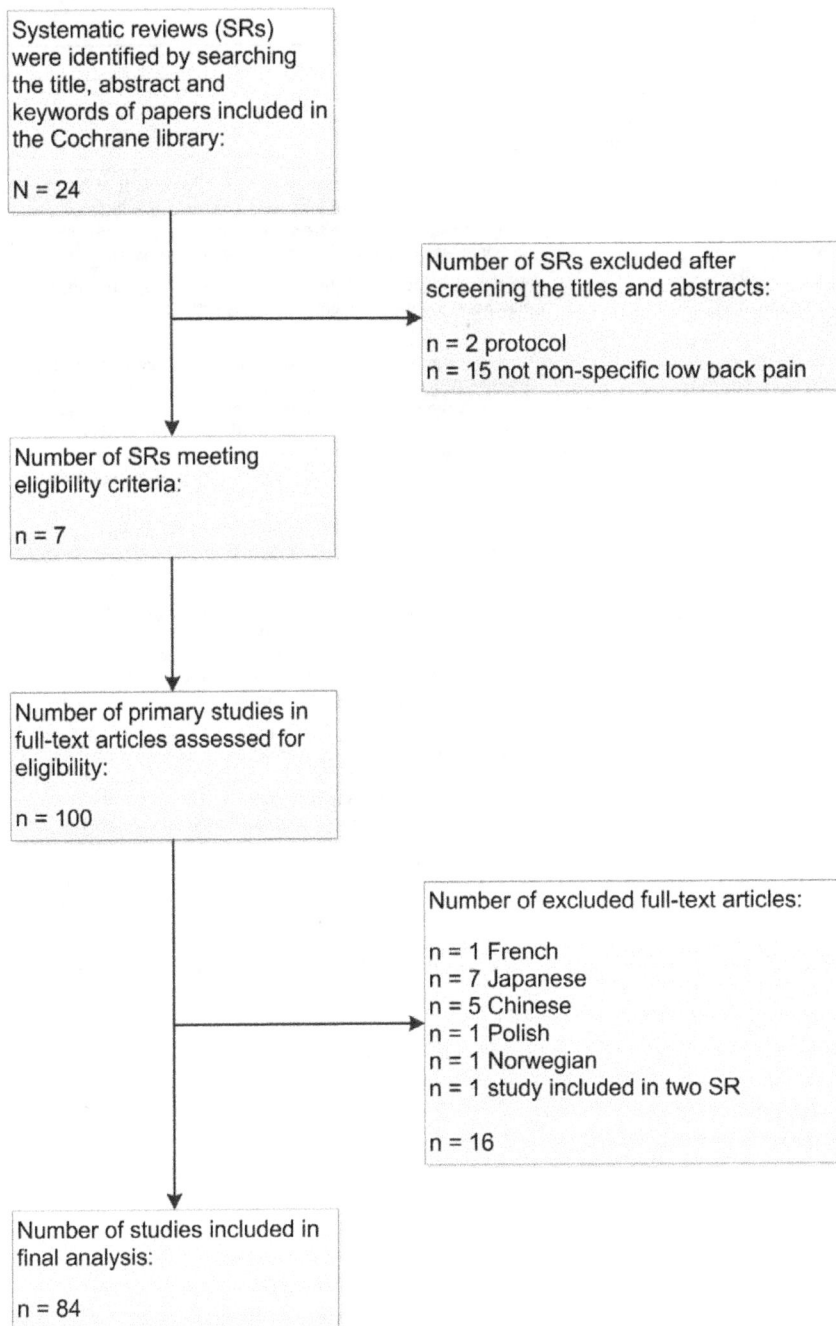

Figure 1. Study flow chart. The Cochrane Database of Systematic Reviews was searched in November, 2010.

No/Don't know," and studies were divided into "Yes", "No", or "Can't tell" categories depending on the answer to that question. The updated Method Guidelines in 2003 [9] further stated, "In order to qualify for a "Yes," groups have to be similar at baseline regarding demographic factors, duration and severity of complaints, percentage of patients with neurologic symptoms." When not enough information is reported, the study must be classified as "Can't tell". We would expect that for primary studies with low SQRs, the answer to the above question would be "Can't tell." We also investigated whether studies with low SQR or that were classified as "Can't tell" were included in the meta-analysis.

Statistical Analysis

Descriptive statistics were used to summarize findings across the entire set of RCTs. We wished to evaluate changes in the quantity of reporting over time, particularly after the publication of the CONSORT statement in 1996 [1], which aimed to improve the quality of reporting in RCTs. Toward this end, the mean number of reported subdomains before and after 1998 (to allow one year for implementation of CONSORT suggestions) was compared using the t-test. Analyses were conducted with SPSS for Windows version 19 (IBM SPSS; Chicago, IL USA) and R statistical software for Windows (http://www.R-project.org/).

Table 2. Summaries of the systematic reviews in our analysis.

Author	Year	Objective	Number of studies analysed	Conclusion
Furlan et al. [32]	2005	To assess the effects of AC for the treatment of NSLBP and the effects of dry-needling for myofascial pain syndrome in the low-back region.	20	Acute LBP: no firm conclusions about the effectiveness of AC. Chronic LBP: AC more effective for pain relief and functional improvement than no treatment or sham treatment and in the short-term only. AC is not more effective than other conventional treatments.
Urquhart et al. [33]	2008	To determine whether antidepressants are more effective than placebo for the treatment of NSLBP	9	No clear evidence that antidepressants are more effective than placebo in the management of patients with CLBP.
Henschke et al. [14]	2010	To determine the effects of behavioural therapy for CLBP and the most effective behavioural approach	32	Short-term: moderate quality evidence that operant therapy is more effective than being placed on a waiting list and that behavioural therapy is more effective than usual care for pain relief. No specific type of behavioural therapy is more effective than another. Intermediate- to long-term: Little or no difference between behavioural therapy and group exercises for pain or depressive symptoms.
Staal et al. [34]	2008	To determine if injection therapy is more effective than placebo or other treatments for patients with subacute or chronic LBP.	10	Insufficient evidence to support the use of injection therapy in subacute and chronic LBP. Insufficient data to answer whether specific subgroups of patients respond to a specific type of injection therapy.
Deshpande et al. [35]	2007	To determine the efficacy of opioids in adults with CLBP.	4	Quality remark: Although high internal validity scores, the study showed a lack of generalizability, inadequate description of study populations, a poor intention-to-treat analysis, and limited interpretation of functional improvement. The benefits of opioids in clinical practice for the long-term management of CLBP remain questionable.
Dagenais et al. [36]	2007	To determine the efficacy of prolotherapy in adults with CLBP.	5	When used alone, prolotherapy is not an effective treatment for CLBP. When combined with spinal manipulation, exercise, and other co-interventions, prolotherapy may improve CLBP and disability. Quality remark: Conclusions are confounded by clinical heterogeneity amongst studies and by the presence of co-interventions.
Khadilkar et al. [37]	2008	To determine whether TENS is more effective than placebo for the management of CLBP.	4	The current evidence from a small number of placebo-controlled trials does not support the use of TENS in the routine management of CLBP.

CLBP/NSLBP: chronic low back pain/nonspecific low back pain; LBP: low back pain; AC: acupuncture; UC: usual care; TENS: transcutaneous electrical nerve stimulation.

Ethics Statement

For this study no ethical approval was required. No protocol was published or registered. All methods were determined a priori.

Results

Study Selection

Seven systematic reviews met the eligibility criteria (Figure 1). The reviews were published between 2005 and 2010 and included 100 primary studies. A total of 84 primary studies (RCTs) were included in the analysis. The main reason for exclusion was publication in a language other than English (n = 16). Figure 1 shows a flow diagram of the study selection process.

Study Characteristics

Table 2 summarizes the objectives, the number of included RCTs, and the conclusions of each systematic review. Most RCTs aimed to investigate treatments only for chronic low back pain; few studies included patients with subacute and acute low back pain. The number of RCTs included in each systematic review ranged from four [13] to thirty-two [14] trials. The RCTs were published between 1971 and 2009. More than half of the studies assessed the effects of acupuncture (n = 18, 21.4%) or cognitive behavioural therapy (n = 27, 32.1%). Most patients in the control groups received placebo (n = 26, 30%), sham procedures (n = 12, 14%), or usual care (n = 12, 14%), or the patients were placed on a waiting

list (n = 13, 15%). In most studies, the follow-up time was about 6 months (median 6 months, range 1 hour to 5 years). Details are shown in Table 3.

Reporting of Important Prognostic Factors in Primary Studies

The information reported for the domains and subdomains is summarized in Table 4. The data reported most often were data about socio-demographic status and the history of the current LBP. Information about the patient's general health status, social support, and work-related information was rarely reported. Although statistically significant (p-value = 0.01), the mean number of subdomains with reported information increased after 1998 by fewer than two subdomains (from a mean of 5.4 subdomains to 7.0 subdomains). In studies published after 2001, the median number of subdomains with reported information increased to 8 (of a possible total of 16 subdomains), reflecting a trend towards improved reporting of prognostic important information in recent years (Figure 2).

In 17 of the 84 studies (20%), information was reported for all six of the main domains (high SQR). Information was reported for five of the six main domains (moderate SQR) in 30 studies (36%) and for four or fewer domains (low SQR) in 37 studies (44%). The 27 studies investigating cognitive behavioural or educational therapy (termed CBT) provided information for more domains on average (high or moderate SQR for 82%) than studies of other

Table 3. Characteristics of primary studies included in the systematic reviews.

Systematic review	Year	Patient population (number of studies)	Recruitment and setting (number of studies)	Duration of LBP (years): mean* (range)	Follow-up (months) mean* (range)	Subjects (n) mean* (range)	Age (years) mean* (range)	Outcomes	Data-pooling
Furlan et al.	2005	Chronic SLBP +NSLBP (1), spinal pain syndrome (1), disabling LBP (1), NSLBP (17)	Specialized Unit (13), GP based (2), GP referral (1), Advertisement (3)	8.95 (0.5–12), 12 n.r.	4.15 (13 days–12 months)	74.5 (17–262)	49.67 (38–73)	VAS (9), McGill (2), ODI (2), others (7)	Yes
Urquhart et al.	2008	NSLBP (6), SPLBP+NSLBP (2)	Specialized Unit (3), Advertisement+Specialized Unit (5), GP based (1)	13.94 (3 months–20.3 years)	2.19 (6 weeks–8 months)	65.56 (16–121)	43.9 (26–53)	McGill (1), VAS (2), RMQ (1) others (7)	Yes
Henschke et al.	2010	SP: non-working disabling (1), chronic NSLBP (17), SLBP+NSLBP (1), Quebec taskforce (1), Topographic criteria of Kuorinka et al. (2), hospitalized (2); LBP: employees on sick leave (1), mildly dysfunctional (3), high paraspinal EMG level (1), FAB (1)	Advertisement (4), GP referral (7), GP referral+Advertisement (5), PT (1), Insurance (2), Specialized Unit (11)	7.46 (1.5–12)	12.49 (3 weeks–5 years)	112.19 (20–409)	43.39 (38–50)	NRS (3), McGill (5,) RMQ (4), VAS (2), SF-36 (1), others (12)	Yes
Staal et al.	2008	Chronic SLBP+NSLBP (3), Radiologic severity of Osteoarthritis (Kellgren) (1), NSLBP (6)	Specialized Unit (7), GP setting+Specialized Unit (1), 2 no information (2)	3.29 (1–8.5)	2.32 (after treatment–6 months)	84.5 (16–206)	47 (40–65)	VAS (4), Mc Gill (1), RMQ (1), others (4)	No
Deshpande et al.	2007	Chronic NSLBP (4)	3 GP setting+Specialized Unit, 1 Specialized Unit	Only in one reported (6.6)	3.73 (6 weeks–6 months)	239 (48–336)	50.3 (42–57)	VAS (2), McGill (2), others (2)	Yes
Dagenais et al.	2007	Chronic NSLBP (3), SPLBP+NSLBP (1), SLBP (1)	GP referral (2), Specialized Unit (1), no information (2)	9.55 (0 days–14 years)	9 (624)	171.4 (74–513)	44.4 (39–50)	VAS (4), McGill (1), RMQ (3), NRS (1)	No
Khadilkar et al.	2008	CLBP: nonspecific (3), acute+chronic LBP (1)	GP-based (1), Advertisement (1), Specialized Unit (1)	3.84 (1.4–6)	1.13 (after treatment–3 months)	133.5 (30–324)	42.88 (31–51)	VAS (3), McGill (1), ODI (1), others (2)	No

LBP: low back pain; SPLBP: specific low back pain; NSLBP: non-specific low back pain; SP: spine pain; EMG: electromyography; GP: general practitioner; Specialized unit: specialist, specialized unit at a hospital; VAS: visual analogue scale; RMQ: Roland Morris Disability Questionnaire; SF-36: Multi-purpose short-form health survey; McGill: McGill Pain Questionnaire; ODI: Oswestry Disability Index; FAB: fear avoidance beliefs.
*Values are calculated as the mean of the mean values reported in the primary trials; the range of the mean values are shown.

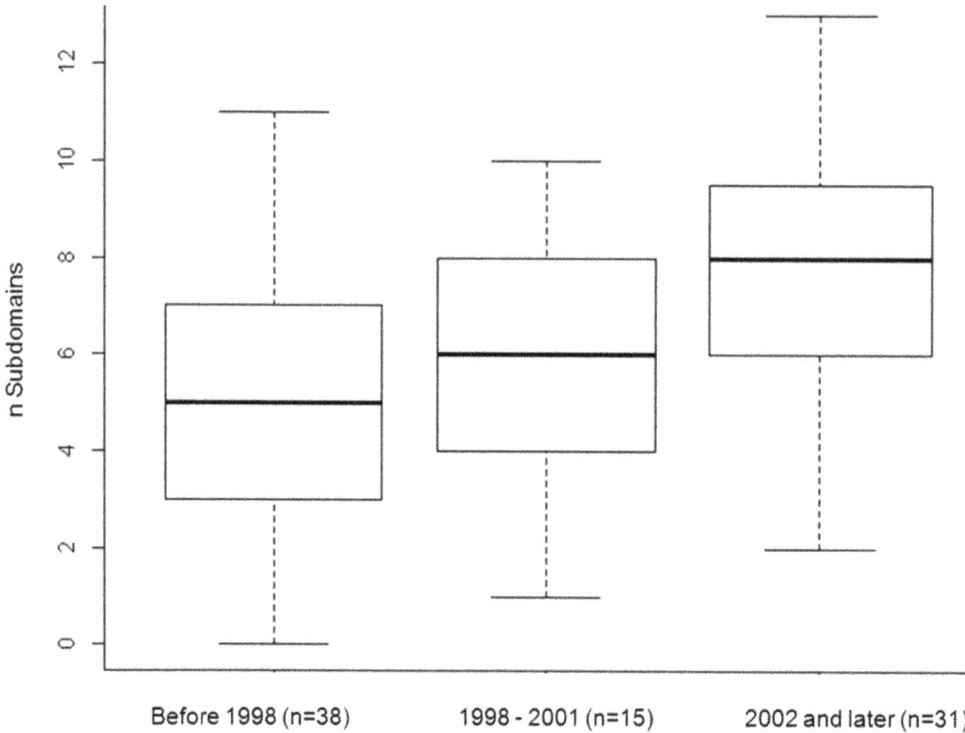

Figure 2. Boxplot showing the number of reported subdomains per primary study over time before and after publication of the CONSORT statement (1996).

Table 4. Quantity of information in the prognostic subdomains in the 84 RCTs.

Domain	Subdomain	Total	%
General patient characteristics	Sociodemographic information	80	95
	Social support	8	10
Baseline health status	Overall health	22	26
	Overall psychological health	47	56
	Previous LBP	33	39
Work-related factors	Work: psychosocial demands	1	1
	Work: physical demands	6	7
	Work history	39	46
	Work place attributes	3	4
Current LBP	Clinical history	67	80
	Disability related to the complaint	48	57
	Changes related to complaint over time	38	46
Clinical examination findings	Physical examination findings	25	30
	Definition of NSLBP diagnosis	56	67
	Change found during the physical exam	21	25
Interactions with work/society	Compensation issues related to LBP	36	43

LBP: low back pain; NSLBP: non-specific low back pain.

interventions. There was poor reporting in the main domains in studies investigating acupuncture, injection therapy, antidepressants, and opioids (SQR poor in 72–100% of the RCTs) (Table 5).

Table 5. Summary of the Score for Quantity of reporting (SQR) types for the RCTs.

	SQR high	SQR moderate	SQR low
All studies (n=84, 100%)	17 (20%)	30 (36%)	37 (44%)
Acupuncture (n=18, 21%)	0 (0%)	5 (28%)	13 (72%)
Antidepressants (n=9, 11%)	1 (5.5%)	1 (5.5%)	8 (89%)
Opioids (n=4, 5%)	0 (0%)	0 (0%)	4 (100%)
CBT (n=27, 32%)	11 (41%)	11 (41%)	5 (18%)
TENS: (n=5, 6%)	1 (20%)	1 (20%)	3 (60%)
EMG (n=4, 5%)	0 (0%)	2 (50%)	2 (50%)
Reflexology (n=1, 1%)	0 (0%)	1 (100%)	0 (0%)
Injection Therapy (n=11, 13%)	2 (18%)	0 (0%)	9 (82%)
Prolotherapy (n=5, 6%)	2 (40%)	0 (0%)	3 (60%)

CBT: cognitive behavioural therapy or educational therapy; TENS: transcutaneous electrical nerve stimulation; EMG: electromyography; Prolotherapy: Repeated injections of irritant solutions to strengthen lumbosacral ligaments; SQR: Score for quantity of reporting, scoring SQR high: information reported in one or more subdomains for all six main domains; SQR moderate: information reported in one or more subdomains for five main domains; SQR low: information reported in one or more subdomains for four or fewer main domains.

Table 6. Comparison of the Score for Quantity of Reporting (SQR) categories (high/moderate/low) for the 84 RCTs and the Cochrane Collaboration Guideline-baseline characteristics (CCG-baseline) categories (Similar/Not similar/Can't tell).

All RCTs (n = 84, 100%)	CCG-baseline: Similar or Not similar (n = 67, 80%)	CCG-baseline: "Can't tell" (n = 17, 20%)
SQR high (n = 17, 20%)	17 (20%)	0 (0%)
SQR moderate (n = 20, 24%)	16 (19%)	4 (5%)
SQR low (n = 47, 56%)	34 (40%)	13 (15%)

Comparison of the Classification Systems for Reporting Prognostic Factors Using SQR and the Cochrane Collaboration Guidelines for Baseline Characteristics (CCG-baseline)

In the systematic reviews, the reporting of baseline characteristics was classified as "Can't tell" in 17 of the 84 studies (20%). The CCG-baseline rating was "Similar" for 59 studies and "Not similar" for 8 studies, indicating that sufficient information for classification was available in most of the studies. The baseline characteristics were classified by the reviewers either as "Similar" or "Not similar" in almost two thirds of the studies with low SQRs (34 studies, 40%) (Table 6). There was thus moderate agreement between the two rating systems, i.e. SQR and CCG-baseline.

Of the 44 studies pooled for meta-analysis, the SQR was low in 22 studies (50%), and 8 (18%) of the studies were classified as "Can't tell" according to the CGC-baseline system (Table 7). Five (11%) of the 44 pooled studies were classified as low SQR and "Can't tell" according to the CGC-baseline system.

Discussion

Main Findings

In a selection of RCTs that examined various treatments for LBP, there was sparse reporting of relevant baseline characteristics and of prognostic information in particular. This information is needed by clinicians who wish to extrapolate the results to individual patients and by those who conduct meta-analyses who must decide whether it makes sense to pool the results of different studies. The reporting of important prognostic variables could have been more complete in almost half of the assessed trial reports. Even information that could be obtained without great effort and expense, e.g., information on general health status, social support, and work-related conditions, was rarely reported. Half of the studies included in one of the meta-analyses failed to provide enough information for the reader to make an informed decision about whether patients in the primary trials were comparable.

Comparison with Other Studies

To our knowledge, this is the first study to focus on the reporting of baseline characteristics in RCTs of patients with chronic LBP and to focus on how this issue is addressed in systematic reviews. Baseline patient characteristics are mainly prognostic factors. A comprehensive description of the distribution of these prognostic factors is relevant for determining the applicability of the study results to various patient populations. Comparable analyses have been performed for systematic reviews of prognostic cohort studies [2,15] and non-randomized intervention studies [16]. The authors of those studies identified incomplete reporting of prognostic factors and recommended a more detailed description of the included patients. Regardless of study design, an incomplete description of patient characteristics increases the risk for bias in interpreting the results of single studies and systematic reviews. A detailed description of the study population helps researchers decide whether it makes sense to pool results from different studies and helps them perform subgroup analyses. The guidelines for conducting systematic reviews mention, without providing detailed instructions, evaluating the comparability of patient populations between primary studies [10,17,18,19]. We found no studies that evaluated the consequences of incomplete reporting of baseline characteristics on the ability of physicians and researchers to interpret RCTs, systematic reviews and meta-analyses.

Clinical Implications

Many current guideline recommendations are based on the results of systematic reviews and meta-analyses, which are ranked highest in the hierarchy of evidence [20]. A thorough and careful synthesis of primary studies is crucial to warrant this ranking. Critique has been raised on the appraisal of systematic reviews and consequentially on the justification of recommendations in the guidelines. There is a controversy for example about the differences in the rating of the methodological quality of systematic reviews [21]. Another issue of concern physicians repeatedly bring up in educational meetings is the inclusion of RCTs in systematic reviews with conflicting or even contradictory results. Physicians question the comparability of patient populations included in systematic reviews and meta-analyses. Conflicting results in RCTs

Table 7. Comparison of the Score for Quantity of Reporting (SQR) categories (high/moderate/low) for the 44 RCTs included in meta-analyses and the Cochrane Collaboration Guideline-baseline characteristics (CCG-baseline) categories (Similar/Not similar/Can't tell).

All RCTs (n = 44, 100%)	CCG-baseline: Similar or Not similar (n = 36, 81%)	CCG-baseline "Can't tell" (n = 8, 19%)
SQR high (n = 11, 25%)	9 (20%)	2 (5%)
SQR moderate (n = 11, 25%)	10 (23%)	1 (2%)
SQR low (n = 22, 50%)	17 (39%)	5 (11%)

could reflect a heterogeneous patient population with a range of prognostic profiles [22]. Other explanations for heterogeneity in the results between primary studies on LBP might be, e.g., varying drug dosages or different numbers of training units in exercise therapy, differences in the measurement of the outcome, and outcome measurement at different time points.

While the problem of heterogeneity has been recognized, there is not much research on this issue in conservative treatment for low back pain [23]. However, in clinical practice it is important to know to which degree patient characteristics at baseline affects treatment efficacy. From a clinician's perspective it seems reasonable to assume that certain treatments (e.g., cognitive behavioral therapy) are more effective in patients presenting with yellow flags (e.g., fear avoidance beliefs, distress) or depression. It is therefore relevant to know about specific treatment effects in subgroups of patients. Clinicians expect from researchers that this heterogeneity in treatment effects is scrutinized and relevant prognostic patient characteristics are considered in the synthesis of RCTs in order to offer an evidence-based and goal oriented health care to the patients [24].

Various concerns on the value of systematic reviews and meta-analyses have been raised in the past years that are beyond the scope of this analysis [20,25,26,27,28]. Systematic reviews offer the possibility to exploit the heterogeneity of prognostic profiles and to conduct subgroup analyses. Thus, reporting the relevant baseline characteristics in primary studies is critical for the quality of the systematic review. Further, collaboration between clinicians and methodologists allows for a meaningful pooling of data in meta-analyses and to examine treatment effects in different groups of patients with LBP. A striking example that underlines the importance of clinical knowledge and subgroup analyses is a recent systematic review investigating vitamin D supplementation for the protection of hip fracture [29]. While the overall effect in this systematic review including all patients, irrespective of their vitamin D blood level at baseline, was not different to placebo, vitamin D protected against hip fractures in individuals with low vitamin D levels at the time of inclusion in the trials.

Limitations of the Study

While we applied robust methodology and a systematic approach to assess the reporting of prognostic information in RCTs, the current study has some limitations. In using a score based on domains, all prognostic information was given equal

weight. We are aware that this may be an over-simplification. The cut-off for 'low SQR' used in the current study was chosen arbitrarily, and more studies would have fulfilled the quality criteria if the cut-off was lower. Because we accepted that any reported information was sufficient to fulfil a domain, we think the cut-off we used was reasonable. Accordingly, non-reporting of information in two or more main domains represents a risk for misinterpretation of results not only in primary studies but also in systematic reviews. We support current efforts to standardize measurements of prognostic factors and reporting in back pain research that will make it easier to compare studies in the future [3,30].

Another limitation of our study is the focus was only on RCTs that were included in systematic reviews published in the Cochrane library. Inclusion of RCTs in systematic reviews published in other databases might give different results. We chose the Cochrane systematic reviews as they are widely recognized as setting the standard for the evaluation of healthcare interventions [31]. Furthermore, the standardized risk of bias assessment in all systematic reviews ensures similar assessment in the different reviews. While the Cochrane reviews are relatively recent, the most recent trial included in our analysis was published in 2009, and more important prognostic information might be reported in more recent studies. Our analysis of changes in reporting over time showed a small but statistically significant increase in reporting in the ten years after publication of the CONSORT statements.

Conclusion

Missing prognostic information potentially threatens the external validity (i.e. generalizability or applicability) not only of primary studies but also of systematic reviews that evaluate treatments for LBP. A detailed description of baseline characteristics, including important prognostic information, will help clinicians and researchers make informed decisions about whether the results of a study or a systematic review apply to their patients.

Author Contributions

Extracted the information and assigned them into predefined categories: MW MS. Conceived and designed the experiments: MW MS FB JS. Performed the experiments: MW MS. Analyzed the data: MW MS FB JS. Contributed reagents/materials/analysis tools: MW MS FB JS. Wrote the paper: MW MS FB JS.

References

1. Schulz KF, Altman DG, Moher D, Group C (2010) CONSORT 2010 statement: updated guidelines for reporting parallel group randomized trials. Ann Intern Med 152: 726–732.

2. Hayden JA, Chou R, Hogg Johnson S, Bombardier C (2009) Systematic reviews of low back pain prognosis had variable methods and results: guidance for future prognosis reviews. J Clin Epidemiol 62: 781–796. e781.

3. Pincus T, Santos R, Breen A, Burton AK, Underwood M, et al. (2008) A review and proposal for a core set of factors for prospective cohorts in low back pain: a consensus statement. Arthritis Rheum 59: 14–24.

4. Nour K, Laforest S, Gauvin L, Gignac M (2006) Behavior change following a self-management intervention for housebound older adults with arthritis: an experimental study. International Journal of Behavioral Nutrition and Physical Activity 3: 12.

5. Laupacis A, Wells G, Richardson W (1994) Users' Guides to the Medical Literature: V. how to use an article about prognosis. JAMA: The Journal of the American Medical Association 272: 234–237.

6. Balagu F, Mannion A, Pellis F, Cedraschi C (2012) Non-specific low back pain. Lancet 379: 482–491.

7. Hayden JA, Dunn KM, van der Windt DA, Shaw WS (2010) What is the prognosis of back pain? Best Practice & Research Clinical Rheumatology 24: 167–179.

8. van Tulder MW, Assendelft WJ, Koes BW, Bouter LM (1997) Method guidelines for systematic reviews in the Cochrane Collaboration Back Review Group for Spinal Disorders. Spine (Philadelphia, Pa 1976) 22: 2323–2330.

9. van Tulder M, Furlan A, Bombardier C, Bouter L, Editorial Board of the Cochrane Collaboration Back Review Group G (2003) Updated method guidelines for systematic reviews in the cochrane collaboration back review group. Spine (Phila Pa 1976) 28: 1290–1299.

10. Furlan AD, Pennick V, Bombardier C, van Tulder M, Editorial Board CBRG (2009) 2009 updated method guidelines for systematic reviews in the Cochrane Back Review Group. Spine (Phila Pa 1976) 34: 1929–1941.

11. Liberati A, Altman DG, Tetzlaff J, Mulrow C, Gøtzsche PC, et al. (2009) The PRISMA statement for reporting systematic reviews and meta-analyses of studies that evaluate healthcare interventions: explanation and elaboration. BMJ 339.

12. Manchikanti L, Singh V, Cash KA, Pampati V, Datta S (2009) A comparative effectiveness evaluation of percutaneous adhesiolysis and epidural steroid injections in managing lumbar post surgery syndrome: a randomized, equivalence controlled trial. Pain Physician 12: E355–368.

13. Trigkilidas D (2010) Acupuncture therapy for chronic lower back pain: a systematic review. Ann R Coll Surg Engl 92: 595–598.

14. Henschke N, Ostelo RW, van Tulder MW, Vlaeyen JW, Morley S, et al. (2010) Behavioural treatment for chronic low-back pain. Cochrane Database Syst Rev: CD002014.

15. Hayden JA, Côté P, Bombardier C (2006) Evaluation of the Quality of Prognosis Studies in Systematic Reviews. Annals of Internal Medicine 144: 427–437.

16. Deeks JJ, Dinnes J, D'Amico R, Sowden AJ, Sakarovitch C, et al. (2003) Evaluating non-randomised intervention studies. Health Technol Assess 7: iii–x, 1–173.

17. Research CoSfSRoCE, Medicine Io (2011) Finding What Works in Health Care: Standards for Systematic Reviews; Eden J, Levit L, Berg A, Morton S, editors: The National Academies Press.

18. Higgins JPT, Green S (2011) Cochrane Handbook for Systematic Reviews of Interventions Version 5.1.0 The Cochrane Collaboration.

19. Dissemination CfRa (2009) CRD's guidance for undertaking reviews in health care. Third Edition ed: CRD, University of York.

20. Egger M, Ebrahim S, Smith GD (2002) Where now for meta-analysis? Int J Epidemiol 31: 1–5.

21. Chou R, Atlas SJ, Loeser JD, Rosenquist RW, Stanos SP (2011) Guideline Warfare Over Interventional Therapies for Low Back Pain: Can We Raise the Level of Discourse? The Journal of Pain 12: 833–839.

22. Jane wit D, Horwitz R, Concato J (2010) Variation in results from randomized, controlled trials: stochastic or systematic? J Clin Epidemiol 63: 56–63.

23. Fourney D, Andersson G, Arnold P, Dettori J, Cahana A, et al. (2011) Chronic low back pain: a heterogeneous condition with challenges for an evidence-based approach. Spine (Philadelphia, Pa 1976) 36: S1–S9.

24. Ostelo R, Croft P, van der Weijden T, van Tulder M (2010) Challenges in using evidence to inform your clinical practice in low back pain. Best Practice & Research Clinical Rheumatology 24: 281–289.

25. Freeman MD (2010) Clinical practice guidelines versus systematic reviews; which serve as the best basis for evidence-based spine medicine? The Spine Journal 10: 512–513.

26. Willis B, Quigley M (2011) The assessment of the quality of reporting of meta-analyses in diagnostic research: a systematic review. BMC Medical Research Methodology 11: 163.

27. Pambrun E, Bouteloup V, Thibaut R, Asselineau J, de-Ldinghen V, et al. (2010) On the validity of meta-analyses: exhaustivity must be warranted, exclusion of duplicate patients too. J Clin Epidemiol 63: 342–343.

28. Kirkham JJ, Dwan KM, Altman DG, Gamble C, Dodd S, et al. (2010) The impact of outcome reporting bias in randomised controlled trials on a cohort of systematic reviews. BMJ 340.

29. Bischoff-Ferrari HA, Willett WC, Orav EJ, Lips P, Meunier PJ, et al. (2012) A pooled analysis of vitamin D dose requirements for fracture prevention. N Engl J Med 367: 40–49.

30. Dionne C, Dunn K, Croft P, Nachemson A, Buchbinder R, et al. (2008) A consensus approach toward the standardization of back pain definitions for use in prevalence studies. Spine (Philadelphia, Pa 1976) 33: 95–103.

31. Tricco A, Tetzlaff J, Pham B, Brehaut J, Moher D (2009) Non-Cochrane vs. Cochrane reviews were twice as likely to have positive conclusion statements: cross-sectional study. J Clin Epidemiol 62: 380–386. e381.

32. Furlan AD, van Tulder MW, Cherkin DC, Tsukayama H, Lao L, et al. (2005) Acupuncture and dry-needling for low back pain. Cochrane Database Syst Rev: CD001351.

33. Urquhart DM, Hoving JL, Assendelft WW, Roland M, van Tulder MW (2008) Antidepressants for non-specific low back pain. Cochrane Database Syst Rev: CD001703.

34. Staal JB, de Bie R, de Vet HC, Hildebrandt J, Nelemans P (2008) Injection therapy for subacute and chronic low-back pain. Cochrane Database Syst Rev: CD001824.

35. Deshpande A, Furlan A, Mailis-Gagnon A, Atlas S, Turk D (2007) Opioids for chronic low-back pain. Cochrane Database Syst Rev: CD004959.

36. Dagenais S, Yelland MJ, Del Mar C, Schoene ML (2007) Prolotherapy injections for chronic low-back pain. Cochrane Database Syst Rev: CD004059.

37. Khadilkar A, Odebiyi DO, Brosseau L, Wells GA (2008) Transcutaneous electrical nerve stimulation (TENS) versus placebo for chronic low-back pain. Cochrane Database Syst Rev: CD003008.

Adherence of French GPs to Chronic Neuropathic Pain Clinical Guidelines: Results of a Cross-Sectional, Randomized, "e" Case-Vignette Survey

Valéria Martinez[1,2]*, Nadine Attal[2,3], Bertrand Vanzo[4], Eric Vicaut[5], Jean Michel Gautier[6], Didier Bouhassira[2,3], Michel Lantéri-Minet[7,8]

1 Anesthésiologie-Réanimation, Hôpital Raymond-Poincaré, Garches, France, 2 INSERM U-987, Centre d'Evaluation et de Traitement de la Douleur, CHU Ambroise Paré, Boulogne-Billancourt, France, 3 Université Versailles-Saint-Quentin, Versailles, France, 4 General Practitioner, Athis Mons, France, 5 Unité de Recherche Clinique - Hôpital Fernand Widal, Paris, France, 6 Réseau InterCLUD Languedoc Roussillon, CHRU Montpellier, Montpellier, France, 7 CHU de Nice, Centre d'Evaluation et Traitement de la Douleur, Nice, France, 8 INSERM/UdA, U1107, Neuro-Dol, Université de Clermont-Ferrand, Clermont-Ferrand, France

Abstract

Background and aims: The French Pain Society published guidelines for neuropathic pain management in 2010. Our aim was to evaluate the compliance of GPs with these guidelines three years later.

Methods: We used "e" case vignette methodology for this non interventional study. A national panel of randomly selected GPs was included. We used eight "e" case-vignettes relating to chronic pain, differing in terms of the type of pain (neuropathic/non neuropathic), etiology (cancer, postoperative pain, low back pain with or without radicular pain, diabetes) and symptoms. GPs received two randomly selected consecutive "e" case vignettes (with/without neuropathic pain). We analyzed their ability to recognize neuropathic pain and to prescribe appropriate first-line treatment.

Results: From the 1265 GPs in the database, we recruited 443 (35.0%), 334 of whom logged onto the web site (26.4%) and 319 (25.2%) of whom completed the survey. Among these GPs, 170 (53.3%) were aware of the guidelines, 136 (42.6%) were able to follow them, and 110 (34.5%) used the DN4 diagnostic tool. Sensitivity for neuropathic pain recognition was 87.8% (CI: 84.2%; 91.4%). However, postoperative neuropathic pain was less well diagnosed (77.9%; CI: 69.6%; 86.2%) than diabetic pain (95.2%; CI: 90.0%; 100.0%), cancer pain (90.6%; CI: 83.5%; 97.8%) and typical radicular pain (90.7%; CI: 84.9%; 96.5%). When neuropathic pain was correctly recognized, the likelihood of appropriate first-line treatment prescription was 90.6% (CI: 87.4%; 93.8%). The treatments proposed were pregabaline (71.8%), gabapentine (43.9%), amiptriptylline (23.2%) and duloxetine (18.2%). However, ibuprofen (11%), acetaminophen-codeine (29.5%) and clonazepam (10%) were still prescribed.

Conclusions: The compliance of GPs with clinical practice guidelines appeared to be satisfactory, but differed between etiologies.

Editor: Laxmaiah Manchikanti, University of Louisville, United States of America

Funding: This study was supported by Pfizer. The sponsor financed the data collection and statistical analysis of the data, which was performed by an independent clinical research organization (ITEC, Bordeaux, France). The funders had no role in the study design and analysis, decision to publish or preparation of the manuscript.

Competing Interests: The authors received honoraria from Pfizer for their participation in the scientific committee of the study.

* E-mail: valeria.martinez.aphp@gmail.com

Introduction

Neuropathic pain constitutes a significant burden for society in terms of impaired quality of life, comorbidities and cost [1–3]. Classical causes of neuropathic pain include diabetes, shingles, spinal cord injury, stroke, multiple sclerosis, cancer and HIV infection, but also more common conditions, such as radicular pain related to radiculopathy, and traumatic or postsurgical nerve injuries [4].

Several large epidemiological surveys have highlighted the under-treatment of neuropathic pain in France in either the general population [5] or in specialist settings [6]. Screening tools have been developed to increase the awareness and recognition of neuropathic pain, particularly by non-specialists [7–9]. The use of these tools may also contribute to reduce false positive diagnoses, which are probably also common in clinical practice.

Evidence-based recommendations for the assessment and management of neuropathic pain have also been developed in recent years [10–13]. In France, the French Pain Society (*Société Française d'Etude et Traitement de la Douleur*/SFETD), in particular, has proposed and disseminated evidence-based recommendations targeting all health professionals, with the aim of facilitating neuropathic pain recognition and management in the ambulatory care setting [14]. These recommendations emphasize the importance of screening tools (particularly the DN4, which was developed in France [7]) as a first step in the diagnosis of neuropathic pain, and propose first- and second-line drug treatments for neuropathic pain, regardless of its etiology, akin to European or international recommendations.

However, very few studies have investigated the real-life impact of evidence-based recommendations on physicians' practices. In the USA, a study by Dworkin and colleagues [15] suggested that the drug treatment of post-herpetic neuralgia by primary care physicians was roughly consistent with the US recommendations issued some years before. However, this study was retrospective and restricted to post-herpetic neuralgia, a condition that is easier for non-specialists to diagnose than many other neurological pain conditions.

Our aim in this study was to describe chronic neuropathic pain management practices among general practitioners (GPs), focusing on the criteria used in decision-making processes and compliance with current French recommendations. We used "case vignettes", a valid and reliable method that is gaining widespread acceptance for quality-of-care assessments in current clinical practice [16–20]. This method provides an effective evaluation of the behavior of physicians in the setting of diagnosis or treatment decisions, and of their compliance with recommendations. It therefore appeared an appropriate method in the context of the objectives of this study.

Materials and Methods

Ethics statement

This study was conducted in accordance with French regulatory requirements. The protocol and all administrative documents, including the financial agreement, with investigators paid for their participation, were approved by the National Medical Council (*Conseil National de l'Ordre des Médecins*; CNOM). The database was declared to the National Data Protection Authority (*Commission Nationale de l'Informatique et des Libertés*; CNIL). Submission to an ethics committee was not required under French law.

Selection of participants

We calculated that a sample of 300 GPs would be required to estimate any percentage with a maximum 95% CI of ±6.5%, taking into account a design effect related to the non-independence of observations made by the same physician. The rate of participation in e-CRF studies is generally about 30%, with 75% of participants being highly active. We therefore decided to select a representative random sample of 1,332 GPs for this study. To this end, we sent a questionnaire, by mail, to the 84,832 GPs practicing in mainland France (listed in the CEGEDIM database), on January 2nd, 2012, asking them whether they would be interested in participating in a non-interventional study. We selected a random sample of 1,332 physicians from the 4,299 GPs who expressed interest in participating in this study between January and July 2012. Contact information was incorrect for 67 GPs, so 1,265 GPs were finally included in our database. In October 2012, we sent these GPs a proposal for participation in this survey. Any physician who did not respond to this mailing was contacted by telephone two weeks later, and attempts at contact were continued until the planned number of participants was reached. In total, 465 GPs agreed to take part in this survey, of whom 443 signed a contract for participation and were issued with a center number. The flow chart for GP selection is summarized in Figure 1.

Construction of case-vignettes

Case vignettes were developed by a multidisciplinary panel of experts (authors of this paper) in the field of neuropathic pain, practicing as GPs, clinicians or nurses in neurology or anesthe-

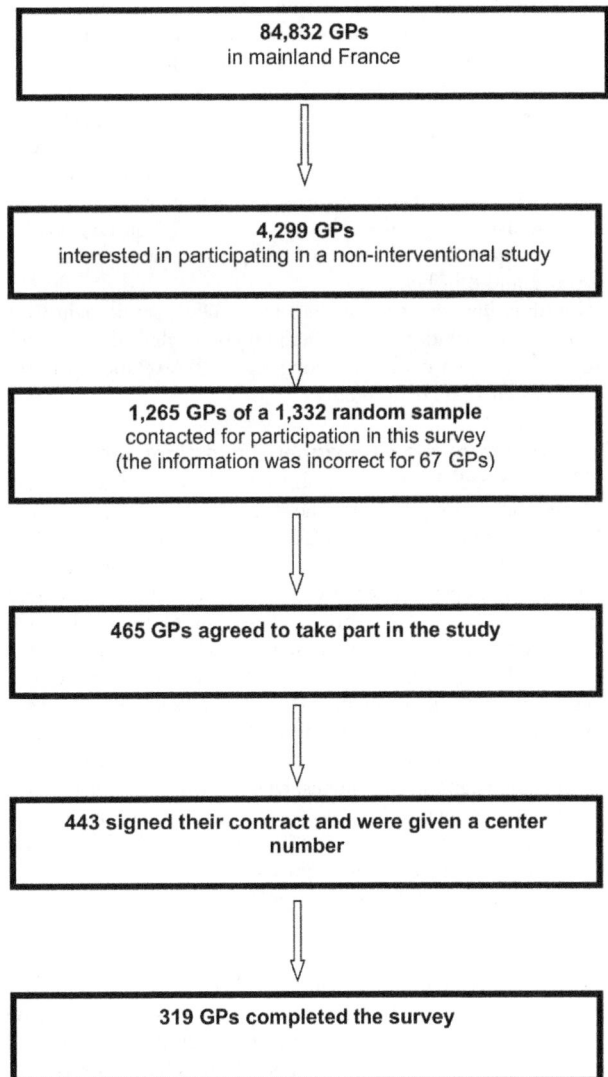

Figure 1. Flow chart of the study.

siology. The description of clinical cases was based on epidemiological and descriptive data characterizing neuropathic pain [21]. Each clinical case was designed to be realistic and concrete, matching as closely as possible the cases observed in clinical practice. We focused on four etiologies of peripheral neuropathic pain frequently encountered in general medical practice: painful diabetic polyneuropathy, cancer chemotherapy-induced peripheral neuropathy [22], typical radicular pain [23] and post-operative neuropathic pain [24–26]. In assessments of performance for the identification of neuropathic pain, we considered two types of chronic pain for each etiology: nociceptive chronic pain and peripheral neuropathic pain. Based on these conditions, we constructed eight case-vignettes, each with a different scenario. The eight case-vignettes are given in File S1.

The scenario needed to be simple, brief (length <15 lines-200 words), with no potential pitfalls. Each case-vignette was constructed in the same way: age, sex, patient's history, chronic pain history, reason for consultation, clinical symptoms, data from clinical examination, with or without results from additional investigations.

Scenarios differed in terms of both symptoms (e.g. burning pain *vs* aching pain) and elements of clinical examination (e.g. allodynia *vs* pain triggered by joint mobilization). The symptoms and clinical examination findings leading to the diagnosis of neuropathic pain were chosen from among the most discriminative, although none of them is specific [7,11,27] and were consistent with those used in validated screening tools, such as the DN4 (*Douleur neuropathique en 4 questions*) [7]. Clinical cases of neuropathic pain included at least six discriminative neuropathic elements, whereas non-neuropathic cases presented fewer than two neuropathic characteristics (see cases n°7 and 8 in File S1).

Non-discriminative clinical elements of neuropathic pain were systematically included in the description of all clinical cases: high pain intensity on a numerical rating scale (>7/10) and comorbid conditions (anxiety, depression).

Construction of the case-vignette questionnaire

The proposed questions and their corresponding items dealt with the different elements for the diagnosis and management of neuropathic pain set out in SFETD recommendations (see Key points in File S1). The construction of this closed-ended questionnaire superimposed over the recommendations made it possible to carry out a relevant assessment of knowledge and facilitated the analysis of responses. The number of questions and items was the same for each case. The knowledge of the GPs was assessed through four multiple-choice questions: i) diagnostic elements, four items, ii) elements from the patient's clinical history guiding diagnosis, four items, iii) elements from clinical examination guiding diagnosis, three items, iv) drugs proposed for first-line treatment, seven items.

The case-vignette questionnaire is shown in in File S1. The list of first-line drugs includes duloxetine, which is authorized only for the treatment of painful diabetic peripheral neuropathy in France.

Procedure

Eight case-vignettes were constructed, corresponding to four neuropathic cases and four non-neuropathic cases (Table 1). By combining these vignettes two-by-two (one neuropathic case and one non-neuropathic case), we obtained 12 possible combinations, which we tested on 20 GPs, to evaluate their comprehensibility. This testing step identified two combinations as too similar to each other (diabetic polyneuropathy and cancer chemotherapy-induced polyneuropathy), and these combinations were therefore removed. Each GP had to provide a response for a set of two case-vignettes randomly selected from the 10 remaining combinations. GPs were blind to the mode of case distribution.

The case-vignettes were stored in a database on a dedicated server for this survey (a web-based application). GPs could access their two assigned case-vignettes at any time, *via* a personal online account protected by a specific and confidential login and password assigned to them after validation of the financial agreement. Once all fields of the case-vignette questionnaire had

Table 1. The eight case-vignettes.

	Neuropathic pain	Non-neuropathic pain
Diabetes	Case 1	Case 2
Cancer	Case 3	Case 4
Low back pain	Case 5	Case 6
Postoperative pain	Case 7	Case 8

been completed, the questionnaire was saved automatically on the administrator's account, preventing any further modification.

In the event of an incorrect diagnosis after the response to the first three questions, GPs were given the correct diagnosis so that they could answer the question relating to therapeutic strategy with the correct diagnosis in mind.

Before completing the case-vignette questionnaires, the participants provided the following information: their age, sex, duration of practice, practice in an urban/rural area, number of chronic pain patients seen per week (and the percentage of these patients with neuropathic pain). After validation of the responses, they were also asked the following questions: *"Are you aware of the SFETD recommendations? Do you implement them? Are you aware of the DN4 tool (Douleur Neuropathique en 4 questions)? Do you use it?"*

Statistical analysis

For continuous variables, we determined the mean and standard deviation. For categorical variables, the number and percentage of subjects in each category are summarized. We used Student's *t* test to assess differences for continuous variables. Chi^2 tests of association were used to test for sequence order differences for categorical variables. The threshold for significance was set at $p = 0.05$.

We determined the percentage of cases correctly diagnosed, with its 95% confidence interval (CI). A similar analysis was performed for each of the eight case-vignettes, according to the type of pain (neuropathic or non-neuropathic) and the underlying disease. The percentages of GPs making 0, 1 and 2 corrected diagnoses were determined.

The elements of the patient's history and clinical examination used to reach the diagnosis were described separately for each of the eight case-vignettes, according to the type of pain (neuropathic or non-neuropathic) and the disease, and for the following subgroups: correct diagnosis/misdiagnosis, knowledge of recommendations (YES/NO) and their implementation (YES/NO), knowledge of the DN4 tool (YES/NO) and its use (YES/NO). The results obtained were compared with the expected responses.

Prescriptions of analgesic treatments were described separately for each of the eight case-vignettes and according to: the type of pain (neuropathic or non-neuropathic), knowledge of the recommendations (YES/NO) and their implementation (YES/NO).

We aimed to evaluate compliance with SFETD guidelines. Thus, for each question on the case-vignette questionnaire, we analyzed the number of correct answers and the number of answers containing at least one element of the correct answer, without any element wrongly ticked.

Analyses were performed with SAS version 9.3 (SAS Institute, Cary, NC).

Results

In total, 443 GPs signed a contract and received a center number, but only the 319 duly completing the e-CRF were included in the analysis. We thus evaluated responses for a total of 638 case-vignettes.

Characteristics of connections

An analysis of connection times showed that the participants remained connected for a median of 17 minutes and that the minimum connection time was four minutes. A few extreme values were obtained, probably due to participants forgetting to sign out.

Table 2. GPs' characteristics.

	Statistics	N = 319
Sex		
Male	n(%)	254 (79.6%)
Female	n(%)	65 (20.4%)
Pattern of medical practice		
Alone	n(%)	125 (40.1%)
Group practice	n(%)	187 (59.9%)
	Missing (n - %)	7 (2.2%)
Urban/Rural		
Rural	n(%)	191 (59.9%)
Urban	n(%)	128 (40.1%)
Age (years)	MeanSD	52.3
	Median	8.4
	Q1;Q3	53.0
	[Min; Max]	[47.0;59.0]
		[31.0;69.0]
Duration of practice		
<10 years	n(%)	33 (10.3%)
> = 10 years	n(%)	286 (89.7%)
Number of chronic pain patients per month	Mean	52.8
	SD	46.7
	Median	45.0
	Q1;Q3	[20.0;70.0]
	[Min; Max]	[2.0;400.0]
Number of chronic pain patients with neuropathic pain per month	Mean	8.6
	SD	10.8
	Median	5.0
	Q1;Q3	[2.5;10.0]
	[Min; Max]	[0.1;100.0]

SD, standard deviation; Q1–Q3, first and third quartiles; min, minimum; max, maximum.

Characteristics of the participants

The demographic features of the 319 GPs completing the questionnaires for both the clinical cases assigned to them are reported in Table 2.

This sample of physicians was representative of the general population of GPs in terms of their nationwide distribution (with a slight underrepresentation of Ile-de-France) and mean age. Men were overrepresented (79.6% vs the expected 59%, based on GP numbers) as frequently reported in studies of this type. Representativeness was assessed on the basis of the French atlas of medical demography (Atlas National CNOM 2012).

Of the 319 GPs completing the questionnaires for both case-vignettes, 53.3% (170/319) were aware of guidelines and 42.6% (136/319) said that they implemented them. The principal reason for not following the recommendations was insufficient knowledge of these recommendations. For the DN4 diagnostic tool, 60.8% of the GPs (194/319) stated that they were aware of it and 34.5% (110/319) reported using it. The main reason for not using this tool was a lack of memorized knowledge.

Evaluation of case-vignettes: diagnosis and therapeutic strategy

Global results. *Of the 319 GPs*, 58.9% made the correct diagnosis for both the allocated case vignettes. The proportion of GPs giving two correct diagnoses did not between the sexes (58.7% men vs 60.0% women; p = 0.845) or between types of practice are (56.0% rural vs 63.3% urban; p = 0.434). The number of accurate diagnoses did not depend on whether the doctors were aware of or implemented the recommendations; similar results were obtained concerning knowledge and use of the DN4 tool. Several case combinations were identified less well than others. The proportions of GPs giving the correct diagnosis for both case vignettes was lowest (Figure 2) when one of the allocated vignettes was a case of cancer with non-neuropathic pain (case no. 4, with case no. 7: 22.6%, or with case no. 5: 34.4%). Postoperative neuropathic pain (case no. 7) also appeared to be difficult to identify, as shown for its combination with case no. 6 (43.8%) or case no. 2 (46.9%).

For the 638 vignettes examined, the correct diagnosis was made in 77.3% of cases. The percentage of correct diagnoses differed considerably between etiologies and was lowest for cancer cases (p = 0.0002; Figure 3).

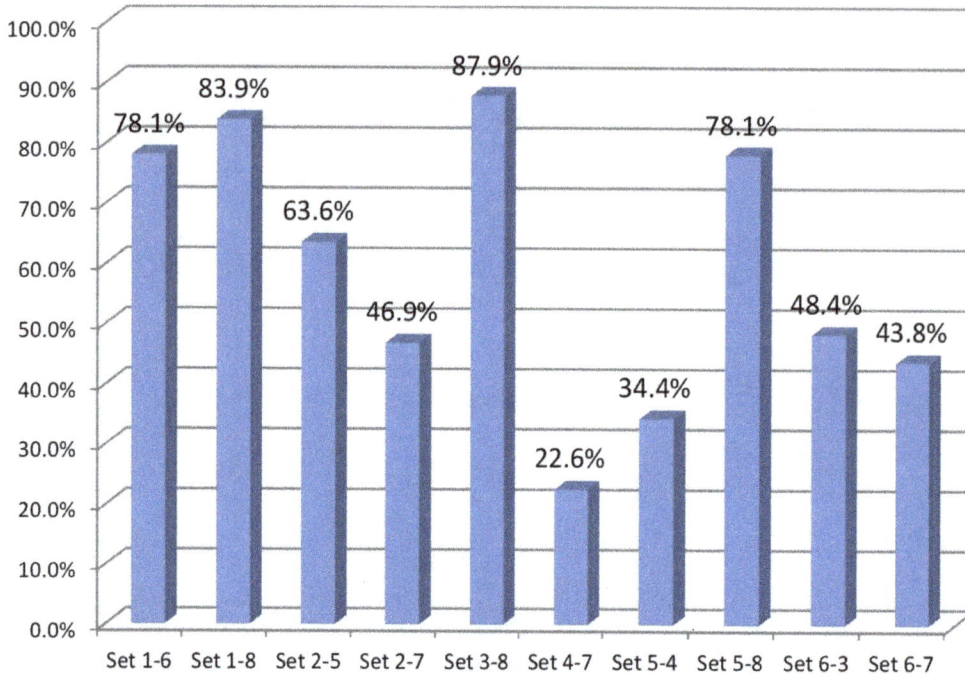

Figure 2. Proportion of investigators (N=319) with 2 correct diagnoses.

Neuropathic pain was well diagnosed in 87.8% (95%CI: 84.2%; 91.4%) of cases (Figure 4), but the frequency of correct diagnosis differed between etiologies (Figure 5). The probability of correct diagnosis seemed to be lower for postoperative neuropathic pain (case no. 7) (77.9%; 95%CI [69.6%; 86.2%]) than for other etiologies (92.0%; 95%CI [88.4%; 95.5%]). Thus, misdiagnosis was 2.8 times more frequent for postoperative neuropathic pain than for other etiologies (22.1% *vs* 8.0%; $p = 0.0005$).

Our analysis of the criteria on which GPs based their diagnosis of neuropathic pain indicated that all items from the patient's history and all items from the clinical examination characterizing this type of pain were recognized in 53.9% and 51.8% of cases, respectively (Table 3). For the 280 GPs making the correct diagnosis, 112 (40%) had ticked at least four correct answers among the seven items proposed; this percentage was significantly lower among the GPs giving the wrong diagnosis (9 of 39 GPs i.e. 23.1%; $p = 0.041$). A case-by-case analysis of the results highlighted differences in the identification of key diagnostic elements as a function of etiology. Indeed, for diabetic neuropathic pain (case no. 1), diagnosis was based mostly on the patient's history rather than clinical examination, whereas, for postoperative neuropathic pain (case no. 7) the key diagnostic elements were more easily identified from clinical examination than from the patient's history. These results are summarized in Table 4.

We found that 53.6% GPs faced with a case of neuropathic pain of any etiology prescribed at least one first-line treatment

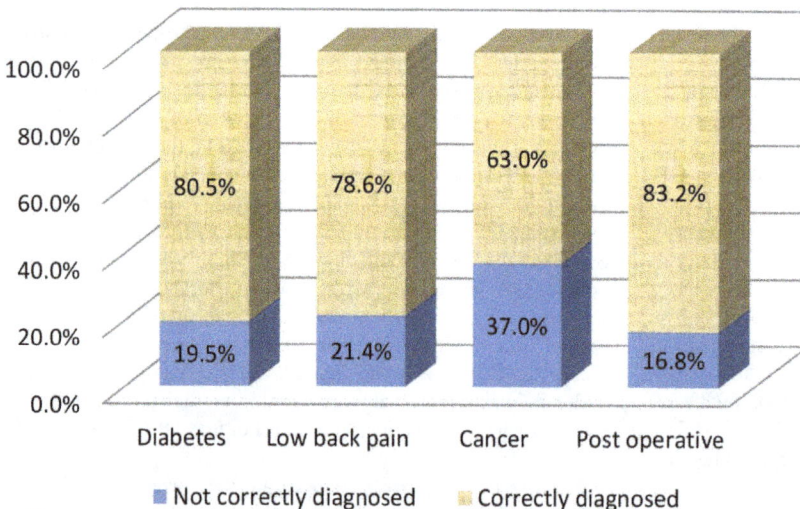

Figure 3. Frequency of correct/incorrect diagnoses by etiology (N=638).

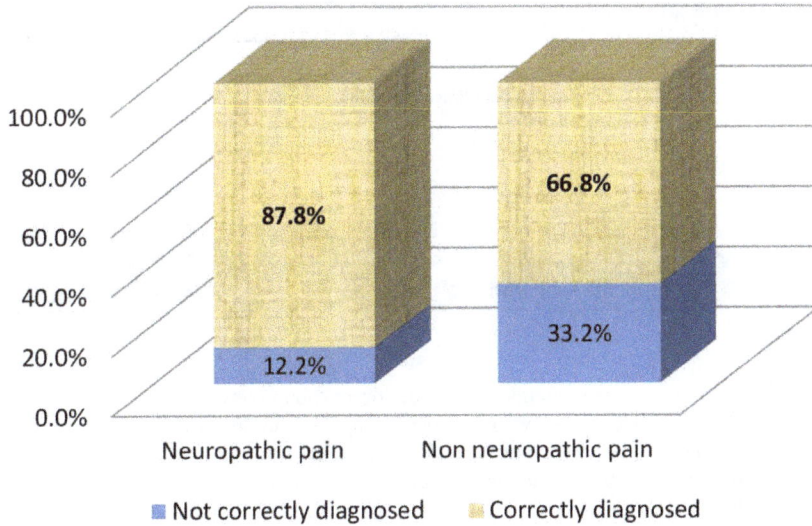

Figure 4. Frequency of correct/incorrect diagnoses by type of pain (N=638).

recommended for this type of pain. Significant differences in prescriptions were observed as a function of etiology. Indeed, a first-line treatment was prescribed for 73.0% of diabetes cases but only 48.8% cases of neuropathic pain of other etiologies ($p = 0.0006$). Only 4.7% of the GPs identified all the drugs that could be used as first-line treatments for neuropathic pain. A significant disparity in drug prescriptions was observed, with pregabalin prescribed in 71.8% of cases, gabapentin in 43.9% and amitriptyline in 23.2%. The orders of the prescription rates for these three drugs did not depend on etiology. However, for diabetic polyneuropathy, duloxetine replaced amitriptyline as the third most frequently prescribed drug. The questions relating to therapeutic approaches also revealed that many doctors would prescribe inappropriate drugs, such as acetaminophen/codeine, ibuprofen and clonazepam, which were prescribed in 29.5%, 11% and 10% of cases, respectively. Data on drug prescriptions in neuropathic pain are presented in Table 4 and Table 5.

Non-neuropathic pain was well diagnosed in 66.8% of cases. Postoperative pain (case no. 8) was the easiest to identify and cancer pain (case no. 4) proved to be the most difficult. An overdiagnosis of neuropathic pain was observed, with 33.2% of the 319 cases of non-neuropathic pain incorrectly diagnosed as neuropathic pain and a clear predominance of incorrect diagnoses for cancer pain (65.1%). These results are presented in Figures 4 and 5.

Correct diagnosis, with all the correct items ticked for history or clinical examination, was observed in 50.7% and 66.2% of cases, respectively. Other than for postoperative pain, the key elements for a correct diagnosis were more frequently obtained from clinical examination than from history (Table 6).

In terms of therapeutic strategy, regardless of the etiology of non-neuropathic pain, about one third of GPs (36.7%) prescribed both appropriate drugs — ibuprofen and acetaminophen/codeine — and about two thirds (63.6%) prescribed at least one of these

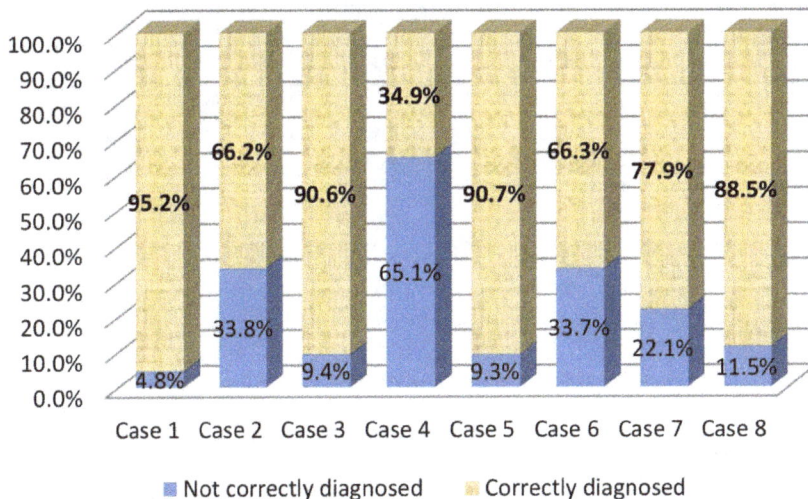

Figure 5. Frequency of correct/incorrect diagnoses for each case-vignette (N=638).

Table 3. Key elements for the correct diagnosis of neuropathic pain.

Etiology	Elements from history-exact response rate-	Elements from clinical examination-exact response rate-	p(Mc Nemar)
Diabetes	66.7% (40/60)	35.0% (21/60)	0.0009
Cancer	55.2% (32/58)	56.9% (33/58)	0.8273
Low back pain	54.5% (48/88)	46.6% (41/88)	0.2967
Postoperative pain	41.9% (31/74)	67.6% (50/74)	0.0038
ALL CASES OF NEUROPATHIC PAIN	53.9% (151/280)	51.8% (145/280)	0.6146

two drugs. Correct prescription rates were similar whether or not the recommendations were applied (Table 7).

For both neuropathic and non-neuropathic pain, knowledge and implementation of the recommendations, and knowledge and use of the DN4 tool, did not appear to affect the likelihood of recognizing key elements from the patient's history or clinical examination for accurate diagnosis.

Case-by-case results. *Painful diabetic polyneuropathy* (case no. 1) was well diagnosed in most cases (95.2%), with 66.7% and 35.0% exact answers for the patient's history and clinical examination, respectively. In terms of therapeutic strategy, the complete list of recommended first-line treatments was rarely given (7.9%), but one of the drugs from this list was proposed in about three in four cases (73.0%). The drug most frequently proposed was pregabalin (73.0% of cases).

Non-neuropathic pain in diabetic patients (case no. 2) was correctly diagnosed in 66.2% of cases, with 46.5% and 97.7% exact answers for the patient's history and clinical examination, respectively. If we considered cases with only one element of the exact answer but with no incorrectly ticked elements, these percentages were 72.1% and 97.7%, respectively. In cases of incorrect diagnosis, no exact answer was obtained for either history or clinical examination. For therapeutic strategy, the two

recommended first-line drugs (ibuprofen and acetaminophen/codeine) were proposed together in less than half the cases (41.5%), but one of these drugs was cited in 70.8% of cases. Acetaminophen/codeine was the most frequently proposed drug (80.0% of cases).

Cancer chemotherapy-induced peripheral neuropathy (case no. 3) was well diagnosed in 90.6% of cases, with 55.2% and 56.9% exact answers for the patient's history and clinical examination, respectively. If we considered answers with at least one correct element, these percentages were 58.6% and 70.7%, respectively. For therapeutic management, very few GPs (3.1%) identified all three recommended first-line drugs, but half (51.6%) proposed one of these drugs. The drug most frequently identified was pregabalin (75.0% of cases).

Non-neuropathic pain in cancer (case no. 4) was diagnosed in only 34.9% of cases, with 45.5% and 81.8% exact answers for the patient's history and clinical examination, respectively. Similar results were obtained if we considered responses with at least one correct element. In cases of incorrect diagnosis, no exact answer was obtained for either the patient's history or for clinical examination. The two recommended first-line drugs (ibuprofen and acetaminophen/codeine) were both proposed in 30.2% of cases, but at least one of these two drugs was cited in 65.1% of

Table 4. Key elements leading to correct diagnosis and choice of therapeutic strategy for each of the 8 case-vignettes.

	Case-vignette							
	1	2	3	4	5	6	7	8
	n=63	n=65	n=64	n=63	n=97	n=95	n=95	n=96
ELEMENTS FROM HISTORY								
Exact answer* (%)	66.7%	46.5%	55.2%	45.5%	54.5%	42.9%	41.9%	60.0%
Correct answer** (%)	71.7%	72.1%	58.6%	45.5%	56.8%	55.6%	45.9%	64.7%
ELEMENTS FROM CLINICAL EXAMINATION								
Exact answer* (%)	35.0%	97.7%	56.9%	81.8%	46.6%	61.9%	67.6%	49.4%
Correct answer (%)	100%***	97.7%	70.7%	81.8%	100%***	61.9%	100%***	77.6%
CORRECT PRESCRIPTIONS								
All first-line drugs proposed	7.9%	41.5%	3.1%	30.0%	5.2%	36.8%	6.3%	37.5%
At least one first-line drug proposed	73.0%	70.8%	51.6%	65.1%	44.3%	62.1%	51.6%	59.4%

* an answer strictly corresponding to the expected answer (the exact answer required all items to be ticked).
** an answer with at least one element of the exact answer, without any element wrongly ticked.

Table 5. Correct prescription rates for neuropathic pain.

Drugs	N=319
Pregabalin/amitryptyline/gabapentin*	15 (4.7%)
Pregabalin	229 (71.8%)
Amitryptyline	74 (23.2%)
Gabapentin	140 (43.9%)
At least one recommended drug**	171 (53.6%)

*all three first-line recommended drugs.
** and no incorrect treatment.

Table 7. Correct prescription rates for non-neuropathic pain.

Drugs	N=319
Ibuprofen/acetaminophen-codeine*	117 (36.7%)
Ibuprofen	200 (62.7%)
Acetaminophen-codeine	248 (77.7%)
At least one recommended drug**	203 (63.6%)

* the two first-line recommended drugs.
** and no incorrect treatment.

cases. Acetaminophen/codeine was the most frequently proposed drug (79.4% of cases).

Typical radicular pain (case no. 5) was correctly identified in 90.7% of cases, with 54.5% and 46.6% exact answers for the patient's history and clinical examination, respectively. Very few GPs (5.2%) identified all three recommended first-line drugs, and only 44.3% proposed one of these drugs. The most frequently cited drug was pregabalin (64.9% of cases).

Non-neuropathic low back pain (case no. 6) was correctly diagnosed in 66.3% of cases, with 42.9% and 61.9% exact answers for the patient's history and clinical examination, respectively. If we considered answers with at least one correct element, these percentages were 55.6% and 61.9%, respectively. In cases of incorrect diagnosis, exact answers for history and clinical examination were observed in only 9.4% and 3.1% of cases, respectively. The two recommended first-line drugs (ibuprofen and acetaminophen/codeine) were both proposed by 36.8% of GPs, and one of these drugs was proposed by 62.1% of GPs. Acetaminophen/codeine was the most frequently proposed drug (83.2% of cases).

Postoperative neuropathic pain (case no. 7) was well diagnosed in 77.9% of cases, with 41.9% and 67.6% exact answers for the patient's history and clinical examination, respectively. In cases of incorrect diagnosis, exact answers from the patient's history and clinical examination were obtained in 33.3% and 28.6% of cases, respectively. For therapeutic strategy, all three recommended first line treatments was rarely ticked together (6.3%), but one of these drugs was proposed in about half the cases (51.6%). The most frequently cited drug was pregabalin (75.8% of cases).

Postoperative non-neuropathic pain (case no. 8) was diagnosed in 88.5% of cases, with 60.0% and 49.4% exact answers for the patient's history and clinical examination, respectively. If we considered answers with at least one correct element, these percentages were 64.7% and 77.6%, respectively.

In cases of wrong diagnosis, no exact answer was given for either history or clinical examination. The two recommended first-line drugs (ibuprofen and acetaminophen/codeine) were both proposed by 37.5% of GPs, and one of these drugs was proposed by 59.4% of GPs.

Discussion

This study is the first to address the issue of the compliance of French general practitioners with current recommendations for the diagnosis and first-line treatment of neuropathic pain [14]. Three years after the publication of French recommendations on neuropathic pain, this study found that only 58.9% of GPs made the correct diagnosis for both the allocated case vignettes. Neuropathic pain was well diagnosed in 87.8% of cases, but only 53.6% of GPs proposed an appropriate first-line treatment. Based on these figures, less than one in two patients (47.1%) consulting for neuropathic pain would receive appropriate treatment.

Diagnosis of neuropathic pain

Accurate diagnosis is the crucial first step toward the successful management of neuropathic pain. We were surprised by the high percentage of correct diagnoses of neuropathic pain obtained in this study (87.8%), given the difficulties encountered in the recognition of this type of pain real life [28,29]. However, the clinical cases submitted to the GPs in this study were simple and somewhat caricatured. Our cases of neuropathic pain included at least seven characteristic features of such pain, whereas four elements are sufficient for the diagnosis of NP with the DN4 tool [7]. Moreover, it has been shown that the use of closed-ended questionnaires with cued items leads to an overestimate of the performance of physicians [30]. The sponsorship of this study by a laboratory heavily involved in research on neuropathic pain may also have resulted in a higher proportion of GPs making the correct diagnosis for neuropathic pain. Thus, although the overall figures appear to be highly satisfactory, further analyses of diagnostic failures can provide us with useful information. Indeed,

Table 6. Key elements for the correct diagnosis of non-neuropathic pain.

Etiology	Elements from history-exact response rate-	Elements from clinical examination-exact response rate-	p(Mc Nemar)
Diabetes	46.5% (20/43)	97.7% (42/43)	<0.0001
Cancer	45.5% (10/22)	81.8% (18/22)	0.0047
Low back pain	42.9% (27/63)	61.9% (39/63)	0.0233
Postoperative pain	60.0% (51/85)	49.4% (42/85)	0.1797
All cases of neuropathic pain	50.7% (108/213)	66.2% (145/213)	0.0011

this detailed analysis identified certain diagnostic difficulties in particular conditions.

Firstly, the large range of answers obtained, depending on the set of two case-vignettes assigned to the GPs, suggested that diagnosis was not always easy. Some cases, such as painful diabetic polyneuropathy, seemed to be much better diagnosed than others, such as postoperative neuropathic pain. We also observed an overdiagnosis of neuropathic pain in cancer patients. Only one in five GPs recognized both non-neuropathic cancer pain and postoperative neuropathic pain. The overdiagnosis of neuropathic pain in some etiologies and its underdiagnosis in others may reflect GPs continuing to think that the nature of pain depends on either its context or its etiology. Parsons et al. recently showed that mean time from the onset of postoperative neuropathic pain symptoms to diagnosis was 9.7 months [29]. Indeed, postoperative pain had long been considered purely, until the widespread recognition about 10 years ago of the neuropathic origin of some postoperative pains [31]. By contrast, diabetic neuropathy has been the subject of extensive academic, scientific communication and marketing, potentially accounting for the high frequency of correct diagnosis (92.2%). GPs overdiagnosed neuropathic pain in cancer patients, probably because they were influenced by the background of previous chemotherapy and the presence of two neuropathic elements (e.g. tingling and hypoesthesia) without taking into account clinical presentation (e.g. location of pain away from nerve damage symptoms).

Overall, these results suggest that limited use is made of the findings of clinical examinations in the diagnosis of neuropathic pain. This hypothesis was confirmed by the analysis of answers relating to the elements of the patient's history and clinical examination leading to the diagnosis of neuropathic pain, which provided us with new insight into the decision-making processes of physicians. Indeed, our results indicate that the elements used to arrive at the correct diagnosis differed between etiologies. In diabetic patients, pain descriptors were used for the identification of neuropathic pain, whereas, in postoperative pain, correct diagnoses were based largely on clinical examination. This is a key point, highlighting the essential nature of clinical examination for the diagnosis of neuropathic pain in general practice. This finding closes the debate about whether clinical examinations should be counted among the screening tools helping non-specialists to identify patients with possible neuropathic pain.

Therapeutic management

The management of patients with chronic neuropathic pain is challenging, despite attempts to develop a more rational therapeutic approach [32]. In our study, only one in two GPs proposed at least one of the recommended first-line treatments when faced with a case of confirmed neuropathic pain. This poor result applied to neuropathic pain of all etiologies. Indeed, when multiplied with the probability of prescription of one appropriate first-line treatment, only 69.5%, 46.7%, 40.2% and 40.2% of patients with diabetes, cancer, radicular pain and postoperative pain, respectively, would receive appropriate medical care. These low rates highlight the large proportion of patients that would not have been correctly treated despite the caricatured description of neuropathic pain in the vignettes, its high intensity (7/10 on VAS) and association with sleep disorders and anxiety in all the case-vignettes assigned to the GPs. These findings suggest that the corresponding figures may be even worse in "real life". As for diagnosis, we observed differences according to etiology with neuropathic pain in diabetic patients much better managed than that in patients presenting with low back pain or postoperative pain.

Another key finding of our results is the lack of knowledge of evidence-based therapy, with less than 5% of GPs being able to list all the first-line drugs recommended for the treatment of neuropathic pain. This suggests that physicians have a very superficial knowledge of recommendations, such that patients with contraindications or treatment failure might not necessarily receive appropriate treatment. It is probably easier for GPs to remember one drug per disease, even if further inquiries must subsequently be made, rather than remembering algorithms of various complexities. Pregabalin was by far the most frequently cited drug, regardless of etiology, followed by gabapentin and amitriptyline. This finding may be accounted for by the risk-benefit profile of pregabalin, which is better tolerated and requires fewer precautions for use than amitriptyline [14]. Finally, this study revealed the persistence of non-recommended drug prescriptions, such as acetaminophen/codeine, ibuprofen or clonazepam. Clonazepam, which belongs to the benzodiazepine class, has been misused and abused and has been subject to prescription limitations imposed by the French authorities since January 2012 [33]. The other drugs in this non-recommended list are very often wrongly prescribed, to one inthree patients for ibuprofen and one in five patients for acetaminophen/codeine. Nevertheless, non-recommended drug prescriptions were less frequent than reported in a recent study investigating the treatment of neuropathic pain in the UK general population [34]. An opioid, or a combination of opioid and non-opioid analgesics, was prescribed as a first-line treatment for 25.4% of patients with diabetic neuropathy and 64.0% of patients with neuropathic back pain. By contrast, no benzodiazepine was prescribed. Our results highlight specific issues that should be addressed in the future to optimize the therapeutic management of neuropathic pain in general practice.

Knowledge of SFETD recommendations

In our study, one in two GPs declared that they knew the recommendations for neuropathic pain. This proportion is similar to published findings from surveys carried out in general practice to assess knowledge about recommendations for six common diseases. However, the percentage of GPs stating that they applied recommendations (42%) was much higher in our study than reported for other diseases (17%) [35]. This led us to question the veracity of the GPs' statements, particularly because we were unable to detect any impact on the recognition of neuropathic pain and its therapeutic management. The remuneration of participation by a pharmaceutical company with considerable involvement in pain management might have favored complaisant responses. We therefore considered the reported implementation of the recommendations by GPs to be too dubious for a relevant assessment of the impact of recommendations on medical practice. Other methodological approaches, such as the assessment of practices before/after the publication of recommendations, or before/after training, would be more appropriate for such an analysis.

Strengths and limitations of case-vignettes

Case-vignettes have been used for years to evaluate of the behavior of physicians in the setting of diagnostic testing or treatment decisions. We chose to use this method for our study as it has been shown to be an accurate, valid, feasible and inexpensive tool for measuring the quality of health care [16,17,19,36,37]. Previous studies have demonstrated the utility of case-vignettes for assessing compliance with recommendations, for measuring physicians' practice performance, particularly for comparisons of different groups of physicians, for identifying deviations from guidelines and physicians with non-ideal approaches to patients due to a lack of knowledge, and for defining areas in which scientific knowledge could be strengthened [19,38,39].

This study had several methodological strengths. Case-vignette design was based on epidemiological and descriptive data for neuropathic pain, which we used to create an initial scenario matching current clinical practice in ambulatory care as closely as possible. Case-vignettes were constructed by an expert panel with six members and were further refined after successful testing on a sample of 20 GPs. The assessment criterion was the recognition of neuropathic pain, and the various items proposed in the questionnaire corresponded to the different diagnostic and therapeutic elements addressed in the French recommendations (pain description, clinical examination, first-line medication).

However, our study also had a number of limitations. Men were overrepresented, introducing a selection bias. Nevertheless, the likelihood of recognizing or correctly managing neuropathic pain is unlikely to differ between the sexes, and no significant difference according to sex was identified in this study. This research was sponsored by Pfizer, and we cannot rule out the possibility that this influenced GPs' answers, particularly given the overdiagnosis of neuropathic pain observed.

We selected case-vignettes relating to only four etiologies of chronic pain. The inclusion of a broader range of etiologies would have increased the difficulty of diagnosis and might have generated different results. We presented cases of pure chronic pain that was either neuropathic or nociceptive. The introduction of mixed pain would probably have increased the percentage of misdiagnoses, given the greater complexity of the possible choices.

Despite the great care that we took to ensure that case-vignettes were similar in terms of difficulty (particularly as concerns the number and quality of neuropathic descriptors included in the cases of neuropathic pain), we cannot rule out the possibility that other difficulties influenced the results. For example, case no. 4, "non-neuropathic cancer pain", which was one of the worst diagnosed cases, had specific features. It was the only case among

the four cases of non-neuropathic pain presenting two neuropathic elements. Moreover, these elements appeared ahead of all the other items proposed whereas, in other cases, they were presented at the end of the list of items. These various aspects highlight the difficulties involved in drawing up case-vignettes. Thus, case-vignettes seem to be a tool that is more useful for highlighting weaknesses on which communication efforts should focus, rather than providing figures concerning medical practice. As previously reported, it is not possible with the case-vignette method to ensure that the responses obtain reflect the way that the GPs would behave in everyday patient care, even if the design and wording of the vignettes are kept as close as possible to real conditions [40]. Indeed, this method does not take into account either doctor-patient interactions or the relational aspects involved in real life.

Conclusions

The complexity of neuropathic chronic pain poses challenges for both management and diagnosis for primary care physicians. Taking into account our findings and the limitations outlined above, this study highlights to poor adoption of SFETD recommendations, with difficulties recognizing neuropathic pain for certain etiologies, insufficient consideration of clinical examination findings, and the paucity of appropriate first-line drugs recalled by GPs. These results may facilitate the design of specific educational programs and interventions aiming to improve the management of neuropathic pain by GPs in France.

Author Contributions

Conceived and designed the experiments: VM NA BV EV JMG DB MLM. Analyzed the data: VM NA BV EV JMG DB MLM. Wrote the paper: VM NA BV EV JMG DB MLM.

References

1. Treede RD, Jensen TS, Campbell JN, Cruccu G, Dostrovsky JO, et al. (2008) Redefinition of neuropathic pain and a grading system for clinical use: consensus statement on clinical and research diagnostic criteria. Neurology 70: 1630–1635.
2. Haanpää ML, Backonja MM, Bennett MI, Bouhassira D, Cruccu G, et al. (2009) Assessment of neuropathic pain in primary care. Am J Med 122 (10 Suppl): S13–21.
3. Radat F, Margot-Duclot A, Attal N (2013) Psychiatric co-morbidities in patients with chronic peripheral neuropathic pain: A multicentre cohort study. Eur J Pain 17: 1547–1557.
4. Attal N, Fermanian C, Fermanian J, Lanteri-Minet M, Alchaar H, et al. (2008) Neuropathic pain: are there distinct subtypes depending on the aetiology or anatomical lesion? Pain 138: 343–353.
5. Attal N, Lanteri-Minet M, Laurent B, Fermanian J, Bouhassira D (2011) The specific disease burden of neuropathic pain: results of a French nationwide survey. Pain 152: 2836–2843.
6. Bouhassira D, Letanoux M, Hartemann A (2013) Chronic pain with neuropathic characteristics in diabetic patients: a French cross-sectional study. PLoS One 8: e74195.
7. Bouhassira D, Attal N, Alchaar H, Boureau F, Brochet B, et al. (2005) Comparison of pain syndromes associated with nervous or somatic lesions and development of a new neuropathic pain diagnostic questionnaire (DN4). Pain 114: 29–36.
8. Bennett MI, Attal N, Backonja MM, Baron R, Bouhassira D, et al. (2007) Using screening tools to identify neuropathic pain. Pain 127: 199–203.
9. Bouhassira D, Attal N (2011) Diagnosis and assessment of neuropathic pain: the saga of clinical tools. Pain 152(3 Suppl): S74–83.
10. Finnerup NB, Otto M, McQuay HJ, Jensen TS, Sindrup SH (2005) Algorithm for neuropathic pain treatment: an evidence based proposal. Pain 118: 289–305.
11. Dworkin RH, O'Connor AB, Backonja M, Farrar JT, Finnerup NB, et al. (2007) Pharmacologic management of neuropathic pain: Evidence-based recommendations. Pain 132: 237–251.
12. Centre for Clinical Practice at NICE (UK) (2010) Neuropathic pain: the pharmacological management of neuropathic pain in adults in non-specialist settings. London: National Institute for Health and Clinical Excellence (UK).
13. Attal N, Cruccu G, Baron R, Haanpaa M, Hansson P, et al. (2010) European Federation of Neurological Societies: EFNS guidelines on the pharmacological treatment of neuropathic pain: 2010 revision. Eur J Neurol 17: e1113–e1188.
14. Martinez V, Attal N, Bouhassira D, Lantéri-Minet M for the French Society for the Study and Treatment of Pain (2010) Chronic neuropathic pain: diagnosis, evaluation and treatment in outpatient services. Guidelines for clinical practice of the French Society for the Study and Treatment of Pain. Douleur analg 23: 51–66.
15. Dworkin RH, Panarites CJ, Armstrong EP, Malone DC, Pham SV (2012) Is treatment of postherpetic neuralgia in the community consistent with evidence-based recommendations? Pain 153: 869–875.
16. Peabody JW, Luck J, Glassman P, Dersselhaus TR, Lee M (2000) Comparison of vignettes, standardized patients, and chart abstraction: a prospective validation study of 3 methods for measuring quality. JAMA 283: 1715–1722.
17. Peabody JW, Luck J, Glassman P, Jain S, Hansen J, et al. (2004) Measuring the quality of physician practice by using clinical vignettes: a prospective validation study. Ann Intern Med 141: 771–780.
18. Peabody JW, Tozija F, Munoz JA, Nordyke RJ, Luck J (2004) Using vignettes to compare the quality of clinical care variation in economically divergent countries. Health Serv Res 39: 1951–1970.
19. Veloski J, Tai S, Evans AS, Nash DB (2005) Clinical vignette-based surveys: a tool for assessing physician practice variation. Am J Med Qual 20: 151–157.
20. Bachmann LM, Muehleisen A, Bock A, ter Riet G, Held U, et al. (2008) Vignette studies of medical choice and judgement to study caregivers' medical decision behaviour: systematic review. BMC Med Res Methodol 8: 50.
21. Bouhassira D, Attal N (2012) Douleurs neuropathiques, Collection: Références en douleur et analgésie, Arnette Editors.

22. Bennett MI, Rayment C, Hjermstad M, Aass N, Caraceni A, et al. (2012) Prevalence and aetiology of neuropathic pain in cancer patients: a systematic review. Pain 153: 359–365.
23. Freynhagen R, Baron R, Gockel U, Tölle TR (2006) painDETECT: a new screening questionnaire to identify neuropathic components in patients with back pain. Curr Med Res Opin 22: 1911–1920.
24. Martinez V, Baudic S, Fletcher D (2013) Chronic postsurgical pain. Ann Fr Anesth Reanim 32: 422–435.
25. Perkins FM, Kehlet H (2000) Chronic pain as an outcome of surgery. A review of predictive factors. Anesthesiology 93: 1123–1133.
26. Johansen A, Romundstad L, Nielsen CS, Schirmer H, Stubhaug A (2012) Persistent postsurgical pain in a general population: prevalence and predictors in the Tromso study. Pain 153: 1390–1396.
27. Woolf CJ, Mannion RJ (1999) Neuropathic pain: aetiology, symptoms, mechanisms, and management. Lancet 353 (9168): 1959–1964.
28. Torrance N, Ferguson JA, Afolabi E, Bennett MI, Serpell MG, et al. (2013) Neuropathic pain in the community: more under-treated than refractory? Pain 154: 690–699.
29. Parsons B, Schaefer C, Mann R, Sadosky A, Daniel S, et al. (2013) Economic and humanistic burden of post-trauma and post-surgical neuropathic pain among adults in the United States. J Pain Res 6: 459–469.
30. Pham T, Roy C, Mariette X, Lioté F, Durieux P, et al. (2009) Effect of response format for clinical vignettes on reporting quality of physician practice BMC Health Serv Res 9: 128.
31. Kehlet H, Jensen TS, WJ (2006) Persistent postsurgical pain: risk factors and prevention. Lancet 367: 1618–1625.
32. Finnerup NB, Sindrup SH, Jensen TS (2010) The evidence for pharmacological treatment of neuropathic pain. Pain 150 (3): 573–581.
33. AFFSAPS (2011) Modification des modalités de prescription et de délivrance du Rivotril. Communiqué de presse.
34. Hall GC, Morant SV, Carroll D, Gabriel ZL, McQuay HJ (2013) An observational descriptive study of the epidemiology and treatment of neuropathic pain in a UK general population. BMC Fam Pract 14: 28.
35. Clerc I, Ventelou B, Guerville MA, Paraponaris A, Verger P (2011) General practitioners and clinical practice guidelines: a reexamination. Med Care Res Rev 68:504–518.
36. Veloski JJ, Fields SK, Boex JR, Blank LL (2005) Measuring professionalism: a review of studies with instruments reported in the literature between 1982 and 2002. Acad Med 80: 366–370.
37. Peabody JW, Liu A (2007) A cross-national comparison of the quality of clinical care using vignettes. Health Policy Plan 22: 294–302.
38. Norcini J (2004) Back to the future: clinical vignettes and the measurement of physician performance. Ann Intern Med 141: 813–814.
39. Dresselhaus TR, Peabody JW, Lee M, Wang MM, Luck J (2000) Measuring compliance with preventive care guidelines: standardized patients, clinical vignettes, and the medical record. J Gen Intern Med 15: 782–788.
40. Dumesnil H, Cortaredona S, Verdoux H, Sebbah R, Paraponaris A, et al. (2012) General practitioners' choices and their determinants when starting treatment for major depression: a cross-sectional, randomized case-vignette survey. PLoS One 7 (12): e52429.

10

Velocity of Lordosis Angle during Spinal Flexion and Extension

Tobias Consmüller[1], Antonius Rohlmann[2]*, Daniel Weinland[1], Claudia Druschel[3], Georg N. Duda[2], William R. Taylor[2]

1 Epionics Medical GmbH, Potsdam, Germany, 2 Julius Wolff Institute, Charité – Universitätsmedizin Berlin, Berlin, Germany, 3 Center for Musculoskeletal Surgery, Charité – Universitätsmedizin Berlin, Berlin, Germany

Abstract

The importance of functional parameters for evaluating the severity of low back pain is gaining clinical recognition, with evidence suggesting that the angular velocity of lordosis is critical for identification of musculoskeletal deficits. However, there is a lack of data regarding the range of functional kinematics (RoKs), particularly which include the changing shape and curvature of the spine. We address this deficit by characterising the angular velocity of lordosis throughout the thoracolumbar spine according to age and gender. The velocity of lumbar back shape changes was measured using Epionics SPINE during maximum flexion and extension activities in 429 asymptomatic volunteers. The difference between maximum positive and negative velocities represented the RoKs. The mean RoKs for flexion decreased with age; 114°/s (20–35 years), 100°/s (36–50 years) and 83°/s (51–75 years). For extension, the corresponding mean RoKs were 73°/s, 57°/s and 47°/s. ANCOVA analyses revealed that age and gender had the largest influence on the RoKs ($p < 0.05$). The Epionics SPINE system allows the rapid assessment of functional kinematics in the lumbar spine. The results of this study now serve as normative data for comparison to patients with spinal pathology or after surgical treatment.

Editor: Steve Milanese, University of South Australia, Australia

Funding: This study was supported by Epionics Medical GmbH, Potsdam, Germany (www.epionics.de/), the EU (VPHOP ICT-2-5.3) (http://www.vphop.eu/), and the BiSP project "Rückenfit" (www.bisp.de/). The funders had no role in interpretation of the results, decision to publish, or preparation of the manuscript.

Competing Interests: T. Consmüller is, and D. Weinland was an employee of Epionics Medical GmbH, a commercial funder of this research. A. Rohlmann was a consultant of Epionics Medical GmbH.

* E-mail: Antonius.Rohlmann@charite.de

Introduction

Low back pain is one of the most common diseases in western industrialised countries [1;2]. Besides the relief of pain, therapeutical measures focus on the conservation and improvement of the subject's functional capacity. Recently, clinical attention has been drawn to assessing the kinematics of changes in spinal shape, which have been shown to provide a greater distinction between patients with low back pain pathology and asymptomatic subjects than measures of e.g. range of motion alone. In this respect, Marras and co-workers demonstrated the importance of dynamics during functional activities by investigating 16 low back pain patients and 18 asymptomatic volunteers using the Ady-Hall lumbar monitor [3]. While they found a reduction of 10% in the range of motion during flexion in low back pain patients compared to healthy volunteers, the significant reduction of 50% in angular velocity indicated a much clearer biomarker for low back pain. More importantly, during extension, the angular velocity of patients was reduced by more than 90%. Further evidence demonstrating the importance of dynamic measures was provided by McGregor and co-workers [4], who examined 20 low back pain patients and 20 healthy volunteers using the CA-6000 [5], similarly concluding that the velocity of spinal flexion in the sagittal plane was a clear target for functional identification of pathology.

A number of measurement tools exist for the objective estimation of the lumbar spines range of motion (RoM), with some offering the change of back shape with respect to time, including Vicon [6], ZooMS [7], Formetric 4D [8], 3space [9], 3D-SpineMoveGuard [10], fibre-optic sensor [11] and inertial measurement units [12]. However, numeric data for dynamic measures of spinal kinematics are only available for the Ady-Hall lumbar monitor, the CA-6000 and the lumbar motion monitor [3;4;13–15]. Widespread accessibility to rapid and mobile approaches for assessing spinal kinematics is, however, critical for these important measures to be considered for aiding clinical decision making.

The so-called range of functional kinematics (RoKs) provides a measure of the maximum and minimum flexion and extension velocities. Normative data has been published for the measurement tools CA-6000 and lumbar motion monitor [16;17]. While the potentiometer link arm of the CA-6000 is positioned at the thoracolumbar joint and at the level of the spina iliaca superior posterior, the lumbar motion monitor uses an electro-goniometer that is attached to the shoulder and pelvis. Thus, these devices measure the velocity for different regions of the back, but are unable to consider the dynamic shape of the back, including the changing curvature at different regions of the spine. In order to allow the formation of normative reference data for clinical usage, where pain and musculoskeletal deficits occur at different heights, complete datasets of dynamic back shape are required, but remain to be established.

The measurement tool Epionics SPINE is an advancement of the former SpineDMS system [18], and allows the dynamic assessment of the shape of the thoracolumbar spine in a rapid and subject specific manner based on strain gauge technology. While age, gender and body-height dependent normative data for back shape and RoM have been determined for this device, no repository of normative data exists for the maximum velocities of lumbar spine movements in the sagittal plane, i.e. flexion and extension.

With the goal of establishing normative data for comparison against patients with spinal pathology or after surgical treatment, the aim of this study was to determine the velocities during changes of lordosis angle for movements in the sagittal plane in healthy volunteers, and therefore quantify changes in dynamic back shape. Furthermore, we aimed to characterise back shape such that parameters of the lumbar functional capacity with respect to individual factors such as age and gender can be derived.

Materials and Methods

Ethics Statement

The study was approved by the Ethics Committee of the Charité – Universitätsmedizin Berlin (registry number EA4/011/10), and each volunteer provided written informed consent to participate.

Subjects

The lumbar spine movements of 429 asymptomatic volunteers (231 females, mean age 40.0±15.2, 198 males, mean age 39.3±13.6 years) were assessed. Inclusion criteria for the study were an age between 20 and 75 years, the absence of back pain in the previous 6 months, and no previous spinal surgery. For the analysis of age dependency, volunteers were divided into classes of 20–35, 36–50 and 51–75 years (189, 146 and 94 persons respectively).

Measuring system

Measurements were conducted using Epionics SPINE (Epionics Medical GmbH, Potsdam, Germany), which allows the temporal assessment of back shape in the region of the thoracolumbar spine for motions in the sagittal plane [19]. The system has been described in detail elsewhere [19], but a brief summary is provided here: Two flexible sensor strips are fixed paravertebrally to the spine using special hollow plasters (Figure 1, left). The strips are placed a distance of 5 cm from the mid-sagittal plane and the lowest sensor segment is positioned relative to the spina iliaca posterior superior. Each sensor strip assesses the curvature of the back shape along the 12 connected segments by measuring bending of the segments relative to one another using a series of strain gauge measurements (Figure 1, right). The sensors are connected via cables to a memory unit, which provides storage of the data, which is collected at 50 Hz, as well as a power supply. The validity and reliability of the measurement tool, as well as normative data for spinal RoMs, have been published elsewhere [18;19].

Measurement protocol

The volunteers performed standard upper body movement choreographies after watching a video, which explained and demonstrated the requested movements. Each subject was asked to perform maximum spinal flexion and extension exercises with extended knees each five times. Between the exercises, each subject's upright standing posture was assessed as a reference position. No instructions were provided to the subjects concerning the velocity of the upper body movements. Thus, all volunteers performed the movements at their preferred speed, which is known to produce more consistent results of motion characteristics (RoM as well as RoKs) than pre-defined slow or maximum speeds [20].

Data analysis

In this study, measurement results were averaged over the left and right sensor strip since only movements in the sagittal plane were considered and the sensor strips were attached symmetrically to the spine [19]. The area of the sensor strips that covered the lumbar lordosis was identified individually for each volunteer as the range of segments that have negative bending during upright standing. The angles of these segments were then summed at every time frame, and the derivative with respect to time, calculated using the Savitzky-golay differentiation filter in the Matlab suite (The Mathworks Inc., Natick, MA, USA), was used to compute the angular velocities. The velocities presented are the mean peak velocities reached during the five repetitions of descending or ascending movement.

Description of the functional capacity

The functional capacity was considered to consist of a combination of the maximum RoM and the maximum RoKs. At each measurement time point, the lordosis angle was therefore computed and the corresponding velocities were calculated using the derivative with respect to time. Velocities were considered positive during movement in anterior direction (descending during flexion and ascending during extension) and negative during movement in the posterior direction (ascending during flexion and descending during extension).

In order to understand the variation of dynamic metrics, an average curve of the volunteers in different age classes was constructed by applying a dynamic time warping procedure to the curves of each volunteer [21]. This temporal standardisation allowed a comparison of the repeated movements for different volunteers at individual instances of time.

The lordosis variation for the RoM was computed as the difference of the lordosis angle at maximum flexion and maximum extension respectively, and for the RoKs as the difference between the maximum (+ve) and minimum (−ve) velocities during flexion and extension.

Statistics

For the determination of number of volunteers required to determine spinal RoKs representative of the population, a power analysis was conducted with nQuery 7.0 (Statistical Solutions Inc., Saugus, MA, USA), using 2-sided 95% confidence interval. Mean RoKs of 106°/s and a standard deviation of 33°/s, obtained from the results of the pilot study, indicated that at least 336 volunteers are required to create a normative database for lumbar RoKs. A covariance analysis (ANCOVA) was used to identify which of the individual parameters (age, gender, BMI (body mass index), body height and weight) played a dominant role on the maximum velocities reached during flexion and extension. Analyses of variance (two-way ANOVA) were used to examine interactions and the statistical variation between groups. The significance level was set to 0.05. The arithmetic means and standard deviations were computed from the maximum velocities for each of the different volunteer groups. Statistical analyses were performed using Matlab (The Mathworks Inc., Natick, MA, USA) and SPSS 19 (IBM, Armonk, NY, USA).

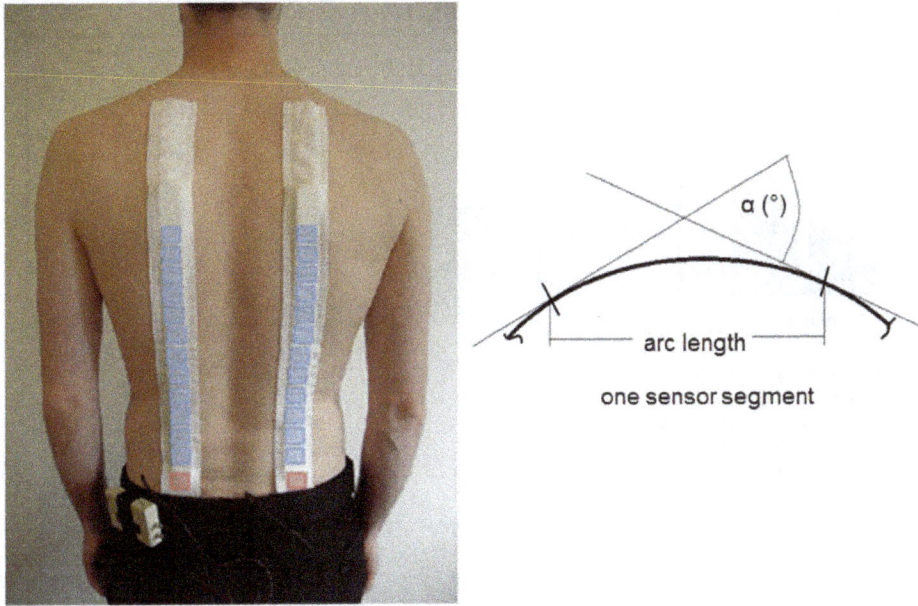

Figure 1. Measurement system. Epionics SPINE system with schematic positions of bending sensor segments (blue) and acceleration sensors (red), (left). A schematic display of the definition of angle α is shown for a single exemplary bending sensor segment (right).

Results

Flexion and Extension

All 429 subjects were able to complete the full movement analysis program without incident. During the flexion movement in general, the magnitude of the negative lordosis angle reduced initially and reached a positive angle before returning to approximately its initial value in the static standing position (Figure 2, left). During the extension activity, the magnitude of the lordosis angle first increased to a maximum angle before returning to the baseline (Figure 2, right). Variations in the repetitions are visible during upright standing, particularly during the over-swing and maximum deflection phases.

The slope of these flexion-extension curves were determined to provide the corresponding angular velocity, where a larger slope was associated with a higher velocity. During the flexion and extension exercises, two extreme values arose: the first during movement into maximum deflection (descending) and the second while returning to the initial position (ascending). For flexion, the average velocity during the descending movement was significantly higher ($p < 0.05$) than during the ascending movement (Figure 3). During the extension activity, the relative velocity of extension and flexion were reversed such that the velocity during the ascending movement was higher ($p < 0.05$). Significant differences were also found when comparing the velocities of descending flexion and extension and ascending flexion and extension.

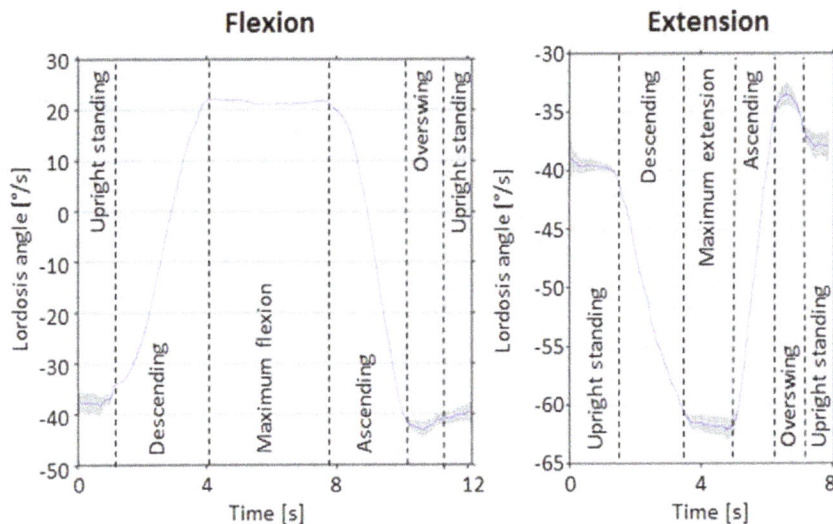

Figure 2. Lordosis angle versus time. Exemplary mean curvature of lordosis angle versus time for one volunteer during a flexion (left) and extension exercise (right). The grey area represents one standard deviation of repeated movements.

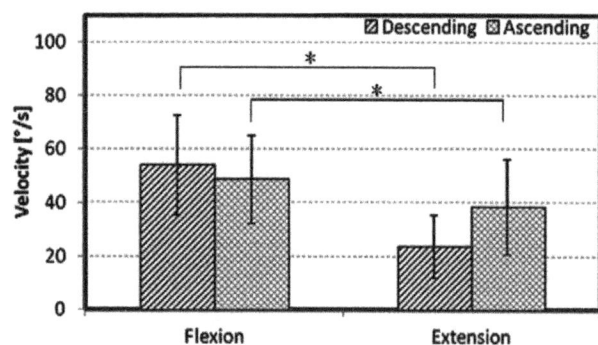

Figure 3. Maximum lordosis angle velocities during flexion and extension. Means and standard deviations of the maximum reached lordosis angle velocities at descending and ascending movement during maximum flexion and extension for all volunteers. Significant differences (* p<0.05) appear between flexion descending-ascending, extension descending-ascending, flexion descending-extension descending, and flexion ascending-extension ascending.

Age and gender differences during flexion

The maximum velocities for both the descending and ascending movements during flexion decreased significantly with increasing age (Figure 4, top, p<0.05). In the youngest age group, females showed higher velocities during flexion (both descending and ascending) compared to the corresponding velocities in males (p<0.05). However, the angular velocities during flexion for females aged between 36 and 50 were higher than in the corresponding males for ascending movements only (p<0.05). No significant differences were found in the oldest age groups.

Age and gender differences during extension

During extension, a progressive decrease of the angular velocities during both descending and ascending movements was also observed with increasing age (Figure 4, bottom, p<0.05). Males aged between 20 and 35, as well as 36 and 50 years were significantly slower in both descending and ascending (p<0.05). Again, for the highest age group no significant differences were apparent.

Description of functional capacity

An analysis of the lordosis angle compared to the angular velocity resulted in circular patterns for the flexion and extension exercises (Figure 5). By normalizing the lordosis angle to the upright standing position, the curves began at 0° and 0°/s. For the maximum flexion/extension angle, the velocity was also zero. The maximum magnitude of the velocity occurred mostly in the middle region of each movement. With increasing age, the maximum angles as well as the maximum velocities became smaller for both flexion and extension exercises. When returning to the initial position after each activity, an over-swing was normally observed, in which the motion was slightly more than required to return to their baseline position. The RoM and RoKs for the different age groups is provided in Table 1.

ANCOVA and ANOVA analyses

The ANCOVA analysis revealed that age and gender had the main influence on the maximum angular velocities reached during flexion and extension exercises for both descending as well as for ascending (Table 2). The ANOVA analysis to determine the interactions between the variables with a major influence on the maximum velocities (age and gender) showed a significant in-

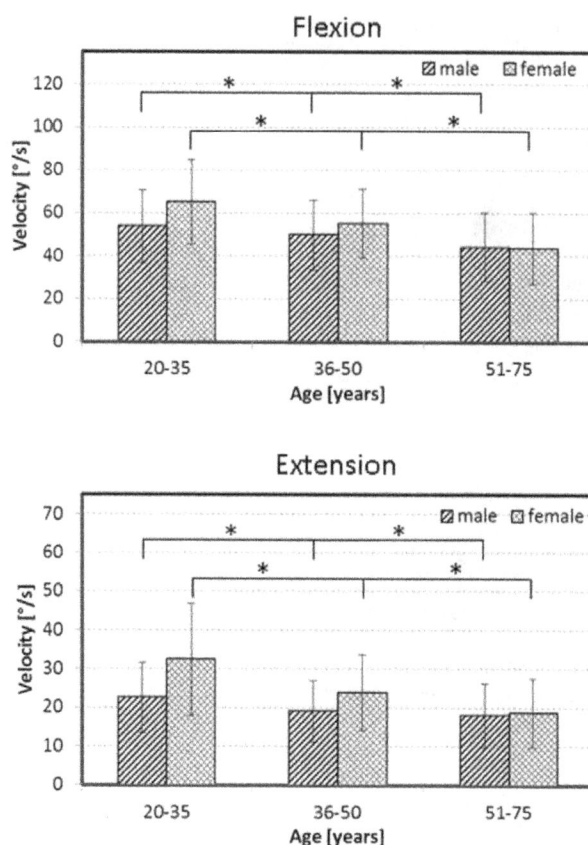

Figure 4. Influence of age and gender on maximum lordosis angle velocity. Means and standard deviations of the maximum lordosis angle velocities during the descending movement into maximum flexion (top) and extension (bottom), displayed according to age and gender. An asterisk (*) indicates statistical significance at the 5% level.

teraction between all velocities except the minimum velocity during flexion (Table 3).

Discussion

Low back pain is often associated with dynamic activities of patients, however the characteristics of dynamic movements, specifically their velocities and changes of velocities are not well known. Differences in dynamic metrics during spinal motion, particularly the angular velocity during flexion and extension movement, are known to play a critical role for differentiating asymptomatic subjects from those with pathological low back pain [3;4]. The use of novel technologies for the assessment of dynamic back shape [5;17] now allows quantification of the key kinematic characteristics between these groups and can aid towards understanding the role of pathology on functional outcome. This study has presented normative data measured in a collective of 429 asymptomatic volunteers, and provides clear evidence that age and gender have a dominant influence on the maximum angular velocity of the lumbar spine, as well as the range of functional dynamics.

The parameters age and gender had the main influence on the variation of maximum angular velocity during flexion and extension exercises. These parameters were also identified to have the main influence on the variation of range of motion in the

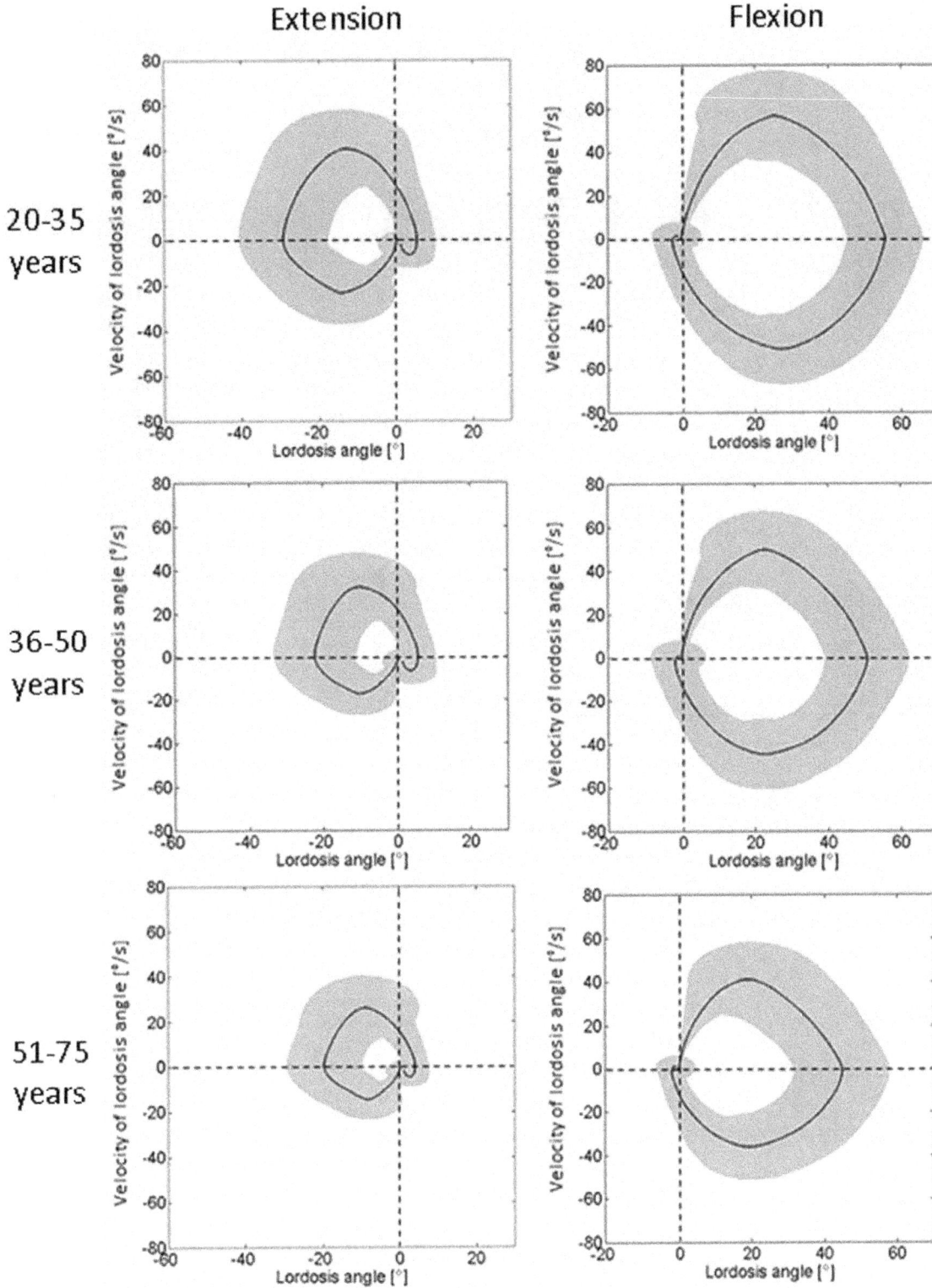

Figure 5. Lordosis angle versus velocity of lordosis angle. Averaged lordosis angle, normalized to the upright standing lordosis, versus the velocity of lordosis angle for extension (left) and flexion (right) depending on age. All figures progress in a clockwise direction. The grey area represents one standard deviation.

sagittal plane [19], which agrees well with earlier findings [17]. Furthermore, interactions between age and gender at different RoMs have been documented previously [22]. The youngest and

mid-aged females showed surprisingly higher angular velocities during flexion and extension than their male counterparts, even though there were no gender specific significant differences in age

Table 1. Means of range of motion (RoM) and range of functional kinematics (RoKs) for flexion and extension dependent upon age grouping.

Age	RoM Extension [°]	RoM Flexion [°]	RoKs Extension [°/s]	RoKs Flexion [°/s]
20–35 years	29.7±11.0	54.0±9.3	73.2±31.1	114.1±34.6
36–50 years	22.4±11.2	50.3±10.1	57.4±25.3	100.3±31.8
51–75 years	19.5±9.3	45.1±12.6	47.1±23.1	82.7±30.9

groupings (20–35 years: p = 0.523, 36–50 years: p = 0.647, 51–75 years: p = 0.041). Furthermore, the RoKs of males and females converged with increasing age. Here, while a comparison with pathological movement patterns was not possible within the confines of this study, these normative data do provide a basis for understanding pathology and the expected limitations in patient cohorts.

The resulting velocities for movements in the sagittal plane are very similar to the results of Marras and co-workers [3]. Their volunteers, which were comparable to the youngest and middle aged groups of the current collective, also moved faster in the

Table 2. Results of the ANCOVA analysis showing the importance of age, gender, body mass index (BMI), height, and weight in determining the maximum velocities during flexion and extension exercises, bold values indicate statistical significance at p<0.05.

	F	p	Eta-squared
Maximum velocity during flexion (descent)			
Age	**52.32**	**<0.01**	**0.110**
Gender	4.05	0.05	0.009
Height	0.16	0.69	0.000
BMI	0.14	0.70	0.000
Weight	0.03	0.86	0.000
Minimum velocity during flexion (ascent)			
Age	**51.66**	**<0.01**	**0.109**
Gender	**8.03**	**<0.01**	**0.019**
Height	0.21	0.64	0.001
Weight	0.08	0.78	0.000
BMI	0.01	0.94	0.000
Maximum velocity during extension (descent)			
Age	**71.55**	**<0.01**	**0.145**
Gender	**9.34**	**<0.01**	**0.022**
BMI	0.27	0.61	0.001
Weight	0.17	0.68	0.000
Height	0.09	0.77	0.000
Minimum velocity during extension (ascent)			
Age	**60.63**	**<0.01**	**0.125**
Gender	**18.44**	**<0.01**	**0.042**
Height	0.79	0.38	0.002
Weight	0.66	0.42	0.002
BMI	0.60	0.44	0.001

The ANCOVA degree of freedom was 1 in all cases.

anterior than in the posterior direction. Moreover, volunteers descended into maximum extension slower than they ascended to upright standing from full flexion. One possible explanation for this relative difference in velocity is that the volunteers maintained slower movement patterns during their approach towards maximum extension in order to reduced their out of balance forces and therefore their risk of falling [23]. Any subsequent movements in the forwards direction to return to upright standing could then happen faster, possibly due to the lever arm offered by the feet for maintaining balance. Although these findings are partly contrary to the findings of McGregor and co-workers [4;17] whose volunteers for the most part reached higher velocities during backward motion towards maximum extension than during forward motion to upright standing, no age dependent normative data has been published until now for movements without resistance. From the results of the current study, it seems that this important factor in modifying the speed of spinal movement patterns might be the key to understanding differences between study cohorts [16].

The quantification of the lordosis angle and velocity of lordosis angle offers a multidimensional evaluation of the spinal functional capacity. The computation of differences between minimum and maximum allows the evaluation of a subject's function on the basis of just a few parameters. Although no patients have been examined in this study, the characterisation of functional and kinematic data presented here and previously [5;17] will now allow a reference for assessing patients (Figure 4), where it is expected that deficits in RoM and RoKs will be detectable [3;4]. Whether the analysis of functional and kinematic data alone will be sufficient to determine e.g. location or extent of a musculoskeletal deficit of the spine, remains to be investigated, but current indications are that such non-invasive data could indeed aid clinical diagnosis and decision making processes.

Table 3. Results of the two-way ANOVA analysis showing the interaction effects of different velocity measures.

	F	p	Eta-squared
Maximum velocity during flexion (descent)	3.77	0.02*	0.018
Minimum velocity during flexion (ascent)	2.83	0.60	0.013
Maximum velocity during extension (descent)	5.10	<0.01*	0.024
Minimum velocity during extension (ascent)	6.41	<0.01*	0.029

A major influence was observed for the maximum velocities of flexion and extension. The degree of freedom was 2 in all cases. * indicates statistical significance at p<0.05.

In this study, no information about the targeted velocity of motion was provided to the volunteers prior to the measurements. As a result, some asymptomatic volunteers conducted the exercises slowly and with caution. Here, this subject specific response might have proved beneficial to the reliability of the study, since each volunteer's preferred pace is known to be the best choice for consistent results [20]. Furthermore, the Epionics SPINE measurement tool is attached to the back in the thoracolumbar region. As a consequence, it could be expected that subjects with a high BMI will produce large variations, but the results of this study indicate that BMI is consistently a non-dominant factor in determining differences between RoKs (Table 2). On the other hand, repetitions of exercises seemed to be highly reproducible between measurements (Figure 2), with greater levels of variation observed when reaching maximum extension – a result that is presumably associated with greater instability in this position. In this respect, additional studies into the reproducibility of movement patterns, particularly the extremes of motion, will be addressed in future studies.

The assessment of RoM and RoKs of the upper body, and therefore an evaluation of physical function, has been enabled using Epionics SPINE in an easy and non-invasive manner. It is expected that the functional assessment of the upper body, especially dynamic variables, can provide additional information for complementing diagnostic imaging and decision making during clinical daily routine.

Acknowledgments

The authors would like to thank the volunteers for their contribution to this study.

Author Contributions

Conceived and designed the experiments: AR GND WRT. Performed the experiments: TC CD. Analyzed the data: TC AR DW WRT. Contributed reagents/materials/analysis tools: CD GND. Wrote the paper: TC AR DW CD GND WRT. Statistics: DW TC.

References

1. Dagenais S, Caro J, Haldeman S (2008) A systematic review of low back pain cost of illness studies in the United States and internationally. Spine J 8(1): 8–20.
2. Frymoyer JW, Cats-Baril WL (1991) An overview of the incidences and costs of low back pain. Orthop Clin North Am 22(2): 263–271.
3. Marras WS, Wongsam PE (1986) Flexibility and velocity of the normal and impaired lumbar spine. Arch Phys Med Rehabil 67(4): 213–217.
4. McGregor AH, McCarthy ID, Hughes SPF (1995) Motion characteristics of normal subjects and people with low back pain. Physiotherapy 81(10): 632–637.
5. Dvorak J, Vajda EG, Grob D, Panjabi MM (1995) Normal motion of the lumbar spine as related to age and gender. Eur Spine J 4(1): 18–23.
6. Schache AG, Blanch P, Rath D, Wrigley T, Bennell K (2002) Three-dimensional angular kinematics of the lumbar spine and pelvis during running. Hum Mov Sci 21(2): 273–293.
7. Ciavarro GL, Andreoni G, Negrini S, Santambrogio GC (2006) Functional assessment of the lumbar spine through the optoelectronic ZooMS system. Clinical application. Eura Medicophys 42(2): 135–143.
8. Betsch M, Wild M, Jungbluth P, Hakimi M, Windolf J, et al. (2011) Reliability and validity of 4D rasterstereography under dynamic conditions. Comput Biol Med 41(6): 308–312.
9. Pearcy MJ, Hindle RJ (1989) New method for the non-invasive three-dimensional measurement of human back movement. Clin Biomech 4: 73–79.
10. Wunderlich M, Ruther T, Essfeld D, Erren TC, Piekarski C, et al. (2011) A new approach to assess movements and isometric postures of spine and trunk at the workplace. Eur Spine J 20(8): 1393–1402.
11. Williams JM, Haq I, Lee RY (2010) Dynamic measurement of lumbar curvature using fibre-optic sensors. Med Eng Phys 32(9): 1043–1049.
12. Goodvin C, Park EJ, Huang K, Sakaki K (2006) Development of a real-time three-dimensional spinal motion measurement system for clinical practice. Med Biol Eng Comput 44(12): 1061–1075.
13. Allread WG, Marras WS, Burr DL (2000) Measuring trunk motions in industry: variability due to task factors, individual differences, and the amount of data collected. Ergonomics 43(6): 691–701.
14. Lindsay D, Horton J (2002) Comparison of spine motion in elite golfers with and without low back pain. J Sports Sci 20(8): 599–605.
15. Marras WS, Fathallah FA, Miller RJ, Davis SW, Mirka GA (1992) Accuracy of a Three Dimensional Lumbar Motion Monitor for Recording Dynamic Trunk Motion Characteristics. International Journal of Industrial Ergonomics 9(1): 75–87.
16. Marras WS, Parnianpour M, Ferguson SA, Kim JY, Crowell RR, et al. (1995) The classification of anatomic- and symptom-based low back disorders using motion measure models. Spine (Phila Pa 1976) 20(23): 2531–2546.
17. McGregor AH, McCarthy ID, Hughes SP (1995) Motion characteristics of the lumbar spine in the normal population. Spine (Phila Pa 1976) 20(22): 2421–2428.
18. Taylor WR, Consmuller T, Rohlmann A (2010) A novel system for the dynamic assessment of back shape. Med Eng Phys 32(9): 1080–1083.
19. Consmuller T, Rohlmann A, Weinland D, Druschel C, Duda GN, et al. (2012) Comparative evaluation of a novel measurement tool to assess lumbar spine posture and range of motion. Eur Spine J 22.
20. McGregor AH, Hughes SPF (2000) The effect of test speed on the motion characteristics of the lumbar spine during an A-P flexion-extension test. Journal of Back and Musculoskeletal Rehabilitation 14: 99–104.
21. Bender A, Bergmann G (2012) Determination of typical patterns from strongly varying signals. Comput Methods Biomech Biomed Engin 15(7): 761–769.
22. Battié MC, Bigos SJ, Sheehy A, Wortley MD (1987) Spinal flexibility and individual factors that influence it. Phys Ther 67:653–658.
23. Hamacher D, Singh NB, Van Dieen JH, Heller MO, Taylor WR (2011) Kinematic measures for assessing gait stability in elderly individuals: a systematic review. J R Soc Interface 8(65): 1682–1698.

11

Predictors of Occurrence and Severity of First Time Low Back Pain Episodes: Findings from a Military Inception Cohort

Steven Z. George[1]*, John D. Childs[2], Deydre S. Teyhen[2], Samuel S. Wu[3], Alison C. Wright[2], Jessica L. Dugan[2], Michael E. Robinson[4]

1 Department of Physical Therapy and Center for Pain Research and Behavioral Health, University of Florida, Gainesville, Florida, United States of America, 2 U.S. Army-Baylor University Doctoral Program in Physical Therapy (MCCS-HGE-PT), Army Medical Department Center and School, Fort Sam Houston, Texas, United States of America, 3 Department of Biostatistics, University of Florida, Gainesville, Florida, United States of America, 4 Department of Clinical and Health Psychology and Center for Pain Research and Behavioral Health, University of Florida, Gainesville, Florida, United States of America

Abstract

Primary prevention studies suggest that additional research on identifying risk factors predictive of low back pain (LBP) is necessary before additional interventions can be developed. In the current study we assembled a large military cohort that was initially free of LBP and followed over 2 years. The purposes of this study were to identify baseline variables from demographic, socioeconomic, general health, and psychological domains that were predictive of a) occurrence; b) time; and c) severity for first episode of self-reported LBP. Baseline and outcome measures were collected via web-based surveillance system or phone to capture monthly information over 2 years. The assembled cohort consisted of 1230 Soldiers who provided self-report data with 518 (42.1%) reporting at least one episode of LBP over 2 years. Multivariate logistic regression analysis indicated that gender, active duty status, mental and physical health scores were significant predictors of LBP. Cox regression revealed that the time to first episode of LBP was significantly shorter for Soldiers that were female, active duty, reported previous injury, and had increased BMI. Multivariate linear regression analysis investigated severity of the first episode by identifying baseline predictors of pain intensity, disability, and psychological distress. Education level and physical fitness were consistent predictors of pain intensity, while gender, smoking status, and previous injury status were predictors of disability. Gender, smoking status, physical health scores, and beliefs of back pain were consistent predictors of psychological distress. These results provide additional data to confirm the multi-factorial nature of LBP and suggest future preventative interventions focus on multi-modal approaches that target modifiable risk factors specific to the population of interest.

Editor: Jos H. Verbeek, Finnish Institute of Occupational Health, Finland

Funding: The POLM trial was supported by the Peer-Review Medical Research Program of the Department of Defense (PR054098). All authors were independent from this funding program. Publication of this article was funded in part by the University of Florida Open-Access Publishing Fund. The funders had no role in study design, data collection and analysis, decision to publish, or preparation of the manuscript.

Competing Interests: The authors have declared that no competing interests exist.

* E-mail: szgeorge@phhp.ufl.edu

Introduction

In general populations low back pain (LBP) is the most prevalent form of chronic musculoskeletal pain [1] often leading to disability [2,3]. In military populations musculoskeletal pain has an adverse effect by frequently causing medical evacuation [4] and LBP in particular a common reason for long term disability [5]. As a result of its negative impact prevention of LBP has remained a research priority for both general [6] and military populations [4,7].

Factors involved in the transition from acute to chronic LBP have been a recent focus of disability prevention research. Such an approach is consistent with secondary prevention [8], and studies in this area have provided important information on effective management of acute LBP. Secondary prevention studies have highlighted psychological influence on the development of chronic LBP [9] and identified patient subgroups that have larger treatment effects when matched treatment is applied [10,11]. The focus on secondary prevention has been productive in

reducing disability from acute episodes of LBP, but there remains the potential of primary prevention for limiting the negative impact of LBP.

The goal in primary prevention is to reduce the overall number of LBP episodes experienced by a population [12]. In contrast to secondary prevention, primary prevention attempts to reduce those that transition from a pain free state to one of experiencing LBP. Back schools, lumbar supports, and ergonomic interventions have all been studied for primary prevention of LBP, but with limited success [13,14,15]. These primary prevention studies suggest that more work needs to be completed in determining what factors are predictive of developing LBP before additional preventative interventions can be developed. For example, if modifiable factors are identified as being predictive of LBP then they may provide logical treatment targets for future LBP prevention trials [6].

The purpose of this paper was to report predictors of first time LBP episodes self-reported during 2 years of military duty. This purpose is consistent with primary prevention priorities highlighted in the literature [6,14]. To best study the development of LBP it is necessary to recruit a group of healthy subjects and follow these subjects until some develop LBP. Furthermore, development of LBP is believed to be multi-factorial in nature so consideration of a range of potential predictors is warranted. In the current study we assembled a large military cohort that was initially free of LBP and included potential predictors from demographic, socioeconomic, general health, and psychological domains. The primary purposes of this study were to identify variables from these domains that were predictive of a) occurrence and b) time to first episode of LBP. Our secondary purposes were to identify variables that were predictive of a) higher pain intensity; b) disability; or c) psychological distress during the first LBP episode.

Methods

Ethics Statement

The institutional review boards at the Brooke Army Medical Center (Fort Sam Houston, Texas) and the University of Florida (Gainesville, FL) granted ethical approval for this project. All subjects provided written informed consent prior to their participation.

Overview

This study was part of the Prevention of Low Back Pain in the Military (POLM) cluster randomized trial [16]. The POLM trial has been registered at ClinicalTrials.gov (http://clinicaltrials.gov) under NCT00373009.

The primary aim of the POLM trial was to determine if core-stabilization exercise and psychosocial education resulted in decreased LBP incidence during 2 years of military duty. POLM trial results indicated that psychosocial education was found to be preventative of seeking healthcare for LBP [17]. This study reports on a secondary aim of the POLM trial which was to determine what factors were predictive of self-reported LBP for Soldiers that responded to a web-based or phone survey tools.

Subjects

Consecutive subjects entering a training program at Fort Sam Houston, TX to become a combat medic in the U.S. Army were considered for participation from February 2007 to March 2008. Research staff at Fort Sam Houston, Texas introduced the study to individual companies of Soldiers and screened potentially eligible Soldiers.

Subjects were required to be 18–35 years of age (or 17 year old emancipated minor), participating in training to become a combat medic, and be able to speak and read English. Subjects with a prior history of LBP were excluded. In this study a prior history of LBP was operationally defined as a previous episode of LBP that limited work or physical activity, lasted longer than 48 hours, and caused the subject to seek health care. Subjects were also excluded if they were currently seeking medical care for LBP; unable to participate in unit exercise due to other musculoskeletal injury; had a history of lower extremity fracture (stress or traumatic); were pregnant; or if they had transferred from another training group. Other possible exclusions included Soldiers who were being accelerated into a company already randomized or Soldiers who were being re-assigned to a different occupational specialty.

Exercise and Education Programs

Companies of Soldiers were randomly assigned to exercise and/or education programs as part of the cluster randomized trial [16]. The assigned exercise and education programs are not a focus of this current paper, but are briefly reviewed as we included these as predictive variables in our statistical analyses. All exercise programs were performed in a group setting under the direct supervision of their drill instructors as part of daily unit physical training. The traditional exercise program (TEP) was selected from commonly performed exercises that target the rectus abdominus and oblique abdominal muscles. The core stabilization exercise program (CSEP) was selected from exercises that target deeper trunk muscles that attach to the spine; such as the transversus abdominus, multifidus, and the erector spinae. The TEP and CSEP are described in more detail in previous POLM publications [18,19].

The brief psychosocial education program (PSEP) involved attendance at 1 session during the first week of training. The session involved an interactive lecture led by study personnel (ACW, JLD) lasting approximately 45 minutes. The lecture consisted of a visual presentation followed by a question and answer session. The PSEP provided Soldiers current, evidence based information on LBP such as stressing that anatomical causes of LBP are not likely and encouraging active coping in response to LBP. Educational material was also provided to the Soldiers by issuing each *The Back Book* as has been done in other LBP trials [20,21,22]. The PSEP is described in more detail in a previous publication [23].

Measures

Baseline measures were collected under supervision of study personnel. Outcome measures were collected via web-based surveillance system or phone to capture monthly information over 2 years.

Baseline measures. Soldiers completed standard questionnaires to assess variables consistent with demographic and socioeconomic domains. The information collected included such variables as age, sex, education, income level, smoking history, previous activity level, previous injury, physical fitness scores, and military status. Soldiers also completed self-report measures to assess general health and psychological domains. The Medical Outcomes Survey 12-Item Short-Form Health Survey was used as a self-report of health status for physical (SF-12 PCS) and mental function (SF-12 MCS) [24]. The Back Beliefs Questionnaire (BBQ) was used to quantify beliefs about LBP related to management and outcome [25]. The State-Trait Anxiety Questionnaire (STAI) [26] and Beck Depression Inventory (BDI) [27,28,29] were used to measure negative affect from generalized anxiety and generalized depression, respectively. Finally, 9 items from the Fear of Pain Questionnaire (FPQ-III) were used to measure fear about specific situations that normally produce pain [30,31,32].

Outcome measures. Soldiers were trained in a computer lab on how to use the POLM web-based outcome surveillance system and all assessments were provided through a secure web-site that protected Soldier confidentiality. Access to the system was prompted by an email which was sent to the Soldier's official military email address on the 1st of each month. Additional emails were sent on the 3rd of the month, and again on the 7th of the month if the Soldier still had not responded. Soldiers were queried whether they had experienced any LBP in the last calendar month by email, and this information was used to determine the initial episode of LBP after completing training. Soldiers not responsive to multiple email requests were contacted by phone at the end of 12 and 24 months to determine if LBP had occurred in the past year. Those Soldiers responding to the phone interview were included with the email survey results because the structure of the phone interview was parallel to the email survey. Soldiers

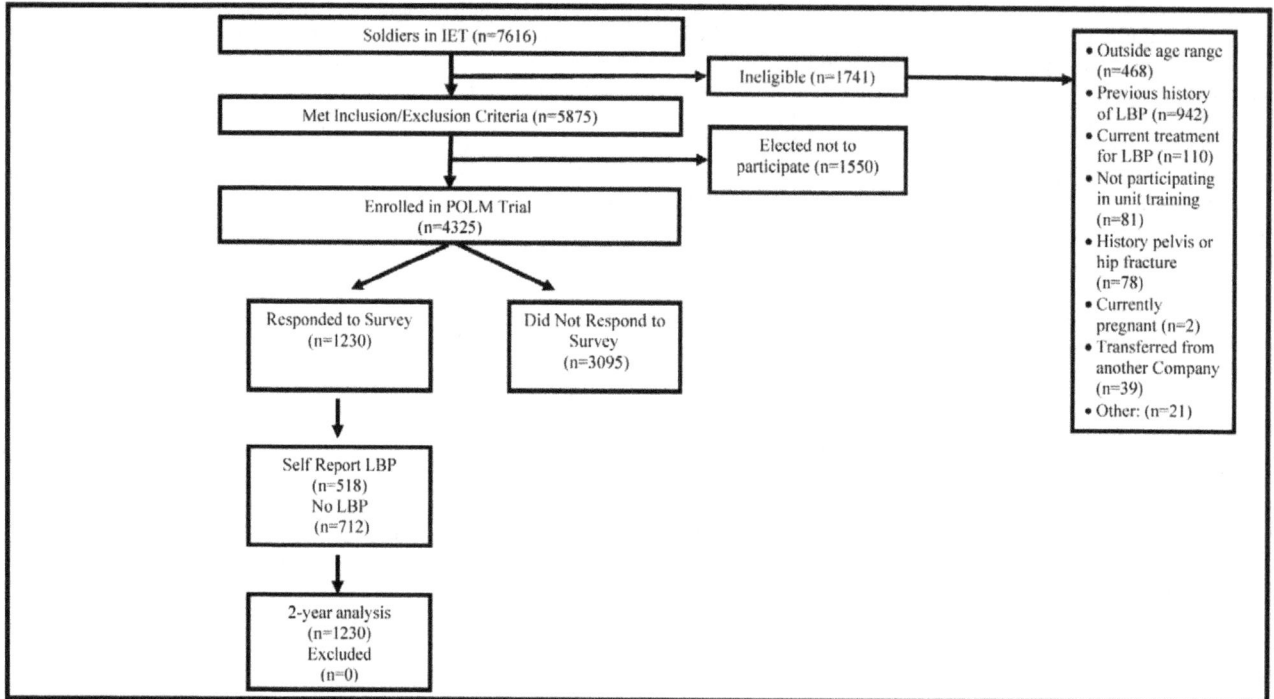

Figure 1. Flow diagram for inception cohort and responders to email surveys. Initial Entry Training (IET), Low Back Pain (LBP), Prevention of Low Back Pain in the Military (POLM), n = total number of soldiers.

successfully contacted by phone completed the same information as they would have if using the web-based system. These self reported incidence data were used as outcomes of interest for our primary purpose – determining baseline predictors for the occurrence and time to first LBP episode.

Soldiers reporting any LBP answered additional questionnaires so that the severity of the first episode could be determined. These measures included pain intensity with a numerical 0–10 rating scale (NRS) [33], disability with the Oswestry Disability Questionnaire (ODQ) [34,35], physical activity and work fear-avoidance beliefs with the Fear-Avoidance Beliefs Questionnaire (FABQ-PA and FABQ-W) [36], and pain catastrophizing by the Pain Catastrophizing Scale (CAT) [37]. Soldiers were also asked to report days of limited military duty in the past 30 days associated with the initial episode of LBP. These data were used as outcomes of interest for our secondary purpose – determining baseline predictors for the severity of LBP episodes.

Data analysis

All statistical analyses were performed using the SAS software, version 9 (SAS Institute Inc, 1996) with a type I error rate of 0.05. All authors had full access to all of the data reported in the study and can take responsibility for data integrity and accuracy. Descriptive data for the baseline variables were computed. Then multivariate logistic regression analysis was used to determine baseline predictors of reporting the first episode of LBP and multivariate Cox regression analysis was used to determine baseline predictors of time to reporting first episode of LBP. In the severity analyses, multivariate linear regression was used to determine baseline predictors of pain intensity, disability, and psychological distress. In the regression analyses baseline predictors were considered from all the individual variables from the demographic, socioeconomic, general health, and psychological

domains. All variables were entered simultaneously into the regression models to determine which were predictive of the outcome of interest while controlling for other potential variables. Therefore, only adjusted estimates are reported in the results.

Results

Figure 1 describes the recruitment and follow up for the POLM cohort, with 1230/3095 (28.4%) responding to the monthly surveys. Of those responding to the surveys, 518/1230 (42.1%) reported at least one episode of LBP during the 2-year follow up period. Specifically, 420 (48.6%) of 865 Soldiers who responded to the monthly web-based survey had at least one episode of LBP, and corresponding numbers for the phone survey were 129 (24.6%) out of 525 responders. Accompanying descriptive data for the POLM cohort is reported in Tables 1 and 2. Soldiers who responded to the phone or web-based surveys over the 2 years differed from the non-responders in age, race, education level, military status, time in military, negative affect (depressive symptoms and anxiety), back beliefs, mental function, smoking prior to military service, exercising routinely prior to military service, and military fitness scores (Tables 1 and 2). In analyses directly relevant for the purposes of this paper, comparisons of baseline characteristics between those who reported LBP and those who did not report LBP revealed differences in gender, activity duty status, BDI, FPQ, SF-12 PCS, SF-12 MCS, and reporting a previous non LBP related injury (Tables 1 and 2).

Factors Predictive of First Episode of Self-Reported LBP

Multivariate logistic regression analysis indicated that gender, active duty status, SF-12 PCS, and SF-12 MCS scores were significant predictors of LBP (Table 3). Specifically, protective factors for developing LBP were being male (OR = 0.644, 95% CI = [0.490, 0.846]), and having better SF-12 PCS scores

Table 1. Comparison of baseline innate and psychological characteristics between those who had LBP and those who had no LBP.

Variable	Label	Responders	LBP	No LBP	P-Value*	Non-responders	P-Value#
		n = 1230	n = 518	n = 712		n = 3095	
Innate Characteristics							
Age (N = 4319)		22.3±4.5	22.6±4.6	22.1±4.3	0.080	21.9±4.1	**0.001**
Gender	Male	852 (69.6%)	329 (63.9%)	523 (73.7%)	**0.0002**	2230 (72.3%)	0.068
	Female	373 (30.4%)	186 (36.1%)	187 (26.3%)		853 (27.7%)	
Race	Black or Africa	109 (8.9%)	58 (11.2%)	51 (7.2%)	0.059	311 (10.1%)	**0.020**
	Hispanic	100 (8.1%)	37 (7.1%)	63 (8.9%)		326 (10.6%)	
	White or Caucas	927 (75.5%)	381 (73.6%)	546 (76.9%)		2263 (73.3%)	
	Other	92 (7.5%)	42 (8.1%)	50 (7.0%)		187 (6.1%)	
EDUCATION	High school or lower	448 (36.4%)	193 (37.3%)	255 (35.8%)	0.204	1487 (48.1%)	**<0.0001**
	Some college	622 (50.6%)	249 (48.1%)	373 (52.4%)		1376 (44.5%)	
	College or higher	160 (13.0%)	76 (14.7%)	84 (11.8%)		231 (7.5%)	
INCOME	Less than $20,000	609 (49.7%)	249 (48.3%)	360 (50.6%)	0.430	1516 (49.1%)	0.738
	Greater than $20,000	617 (50.3%)	266 (51.7%)	351 (49.4%)		1571 (50.9%)	
Active Duty	Active	568 (46.2%)	263 (50.8%)	305 (42.8%)	**0.012**	1964 (63.5%)	**<0.0001**
	Reserve	660 (53.7%)	255 (49.2%)	405 (56.9%)		1122 (36.3%)	
	Other	2 (0.2%)		2 (0.3%)		6 (0.2%)	
Time In Army	<5 months	684 (55.6%)	287 (55.4%)	397 (55.8%)	0.968	2007 (64.9%)	**<0.0001**
	5 months–1 year	315 (25.6%)	132 (25.5%)	183 (25.7%)		654 (21.2%)	
	More than 1 year	231 (18.8%)	99 (19.1%)	132 (18.5%)		430 (13.9%)	
Company Instructor	Delta	295 (24.0%)	117 (22.6%)	178 (25.0%)	0.482	674 (21.8%)	0.286
	Foxtrot	130 (10.6%)	49 (9.5%)	81 (11.4%)		393 (12.7%)	
	Echo	194 (15.8%)	85 (16.4%)	109 (15.3%)		471 (15.2%)	
	Alpha	185 (15.0%)	79 (15.3%)	106 (14.9%)		442 (14.3%)	
	Charlie	169 (13.7%)	68 (13.1%)	101 (14.2%)		441 (14.2%)	
	Bravo	257 (20.9%)	120 (23.2%)	137 (19.2%)		674 (21.8%)	
Height		68.3±3.9	68.0±3.9	68.4±3.9	0.080	68.3±3.9	0.585
Weight		164.0±27.8	164.0±28.0	164.0±27.7	0.992	165.2±27.6	0.207
BMI		24.7±3.1	24.8±3.1	24.6±3.2	0.184	24.8±3.1	0.194
Psychological Characteristics							
BDI Total		6.0±6.1	6.6±5.9	5.5±6.2	**0.002**	6.6±6.7	**0.003**
FPQ Total		18.2±5.7	18.5±5.9	17.9±5.5	**0.040**	18.0±6.0	0.476
BBQ Total		43.9±7.2	43.8±7.2	44.0±7.1	0.610	43.2±7.0	**0.002**
STAI		35.3±9.0	35.9±9.4	34.9±8.6	0.055	36.3±9.2	**0.001**

Responders = those responding to online survey, Non-responders = those not responding to survey, LBP = low back pain,
* = p-values for comparison of those with LBP and those without LBP (responders only),
# = p-values for comparison of those responding to survey and those not responding to survey,
BMI = Body Mass Index, BDI = Beck Depression Inventory, FPQ = Fear of Pain Questionnaire (9 items), BBQ = Back Beliefs Questionnaire, STAI = State Trait Anxiety Inventory (state portion only). Bold font indicates p-value less than 0.05.

(OR = 0.960 for each additional point, 95% CI = [0.935, 0.987]) and better SF-12 MCS scores (OR = 0.964 for each additional point, 95% CI = [0.943, 0.985]). Increased risk of reporting LBP was noted for Soldiers on active duty (OR = 1.441 times the odds for soldiers on reserve, 95% CI = [1.094, 1.899]). Figure 2 presents the ROC curve for the fitted logistic regression model, which has an area under curve (AUC) of 0.64. Due to correlation between MCS score, STAI and BDI (with correlation coefficients approximately equal 0.60), we compared the above results with those from a reduced model attained through backward variable selection. All four factors remained statistically significant with

ORs of 0.626, 0.960, 0.973 and 1.392, respectively. The reduced model also identified BMI as a risk factor (OR = 1.044 for each additional point, 95% CI = [1.005, 1.084]), and it has AUC of 0.61 for its ROC curve. Furthermore, similar sensitivity and specificity were found from 100 repetitions of cross-validations that left out one-third randomly selected samples in the model fitting.

Cox regression revealed that the time to first episode of LBP was significantly shorter for female, active duty, profiled soldiers and increasing BMI, with corresponding hazard ratios of 1.497 (95% CI = [1.238, −1.809]), 1.366 (95% CI = [1.120, 1.665]), 1.271

Table 2. Comparison of baseline health status, activity, and attention effects between those who had LBP and those who had no LBP.

variable	Label	Responders n = 1230	LBP n = 518	No LBP n = 712	P-Value*	Non-responders n = 3095	P-Value#
Baseline Health Status & Physical Activity							
PCS Total		53.6±5.0	53.0±5.5	54.0±4.6	**0.001**	53.3±5.2	0.191
MCS Total		49.8±8.0	49.0±8.4	50.4±7.5	**0.002**	48.9±8.8	**0.002**
Smoke Prior to Army	Yes	333 (27.1%)	150 (29.0%)	183 (25.7%)	0.205	1219 (39.4%)	**<0.0001**
	No	897 (72.9%)	368 (71.0%)	529 (74.3%)		1874 (60.6%)	
Exercise Routinely	Yes	670 (54.5%)	278 (53.7%)	392 (55.1%)	0.629	1550 (50.1%)	**0.010**
	No	560 (45.5%)	240 (46.3%)	320 (44.9%)		1542 (49.9%)	
Last APFT Score	Below 150	4 (0.3%)	1 (0.2%)	3 (0.4%)	0.191	20 (0.6%)	**0.021**
	150–200	260 (21.2%)	125 (24.2%)	135 (19.0%)		750 (24.2%)	
	200–250	567 (46.2%)	233 (45.1%)	334 (47.0%)		1461 (47.2%)	
	250–300	369 (30.0%)	149 (28.8%)	220 (30.9%)		808 (26.1%)	
	Above 300	28 (2.3%)	9 (1.7%)	19 (2.7%)		55 (1.8%)	
Profiled	Yes	231 (18.8%)	118 (22.8%)	113 (15.9%)	**0.002**	664 (21.5%)	0.050
	No	999 (81.2%)	400 (77.2%)	599 (84.1%)		2430 (78.5%)	
Attention/Relational Effect							
Physical/USI Exam	No	1102 (89.6%)	458 (88.4%)	644 (90.4%)	0.249	2849 (92.1%)	**0.010**
	Yes	128 (10.4%)	60 (11.6%)	68 (9.6%)		246 (7.9%)	
PSEP	No	642 (52.2%)	269 (51.9%)	373 (52.4%)	0.874	1670 (54.0%)	0.294
	Yes	588 (47.8%)	249 (48.1%)	339 (47.6%)		1425 (46.0%)	
Exercise Group	TEP only	334 (27.2%)	148 (28.6%)	186 (26.1%)	0.622	882 (28.5%)	0.747
	TEP+PSEP	277 (22.5%)	119 (23.0%)	158 (22.2%)		675 (21.8%)	
	CSEP	308 (25.0%)	121 (23.4%)	187 (26.3%)		788 (25.5%)	
	CSEP+PSEP	311 (25.3%)	130 (25.1%)	181 (25.4%)		750 (24.2%)	

Responders = those responding to online survey, Non-responders = those not responding to survey, LBP = low back pain,
* = p-values for comparison of those with LBP and those without LBP (responders only),
# = p-values for comparison of those responding to survey and those not responding to survey,
PCS (SF-12) = Physical Component Summary Score from the Short Form Medical Survey (12 items), MCS (SF-12) = Mental Component Summary Score from the Short Form Medical Survey (12 items), APFT = Army Physical Fitness Test, Profiled = injured during training, USI = ultrasound imaging, PSEP = psychosocial education program, TEP = traditional exercise program, CSEP = core stabilization exercise program. Bold font indicates p-value less than 0.05.

(95% CI = [1.026, 1.573]) and 1.031 (95% CI = [1.002, 1.060]), respectively.

Factors Predictive of LBP Severity – Pain Intensity

Descriptive statistics for pain intensity reported during first LBP episode were 2.0 (sd = 1.9) for the current pain intensity rating, 3.2 (sd = 2.5) for the highest pain intensity rating in past 24 hours, and 0.8 (sd = 1.4) for the lowest pain intensity rating in the past 24 hours. Multivariate linear regression analysis identified baseline predictors of current ($R^2 = 7.4\%$), highest ($R^2 = 9.9\%$), and lowest ($R^2 = 9.7\%$) NRS pain intensity ratings during the first episode of LBP. Only education level and last physical fitness score were predictors of all NRS pain intensity ratings. Duration of service and better SF-12 MCS score were also predictors for highest NRS pain intensity ratings. Specifically, highest pain intensity ratings for soldiers with high school or lower education levels were 1.121 higher (95% CI = [0.239, 2.003] on average than ratings for soldiers with college degrees, 0.948 higher (95% CI = [0.186, 1.710]) for soldiers with 5 months to 1 year of service compared to those with more than 1 year of service, and 5.560 higher (95% CI = [0.117, 11.003]) on average than ratings for soldiers with physical fitness scores

below 150 when compared to those above 300. SF-12 MCS scores were protective of highest pain intensity ratings, with a decrease of 0.043 for each additional point (95% CI = [−0.086, 0.001]).

Factors Predictive of LBP Severity – Disability

Descriptive statistics for disability reported during first LBP episode were 9.8 (sd = 11.7) for ODQ score and 1.3 (sd = 4.5) for number of days with limited work duties in the past 30 days. Multivariate linear regression analysis revealed gender, smoking status, and previous injury status as baseline predictors of ODQ score ($R^2 = 11.4\%$) and days of limited work duty ($R^2 = 6.2\%$). Specifically, men on average scored 3.118 points lower on the ODQ than women (95% CI = [−5.646, −0.590]) while Soldiers who smoked prior to entering the Army scored on average 2.671 higher than those who did not (95% CI = [0.0270, 5.315]). Soldiers who had a previous non LBP related injury scored on average 3.394 higher on the ODQ than soldiers who had not (95% CI = [0.505, 6.283]). The number of days of limited duty, on average, was 1.6 less for Soldiers in the TEP only group than for soldiers receiving combined CSEP+PSEP group (95% CI = [−2.858, −0.342]).

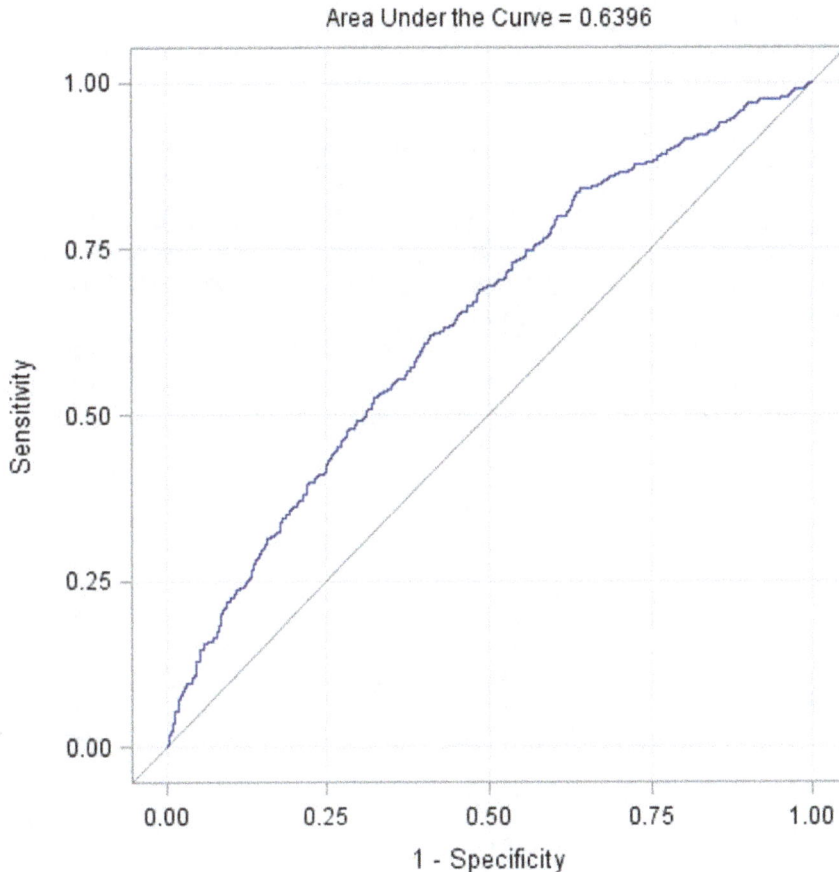

Figure 2. ROC curve for the multivariate logistic regression model predicting initial low back pain occurrence.

Factors Predictive of LBP Severity – Psychological Distress

Descriptive statistics for psychological distress reported during first LBP episode were 9.7 (sd = 6.1) for FABQ-PA scores, 10.6 (sd = 9.1) for FABQ-W scores, and 5.5 (sd = 9.5) for CAT scores. Multivariate linear regression analysis indicated that gender, smoking status, and SF-12 PCS scores were predictive of FABQ-PA scores (R^2 = 14.2%) while BMI, SF-12 PCS, and BBQ scores were predictive of FABQ-W scores (R^2 = 10.6%). For the FABQ-PA men on average scored 1.639 lower than women (95% CI = [−2.952, −0.326]) and Soldiers who smoked scored on average 1.700 higher than those who did not smoke (95% CI = [0.332, 3.068]). FABQ-PA scores decreased on average by 0.183 points for each additional point of SF-12 PCS (95% CI = [−0.303, −0.0634]). FABQ-W scores decreased on average by 0.590 for each unit increase in BMI (95% CI = [−0.911, −0.269]) and by 0.224 points for each additional point of SF-12 PCS (95% CI = [−0.406, −0.0417]). FABQ-W scores also decreased on average by 0.133 for each additional point of BBQ (95% CI = [−0.260, −0.0056]).

Multivariate linear regression analysis indicated that exercising routinely before entering the military, SF-12 PCS, and the BBQ were predictive of CAT scores (R^2 = 8.6%) during first episode of LBP. Specifically, we estimated that CAT scores are 2.380 points higher on average for soldiers who exercised routinely (95% CI = [0.347, 4.413]), while CAT scores decreased by 0.239 for each additional point of SF-12 PCS (95% CI = [−0.433, −0.0450], p = 0.016). CAT scores also decreased by 0.143 for

each additional point of BBQ score (95% CI = [−0.280, −0.0058], p = 0.040).

Discussion

Rigorous studies reporting predictors for the development of LBP are rarely reported in the literature because of the difficulty of assembling pain free cohorts and following them until LBP occurs. Strengths of the current study were the recruitment of a large inception cohort of Soldiers without previous history of LBP, consideration of a range of potentially relevant baseline predictors, and collection of follow up data over a 2 year period. Results from this study suggest that active duty (i.e. not reserve or national guard) status increased risk of LBP occurrence, while better mental and physical health scores and being male were protective. Being female and active duty status were also predictive of shorter time to first episode of LBP, as well as experiencing a previous non LBP related injury and having higher BMI. In studies that used a similar prospective design we found agreement with better physical health [38,39,40] as being protective for the development of LBP. Other studies reported risk factors that were not predictive of occurrence in this cohort including age [41,40], body weight [39,40], smoking status [42], and psychological or psychosocial factors [43,42,44]. Our military cohort was of a relatively homogenous age range, with low baseline levels of psychological and psychosocial factors. Obviously cohort differences could account for the discrepancies in identified predictors of LBP occurrence, as there is limited consistency among these studies.

Table 3. Logistic regression for baseline prediction of reporting first episode of low back pain.

Factor	Level	Odds Ratio Estimates				P-value
		Compare to	Point Estimate	95% Confidence Limits		
Gender	Male	Female	0.644	0.49	0.846	**0.002**
Race	Black or Africa	Other	1.324	0.729	2.405	0.357
	Hispanic	Other	0.761	0.41	1.414	0.389
	White or Caucas	Other	0.949	0.592	1.522	0.829
Education	High school or lower	College or higher	1.013	0.65	1.58	0.954
	Some college	College or higher	0.845	0.573	1.247	0.398
INCOME	Less than $20,000	Greater than $20,000	1.048	0.807	1.361	0.727
Active Duty Status	Active	Reserve	1.441	1.094	1.899	**0.009**
Smoke Prior to entering Army	Yes	No	1.098	0.833	1.448	0.508
Time In Army	<5 months	More than 1 year	0.914	0.654	1.279	0.601
	5 months–1 year	More than 1 year	1.075	0.746	1.551	0.697
Exercise Routinely	Yes	No	1.074	0.834	1.382	0.582
Last APFT Score	Below 150	Above 300	0.357	0.029	4.439	0.423
	150–200	Above 300	1.471	0.603	3.59	0.397
	200–250	Above 300	1.122	0.475	2.654	0.793
	250–300	Above 300	1.163	0.491	2.756	0.731
Previous Injury	Yes	No	1.224	0.891	1.683	0.213
Age			1.012	0.978	1.046	0.498
BMI			1.039	0.998	1.082	0.061
PCS (SF-12)			0.96	0.935	0.987	**0.003**
MCS (SF-12)			0.964	0.943	0.985	**0.001**
FPQ			1.008	0.986	1.031	0.468
STAI			0.982	0.961	1.003	0.089
BDI			1.01	0.982	1.039	0.497
BBQ			1	0.983	1.017	0.966
Exercise and Education Groups	TEP	CSEP	1.372	0.985	1.91	0.061
	TEP+PSEP	CSEP	1.297	0.911	1.845	0.149
	TEP	TEP+PSEP	1.058	0.751	1.489	0.748

LBP = low back pain, BMI = body mass index, BDI = Beck Depression Inventory, FPQ = Fear of Pain Questionnaire (9 items), BBQ = Back Beliefs Questionnaire, STAI = State Trait Anxiety Inventory (state portion only), PCS (SF-12) = Physical Component Summary Score from the Short Form Medical Survey (12 items), MCS (SF-12) = Mental Component Summary Score from the Short Form Medical Survey (12 items), TEP = traditional exercise program, PSEP = psychosocial education program, CSEP = core stabilization exercise program. Bold font indicates p-value less than 0.05.

A novel aspect of the current study was that we were also able to identify predictors of severity for the first LBP episode by collecting data on pain intensity, disability, and psychological distress. Collectively our results indicated that lower educational and fitness levels were predictive of higher pain intensity scores. Smoking and history of previous non LBP related injury were predictive of having more disability, while being male was predictive of less disability. Only the type of exercise program was predictive of number of days of missed duty. Lower education and fitness levels consistently predicted higher psychological distress, while better physical health scores and beliefs about back pain were predictive of lower psychological distress. There were two counterintuitive findings for psychological distress noted. Higher BMI was predictive of lower work fear-avoidance beliefs and exercising routinely was predictive of higher pain catastrophizing. Overall these results considering severity of first LBP episode may provide important new data on prevention strategies, as previous studies in this area have focused exclusively on incidence or occurrence of LBP [39,43,41,42,38,44,40]. Data from the current study extends

previous work by highlighting factors that may predict severity of first LBP episode. These factors may be especially important for future prevention studies because severity appears to be a key factor in the decision to seek healthcare for LBP [45,46,47]. Comparison of these factors to others reported in the literature was not possible because incidence studies have not typically included severity measures. Therefore these predictors of severity should be considered as preliminary with future research necessary to replicate these findings.

Although we are reporting baseline predictors of the development and severity of LBP, several caveats should be considered when interpreting these results. First, there were very few consistent predictors identified in this study. Many of the predictors appeared to be specific to the outcome measure. Second, we identified baseline predictors that were statistically significant, but the magnitude of these predictors was often low. For example, the increased risk of being on active duty was associated with an OR of 1.44 (lower bound of 95% CI = 1.09), while the protective factor of being male was associated with an

OR of 0.64 (upper bound of 95% CI = 0.85). Third, we included all participants in our prediction models instead of including only those in a control condition as is more commonly done in prognostic studies. This decision was made because in this setting all Soldiers were undergoing training which included required exercise so there was no option for a "true" control condition of no exercise. Last, not many of the identified predictive factors were modifiable in nature. This was especially true for the factors predicting the occurrence of LBP, with more opportunity for modifiable factors noticed for the severity outcomes. Data from this cohort provide further indication of the multi-factorial nature of the development of LBP as inconsistency in predictors seems to be the norm in the literature, [39,43,41,42,38,44,40]. In the event consistent factors are identified they often lack the magnitude to be considered as "definitive" predictors for the development of LBP.

Effective strategies for preventing LBP remain elusive. Back schools, lumbar supports, and ergonomic interventions have limited evidence for prevention [14,13,15] Education for primary prevention of LBP has received mixed support in trials; with support for psychosocial education [17], but not for biomedical or biomechanical based education programs [14]. Collectively the results from the current study and others investigating predictors of LBP [39,43,41,42,38,44,40] provide guidance for future primary prevention intervention strategies. It is clear from the assembled data that single modality approaches are not likely to be effective in preventing LBP, echoing expert and consensus opinion in this area [6,48]. A recommendation from the current study is that LBP prevention strategies will likely have to be contextual in nature, such that effective LBP prevention strategies for a military population may differ from one used for hospital nurses. For example, results from this military cohort suggest prevention of occurrence of LBP may be futile based on the lack of modifiable predictors, but there were some modifiable factors identified in a study of nurses [44]. Based on our data preventative interventions tailored at decreasing the severity of LBP or visits for health care seem feasible for the military, especially those that utilize general exercise approaches to target improving fitness levels and educational programs to improve back beliefs [17,23].

There are, of course, limitations to consider when interpreting results from this study. The primary limitation is the low follow up rate to our web based survey system (28.4%) which did not allow us to follow the entire cohort. We have identified differences in responders in a preliminary analysis at 1 year follow up [49] and these differences were confirmed in this paper with 2 year follow up. However we do not have specific reasons for the lack of response. It could be due to the wide geographic area of deployment for these Soldiers including areas that would not have ready email access. We did consider using estimation or imputation methods to account for these missing data. However our confidence in the validity of these techniques to provide additional information was low due to the follow up rate (not enough complete data to allow for estimation or imputation) and the aforementioned baseline differences between responders (data used for estimating or imputing) and non-responders. Therefore, a decision was made to report only the completed data and note the limitations of doing so, rather than taking on additional limitations inherent in estimating missing data in a situation like this.

The result of the low follow up rate highlights the difficulty of collecting complete data on inception cohorts for the development of LBP. Critical interpretation of our results hinges on the acknowledgment that responder bias may have had a profound impact on these analyses. There are numerous baseline differences in responders and non-responders and this is a concern. Many of these statistical differences were small in magnitude and likely a function of the high statistical power that accompanies a large sample. For example the age difference between responders and non-responders was 0.4 years corresponding to an effect size of 0.09 (Cohen's D). Such a small difference in age between responders and non responders is not likely to reflect responder bias for age, and there were similarly small differences for many of the other variables (Tables 1 and 2). Another issue to consider when determining the impact of the low follow up rate is that our methodology differed from other survey studies in that we had access to the entire sample at baseline (Figure 1). We were then able to determine differences between survey responders and non responders. This type of comparison is not an option in the more commonly incorporated design of surveying a larger group with the researchers only able to analyze data from responders. In the current study we had the advantage of being able to identify characteristics of non-responders so that the reader can make his/her own conclusions about the impact of responder bias. Unfortunately the definite quantitative impact of this responder bias for this study is impossible to estimate. In practical terms it means that these data can only be generalized to individuals that respond to survey requests, which makes it quite consistent with other studies in the literature that using this methodology.

Another consequence of this low follow up rate is that our estimates of LBP occurrence should not be mistaken for a true incidence estimate for this population. It is quite likely that the rate of LBP (42.1%) in this cohort is an overestimate of the actual incidence rate. Another potential limitation is that these analyses focused only on the first time episode of LBP. We did not consider recurrence in these analyses, but acknowledge that LBP is often a recurrent problem [50]. Finally another limitation to consider is the validity of self-report of LBP has been questioned for military populations as discrepancies were identified in indication of ever having LBP and scores on validated questionnaires (like the ODQ) [51]. This concern is mitigated somewhat in the current study because we didn't rely solely on one aspect of self-report, and instead included multiple validated questionnaires.

In conclusion, this military inception cohort provided information on baseline factors that were predictive of occurrence of LBP and severity. Our results confirm the multi-factorial nature of LBP as predictors of LBP occurrence and severity were neither consistent nor definitive. Future attempts at developing preventative strategies should consider these results and focus on multi-modal approaches that target modifiable risk factors specific to the population of interest.

Acknowledgments

The leadership, cadre, and students from the 232nd Medical Battalion and the 32nd Medical Brigade for their support and study participation.

Christopher Barnes, Yang Li, and Erik Henrickson for creation and management of the website and database and Jessica Neff for assistance with data entry and confirmation. Yunfeng Dai for assistance with statistical analyses.

Donna Cunningham for her administrative assistance and various physical therapy students from the U.S. Army-Baylor University, University of Texas Health Science Center at San Antonio, Texas State University, University of Puget Sound, East Tennessee State University, and University of Colorado at Denver and Health Science Center.

Author Contributions

Conceived and designed the experiments: SZG JDC DST MER. Performed the experiments: JDC DST ACW JLD. Analyzed the data: SSW. Wrote the paper: SZG JDC DST SSW MER.

References

1. Mantyselka P, Kumpusalo E, Ahonen R, Kumpusalo A, Kauhanen J, et al. (2001) Pain as a reason to visit the doctor: a study in Finnish primary health care. Pain 89: 175–180.

2. Walker BF, Muller R, Grant WD (2004) Low back pain in Australian adults: prevalence and associated disability. J Manipulative Physiol Ther 27: 238–244.

3. Stewart WF, Ricci JA, Chee E, Morganstein D, Lipton R (2003) Lost productive time and cost due to common pain conditions in the US workforce. JAMA 290: 2443–2454.

4. Cohen SP, Brown C, Kurihara C, Plunkett A, Nguyen C, et al. (2010) Diagnoses and factors associated with medical evacuation and return to duty for service members participating in Operation Iraqi Freedom or Operation Enduring Freedom: a prospective cohort study. Lancet 375: 301–309.

5. Lincoln AE, Smith GS, Amoroso PJ, Bell NS (2002) The natural history and risk factors of musculoskeletal conditions resulting in disability among US Army personnel. Work 18: 99–113.

6. Burton AK, Balague F, Cardon G, Eriksen HR, Henrotin Y, et al. (2005) How to prevent low back pain. Best Pract Res Clin Rheumatol 19: 541–555.

7. Cohen SP, Nguyen C, Kapoor SG, Anderson-Barnes VC, Foster L, et al. (2009) Back pain during war: an analysis of factors affecting outcome. Arch Intern Med 169: 1916–1923.

8. Frank JW, Brooker AS, DeMaio SE, Kerr MS, Maetzel A, et al. (1996) Disability resulting from occupational low back pain. Part II: What do we know about secondary prevention? A review of the scientific evidence on prevention after disability begins. Spine 21: 2918–2929.

9. Nicholas MK, Linton SJ, Watson PJ, Main CJ (2011) Early Identification and Management of Psychological Risk Factors ("Yellow Flags") in Patients With Low Back Pain: A Reappraisal. Phys Ther 91: 737–753.

10. Foster NE, Hill JC, Hay EM (2011) Subgrouping patients with low back pain in primary care: are we getting any better at it? Man Ther 16: 3–8.

11. Fritz JM, Cleland JA, Childs JD (2007) Subgrouping patients with low back pain: evolution of a classification approach to physical therapy. J Orthop Sports Phys Ther 37: 290–302.

12. Frank JW, Kerr MS, Brooker AS, DeMaio SE, Maetzel A, et al. (1996) Disability resulting from occupational low back pain. Part I: What do we know about primary prevention? A review of the scientific evidence on prevention before disability begins. Spine 21: 2908–2917.

13. Linton SJ, van Tulder MW (2001) Preventive interventions for back and neck pain problems: what is the evidence? Spine 26: 778–787.

14. Burton AK, Balague F, Cardon G, Eriksen HR, Henrotin Y, et al. (2006) Chapter 2. European guidelines for prevention in low back pain : November 2004. Eur Spine J 15 Suppl 2: S136–S168.

15. Bigos SJ, Holland J, Holland C, Webster JS, Battie M, et al. (2009) High-quality controlled trials on preventing episodes of back problems: systematic literature review in working-age adults. Spine J 9: 147–168.

16. George SZ, Childs JD, Teyhen DS, Wu SS, Wright AC, et al. (2007) Rationale, design, and protocol for the prevention of low back pain in the military (POLM) trial (NCT00373009). BMC Musculoskelet Disord 8: 92.

17. George SZ, Childs JD, Teyhen DS, Wu SS, Wright AC, et al. (2011) Brief psychosocial education, not core stabilization, reduced incidence of low back pain: results from the Prevention of Low Back Pain in the Military (POLM) cluster randomized trial. BMC Med 9: 128.

18. Childs JD, Teyhen DS, Benedict TM, Morris JB, Fortenberry AD, et al. (2009) Effects of sit-up training versus core stabilization exercises on sit-up performance. Med Sci Sports Exerc 41: 2072–2083.

19. Childs JD, Teyhen DS, Casey PR, Coy-Singh KA, Feldtmann AW, et al. (2010) Effects of traditional sit-up training versus core stabilization exercises on short-term musculoskeletal injuries in US Army soldiers: a cluster randomized trial. Phys Ther 90: 1404–1412.

20. Burton AK, Waddell G, Tillotson KM, Summerton N (1999) Information and advice to patients with back pain can have a positive effect. A randomized controlled trial of a novel educational booklet in primary care. Spine 24: 2484–2491.

21. Coudeyre E, Tubach F, Rannou F, Baron G, Coriat F, et al. (2007) Effect of a simple information booklet on pain persistence after an acute episode of low back pain: a non-randomized trial in a primary care setting. PLoS ONE 2: e706.

22. George SZ, Fritz JM, Bialosky JE, Donald DA (2003) The effect of a fear-avoidance-based physical therapy intervention for patients with acute low back pain: results of a randomized clinical trial. Spine 28: 2551–2560.

23. George SZ, Teyhen DS, Wu SS, Wright AC, Dugan JL, et al. (2009) Psychosocial education improves low back pain beliefs: results from a cluster randomized clinical trial (NCT00373009) in a primary prevention setting. Eur Spine J 18: 1050–1058.

24. Ware J, Jr., Kosinski M, Keller SD (1996) A 12-Item Short-Form Health Survey: construction of scales and preliminary tests of reliability and validity. Med Care 34: 220–233.

25. Symonds TL, Burton AK, Tillotson KM, Main CJ (1996) Do attitudes and beliefs influence work loss due to low back trouble? Occup Med (Lond) 46: 25–32.

26. Spielberger CD, Gorsuch RL, Lushene RE, Vagg PR, Jacobs GA (1983) Manual for the state and trait anxiety inventory (form Y) Consulting Psychologists Press, Palo Alto CA.

27. Whisman MA, Perez JE, Ramel W (2000) Factor structure of the Beck Depression Inventory-Second Edition (BDI-II) in a student sample. J Clin Psychol 56: 545–551.

28. Schotte CK, Maes M, Cluydts R, De Doncker D, Cosyns P (1997) Construct validity of the Beck Depression Inventory in a depressive population. J Affect Disord 46: 115–125.

29. Chibnall JT, Tait RC (1994) The short form of the Beck Depression Inventory: validity issues with chronic pain patients. Clin J Pain 10: 261–266.

30. McNeil DW, Rainwater AJ (1998) Development of the Fear of Pain Questionnaire-III. J Behav Med 21: 389–410.

31. Albaret MC, Munoz Sastre MT, Cottencin A, Mullet E (2004) The Fear of Pain questionnaire: factor structure in samples of young, middle-aged and elderly European people. Eur J Pain 8: 273–281.

32. Osman A, Breitenstein JL, Barrios FX, Gutierrez PM, Kopper BA (2002) The Fear of Pain Questionnaire-III: further reliability and validity with nonclinical samples. J Behav Med 25: 155–173.

33. Jensen MP, Turner JA, Romano JM (1994) What is the maximum number of levels needed in pain intensity measurement? Pain 58: 387–392.

34. Fairbank JC, Pynsent PB (2000) The Oswestry Disability Index. Spine 25: 2940–2953.

35. Roland M, Fairbank J (2000) The Roland-Morris Disability Questionnaire and the Oswestry Disability Questionnaire. Spine 25: 3115–3124.

36. Waddell G, Newton M, Henderson I, Somerville D, Main CJ (1993) A Fear-Avoidance Beliefs Questionnaire (FABQ) and the role of fear-avoidance beliefs in chronic low back pain and disability. Pain 52: 157–168.

37. Sullivan MJL, Bishop SR, Pivik J (1995) The Pain Catastrophizing Scale: development and validation. Psychological Assessment 7: 524–532.

38. Stevenson JM, Weber CL, Smith JT, Dumas GA, Albert WJ (2001) A longitudinal study of the development of low back pain in an industrial population. Spine 26: 1370–1377.

39. Croft PR, Papageorgiou AC, Thomas E, Macfarlane GJ, Silman AJ (1999) Short-term physical risk factors for new episodes of low back pain. Prospective evidence from the South Manchester Back Pain Study. Spine 24: 1556–1561.

40. Elders LA, Burdorf A (2004) Prevalence, incidence, and recurrence of low back pain in scaffolders during a 3-year follow-up study. Spine 29: E101–E106.

41. Park H, Sprince NL, Whitten PS, Burmeister LF, Zwerling C (2001) Risk factors for back pain among male farmers: analysis of Iowa Farm Family Health and Hazard Surveillance Study. Am J Ind Med 40: 646–654.

42. Power C, Frank J, Hertzman C, Schierhout G, Li L (2001) Predictors of low back pain onset in a prospective British study. Am J Public Health 91: 1671–1678.

43. Papageorgiou AC, Macfarlane GJ, Thomas E, Croft PR, Jayson MI, et al. (1997) Psychosocial factors in the workplace–do they predict new episodes of low back pain? Evidence from the South Manchester Back Pain Study. Spine 22: 1137–1142.

44. Yip VY (2004) New low back pain in nurses: work activities, work stress and sedentary lifestyle. J Adv Nurs 46: 430–440.

45. Cote P, Cassidy JD, Carroll L (2001) The treatment of neck and low back pain: who seeks care? who goes where? Med Care 39: 956–967.

46. Mortimer M, Ahlberg G (2003) To seek or not to seek? Care-seeking behaviour among people with low-back pain. Scand J Public Health 31: 194–203.

47. IJzelenberg W, Burdorf A (2004) Patterns of care for low back pain in a working population. Spine 29: 1362–1368.

48. Guzman J, Hayden J, Furlan AD, Cassidy JD, Loisel P, et al. (2007) Key factors in back disability prevention: a consensus panel on their impact and modifiability. Spine (Phila Pa 1976) 32: 807–815.

49. Childs JD, Teyhen DS, Van Wyngaarden JJ, Dougherty BF, Ladislas BJ, et al. (2011) Predictors of web-based follow-up response in the Prevention of Low Back Pain in the Military Trial (POLM). BMC Musculoskelet Disord 12: 132.

50. Carey TS, Garrett JM, Jackman A, Hadler N (1999) Recurrence and care seeking after acute back pain: results of a long-term follow-up study. North Carolina Back Pain Project. Med Care 37: 157–164.

51. Carragee EJ, Cohen SP (2009) Lifetime asymptomatic for back pain: the validity of self-report measures in soldiers. Spine (Phila Pa 1976) 34: 978–983.

Soft Tissue Artefacts of the Human Back: Comparison of the Sagittal Curvature of the Spine Measured Using Skin Markers and an Open Upright MRI

Roland Zemp[1], Renate List[1], Turgut Gülay[1], Jean Pierre Elsig[2], Jaroslav Naxera[3], William R. Taylor[1], Silvio Lorenzetti[1]*

1 Institute for Biomechanics, ETH Zurich, Zurich, Switzerland, **2** Spine Surgery, Küsnacht, Switzerland, **3** Röntgeninstitut Zurich-Altstetten, Zurich, Switzerland

Abstract

Soft tissue artefact affects the determination of skeletal kinematics. Thus, it is important to know the accuracy and limitations of kinematic parameters determined and modelled based on skin marker data. Here, the curvature angles, as well as the rotations of the lumbar and thoracic segments, of seven healthy subjects were determined in the sagittal plane using a skin marker set and compared to measurements taken in an open upright MRI scanner in order to understand the influence of soft tissue artefact at the back. The mean STA in the flexed compared to the extended positions were 10.2±6.1 mm (lumbar)/9.3±4.2 mm (thoracic) and 10.7±4.8 mm (lumbar)/9.2±4.9 mm (thoracic) respectively. A linear regression of the lumbar and thoracic curvatures between the marker-based measurements and MRI-based measurements resulted in coefficients of determination, R^2, of 0.552 and 0.385 respectively. Skin marker measurements therefore allow for the assessment of changes in the lumbar and thoracic curvature angles, but the absolute values suffer from uncertainty. Nevertheless, this marker set appears to be suitable for quantifying lumbar and thoracic spinal changes between quasi-static whole body postural changes.

Editor: Shao-Xiang Zhang, College of Basic Medical Science, Third Military Medical University, China

Funding: The authors have no support or funding to report.

Competing Interests: JN is an employee of Röntgeninstitut Zurich-Altstetten. There are no patents, products in development or marketed products to declare.

* E-mail: sl@ethz.ch

Introduction

Back pain is an increasingly common affliction, with approximately one-third of the population suffering from low back pain at any given time [1]. Kinematic parameters of the lumbar spine, such as the rate of angular rotation and linear displacement at the joints (L3/L4; L4/L5; L5/S1), especially during the onset of lumbar flexion, are useful for discriminating between individuals with and without low back pain [2]. While motion of the lumbar spine is accessible using video fluoroscopy [2–4], the approach is highly invasive and exposes subjects to unnecessary X-ray radiation [4]. Moreover, while novel dynamic and non-invasive approaches now exist for assessing functional motion of the back, even over extended periods of time [5–8], the accuracy of such methods for evaluating the underlying skeletal kinematics remains unknown.

In addition to instability and degeneration of supporting soft tissue structures, overloading is considered a main cause of low back pain due to a combination of cumulative or acute loads [9,10]. However, determination of the internal loading conditions requires knowledge of the spine's position and movement. While bone pins allow direct access to skeletal kinematics [11–13], they are only rarely used due to their invasive nature. Motion analysis, on the other hand, allows the non-invasive investigation of motion patterns [14]. However, while skin markers are easy to apply and rarely limit the subject's movement, they are affected by soft tissue artefact (STA), which results from motion of the skin relative to the underlying bones due to inertial effects, skin elasticity and deformation caused by muscle contraction [15–17]. STA occurs in all directions, and the distributions are known to be non-uniform [18].

To obtain an understanding of the accuracy of skin markers for assessing spinal kinematics, a marker set has been developed that allows global parameters of curvature angles [19–25] and back segment rotations [26–30] to be investigated [31]. However, the accuracy and precision of these analyses remain unknown. Several studies have validated skin markers on different body regions [18,32–38], but validation studies of back markers are rare [26–28,39,40] (Table 1), and few have been validated against global spinal shape, including spinal segment curvature or rotations.

Using open MRI and skin markers, the goal of this study was to determine the magnitude and direction of STA on the back and compare the spinal curvature and segment angles. We then examined whether the shape of the spine (lumbar and thoracic curvature angle and lumbar and thoracic segment rotation in the sagittal plane) can be measured with sufficient accuracy to determine spinal shape between posture changes or during quasi-static movements using skin markers.

Table 1. Literature summary of the soft tissue artefact of different body locations.

Body location	Author	Soft tissue artefact	Motion
Foot	Tranberg and Karlsson [34]	Up to 4.3 mm	Static weight-bearing position
	Maslen and Ackland [35]	Mean marker error up to 14.9 mm	Static weight-bearing position
Shank	Gao and Zheng [18]	Inter-marker movement up to 9.3 mm	Level walking
	Garling et al. [36]	Up to 11 mm	Step up
	Sangeux et al. [32]	Up to 7 mm	Static non-weight-bearing; knee flexion between 0° and 90°
Thigh	Gao and Zheng [18]	Inter-marker movement up to 19.1 mm	Level walking
	Garling et al. [36]	Up to 17 mm	Step up
	Sangeux et al. [32]	Up to 22 mm	Static non-weight-bearing; knee flexion between 0° and 90°
	Akbarshahi et al. [38]	RMSE up to 29.3 mm around the knee joint	Functional activity: open-chain knee flexion, hip axial rotation, level walking, step up
Scapula	Matsui et al. [33]	Mean marker error of about 67 mm	Arm elevation
Finger	Ryu et al. [37]	Up to 10.9 mm	Hand flexion
Back	Morl and Blickhan [39]	Up to 9.86 mm at lumbar levels L3 and L4	Rotated seating: shoulder turned approximately 90° with respect to the pelvis
	Heneghan and Balanos [40]	Up to 16 mm at thoracic levels (T1, T6, T12)	35° of axial rotation in a seated upright position
		Up to 1.5 mm at thoracic levels (T1, T6, T12)	Single arm elevation in a seated upright position
Trunk	This study	Up to 27.4 mm	Static sitting position

Methods

Accuracy of the marker and vertebra positions using MRI

The accuracy of assessing vertebral location using MRI was determined using a plate of acrylic glass with five MRI-visible skin markers (paintballs) and two lamb vertebrae (Figure 1). The paintballs were placed into precision-drilled holes (±0.1 mm) in each of the four corners and middle of the plate. The two vertebrae were glued onto the plate between the markers. The plate was then examined using an open MRI (Upright Multi-Position MRI; 0.6 Tesla; Fonar Corporation, Melville, USA) in horizontal (0°), forward tilted (45°) and vertical (90°) positions in order to quantify the accuracy of the marker and vertebrae locations as well as the orientation of each vertebrae base plate plane (BPP) relative to horizontal.

Subjects

Seven healthy subjects (three female; average age 29 y (range 22–46); height 174 cm (160–184); mass 71 kg (55–96)) provided written informed consent to participate in this pilot study that was approved by the local ethics committee. Subject recruitment was achieved through voluntary participation after public poster advertising. The participant on Figure 2 has seen this manuscript and figure and has provided written informed consent for its use in publication. A wide range of subject height and weight was chosen in order to exemplarily investigate the range of kinematics that could be observed within a broad population. A power analysis (one-tailed paired t-test, $\alpha = 0.05$, $\beta = 0.1$) performed using a statistical software package (G*Power 3.1.3) [41], based on the determined accuracy of the acrylic plate measuring system (SD of the curvature angle due to the measurement system: 3.6°) and one test measurement (difference in lumbar curvature angle between the upright and extended position: 8°) with an effect size dz of

1.571 (where $dz = \dfrac{8°}{\sqrt{2} * 3.6°}$) revealed a minimum subject number of six with a power level of 0.948.

Instrumentation

T2-weighted sagittal images were taken with a repetition time of 2750 ms, an echo time of 110 ms and a layer thickness of 4 mm. The resolution was 240×240 in an image plane of 360×360 mm, providing a voxel size of $1.5*1.5*4$ mm^3. The layers were ranked without any gaps between the marginal markers. As a consequence, the lumbar and thoracic regions required approximately 35 and 50 images respectively, corresponding to a measurement time of approximately seven minutes for each posture.

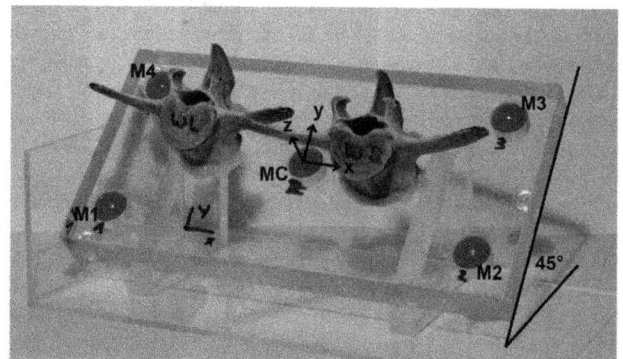

Figure 1. Acrylic glass plate with five MRI visible markers (paintballs: M1, M2, M3, M4, MC, with distances of M1–M2 = 180 mm, M2–M3 = 70 mm) and two lamb vertebrae, shown in the forward tilted position (45°).

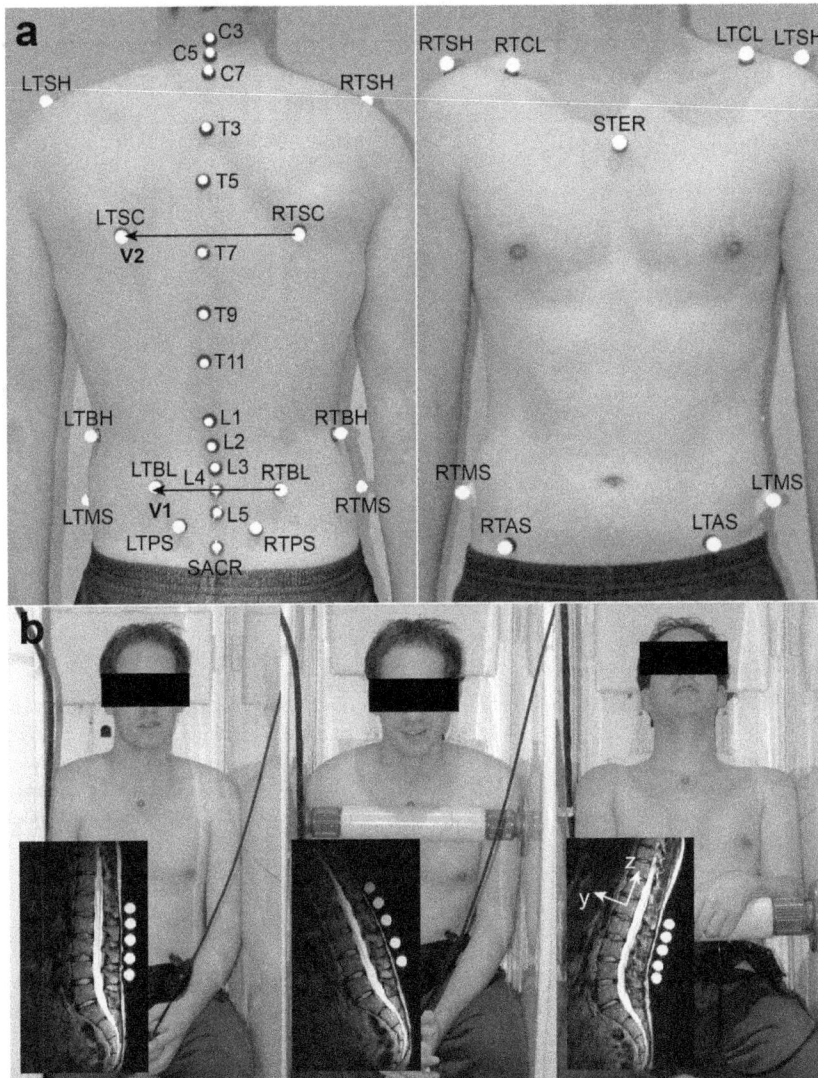

Figure 2. Measurement set-up including (a) the "IfB-marker-set" of the trunk and the pelvis (for explanation of abbreviations and for segmental allocation, see Table 2) and (b) the three analysed seating positions with an example of a corresponding MR image including a local coordinate system of a vertebral body. Upright seating position: lower spine had partial contact with the backrest, and the whole upper body was in an upright position. Flexed seating position: upper body was tilted about 30° forward and supported on a bar, while the arms were rested on their lap. Extended seating position: the subject's bottom was pushed approximately 20 cm forward and the head was supported by the backrest. (from left to right).

Marker set

Based on our whole body "IfB-marker-set" [42–47] (Figure 2a), only the markers for the lumbar and thoracic segments were used (Table 2). The markers were MRI-visible commercial paintballs (BrassEagle Wild Streak Paintballs, diameter 17.3 mm), which consisted of a dyed liquid surrounded by a thin gelatin shell. After palpation, performed in an upright standing position, the markers were mounted on washers and were fixed to the skin using a toupee plaster. In order to provide support during sitting while preventing marker contact with the backrest, two foam tubes were attached to the paraspinal muscle bellies. The subjects' lumbar and thoracic spines were then measured in the MRI in upright, flexed and extended seating positions (Figure 2b).

Data analysis

The MR images were manually segmented using Avizo (v5.1, Mercury Computer Systems Inc., Burlington, USA). Spheres were fitted to the markers (Geomagic Studio, v9, Raindrop Geomagic, USA), and the normal vector of each vertebral body's BPP and centre of gravity (CoG) were determined.

Data analysis was performed using MATLAB (vR2010a, MathWorks Inc., Natick, USA). STA was described by changes in the vectors pointing from the vertebral bodies' CoG to the corresponding marker. The normal vector of the BPP defined the cranial (z) axis of each vertebral body coordinate system. As an exception, due to increased segmentation stability, the z-axis of the fifth lumbar vertebra was determined using the upper plate, and rotated accordingly. The y-axis was the cross-product of the z-vector with the unit vector in the anterior-posterior direction of the

Table 2. Marker placement, segment allocation and abbreviations.

Abbreviations	Marker placement	Segment allocation
RTSH, LTSH	Right and left acromion	Upper trunk segment
RTCL, LTCL	Right and left clavicula	
C7	7th cervical vertebrae	
C3, C5	3rd, 5th cervical vertebrae	
STER	Sternum	Thoracic segment
RTSC, LTSC	Right and left inferior angle of the scapula	
RTBH, LTBH	Right and left most inferior rib	
T3, T5, T7, T9, T11	3rd, 5th, 7th, 9th, 11th thoracic vertebrae	
RTBL, LTBL	Right and left lateral back on height of L4	Lumbar Segment
L1, L2, L3, L4, L5	1st, 2nd, 3rd, 4th, 5th lumbar vertebrae	
RTAS, LTAS	Right and left anterior superior iliac spine	Pelvic segment
RTPS, LTPS	Right and left posterior superior iliac spine	
RTMS, LTMS	Right and left mid superior iliac spine	
SACR	Sacrum	

MRI, and the x-axis was defined by the normalised cross-product of the y and z vectors (Figure 2b). Each local coordinate system was located at the CoG of the respective vertebral body. The vectors from the vertebral bodies' CoG to the corresponding markers were constructed using the local coordinate systems. The differences between this vector in the upright and the flexed or extended seating positions described the magnitude and direction of STA of each marker on the spinous process.

To determine the curvature angles [48] of the lumbar (α_{lumbar}) and thoracic ($\alpha_{thoracic}$) spines, the sagittal planes of the spines were defined normal to the vectors from RTBL to LTBL (V_1) and from RTSC to LTSC (V_2) respectively (Figure 2a). The position vectors of the markers and the vertebral bodies were projected onto this plane. Circles [49] were created for the lumbar and thoracic spines that best fitted the CoGs of L1–L5, and T3, T5, T7, T9 & T11 respectively. α_{lumbar} was then calculated as the angle between the two radius vectors from the circle centre to the CoG of L1 and L5, and $\alpha_{thoracic}$ accordingly as the angle between the radius vectors T3 & T11. The same angles were calculated for the corresponding lumbar and thoracic markers. Kyphosis was defined as a positive angle ($\alpha > 0$).

To analyse the accuracy with which the skin markers were able to represent the rotation of the vertebral bodies, the mean sagittal rotation error (ESR) of the lumbar and thoracic segments (Table 2) was calculated. Marker cloud registration was performed using a least squares method[41]. The sagittal rotation of the lumbar and thoracic segments was calculated between the corresponding marker cloud in the upright and compared to the flexed or extended positions. Here, the rotation of each vertebral section was calculated using a 3D regression line, fitted through the vertebral CoGs, and compared against the rigid rotation of the relevant marker cloud.

Due to the large radius of the paintballs, some lumbar markers of subjects 3, 4, and 7 touched each other in the extended seating position and it was not possible to analyse these MR images. Owing to image blur as a result of body movement during the measurements, the thoracic MR images of subject 2 in the flexed seating position were not taken into account for the analysis.

Statistics

All statistics were determined using IBM SPSS Statistics (v19, SPSS Inc., Chicago, USA). Statistical significance was defined as $p < 0.05$. The absolute marker artefact was analysed using analyses of variance (ANOVA) for the subjects, positions and marker locations. Furthermore, correlations between the curvature angles based on the marker and vertebral body coordinates were investigated using linear regression analysis.

Results

Accuracy of the marker and vertebra positions using MRI

The accuracy of the MRI and the image segmentation was similar to that of a conventional motion capture system. Based on the mean error between different markers on the acrylic plate (0.6 ± 0.5 mm) and between the vertebral CoGs and the markers (1.1 ± 1.1 mm), the direction-related measurement uncertainties (σ_x, σ_y, σ_z) of the markers were (1.0 mm, 0.5 mm, 0.5 mm) and for the vertebral bodies (2.0 mm, 1.0 mm, 1.0 mm). The orientation of the BPP relative to horizontal varied by up to 2.7°. The mean error was 1.6 ± 1.2°.

Subject measurements

The mean STA in the flexed and extended positions were 10.2 ± 6.1 mm (lumbar)/9.3 ± 4.2 mm (thoracic) and 10.7 ± 4.8 mm/9.2 ± 4.9 mm respectively. The largest STA was 27.4 mm for marker SPL5 in the flexed position. The STA was significantly different between subjects ($p < 0.001$ lumbar and thoracic), but no differences were observed for either markers ($p = 0.604$ lumbar, $p = 0.404$ thoracic) or seating positions ($p = 0.428$ lumbar, $p = 0.926$ thoracic) (Table 3). The subject's mean STA of the lumbar and thoracic markers as well as the flexed and extended positions varied between 6.2 mm and 13.2 mm for the seven subjects with a BMI between 20.6 kg/m^2 and 30.3 kg/m^2. However, no clear relationship between STA and BMI was observed.

The lumbar (α_{lumbar}) and thoracic curvature angles ($\alpha_{thoracic}$) calculated using the markers and the vertebral bodies revealed no clear correlation ($R^2 = 0.552$ (lumbar); $R^2 = 0.385$ (thoracic); Figure 3). The root mean square errors (RMSEs) of the differences

Table 3. Direction-related (r_x, r_y, r_z) mean marker artefact (mean) and the absolute values ($|r|$) with their standard deviations (SD) of the lumbar and thoracic skin markers in the flexed and extended positions.

	Marker	Flexion [mm]			
		r_x (mean (SD))	r_y (mean (SD))	r_z (mean (SD))	$|r|$ (mean (SD))
Thoracic	SPT1 (T3)	0.6 (1.8)	0.1 (1.3)	5.1 (2.3)	5.4 (2.0)
	SPT2 (T5)	0.0 (4.4)	0.1 (2.3)	−3.1 (4.8)	6.7 (2.4)
	SPT3 (T7)	0.4 (3.7)	1.4 (2.3)	−8.0 (4.8)	8.9 (5.0)
	SPT4 (T9)	2.9 (4.5)	2.2 (4.2)	−10.4 (1.4)	12.2 (2.7)
	SPT5 (T11)	0.1 (4.8)	1.7 (6.6)	−7.2 (5.1)	10.7 (4.6)
Lumbar	SPL1 (L1)	−1.8 (2.7)	−1.7 (2.7)	−7.1 (3.4)	8.5 (3.0)
	SPL2 (L2)	−2.6 (3.6)	−1.8 (2.2)	−6.2 (5.2)	8.4 (4.4)
	SPL3 (L3)	−3.7 (4.0)	−1.7 (2.9)	−7.1 (7.6)	10.1 (6.4)
	SPL4 (L4)	−3.9 (4.8)	−2.6 (2.7)	−6.2 (9.6)	10.7 (7.7)
	SPL5 (L5)	−4.1 (5.6)	−2.6 (3.8)	−9.1 (10.0)	13.2 (8.2)
	Marker	Extension [mm]			
		r_x (mean (SD))	r_y (mean (SD))	r_z (mean (SD))	$|r|$ (mean (SD))
Thoracic	SPT1 (T3)	2.0 (1.6)	2.2 (3.4)	3.4 (9.1)	8.0 (6.4)
	SPT2 (T5)	−0.6 (3.1)	0.7 (4.9)	2.9 (9.4)	9.3 (5.7)
	SPT3 (T7)	0.2 (6.0)	−3.3 (3.9)	−2.3 (8.9)	10.3 (5.2)
	SPT4 (T9)	2.7 (4.9)	0.8 (2.4)	−5.7 (7.9)	10.0 (5.0)
	SPT5 (T11)	−0.1 (4.3)	1.4 (2.4)	−4.1 (6.4)	8.0 (3.7)
Lumbar	SPL1 (L1)	−1.1 (2.3)	0.8 (1.4)	10.3 (6.3)	10.6 (6.3)
	SPL2 (L2)	−2.2 (2.1)	2.7 (2.6)	8.5 (5.8)	10.1 (4.6)
	SPL3 (L3)	−2.8 (3.3)	2.9 (7.3)	8.2 (7.6)	12.1 (6.2)
	SPL4 (L4)	−3.8 (2.1)	2.4 (2.6)	9.5 (7.7)	11.8 (5.8)
	SPL5 (L5)	−4.8 (2.0)	3.7 (2.9)	1.0 (6.4)	8.8 (1.1)

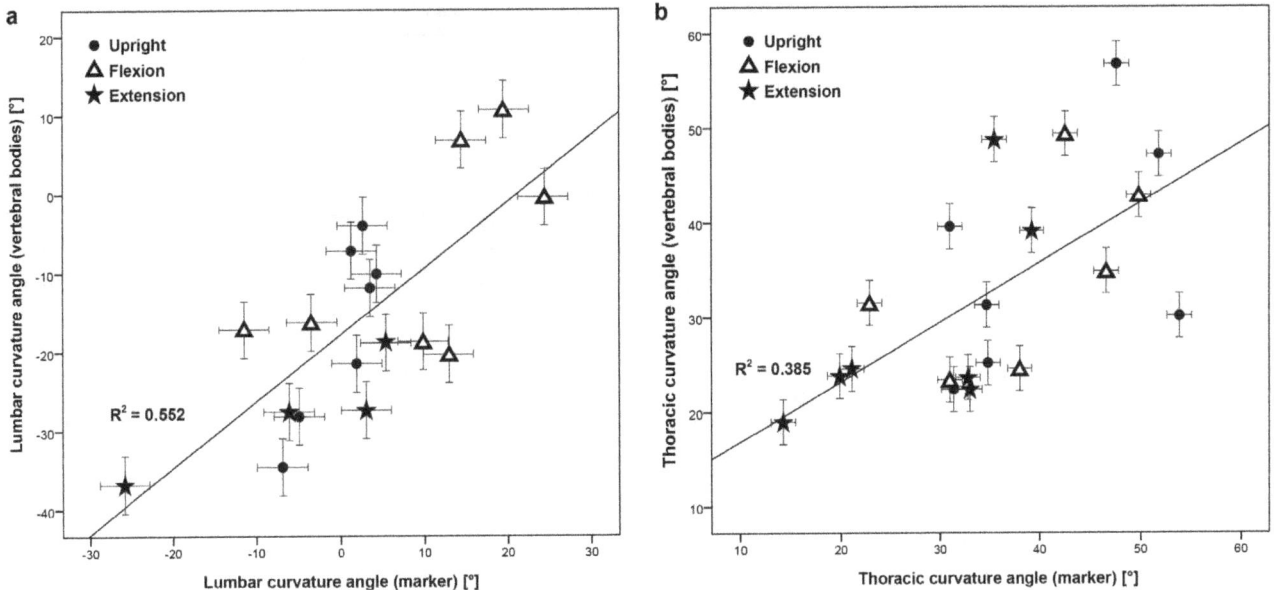

Figure 3. Scatter diagram of the lumbar (a) and thoracic curvature angle (b) in the upright (circle), flexed (triangle) and extended positions (star). The x-axis represents the values calculated from the markers, and the y-axis from the vertebral bodies. The crosses show the open MRI's measurement uncertainty of the curvature angles calculated from the markers (x-axis) and calculated from the vertebral bodies (y-axis).

Table 4. Mean (SD) lumbar (α_{lumbar}) and thoracic curvature angle ($\alpha_{thoracic}$) in the upright, flexed and extended sitting positions calculated with the vertebral bodies and the skin marker, as well as the mean differences (SD; RMSE) between the values from the skin marker and the vertebral bodies.

	Upright		Flexion		Extension	
	Vertebral bodies	**Marker**	**Vertebral bodies**	**Marker**	**Vertebral bodies**	**Marker**
	Difference		**Difference**		**Difference**	
α_{lumbar} [°]	−16.8 (11.5)	0.3 (4.3)	−7.9 (13.2)	9.4 (12.6)	−27.7 (7.3)	−5.9 (14.2)
	17.1 (8.0; 18.6)		17.3 (11.2; 20.2)		21.8 (8.1; 22.9)	
$\alpha_{thoracic}$ [°]	36.0 (12.4)	40.7 (10.0)	34.4 (10.2)	38.5 (10.1)	28.7 (10.9)	27.9 (9.4)
	4.7 (11.4; 11.5)		4.0 (9.4; 9.5)		−0.8 (8.3; 7.8)	

between the curvature angles determined by the markers and by the vertebral bodies were approximately two times higher for the lumbar spine than the thoracic spine (Table 4). The lumbar curvature angles from the upright to the flexed and extended positions showed the same sign in six of the seven subjects and three of the four subjects respectively, whereas the sign of the thoracic curvature angle was the same in all subjects (Figure 4).

The ESR of the lumbar and thoracic segments calculated using the skin markers were $2.5\pm2.7°$ (RMSE: 3.6°) and $-1.1\pm2.9°$ (RMSE: 3.0°) respectively. The largest ESRs were 6.6° (lumbar) and 9.1° (thoracic).

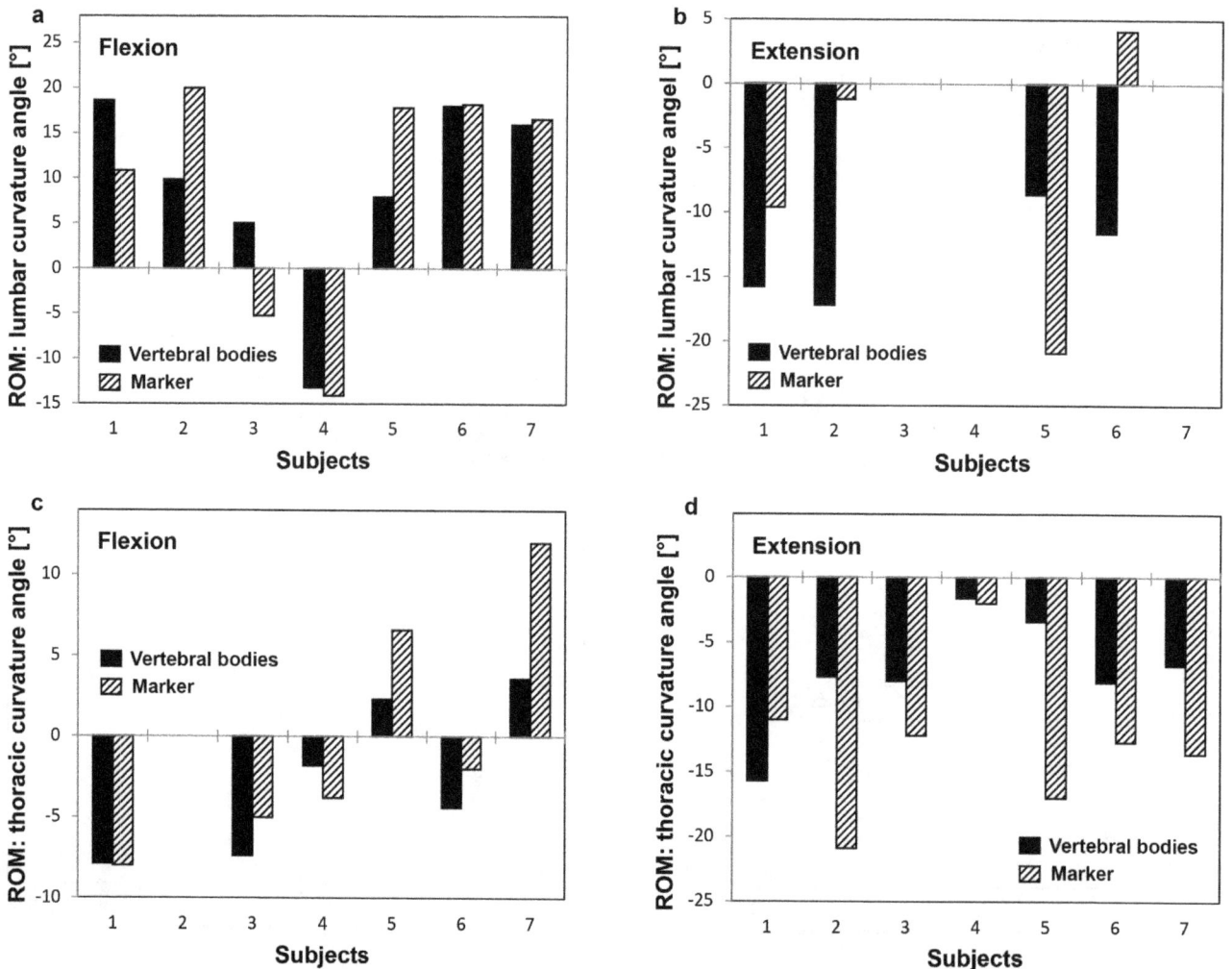

Figure 4. Range of lumbar (a/b) and thoracic (c/d) curvature angle of the subjects, calculated using the vertebral bodies (black) and the skin markers (hatched). The range was defined from the upright to the flexed (a/c) and to the extended positions (c/d).

Discussion

While the exact motion of the vertebrae remains unclear without the use of invasive approaches, knowledge on the accuracy of skin markers for assessing skeletal kinematics provides a baseline for identifying situations where non-invasive approaches are appropriate, and where not [50]. The measurement uncertainty of our MRI-based measurement system was similar to those of a typical motion capture system (1.5 mm) [51], with out-of-plane error about double the in-plane error. Analysis of the back STA produced similar results to those observed in other studies [39,40] and also for other body parts (Table 1). The observed intra- and inter-individual patterns of STA during flexion and extension did not allow the determination of a common correction method by which to estimate the behaviour of single markers. In general, the inter-individual differences were larger than the differences within a single subject - a result that is in agreement with results from studies on the knee joint [36]. Knowledge of the influence of STA when using skin markers is required to ensure compensation for the largest error sources [16,52,53].

The present study only allowed the quantification of STA in a static set-up. However, we must be conscious of the fact that the spinal movement differs from other skeletal joints e.g. the hip or the knee, since the spine consists of several segments that allow movement relative to one another, including a different range of motion (ROM) in several planes. The present study only allowed the quantification of STA in a static set-up. It must be assumed that during dynamic activities, and especially impact situations, STA is even larger. For example, Akbarshahi and co-workers [38] found much larger marker STA during functional activities than Sangeux et al. [32], who used a static set-up (Table 1). Therefore, studies using static measurements seem to underestimate the magnitude of STA, possibly by a factor of two or more.

Due to the fact that the power analysis in this study was based on measurements using lamb vertebrae, the actual study in humans may require additional subjects to ensure sufficient power, due to secondary errors such as unintentional movements during MRI scanning. However, as a result of this power analysis, relatively few subjects were recruited into this study, and it was not possible to observe any clear relationships between STA and e.g. age, gender, height or material properties of the soft tissues. It is, of course, entirely possible that these or other subject-specific factors contribute to the magnitude of STA on the back. Here, it is quite conceivable for example that the individual elastic properties of the soft tissues have a strong influence on the magnitude of STA; such observations have been reported at other regions of the body (thigh) by Kratzenstein and co-workers [52], who also demonstrated locally varying STA, which was mainly attributed to muscle contraction and skin elasticity. In addition, no relationship between the levels of STA and BMI were observed in our study, but this could also be an artefact of the low number of subjects in our cohort. However, this finding is consistent with studies that used fluoroscopy [36] or bone pins [54] to examine the role of soft tissues on the underlying skeletal kinematics. Increasing the number of subjects could allow a better understanding of the relationships between BMI, age, gender, height or material properties of the soft tissues, but this was not the focus of the current study. In order to establish the influence of such subject-specific factors on STA, further research would be required in specific homogenous cohorts.

Since the correlations between the spinal curvature calculated from the skin markers and the vertebral bodies for each position (upright, flexion, extension) as well as for all positions together were low (Figure 3: $R^2 = 0.552$ (lumbar), $R^2 = 0.385$ (thoracic)), results that examine the lumbar and thoracic curvature angles by means of skin markers should be interpreted cautiously. This was possibly due to the fact that the anatomical distance and the material properties of the musculoskeletal tissues between the markers and CoG are generally not constant, resulting in inhomogenous deformation between the different positions. However, the range of curvature angles exhibited the same sign when comparing the upright with the flexed and the extended seating positions in 22 out of the 24 cases (Figure 4). Due to the fact that the range of curvature calculated from the skin markers did not consistently over- or underestimate that calculated from the vertebral bodies within subjects, positions or spinal segment, there is no clear method to enhance the accuracy of skin marker estimations through automated correction.

To summarise, the results of our study indicate that a change of lordotic/kyphotic shape, but not of the absolute amount of curvature, can be estimated using skin markers. Based on these findings, the use of the presented back marker set for analysing spinal motion seems to be as accurate as estimations of skeletal kinematics in the lower extremities (Table 1). Changes of the lumbar and thoracic curvature angle are measurable in the sagittal plane using the presented marker set, but measurement of the absolute curvature angles appears to be limited when using skin markers. These limitations associated with STA must be taken into account during non-invasive assessment of back motion before an improved understanding of the kinematics of subjects with and without back pain can be gained.

Acknowledgments

We would like to thank the technical support of Kerstin Wenker at the Upright MRI Center Zürich. **Ethics**: This study was approved by the ethics committee of the ETH Zürich under the number: EK 2010-N-43.

Author Contributions

Conceived and designed the experiments: RZ SL. Performed the experiments: RZ JPE JN. Analyzed the data: RZ RL TG JN JPE WRT SL. Contributed reagents/materials/analysis tools: JN JPE. Wrote the paper: RZ RL TG WRT SL.

References

1. McBeth J, Jones K (2007) Epidemiology of chronic musculoskeletal pain. Best Pract Res Clin Rheumatol 21: 403–425.
2. Teyhen DS, Flynn TW, Childs JD, Kuklo TR, Rosner MK, et al. (2007) Fluoroscopic video to identify aberrant lumbar motion. Spine (Phila Pa 1976) 32: E220–229.
3. Lee SW, Wong KW, Chan MK, Yeung HM, Chiu JL, et al. (2002) Development and validation of a new technique for assessing lumbar spine motion. Spine (Phila Pa 1976) 27: E215–220.
4. Teyhen DS, Flynn TW, Bovik AC, Abraham LD (2005) A new technique for digital fluoroscopic video assessment of sagittal plane lumbar spine motion. Spine (Phila Pa 1976) 30: E406–413.
5. Consmuller T, Rohlmann A, Weinland D, Druschel C, Duda GN, et al. (2012) Comparative evaluation of a novel measurement tool to assess lumbar spine posture and range of motion. Eur Spine J 21: 2170–2180.
6. Consmuller T, Rohlmann A, Weinland D, Druschel C, Duda GN, et al. (2012) Velocity of lordosis angle during spinal flexion and extension. PLoS One 7: e50135.
7. Consmuller T, Rohlmann A, Weinland D, Schmidt H, Zippelius T, et al. (2013) Automatic distinction of upper body motions in the main anatomical planes. Med Eng Phys.
8. Taylor WR, Consmuller T, Rohlmann A (2010) A novel system for the dynamic assessment of back shape. Med Eng Phys 32: 1080–1083.
9. Kumar S (1990) Cumulative Load as a Risk Factor for Back Pain. Spine 15: 1311–1316.

10. Hoogendoorn WE, van Poppel MNM, Bongers PM, Koes BW, Bouter LM (1999) Physical load during work and leisure time as risk factors for back pain. Scandinavian Journal of Work Environment & Health 25: 387–403.

11. Rozumalski A, Schwartz MH, Wervey R, Swanson A, Dykes DC, et al. (2008) The in vivo three-dimensional motion of the human lumbar spine during gait. Gait Posture 28: 378–384.

12. Kramers-de Quervain IA, Baumgartner W, Stüssi E, Grob D (2001) Segmental motion of L3/4 and L4/5 of the lumbar spine during stair ambulation. 18th Conference of the International Society of Biomechanics Zürich, Switzerland.

13. Baumgartner W, Grob D, Kramers-de Quervain IA, Stüssi E (2001) Novel in vivo motion analysis of the healthy lower lumbar spine during standardized movements and complex daily activities. 18th Conference of the International Society of Biomechanics Zürich, Switzerland.

14. Telfer S, Morlan G, Hyslop E, Semple R, Rafferty D, et al. (2010) A novel device for improving marker placement accuracy. Gait Posture 32: 536–539.

15. Cappozzo A, Catani F, Leardini A, Benedetti MG, Croce UD (1996) Position and orientation in space of bones during movement: experimental artefacts. Clin Biomech (Bristol, Avon) 11: 90–100.

16. Taylor WR, Ehrig RM, Duda GN, Schell H, Seebeck P, et al. (2005) On the influence of soft tissue coverage in the determination of bone kinematics using skin markers. J Orthop Res 23: 726–734.

17. Leardini A, Chiari L, Della Croce U, Cappozzo A (2005) Human movement analysis using stereophotogrammetry. Part 3. Soft tissue artifact assessment and compensation. Gait Posture 21: 212–225.

18. Gao B, Zheng N (2008) Investigation of soft tissue movement during level walking: Translations and rotations of skin markers. Journal of Biomechanics 41: 3189–3195.

19. Leitkam ST, Bush TR, Li M (2011) A methodology for quantifying seated lumbar curvatures. J Biomech Eng 133: 114502.

20. Keller TS, Colloca CJ, Harrison DE, Harrison DD, Janik TJ (2005) Influence of spine morphology on intervertebral disc loads and stresses in asymptomatic adults: implications for the ideal spine. Spine J 5: 297–309.

21. Wojtys EM, Ashton-Miller JA, Huston LJ, Moga PJ (2000) The association between athletic training time and the sagittal curvature of the immature spine. American Journal of Sports Medicine 28: 490–498.

22. Amonookuofi HS (1992) Changes in the Lumbosacral Angle, Sacral Inclination and the Curvature of the Lumbar Spine during Aging. Acta Anatomica 145: 373–377.

23. Norton BJ, Sahrmann SA, Van Dillen LR (2004) Differences in measurements of lumbar curvature related to gender and low back pain. Journal of Orthopaedic & Sports Physical Therapy 34: 524–534.

24. Bae TS, Mun M (2010) Effect of lumbar lordotic angle on lumbosacral joint during isokinetic exercise: a simulation study. Clin Biomech (Bristol, Avon) 25: 628–635.

25. Frigo C, Carabalona R, Dalla Mura M, Negrini S (2003) The upper body segmental movements during walking by young females. Clin Biomech (Bristol, Avon) 18: 419–425.

26. Bull AM, McGregor AH (2000) Measuring spinal motion in rowers: the use of an electromagnetic device. Clin Biomech (Bristol, Avon) 15: 772–776.

27. Wu SK, Lan HH, Kuo LC, Tsai SW, Chen CL, et al. (2007) The feasibility of a video-based motion analysis system in measuring the segmental movements between upper and lower cervical spine. Gait Posture 26: 161–166.

28. Bull AMJ, Holt PJ, Wragg P, McGregor AH (2004) Validation of the use of a skin-mounted device to measure out-of-plane rotations of the spine for a rowing activity. Journal of Musculoskeletal Research 08: 129–132.

29. Syczewska M, Oberg T, Karlsson D (1999) Segmental movements of the spine during treadmill walking with normal speed. Clin Biomech (Bristol, Avon) 14: 384–388.

30. Crosbie J, Vachalathiti R, Smith R (1997) Age, gender and speed effects on spinal kinematics during walking. Gait Posture 5: 13–20.

31. List R, Gülay T, Lorenzetti S (2010) Kinematics of the trunk and the spine during unrestricted and restricted squats - A preliminary analysis. XXVIIIth International Congress of Biomechanics in Sports. Marquette: ISBS. pp. 4 pages.

32. Sangeux M, Marin F, Charleux F, Durselen L, Ho Ba Tho MC (2006) Quantification of the 3D relative movement of external marker sets vs. bones based on magnetic resonance imaging. Clin Biomech (Bristol, Avon) 21: 984–991.

33. Matsui K, Shimada K, Andrew PD (2006) Deviation of skin marker from bone target during movement of the scapula. J Orthop Sci 11: 180–184.

34. Tranberg R, Karlsson D (1998) The relative skin movement of the foot: a 2-D roentgen photogrammetry study. Clin Biomech (Bristol, Avon) 13: 71–76.

35. Maslen BA, Ackland TR (1994) Radiographic Study of Skin Displacement Errors in the Foot and Ankle during Standing. Clinical Biomechanics 9: 291–296.

36. Garling EH, Kaptein BL, Mertens B, Barendregt W, Veeger HE, et al. (2007) Soft-tissue artefact assessment during step-up using fluoroscopy and skin-mounted markers. J Biomech 40 Suppl 1: S18–24.

37. Ryu JH, Miyata N, Kouchi M, Mochimaru M, Lee KH (2006) Analysis of skin movement with respect to flexional bone motion using MR images of a hand. J Biomech 39: 844–852.

38. Akbarshahi M, Schache AG, Fernandez JW, Baker R, Banks S, et al. (2010) Non-invasive assessment of soft-tissue artifact and its effect on knee joint kinematics during functional activity. J Biomech 43: 1292–1301.

39. Morl F, Blickhan R (2006) Three-dimensional relation of skin markers to lumbar vertebrae of healthy subjects in different postures measured by open MRI. Eur Spine J 15: 742–751.

40. Heneghan NR, Balanos GM (2010) Soft tissue artefact in the thoracic spine during axial rotation and arm elevation using ultrasound imaging: a descriptive study. Man Ther 15: 599–602.

41. Faul F, Erdfelder E, Buchner A, Lang AG (2009) Statistical power analyses using G*Power 3.1: tests for correlation and regression analyses. Behav Res Methods 41: 1149–1160.

42. Dettwyler MT (2005) Biomechanische Untersuchungen und Modellierungen am menschlichen oberen Sprunggelenk im Hinblick auf Arthroplasiken. PhD thesis, ETH Zürich.

43. List R (2005) A hybrid marker set: for future basic research and instrumented gait analysis at the Laboratory for biomechanics. Thesis, ETH Zürich.

44. Unternährer S (2005) Entwicklung eines Markersets für Rückfuss und Vorfuss. Thesis, ETH Zürich.

45. Stoop M (2009) Biomechanik der Kniebeuge: Berechnung der Kräfte und Drehmomente am Knie- und Hüftgelelnk in Abhängigkeit der Bewegungsausführung. Thesis, ETH Zürich.

46. Gülay T, List R, Lorenzetti S (2011) Moments in the knee and hip during descent and ascent of squats. 29th Conference of the International Society of Biomechanics in Sports Porto, Portugal.

47. Lorenzetti S, Gulay T, Stoop M, List R, Gerber H, et al. (2012) Comparison of the angles and corresponding moments in the knee and hip during restricted and unrestricted squats. J Strength Cond Res 26: 2829–2836.

48. Baumgartner D, Zemp R, List R, Stoop M, Naxera J, et al. (2012) The spinal curvature of three different sitting positions analysed in an open MRI scanner. ScientificWorldJournal 2012: 184016.

49. Pratt V (1987) Direct Least-Squares Fitting of Algebraic Surfaces. Computer Graphics 21: 145–152.

50. List R, Gulay T, Stoop M, Lorenzetti S (2012) Kinematics of the Trunk and the Lower Extremities during Restricted and Unrestricted Squats. J Strength Cond Res.

51. Barker S, Craik R, Freedman W, Herrmann N, Hillstrom H (2006) Accuracy, reliability, and validity of a spatiotemporal gait analysis system. Med Eng Phys 28: 460–467.

52. Kratzenstein S, Kornaropoulos EI, Ehrig RM, Heller MO, Popplau BM, et al. (2012) Effective marker placement for functional identification of the centre of rotation at the hip. Gait Posture 36: 482–486.

53. Heller MO, Kratzenstein S, Ehrig RM, Wassilew G, Duda GN, et al. (2011) The weighted optimal common shape technique improves identification of the hip joint center of rotation in vivo. J Orthop Res 29: 1470–1475.

54. Holden JP, Orsini JA, Siegel KL, Kepple TM, Gerber LH, et al. (1997) Surface movement errors in shank kinematics and knee kinetics during gait. Gait & Posture 5: 217–227.

A Meta-Analysis of Core Stability Exercise versus General Exercise for Chronic Low Back Pain

Xue-Qiang Wang[1], Jie-Jiao Zheng[2]*, Zhuo-Wei Yu[2], Xia Bi[3], Shu-Jie Lou[4], Jing Liu[1], Bin Cai[5], Ying-Hui Hua[6], Mark Wu[7], Mao-Ling Wei[8], Hai-Min Shen[9], Yi Chen[2], Yu-Jian Pan[2], Guo-Hui Xu[2], Pei-Jie Chen[1]*

1 Department of Sport Rehabilitation, Shanghai University of Sport, Shanghai, China, **2** Department of Rehabilitation Medicine, Huadong Hospital Affiliated to Fudan University, Shanghai, China, **3** Department of Rehabilitation Medicine, Shanghai Gongli Hospital, Shanghai, China, **4** Department of Exercise and Sport Science, Shanghai University of Sport, Shanghai, China, **5** Department of Orthopaedics and Rehabilitation, Ninth People's Hospital Affiliated to Shanghai Jiaotong University Medical School, Shanghai, China, **6** Department of Sport Medicine, Huashan Hospital Affiliated to Fudan University, Shanghai, China, **7** Department of Rehabilitation and Ancillary Services, Gleneagles International Medical and Surgical Center, Shanghai, China, **8** Chinese Evidence-based Medicine, West China Hospital of Sichuan University, Chengdu, China, **9** Department of Orthopaedics and Trauma Surgery, Huadong Hospital Affiliated to Fudan University, Shanghai, China

Abstract

Objective: To review the effects of core stability exercise or general exercise for patients with chronic low back pain (LBP).

Summary of Background Data: Exercise therapy appears to be effective at decreasing pain and improving function for patients with chronic LBP in practice guidelines. Core stability exercise is becoming increasingly popular for LBP. However, it is currently unknown whether core stability exercise produces more beneficial effects than general exercise in patients with chronic LBP.

Methods: Published articles from 1970 to October 2011 were identified using electronic searches. For this meta-analysis, two reviewers independently selected relevant randomized controlled trials (RCTs) investigating core stability exercise versus general exercise for the treatment of patients with chronic LBP. Data were extracted independently by the same two individuals who selected the studies.

Results: From the 28 potentially relevant trials, a total of 5 trials involving 414 participants were included in the current analysis. The pooling revealed that core stability exercise was better than general exercise for reducing pain [mean difference (−1.29); 95% confidence interval (−2.47, −0.11); P = 0.003] and disability [mean difference (−7.14); 95% confidence interval (−11.64, −2.65); P = 0.002] at the time of the short-term follow-up. However, no significant differences were observed between core stability exercise and general exercise in reducing pain at 6 months [mean difference (−0.50); 95% confidence interval (−1.36, 0.36); P = 0.26] and 12 months [mean difference (−0.32); 95% confidence interval (−0.87, 0.23); P = 0.25].

Conclusions: Compared to general exercise, core stability exercise is more effective in decreasing pain and may improve physical function in patients with chronic LBP in the short term. However, no significant long-term differences in pain severity were observed between patients who engaged in core stability exercise versus those who engaged in general exercise.

Systematic Review Registration: http://www.crd.york.ac.uk/PROSPERO PROSPERO registration number: CRD42011001717.

Editor: Sam Eldabe, The James Cook University Hospital, United Kingdom

Funding: This work was supported by the Shanghai Key Lab of Human Performance (SUS) (11DZ2261100); the National Science Foundation for Young Scholars of China (Grant No.81101391); the Science and Technology Foundation Program of Shanghai University of Sport (Grant No. YJSCX201120), and the Science and Technology Development Fund of Shanghai Pudong (Grant No.PKJ2011-Y05. The funders had no role in study design, data collection and analysis, decision to publish, or preparation of the manuscript.

Competing Interests: The authors have declared that no competing interests exist.

* E-mail: chenpeijie@sus.edu.cn (P-JC); zjjcss@126.com (J-JZ)

Introduction

Low back pain (LBP) is one of the two most common types of disability affecting individuals in Western countries (the other is mental illness), and the assessment of LBP-related disabilities represents a significant challenge [1]. LBP affects approximately 80% of people at some stage in their lives [2,3]. In developing countries, the 1-year prevalence of LBP among farmers was 72%

in southwest Nigeria [4], 56% in Thailand [5], and 64% in China [6]. The impact of chronic LBP can be severe and profound because chronic LBP often results in lost wages and additional medical expenses and can even increase the risk of incurring other medical conditions [7,8]. In the United States, the total indirect and direct costs due to LBP are estimated to be greater than $100 billion annually [9,10].

Exercise therapy seems to be an effective treatment to relieve the pain and to improve the functional status of patients with chronic LBP in most clinical practice guidelines [11]. Core stability training has become a popular fitness trend that has begun to be applied in rehabilitation programs and in sports medicine [12]. Many studies [13–15] have shown that core stability exercise is an important component of rehabilitation for LBP. Panjabi [16] proposed a well-known model of the spine stability system that consists of three subsystems: the passive subsystem (which includes bone, ligament and joint capsule), the active subsystem (which includes muscle and tendons), and the neural subsystem (which consists of the central nervous system and peripheral nervous system). According to this model, these three subsystems work together to provide stabilization by controlling spinal movement. Thus, an effective core stability exercise should consider the motor and sensory components of the exercise and how they relate to these systems to promote optimal spinal stability [17]. In addition, core stability training includes the exercise associated with the prior activation of the local trunk muscles and should be advanced to include more intricate static, dynamic, and functional exercises that involve the coordinated contraction of local and superficial spinal muscles.

Although there have been four published systematic reviews [18–21] of core stability training, these articles only include a review of the literature published prior to June 2008. Positive effects have been reported with different forms of exercise used by physical therapists. However, it is currently unclear whether core stability training produces more beneficial effects than conventional exercise for patients with chronic LBP.

Core stability training has a powerful theoretical foundation for the prevention and treatment of LBP, as is evidenced by its widespread clinical use. However, there appears to be no consensus agreement that core stability exercise is better than general exercise for chronic LBP. It is important to ensure that the determination of the most effective exercise for LBP is based on scientific evidence so as not to waste staff time and resources and to avoid unnecessary stress for patients with LBP and their families. The purpose of this paper is to conduct a meta-analysis of the effects of core stability exercise compared to general exercise as a treatment for chronic LBP.

Methods

Search Strategy

We identified randomized controlled trials (RCTs) by electronically searching the following databases: China Biology Medicine disc (1970–October 2011), PubMed (1970–October 2011), Embase (1970–October 2011), and the Cochrane Library (1970–October 2011).

A detailed explanation of the full electronic search strategy for PubMed is presented in Appendix S1. Briefly, the following medical subject headings (MeSH) were included: low back pain, sciatica, lumbosacral region, exercise, and chronic pain. The keywords used were RCTs, double-blind method, single-blind method, random allocation, pelvic girdle pain, motor control, exercise therapy, stability, stabilization, general exercise, tradiional exercise, conventional exercise, specific exercise, and physical therapy. We removed duplicates that were identified in multiple database searches.

Inclusion Criteria

1. Types of studies. Only RCTs examining the effects of core stability exercise versus general exercise for the treatment of patients with chronic LBP were included. No language or publication date limits were set.

2. Types of participants. We included articles with both female and male subjects (over 18 years of age) who had chronic LBP (longer than 3 months). We excluded articles that included participants with LBP evoked by specific conditions or pathologies.

3. Types of interventions. We included articles that compared a control group, which received general exercise, and a treatment group, which received core stability exercise training. A core stability training program could be described as the reinforcement of the ability to insure stability of the neutral spine position [22]. Core stability exercises were usually performed on labile devices, such as an air-filled disc, a low density mat, a wobble board, or a Swiss ball [23].

4. Types of outcome measures. The primary outcomes of interest were pain intensity, back-specific functional status, quality of life, and work absenteeism. Outcomes were recorded for three time periods [11]: long term (1 year or more), intermediate (6 months), and short term (less than 3 months).

Selection of Studies

Two reviewers (Wang XQ, Bi X) used the pre-specified criteria to screen for relevant titles, abstracts and full papers. An article was removed if it was determined not to meet the inclusion criteria. If these two reviewers reached different final selection decisions, a third reviewer (Zheng JJ) was consulted.

Data Extraction

We extracted the following data from the included articles: study design, subject information, description of interventions between the control and experimental group, follow-up period, and outcome measures. These data were then compiled into a standard table. The two reviewers who selected the appropriate studies also extracted the data and evaluated the risk of bias. It was necessary to consult an arbiter (Zheng JJ) to reconcile any disagreements.

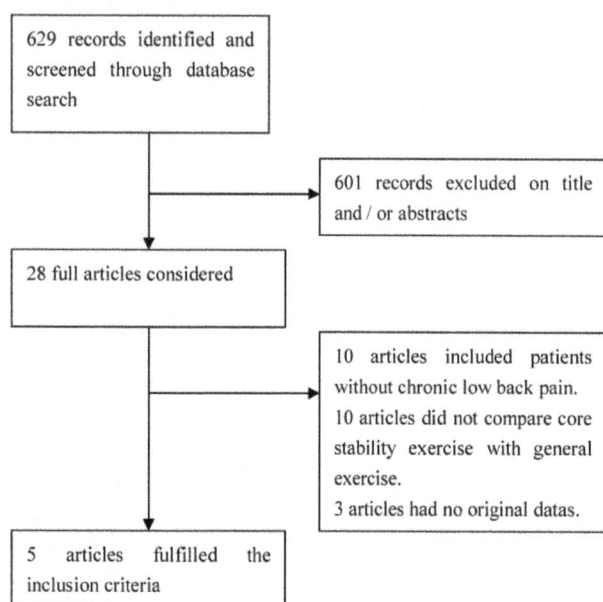

Figure 1. Flow chart of the study selection procedure.

Table 1. Characteristics of Included Studies.

Article	Patient Characteristic, Sample Size, and Duration of Complaint, year	Core stabilization exercise group	General exercise group	Outcomes	Follow up
Manuela 2007 (Brazil)	aged 18–80;n = 240; Duration of LBP>3mon;	n = 80(age: 51.9±15.3); retraining specific trunk muscles using ultrasound feedback; 12 treatment sessions over 8 weeks	n = 80(age: 54.8±15.3); strengthening, stretching and aerobic exercises; 12 treatment sessions over 8 weeks	pain(VAS) and disability (Roland Morris Disability Questionnaire)	8 weeks 6month 12month
Monica 2010 (Norway)	aged 19–60;n = 72; Duration of LBP>3mon;	n = 36(age:40.9±11.5); motor control exercise; once a week for 8 weeks;	n = 36(age:36.0±10.3); trunk strengthening and stretching exercises; once a week for 8 weeks	pain(NRS 0–10) disability (ODI)	8 weeks 12month
Fabio 2010 (Brazil)	n = 30; Duration of LBP>3 month;	n = 15(age: 42.07±8.15); segmental stabilization exercises; twice per week for 6 weeks	n = 15(age: 41.73±6.42); superficial strengthening exercise(n = 15); twice per week for 6 weeks	pain(VAS, McGill) and disability (ODI)	6 weeks
Ottar 2010 (Norway)	aged 19–60;n = 72; Duration of LBP>3mon;	n = 36(age:43.4±10.2); sling exercise; once a week for 8 weeks	n = 36(age:36.0±10.3); trunk strengthening and stretching exercises; once a week for 8 weeks	pain(NRS 0–10) disability (ODI)	8 weeks 12month
Padmini 2008 (India)	aged 18–60;n = 80; Duration of LBP>3mon;	n = 40(age:49±3.6); traditional yoga scriptures; 1 week	n = 40(age:48±4); physical exercises(n = 40); 1 week	disability (ODI)	1 weeks

Abbreviations: LBP, low back pain; ODI, Oswestry Disability Index; VAS, Visual Analog Scale; NRS, Numerical Rating Scale.

Assessing the Risk of Bias

We used the Cochrane Collaboration recommendations [24] to assess the risk of bias for all articles. The following information was evaluated: random sequence generation, allocation concealment, blinding of participants and personnel, blinding of outcome assessments, incomplete outcome data, selective reporting and other bias. Two reviewers (Xu GH, Hua YH) evaluated the methodological quality of all articles examined in the current study. An arbiter was consulted (Chen PJ) to reconcile any disagreements.

Statistical Analysis

Review Manager Software (RevMan5.2) was used for the meta-analysis. Heterogeneity among the studies was evaluated using the I^2 statistic and the chi-squared test. The fixed effects model was used if the heterogeneity test did not reveal statistical significance ($I^2<50\%$; P>0.1). Otherwise, we adopted the random effects model. We conducted a sensitivity analysis if heterogeneity existed among the studies. All of the variables in the studies included in this meta-analysis were continuous, so we used the mean difference (MD) and 95% confidence interval (CI) to analyze the studies. We considered P values less than 0.05 to be statistically significant.

Systematic review registration: http://www.crd.york.ac.uk/ PROSPERO. PROSPERO registration number: CRD42011001717.

Results

Search Results

The process of identifying eligible studies was outlined in figure 1. Six hundred twenty-nine records were initially identified through the Cochrane Library, PubMed, Embase, and China Biology Medicine disc. Of these, 28 potentially eligible articles were included based on their title and abstract. After reviewing these 28 potential articles, only 5 articles [25–29] fulfilled the inclusion criteria. The remaining 23 articles [30–52] were removed because the trials included participants with diagnoses other than chronic LBP, did not compare core stability exercise with general exercise, or the original data were not available from the authors. The characteristics of each included study are described in table 1.

Risk of Bias of Included Studies

According to the Cochrane Collaboration recommendations, each article was at a high risk of bias. Thus, the evidence involved in this meta-analysis had a high overall risk of bias. Each article was described as randomized, but the randomization method was unclear for one study [27]. Four articles used the allocation concealment method, but we could not determine the allocation concealment in the Ottar 2010 article [28]. Three of the included articles attempted to blind the participants to the allocated treatment, and outcome assessors were blinded in five trials. Incomplete outcome data were at a low risk of bias in all articles. The risk of bias assessment of all included studies is described in table 2.

Core Stability Exercise Versus General Exercise on Pain Intensity

In total, four trials assessed pain intensity using a numeric rating scale (NRS) and a visual analog scale (VAS). The data indicated that core stability exercise was better than general exercise for short-term pain relief when the results were combined in a random-effects model [MD (95% CI) = −1.29 (−2.47, −0.11), P = 0.003] [Fig. 2(A)]. However, no significant differences were observed between the effects of core stability exercise and general exercise at 6 months [MD (95% CI) = −0.50 (−1.36, 0.36), P = 0.26] [Fig. 2(B)] or 12 months [MD (95% CI) = −0.32 (−0.87, 0.23), P = 0.25] [Fig. 2(C)].

Table 2. Risk of Bias Assessment of Included Studies.

Article	Random sequence generation	Allocation concealment	Blinding of participants and personnel	Blinding of outcome assessment	Incomplete outcome data	Selective reporting	Other bias	Risk of bias
Manuela 2007(Brazil)	low	low	low	low	low	low	high	high
Monica 2010 (Norway)	low	low	low	low	low	low	high	high
Fabio 2010 (Brazil)	low	low	unclear	low	low	low	high	high
Ottar 2010 (Norway)	low	unclear	low	low	low	low	high	high
Padmini 2008 (India)	low	low	high	low	low	low	high	high

Core Stability Exercise Versus General Exercise on Disability

Five studies included self-reported back-specific functional status. Of these, one used the Roland Morris Disability Questionnaire (RMDQ), and four used the Oswestry Disability Index (ODI). Compared to general exercise, core stability exercise resulted in a significant improvement in functional status by the random-effects model in the short term [MD (95% CI) = −7.14 (−11.64, −2.65), P = 0.002] (Fig. 3).

Discussion

This meta-analysis, which included 414 patients, identified 5 RCTs that compared core stability exercise and general exercise for chronic LBP. The risk of bias was assessed for each article using the Cochrane Collaboration recommendations. In addition, each article contained a high risk of other bias. And it was difficult to evaluate whether the articles described the outcome measures they had originally meant to describe. However, no serious complications were reported in any of the five articles that investigated adverse events. However, the number of included subjects was too small to determine the safety of core stability exercise.

The results of this meta-analysis indicate that core stability exercise is better than general exercise for pain relief and improving back-specific functional status in the short term. However, no significant differences in pain relief were observed in the intermediate- and long-term follow-up periods. The primary results of this review are consistent with the findings of a systematic review [20] of the effects of core stability exercise on nonspecific LBP. The results of the meta-analysis indicated that core stability exercise can be more effective than other types of exercise in improving back-specific functional status in the short term (MD = −5.1points, 95% CI = −8.7 to 1.4). Two other systematic reviews [18,19] also reported that specific stabilization exercise was better than ordinary medical care and treatment by a general practitioner for reducing pain over the short term and intermediate term.

Compared to the prior reviews, approximately four-fifths of the articles included in the current study were new, and all of the articles in the current analysis considered only patients with chronic LBP (duration of pain >12 weeks). In addition, we conducted a meta-analysis of the effects of core stability exercise compared to general exercise. Because of these characteristics, this meta-analysis is considered to be much more robust.

Core stability is the ability to control the position and movement of the central portion of the body [53]. Popular fitness programs, such as Tai Chi, Yoga, and Pilates, are based on core stability exercise principles. There are several different approaches currently in use for core stability exercise for LBP, which could lead to different results. A systematic review and meta-analysis of different core stability exercises for LBP should be conducted to determine the optimal treatment approach.

Limitations

This meta-analysis was characterized by several limitations that should be noted. The first limitation, which is common in many systematic reviews, was that the findings were based on relatively low quality data that had a high risk of bias. Although several of the articles involved in this meta-analysis were published within the last five years, methodologically rigorous articles were still deficient. Second, the total number of subjects involved in the meta-analysis was too small to identify relatively small disparities between the effects of core stability exercise and general exercise.

A

Study or Subgroup	core stability exercise			general exercise			Weight	Mean Difference IV, Random, 95% CI
	Mean	SD	Total	Mean	SD	Total		
Fabio 2010	0.06	0.16	15	2.89	1.45	15	26.7%	-2.83 [-3.57, -2.09]
Manuela 2007	4	2.5	73	4.8	2.4	74	26.3%	-0.80 [-1.59, -0.01]
Monica 2010	1.76	1.54	31	2.73	2.32	26	24.2%	-0.97 [-2.01, 0.07]
Ottar 2010	2.34	2.26	30	2.73	2.32	26	22.8%	-0.39 [-1.59, 0.81]
Total (95% CI)			149			141	100.0%	-1.29 [-2.47, -0.11]

Heterogeneity: Tau² = 1.21; Chi² = 19.72, df = 3 (P = 0.0002); I² = 85%
Test for overall effect: Z = 2.15 (P = 0.03)

B

Study or Subgroup	core stability exercise			general exercise			Weight	Mean Difference IV, Random, 95% CI
	Mean	SD	Total	Mean	SD	Total		
Manuela 2007	4.3	2.6	68	4.8	2.6	71	100.0%	-0.50 [-1.36, 0.36]
Total (95% CI)			68			71	100.0%	-0.50 [-1.36, 0.36]

Heterogeneity: Not applicable
Test for overall effect: Z = 1.13 (P = 0.26)

C

Study or Subgroup	core stability exercise			general exercise			Weight	Mean Difference IV, Fixed, 95% CI
	Mean	SD	Total	Mean	SD	Total		
Manuela 2007	4.9	2.9	65	5.2	2.8	73	32.8%	-0.30 [-1.25, 0.65]
Monica 2010	2.01	1.94	36	2.66	2.03	37	36.0%	-0.65 [-1.56, 0.26]
Ottar 2010	2.7	2.22	36	2.66	2.03	37	31.3%	0.04 [-0.94, 1.02]
Total (95% CI)			137			147	100.0%	-0.32 [-0.87, 0.23]

Heterogeneity: Chi² = 1.03, df = 2 (P = 0.60); I² = 0%
Test for overall effect: Z = 1.15 (P = 0.25)

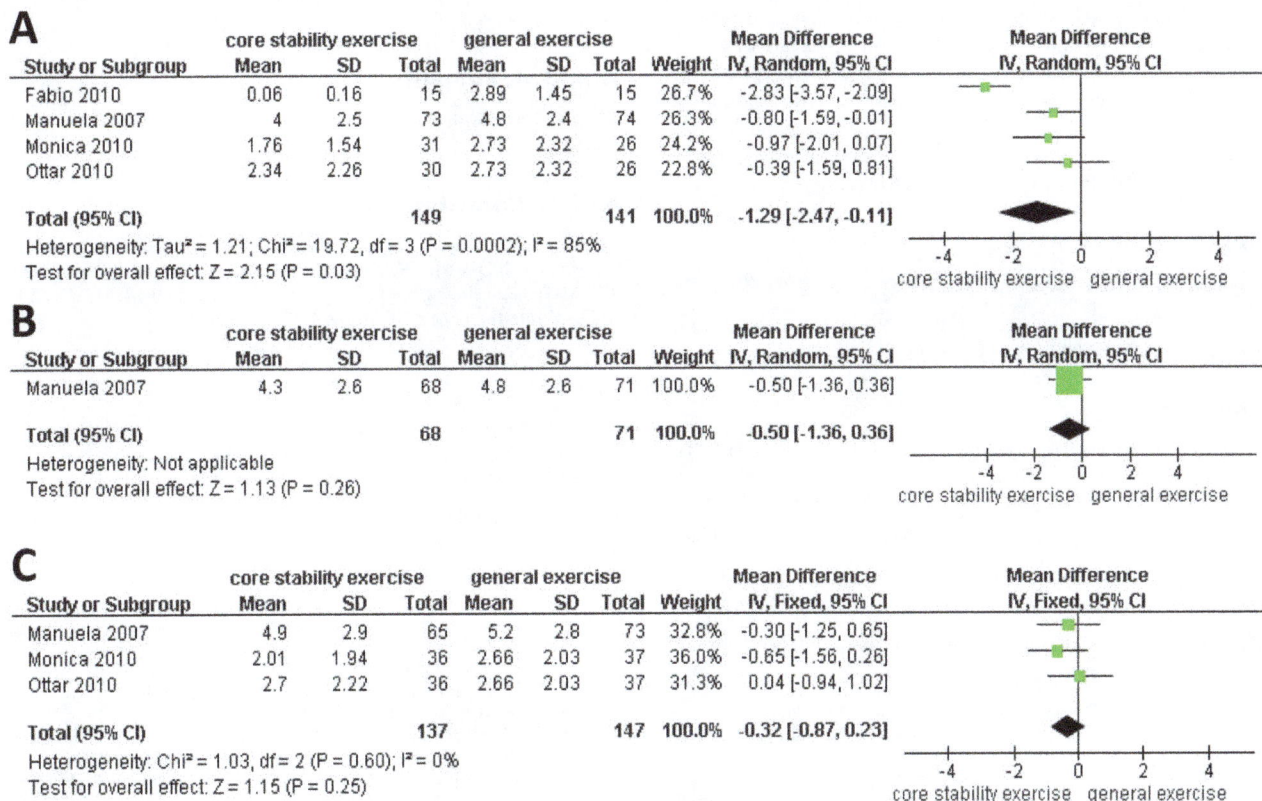

Figure 2. Meta-analyses of core stability exercise versus general exercise effect on pain. A: mean difference (MD) at the end of the intervention (not longer than 3 months). B: MD at six months. C: MD at long-term follow-up (12 months or more).

A third limitation was that numerous articles did not contain sufficient information for evaluating the quality and clinical relevance of the data. Another limitation was the probability of publication bias, which we attempted to diminish via a substantial database search. However, unpublished articles were not searched. Finally, it would have been preferable to conduct multiple outcome measures between the compared treatments in this meta-analysis. However, the primary outcome measures evaluated in the majority of articles were pain intensity and back-specific functional status. Relatively few articles had a significant analysis of quality of life, global improvement, and return to work/absenteeism.

Implications for Practice

In comparison to general exercise, core stability exercise may be more effective in relieving pain and improving back-specific function for patients with chronic LBP in the short term. However, no significant differences were observed between core stability exercise and general exercise in pain and functional status in the long term. However, these conclusions are sustained by low-quality data, and more definitive articles are required to confirm these results.

Implications for Research

Articles that were methodologically sound and sufficiently powered are required to confirm the effects of core stability exercise on pain relief and functional improvements in patients with chronic LBP. The types of outcomes in articles should include

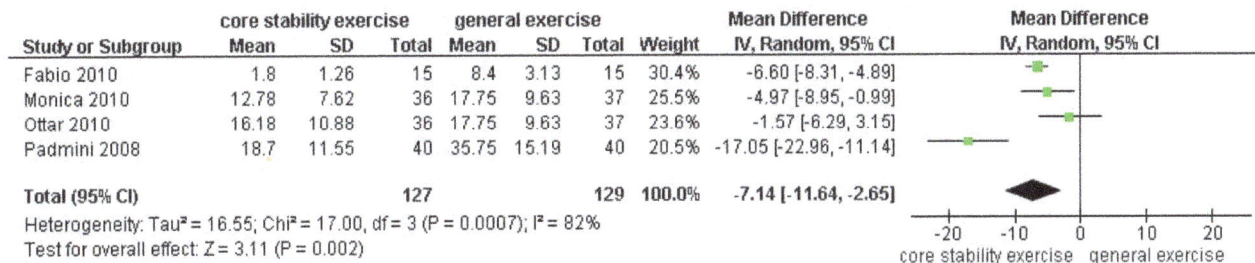

Study or Subgroup	core stability exercise			general exercise			Weight	Mean Difference IV, Random, 95% CI
	Mean	SD	Total	Mean	SD	Total		
Fabio 2010	1.8	1.26	15	8.4	3.13	15	30.4%	-6.60 [-8.31, -4.89]
Monica 2010	12.78	7.62	36	17.75	9.63	37	25.5%	-4.97 [-8.95, -0.99]
Ottar 2010	16.18	10.88	36	17.75	9.63	37	23.6%	-1.57 [-6.29, 3.15]
Padmini 2008	18.7	11.55	40	35.75	15.19	40	20.5%	-17.05 [-22.96, -11.14]
Total (95% CI)			127			129	100.0%	-7.14 [-11.64, -2.65]

Heterogeneity: Tau² = 16.55; Chi² = 17.00, df = 3 (P = 0.0007); I² = 82%
Test for overall effect: Z = 3.11 (P = 0.002)

Figure 3. Meta-analyses of core stability exercise versus general exercise effect on back-specific functional status (Oswestry Disability Index, ODI): mean difference (MD) at the end of the intervention (not longer than 3 months).

proprioception, muscle strength and trunk endurance to provide insight into the potential mechanisms of cooperative action. Comparisons of different core stability exercises would be more reasonable. The effects of core stability exercise should be evaluated over the long term. Eventually, theories regarding the mechanisms by which core stability exercise relieves pain in patients with LBP should be explored further.

Supporting Information

Appendix S1   MEDLINE search strategy.

Checklist S1   PRISMA 2009 Checklist

References

1. Katz RT (2001) Impairment and disability rating in low back pain. Phys Med Rehabil Clin N Am 12: 681–94.
2. Beith ID, Kemp A, Kenyon J, Prout M, Chestnut TJ (2011) Identifying neuropathic back and leg pain: a cross-sectional study. Pain 152: 1511–6.
3. Andersson GB (1999) Epidemiological features of chronic low-back pain. Lancet 354: 581–5.
4. Fabunmi AA, Aba SO, Odunaiya NA (2005) Prevalence of low back pain among peasant farmers in a rural community in South West Nigeria. Afr J Med Med Sci 34: 259–62.
5. Barrero LH, Hsu YH, Terwedow H, Perry MJ, Dennerlein JT, et al (2006) Prevalence and physical determinants of low back pain in a rural Chinese population. Spine (Phila Pa 1976) 31: 2728–34.
6. Taechasubamorn P, Nopkesorn T, Pannarunothai S (2011) Prevalence of low back pain among rice farmers in a rural community in Thailand. J Med Assoc Thai 94: 616–21.
7. Ivanova JI, Birnbaum HG, Schiller M, Kantor E, Johnstone BM, et al (2011) Real-world practice patterns, health-care utilization, and costs in patients with low back pain: the long road to guideline-concordant care. Spine J 11: 622–32.
8. Miller P, Kendrick D, Bentley E, Fielding K (2002) Cost-effectiveness of lumbar spine radiography in primary care patients with low back pain. Spine (Phila Pa 1976) 27: 2291–7.
9. Frymoyer JW, Cats-Baril WL (1991) An overview of the incidences and costs of low back pain. Orthop Clin North Am 22: 263–71.
10. Crow WT, Willis DR (2009) Estimating cost of care for patients with acute low back pain: a retrospective review of patient records. J Am Osteopath Assoc 109: 229–33.
11. Hayden JA, van Tulder MW, Malmivaara A, Koes BW (2005) Exercise therapy for treatment of non-specific low back pain. Cochrane Database Syst Rev CD000335.
12. Akuthota V, Ferreiro A, Moore T, Fredericson M (2008) Core Stability Exercise Principles. Curr Sports Med Rep 7: 39–44.
13. Desai I, Marshall PW (2010) Acute effect of labile surfaces during core stability exercises in people with and without low back pain. J Electromyogr Kinesiol 20: 1155–62.
14. Baerga-Varela L, Abréu Ramos AM (2006) Core strengthening exercises for low back pain. Bol Asoc Med P R 98: 56–61.
15. Sung PS, Yoon B, Lee DC (2010) Lumbar spine stability for subjects with and without low back pain during one-leg standing test. Spine (Phila Pa 1976) 35: E753–60.
16. Panjabi MM (1992) The stabilizing system of the spine. Part II. Neutral zone and instability hypothesis. J Spinal Disord 5: 390–6.
17. Hodges PW (2003) Core stability exercise in chronic low back pain. Orthop Clin North Am 34: 245–54.
18. Ferreira PH, Ferreira ML, Maher CG, Herbert RD, Refshauge K (2006) Specific stabilisation exercise for spinal and pelvic pain: a systematic review. Aust J Physiother 52: 79–88.
19. Rackwitz B, de Bie R, Limm H, von Garnier K, Ewert T, Stucki G (2006) Segmental stabilizing exercises and low back pain. What is the evidence? A systematic review of randomized controlled trials. Clin Rehabil 20: 553–67.
20. Macedo LG, Maher CG, Latimer J, McAuley JH (2009) Motor control exercise for persistent, nonspecific low back pain: a systematic review. Phys Ther 89: 9–25.
21. Hauggaard A, Persson A (2007) Specific spinal stabilisation exercises in patients with low back pain: a systematic review. Phys Ther Rev 12: 233–248.
22. Akuthota V, Ferreiro A, Moore T, Fredericson M (2008) Core Stability Exercise Principles. Curr Sports Med Rep 7: 39–44.
23. Willardson JM (2004) The effectiveness of resistance exercises performed on unstable equipment. Strength and Conditioning Journal 26: 70–74.
24. Higgins JPT, Altman DG (2008) Assessing risk of bias in included studies. In: Higgins JPT, Green S, eds. Cochrane handbook for systematic reviews of interventions. Wiley 187–241.
25. Ferreira ML, Ferreira PH, Latimer J, Herbert RD, Hodges PW, et al (2007) Comparison of general exercise, motor control exercise and spinal manipulative therapy for chronic low back pain: A randomized trial. Pain 131: 31–7.
26. Unsgaard-Tøndel M, Fladmark AM, Salvesen Ø, Vasseljen O (2010) Motor control exercises, sling exercises, and general exercises for patients with chronic low back pain: a randomized controlled trial with 1-year follow-up. Phys Ther 90: 1426–40.
27. França FR, Burke TN, Hanada ES, Marques AP (2010) Segmental stabilization and muscular strengthening in chronic low back pain: a comparative study. Clinics (Sao Paulo) 65: 1013–7.
28. Vasseljen O, Fladmark AM (2010) Abdominal muscle contraction thickness and function after specific and general exercises: a randomized controlled trial in chronic low back pain patients. Man Ther 15: 482–9.
29. Tekur P, Singphow C, Nagendra HR, Raghuram N (2008) Effect of short-term intensive yoga program on pain, functional disability and spinal flexibility in chronic low back pain: a randomized control study. J Altern Complement Med. 14: 637–44.
30. Koumantakis GA, Watson PJ, Oldham JA (2005) Trunk muscle stabilization training plus general exercise versus general exercise only: randomized controlled trial of patients with recurrent low back pain. Phys Ther 85: 209–25.
31. Marshall PW, Murphy BA (2008) Muscle activation changes after exercise rehabilitation for chronic low back pain. Arch Phys Med Rehabil 89: 1305–13.
32. Kumar S, Sharma VP, Negi MP (2009) Efficacy of dynamic muscular stabilization techniques (DMST) over conventional techniques in rehabilitation of chronic low back pain. J Strength Cond Res 23: 2651–9.
33. Cairns MC, Foster NE, Wright C (2006) Randomized controlled trial of specific spinal stabilization exercises and conventional physiotherapy for recurrent low back pain. Spine (Phila Pa 1976) 2006 31: E670–81.
34. O'Sullivan PB, Phyty GD, Twomey LT, Allison GT (1997) Evaluation of specific stabilizing exercise in the treatment of chronic low back pain with radiologic diagnosis of spondylolysis or spondylolisthesis. Spine (Phila Pa 1976) 22: 2959–67.
35. Stuge B, Laerum E, Kirkesola G, Vøllestad N (2004) The efficacy of a treatment program focusing on specific stabilizing exercises for pelvic girdle pain after pregnancy: a randomized controlled trial. Spine (Phila Pa 1976) 29: 351–9.
36. Elden H, Ladfors L, Olsen MF, Ostgaard HC, Hagberg H (2005) Effects of acupuncture and stabilising exercises as adjunct to standard treatment in pregnant women with pelvic girdle pain: randomised single blind controlled trial. BMJ 330: 761.
37. Stuge B, Veierød MB, Laerum E, Vøllestad N (2004) The efficacy of a treatment program focusing on specific stabilizing exercises for pelvic girdle pain after pregnancy: a two-year follow-up of a randomized clinical trial. Spine (Phila Pa 1976) 29: E197–203.
38. Rasmussen-Barr E, Ang B, Arvidsson I, Nilsson-Wikmar L (2009) Graded exercise for recurrent low-back pain: a randomized, controlled trial with 6-, 12-, and 36-month follow-ups. Spine (Phila Pa 1976) 34: 221–8.
39. Kumar S, Negi MP, Sharma VP, Shukla R, Dev R, et al (2009) Efficacy of two multimodal treatments on physical strength of occupationally subgrouped male with low back pain. J Back Musculoskelet Rehabil 22: 179–88.
40. Sherman KJ, Cherkin DC, Cook AJ, Hawkes RJ, Deyo RA, et al (2010) Comparison of yoga versus stretching for chronic low back pain: protocol for the Yoga Exercise Self-care (YES) trial. Trials 11: 36.
41. Elden H, Ostgaard HC, Fagevik-Olsen M, Ladfors L, Hagberg H (2008) Treatments of pelvic girdle pain in pregnant women: adverse effects of standard treatment, acupuncture and stabilising exercises on the pregnancy, mother, delivery and the fetus/neonate. BMC Complement Altern Med 8: 34.
42. Macedo LG, Latimer J, Maher CG, Hodges PW, Nicholas M, et al (2008) Motor control or graded activity exercises for chronic low back pain? A randomised controlled trial. BMC Musculoskelet Disord 9: 65.
43. Sherman KJ, Cherkin DC, Erro J, Miglioretti DL, Deyo RA (2005) Comparing yoga, exercise, and a self-care book for chronic low back pain: a randomized, controlled trial. Ann Intern Med 143: 849–56.

Acknowledgments

We would like to thank American Journal Experts for English language editing.

Author Contributions

Conceived and designed the experiments: XQW JJZ PJC. Performed the experiments: XQW SJL BC ZWY MLW. Analyzed the data: YHH JL XB PJC MW. Contributed reagents/materials/analysis tools: HMS YC YJP GHX. Wrote the paper: XQW JJZ PJC.

44. Kluge J, Hall D, Louw Q, Theron G, Grové D (2011) Specific exercises to treat pregnancy-related low back pain in a South African population. Int J Gynaecol Obstet 113: 187–91.

45. Mohseni-Bandpei MA, Rahmani N, Behtash H, Karimloo M (2011) The effect of pelvic floor muscle exercise on women with chronic non-specific low back pain. J Bodyw Mov Ther 15: 75–81.

46. Koumantakis GA, Watson PJ, Oldham JA (2005) Supplementation of general endurance exercise with stabilisation training versus general exercise only. Physiological and functional outcomes of a randomised controlled trial of patients with recurrent low back pain. Clin Biomech (Bristol, Avon) 20: 474–82.

47. Bentsen H, Lindgärde F, Manthorpe R (1997) The effect of dynamic strength back exercise and/or a home training program in 57-year-old women with chronic low back pain. Results of a prospective randomized study with a 3-year follow-up period. Spine (Phila Pa 1976) 22: 1494–500.

48. Schenkman ML, Jordan S, Akuthota V, Roman M, Kohrt WM, et al (2009) Functional movement training for recurrent low back pain: lessons from a pilot randomized controlled trial. PM R 1: 137–46.

49. Ewert T, Limm H, Wessels T, Rackwitz B, von Garnier K, et al (2009) The comparative effectiveness of a multimodal program versus exercise alone for the secondary prevention of chronic low back pain and disability. PM R 1: 798–808.

50. Kumar S, Sharma VP, Shukla R, Dev R (2010) Comparative efficacy of two multimodal treatments on male and female sub-groups with low back pain (part II) J Back Musculoskelet Rehabil 23: 1–9.

51. Wang Xueqiang, Zheng Jiejiao, Bi Xia, Liu Jing (2012) Effect of core stability training on patients with chronic low back pain. HealthMED 6: 754–759.

52. Guo Xianfeng, Yuan Shuaixiao, Li Xu (2010) Sling exercise therapy on back pain of adults with idiopathic scoliosis. Chin J Rehabil Theory Pract 16: 716–719.

53. Omkar SN, Vishwas S, Tech B (2009) Yoga techniques as a means of core stability training. J Bodyw Mov Ther 13: 98–103.

14

Flexion Relaxation and Its Relation to Pain and Function over the Duration of a Back Pain Episode

Raymond W. McGorry*, Jia-Hua Lin

Liberty Mutual Research Institute for Safety, Hopkinton, Massachusetts, United States of America

Abstract

Background: Relaxation of the erector spinae often occurs in healthy individuals as full trunk flexion is achieved when bending forward from standing. This phenomenon, referred to as flexion relaxation is often absent or disrupted (EMG activity persists) in individuals reporting low back pain (LBP).

Methods and Results: Self-reported pain and disability scores were compared to EMG measures related to the flexion relaxation (FR) phenomenon by 33 participants with LBP at up to eight sessions over a study period of up to eight weeks. Fourteen participants served as a control group. In the protocol, starting from standing participants bent forward to a fully flexed posture, and then extended the trunk to return to standing position. A thoracic inclinometer was used to measure trunk posture. Surface electrodes located at the L2 and L5 levels recorded EMG amplitudes of the erector spinae. Ratios of EMG amplitudes recorded during forward bending to amplitudes at full flexion, and ratios of extension to full flexion were calculated. EMG amplitudes and their ratios were compared between control and LBP groups at the initial visit. No significant differences between groups were found except at the L5 location at full flexion. Correlations of the ratios to pain and function scores recorded in repeated sessions over the LBP episode also were compared between LBP group participants classified as having transient, recurrent or chronic symptoms. In another analysis participants were grouped by whether their symptoms resolved over the study period.

Conclusions: The transient LBP group had significantly stronger correlations between pain and function to both ratios, than did those with more chronic LBP symptoms. Participants who experienced symptom resolution generally had stronger correlations of ratios to both pain and function than those with partial or no resolution. Improved understanding of these relationships may provide insight in clinical management of LBP.

Editor: Natasha M. Maurits, University Medical Center Groningen UMCG, Netherlands

Funding: The authors have no support or funding to report.

Competing Interests: The authors have declared that no competing interests exist.

* E-mail: Raymond.mcgorry@libertymutual.com

Introduction

The observation of electrical silence of the erector spinae (ES) at full trunk flexion was first referred to as flexion relaxation (FR) by Floyd and Silver [1]. Though often studied since, the exact mechanism for FR is not definitively known. One proposed mechanism may be stretch reflex inhibition, a reflexive contraction orchestrated by the muscle spindle in response to passive longitudinal stretching [1,2]. The lumbodorsal fascia and other ligaments might provide the necessary supporting moment for the trunk, reducing the necessity of active muscular contraction to maintain the fully flexed posture [3]. Adams et al. suggested that when the ES is electrically silent at full trunk flexion, passive tension of the muscle tissue could provide some resistance to trunk moment [4].

The literature suggests that FR of the lumbar ES at full trunk flexion is observed in the majority of healthy individuals without back pain, though substantial variability in the behavior exists, likely due to individual differences such as anthropometric variation as well as differences in protocols (e.g. posture, electrode placement) [1,5–10]. It has also been observed that FR may vary with change in the speed of the flexion/extension motion,

prolonged static flexion, muscle fatigue, external load application, and with compound motions [6,9–14]. The sEMG amplitude of the ES during trunk extension against gravity (concentric) is typically greater than during the eccentric trunk flexion phase [8,15].

One method reported for quantifying FR, to best allow comparison of measures repeated over time or between individuals, is to calculate the ratio of the sEMG amplitude of the ES during the trunk flexion phase to that recorded at full static flexion. This technique, commonly referred to the "flexion relaxation ratio," or similar terminology, was first reported by Sihvonen et al. [7], and has been widely adopted as a method for quantifying FR [8,16–22].

In many studies, FR was absent or significantly impaired (sEMG activity persists at full trunk flexion) in those with low back pain (LBP). Absence or impairment of FR has been reported to vary from 41% of cases (in a population of subjects with a history of LBP, but pain free at the time of testing) to as many as 100% of subjects with active LBP [5,7]. Geisser et al. in their meta-analysis reported that FR could discriminate between individuals with and without LBP [18]. Using various FR-related measures of trunk flexion/extension in standing, several reports show differences between normal (pain-free) and LBP groups [7,8,11,16,23].

FR may vary with severity and duration of LBP symptoms, and a re-establishment of FR may reflect clinical improvement. The literature shows that, in some but not all individuals for whom FR was absent (electrical silence did not occur at full flexion) while experiencing an episode of LBP, FR was reestablished when their symptoms resolved [1,24–26]. Paquet et al. in their report on the relationship of muscle activity and lumbar/pelvic coordination concluded "…the lack of relaxation of the ES muscle may be associated with perturbation of movement patterns and the duration of symptoms" [11]. More recently, several studies reported results of pre-treatment – post-treatment evaluations of exercise or functional restoration programs with patients with chronic LBP in a tertiary care setting. These results suggest that some measures related to the FR phenomenon had some ability to discriminate functional improvement in patients with chronic LBP following back rehabilitation programs [21,27–30]. While there is preliminary evidence that FR can be restored, whether partially or fully, more research is needed to evaluate longitudinal changes in FR over time in relation to symptoms.

While the studies cited above have focused on FR-related measures as a method to distinguish individuals with and without LBP, or as a method for documenting or guiding rehabilitation of those with chronic LBP, few studies have attempted to correlate FR with measures of self-reported pain and/or disability [22,24,31]. Further, there are no reports in the literature of the nature of, or changes to FR-related measures using repeated measures over the course of an LBP episode. Toward the goal of improved understanding of how FR changes with changes in pain and function over time, the present study will investigate how these factors relate among a community sample of individuals during a prospective study conducted over the natural course of an episode of nonspecific LBP. These measures and their relationships will also be compared to those obtained in a symptom-free control group. The correlation of FR related measures to self-reported function and the intensity of back pain were evaluated over the a period of up to eight weeks, and the results are compared for participant grouping based on symptom history, and also based on groupings based on resolution of pain symptoms. The results should provide some clinical insight for the practitioner in treatment of the individual experiencing an episode of nonspecific LBP.

Methods

Ethics Statement

All research involving human participants was approved by the institutional review board of the Liberty Mutual Research Institute for Safety. Written informed consent was obtained, and all data was de-identified, kept confidential and analyzed anonymously. The clinical investigation was conducted according to the principles expressed in the Declaration of Helsinki.

Participants

Men and women experiencing a LBP episode were recruited by means of advertisements posted at local clinicians' offices (physical therapists, chiropractors, and physicians) and by newspaper advertisement to participate in a maximum eight-week clinical study. The inclusion criteria for the study were that potential participants be 18 to 65 years of age and presently experiencing LBP. Participants were included whether it was their first experience with LBP, or if they were experiencing a recurrence. The purpose and protocol for the study was explained to all respondents, and those that expressed interest completed a medical history form and were interviewed and examined by a health care provider. Medical exclusion criteria were: major structural abnormalities, significant neurological deficits or evidence of severe nerve root compression, active systemic, inflammatory, musculoskeletal or neoplastic disease or history of previous back surgery. An additional exclusion criterion was having an active worker's compensation claim or related litigation pending, to avoid any potential confounding due to medico-legal concerns. Thirty-four individuals meeting the study criteria for nonspecific back pain were enrolled and assigned to the LBP group. One participant withdrew after the initial visit. Thirty-three participants belonging to the LBP group completed the multi-session protocol.

Eighteen participants were recruited for the Control group. The selection criteria were that participants be 18 to 65 years of age, in good health and had no significant history of back pain. Fourteen from the Control group performed a single session of the experimental protocol. The remaining four participants completed four additional sessions (five sessions in total) performing the experimental protocol at two-week intervals over an eight-week period. This multi-session subset served to provide some indication of the inherent variability in the dependent measures. Participant demographic information for the two groups was collected and is presented in Table 1.

Experimental design

A within-subject repeated measures design was used. The two levels of pain status were LBP and Control (no-LBP). The dependent variables were trunk inclination and sEMG amplitude at four locations on the erector spinae.

Equipment

Trunk inclination. Trunk kinematics were evaluated using an electronic inclinometer (Model #N4, Seika Corp., Tokyo, Japan). The inclinometer was attached to an appropriately sized adjustable harness/vest (small, medium, large). The inclinometer was located dorsally at the mid-thoracic region overlying the sixth thoracic spinous process, and this orientation allowed measurement of gross trunk flexion/extension.

Surface EMG – Four differential surface electrodes and an amplification and conditioning system (Bagnoli-8 EMG System, Delsis Corp., Boston, MA) were used in this study. The electrodes, with an inter-electrode distance of 1 cm, had onboard amplification with a frequency response of 20 to 450 Hz, and a common mode rejection ratio of 92 dB. A gain of 1000 was used. Four sEMG signals and the inclinometer output were sampled at 1000 Hz and stored in computer memory.

Subjective measures (LBP group only)

Daily Pain Score. A numerical pain rating scale (NPRS) was used to quantify the intensity of back pain. Participants rated their pain a 0 to 10 scale, where the anchors at 0 and 10 were "no pain" and "the worst pain imaginable", respectively [32]. At the

Table 1. Participant demographics.

	n	Gender	Age (yr)	Height (cm)	Weight (kg)
Control	18	10 M, 8 F	35.2 (9.4)	168.4 (10.5)	69.7 (11.7)
LBP	33	17 M, 16 F	40.5 (12.8)	168.9 (10.4)	75.0 (15.3)

beginning of each experimental session participants rated the pain intensity they were feeling "right now."

Functional Level. At the start of each experimental session participants also reported on their function in daily activities today using the clinically validated Back Pain Functional Scale (BPFS) [33]. This questionnaire rates impairment on a 0 to 5 scale, with each point anchored by a functional rating ranging from "unable to perform activity" to "no difficulty" for 12 activities, providing a functional continuum from 0 representing total dysfunction to 60, normal function.

Experimental protocol

At the initial experimental session with the LBP participants, the experimental nature of the measurements was discussed and that the protocol was not related to treatment was reinforced. Participants were then educated in pain scoring, and rating function using the BPFS. Participants from both groups were treated as follows. While standing, the sEMG sites were located and marked at the level of L2 and L5 spinous processes, 2.5 cm to the left and right of midline. The electrode placement was selected for consistency with previous reports in the FR literature [e.g. 16, 19, 22, 27]. For the LBP group and the four members of the Control group that participated in the eight-week protocol, the electrode locations and skin landmarks were transferred to a transparent plastic film to permit consistent repositioning during subsequent sessions. The four electrode sites were then prepared with an alcohol scrub, and shaved when necessary. Electrodes were oriented along the long axis of the muscle and attached using skin tape. The reference electrode was placed over the right clavicle. The harness with the inclinometer was donned so that the inclinometer was maintained firmly over the posterior midline at the mid-thoracic level.

The experimental task, a flexion/extension motion starting in standing, was paced by a computer running a custom data acquisition program that produced a series of audible beeps. With feet shoulder-width apart and looking forward the participant was instructed to move in response to the audible cues, keeping the knees straight but not locked and the arms hanging freely, while slowly flexing forward to full flexion over a four-second period, pausing for four seconds at full trunk flexion, and then returning to the upright starting position during a four-second trunk extension period. This protocol is typical of those used in studies of flexion relaxation [e.g. 1, 28, 30]. Figure 1 demonstrates the timing of the experimental task. Three replications of the motion were performed. The first trial was treated as practice and was omitted from analysis to minimize transient effects related to muscle warm-up, or stretching. Data from the last two replications were used in the subsequent analysis.

LBP group participants were scheduled for eight visits distributed over an eight week period scheduled twice a week for the first two weeks, once a week for the third and fourth weeks and once each in the sixth and eighth weeks. A stopping criterion was used for LBP participants whose pain resolved during the course of the experimental protocol. When participants reported a pain score of "0" at two consecutive sessions, participation was discontinued. When the experimental session was scheduled to coincide with a treatment session at a clinic, ratings and measurements were made prior to treatment, to minimize confounding by the effect of the treatment. The subset of four Control participants performed the protocol at five biweekly sessions.

Data reduction

The inclinometer signal for each trial, filtered with a 4th order zero-lag low pass Butterworth filter with an 8 Hz cutoff, was displayed on the computer screen. Using a custom software program one research team member marked four inflection points of the inclinometer tracing dividing the experimental task into three phases: the flexion phase (FL), the static fully flexed or flexion relaxation (FR) phase and the extension phase (EX). The sEMG signals were RMS filtered with a 100 ms centered window. Within the FL and EX phases the peak amplitude of each of the four EMG sites was determined, and the mean for a one-second window about the peak was taken as the sEMG amplitude value. The value for the FR phase was calculated by taking the mean of a one-second window about the midpoint between the end of FL phase and the beginning of EX phase. The mean was taken for each phase for the two replications recorded at each session. The mean was then taken for the means for the left and right L2 sEMG, and the left and right L5 sEMG, yielding six measures used in the analysis: L2 and L5 amplitude during flexion (FL_{L2}, FL_{L5}), L2 and L5 amplitude during the flexion relaxation (FR_{L2}, FR_{L5}) and L2 and L5 amplitude during extension (EX_{L2} and EX_{L5}).

Flexion relaxation ratios. Calculating ratios of sEMG amplitudes between the phases of motion is a technique that allows normalization for repeated measures over time or for between-subject comparisons. The ratio of mean sEMG amplitude during the flexion movement to the mean amplitude during the FR phase for the L2 and L5 locations ($FL-FR_{L2}$ and $FL-FR_{L5}$, respectively) was calculated as previously described by Watson et al. and Ahern et al. [16,23]. This methodology was also used with the mean amplitudes determined for the extension phase ($EX-FR_{L2}$ and $EX-FR_{L5}$). Higher ratios indicate relatively more flexion relaxation (less activation) of the erector spinae at full trunk flexion. As an example, Figure 2 provides graphs of L5 sEMG and trunk angular displacement recorded during the experimental task. When Figure 2a was recorded the participant reported pain

|------------- Flexion -------------| **Full flexion** |------------- Extension -------------|
                                          (static)

    4 seconds   **4 seconds**   **4 seconds**

Figure 1. The experimental motion in standing illustrating the trunk flexion, static flexion, and extension phases, four seconds each.

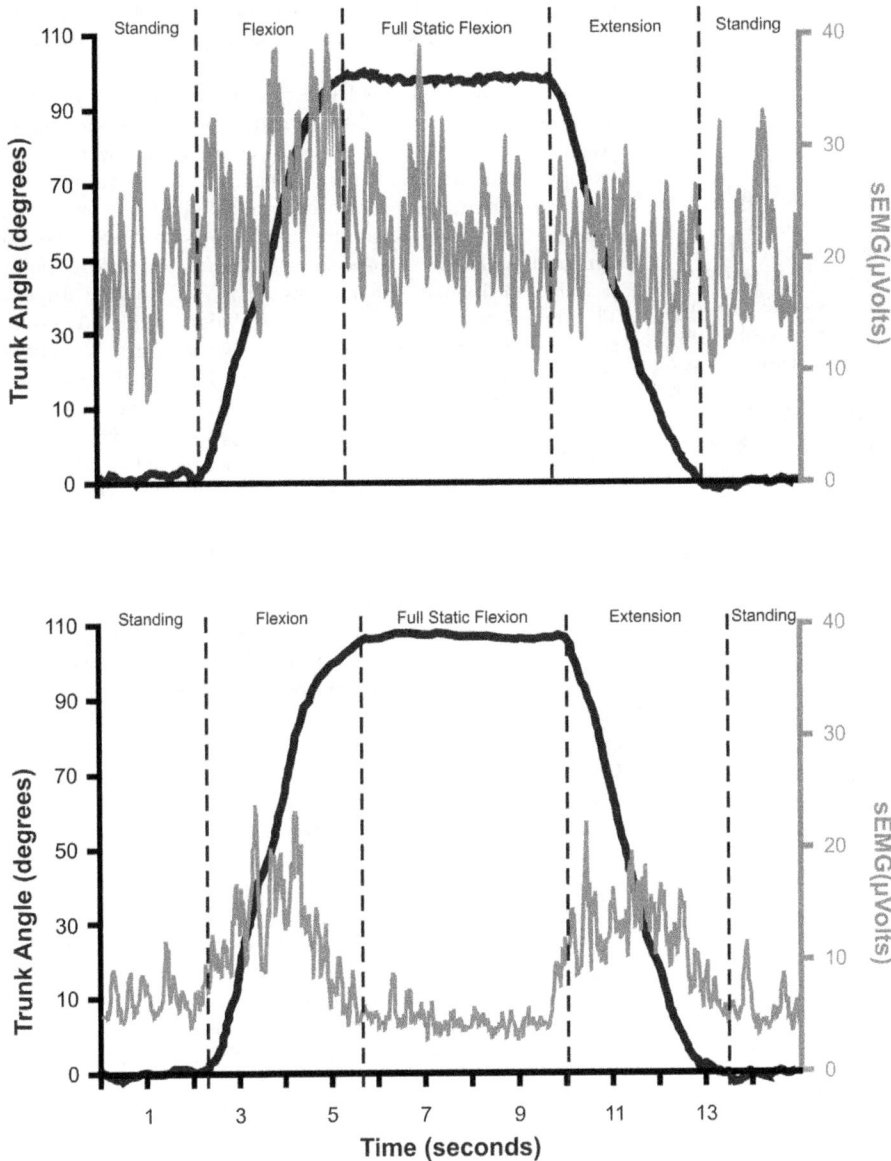

Figure 2. Trunk inclinometer and L5 sEMG tracings demonstrating different flexion relaxation states: 2a) absent flexion relaxation, 2b) normal flexion relaxation.

and functional limitations. The FL-FR_{L5} ratio was 1.2, and the EX-FR_{L5} ratio was 0.9. Figure 2b was recorded at a subsequent session where the participant reported no LBP or functional limitation, and had FL-FR_{L5} and EX-FR_{L5} ratios of 2.7 and 2.3, respectively.

Group assignments. Group assignments were made for participants with LBP based on two factors. The first group assignments were based on their self-reported "pain history," using a criteria proposed by Von Korff [34]. The three group assignments were Transient, Recurrent, and Chronic. Transient group assignment was for those experiencing first episode of LBP, and reporting having pain less than half the days of the past six months. The Recurrent group had a history of LBP greater than six months, but reporting pain on fewer than half the days during that period. The Chronic group reported LBP on greater than half the days of the past six months.

The second grouping was based on the degree of improvement in LBP symptoms, or "pain resolution", reported over the period of study participation. Assignment to the Resolved group was for participants who reported a "0" pain score on the final day of their enrollment. Partial resolution designation was for participants who reported a pain score of "1" on the final visit indicating that the participant was not reporting full resolution, and at least some degree of pain is present. The unresolved group designation was applied those with a "2" or greater score at the final visit.

Statistical analysis

One-way repeated measure ANOVAs were performed with the Control and LBP group initial visit data to test for differences in the four sEMG ratios. Spearman correlation coefficients were calculated for each participant between pairs of pain scores and the sEMG ratios, and between the BPFS function score and the sEMG ratios. Multivariate analysis of variance (MANOVA) was performed to test the effect of group divisions based on both pain history and pain resolution, on the sEMG measures. Tukey's post hoc analysis was employed if the effect was significant. The criterion selected for statistical significance was set at p = 0.05.

Results

At the initial experimental session the 33 LBP group participants reported a mean (standard deviation) of 7.3 (7.5) year history of back pain. At the initial session the LBP group reported a pain score of 3.0 (1.6) and a function score of 43.9 (8.0) on the BPFS scale. LBP group participated in a total 248 study sessions. Twenty-seven participants completed the full eight-session protocol. Based on the stopping criteria ("0" pain scores for two consecutive visits), three participants completed seven sessions, one completed five sessions and two completed three sessions. These six participants remained pain-free for the remainder of the eight-week protocol. Six additional participants gave a "0" pain score on their final visit, for a total of 12 participants reporting resolution of their symptoms by the final visit. The gross trunk flexion range of motion (ROM) during the experimental task was 111.0° (17.0) and 112.8° (16.7) for the Control and LBP groups, respectively.

The sEMG amplitudes recorded at the two lumbar levels for the three phases of the experimental task are presented in Figure 3 for the Control and LBP groups at the initial visit. At the initial visit there was a significant difference between the LBP and Control groups in L5 sEMG amplitude during the FR phase, 7.7 (3.9) μV and 5.7 (1.5) μV, respectively. There were no other significant between-group differences in amplitudes at the initial visit. For both groups sEMG amplitudes were generally greater during the eccentric contraction of trunk flexion phase than the subsequent FR period. The mean amplitudes occurring during trunk extension when returning to the standing posture (concentric contraction) were generally greater than for the observed for the eccentric contraction of the initial flexion phase.

Figure 4 shows bar graphs of FL-FR$_{L2}$ and FL-FR$_{L5}$ and EX-FR$_{L2}$ and EX-FR$_{L5}$ ratios for the Control group and for LBP groups recorded at the initial visit. There were no significant differences in any of the sEMG ratios between LBP and Control groups at the initial visit. The data from the subgroup of Controls was evaluated to provide an indication of the variability of these ratios in repeated measures of pain-free individuals over time. Means of the coefficients of variation between the ratios calculated

for each of the four participant's experimental sessions were FL-FR$_{L2}$ = 0.48, FL-FR$_{L5}$ = 0.33, EX-FR$_{L2}$ = 0.20 and EX-FR$_{L5}$ = 0.18.

ANOVAs were conducted to test for differences between sEMG ratios recorded at the initial visit and final visits for participant groupings based on characteristics of their pain experience. Grouping of participants based on pain history yielded assignment to the three groups in the following proportions: Transient (n = 8), Chronic (n = 7) and Recurrent (n = 18). ANOVA revealed no significant differences between any of the four sEMG ratios recorded on the first and last visits, for any of the three groups. The groupings based on pain resolution produced group assignment in the following proportions: Resolved (n = 12), Partial resolution (n = 8), Unresolved group (n = 13). For the Resolved group the difference in the FL-FR$_{L5}$ ratio approached statistical significance (p = .06) between the first visit, 1.56 (0.68), and last visit, 2.04 (0.48), but no significant differences were found between the first and last visits for any of the four sEMG ratios recorded on, for any of the groups.

The Spearman correlation coefficients calculated between the sEMG ratios and the pain scores were generally negative, with increasing pain scores associated with decreasing ratios. Correlations between function ratings and ratios were generally positive, being indicative of more pronounced FR (and thus greater ratios) with improving function. Correlations between sEMG ratios and pain and function taken for the LBP population as a whole did not exceed 0.20, and no correlations were statistically significant. Correlations were generally stronger for some groups, in the analysis of groups based on history pain behavior and symptom resolution. Table 2 presents Spearman correlation coefficients calculated between the sEMG ratios and both pain scores and function ratings for the analysis of participants grouped based on pain history and on pain resolution.

Correlations for both pain and function to all dependent measures were generally stronger for the L5 ES site than the L2 site. The highest correlations of both pain and function were to EX-FR$_{L5}$ for the Transient group in the pain history analysis, and for the Resolved group of the pain resolution analysis. MANOVA showed significant differences for both pain scores and function ratings, for both the FL-FR$_{L5}$ and EX-FR$_{L5}$ variables. For both variables Tukey's post hoc testing show significantly greater correlations for both pain and function in the Transient group

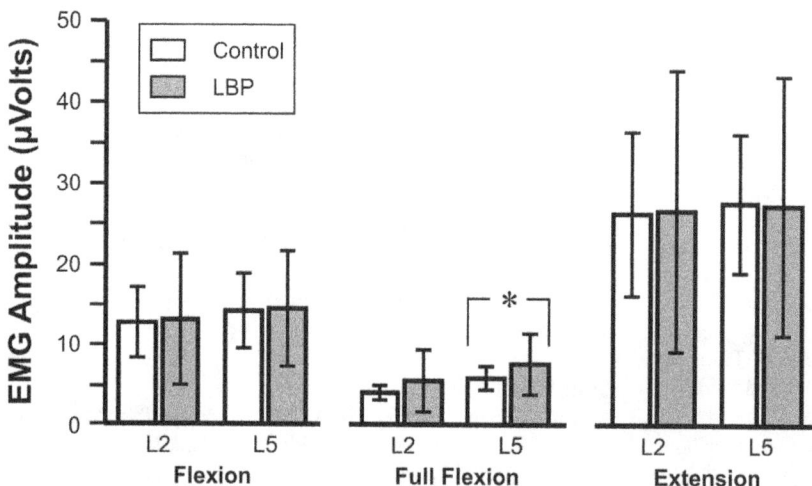

Figure 3. L2 and L5 sEMG amplitudes for the three phases at the initial visit. The asterisk indicates significant differences.

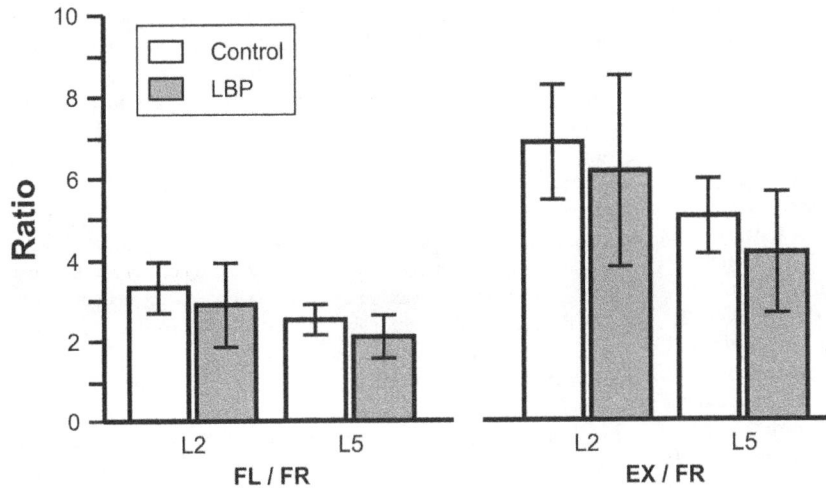

Figure 4. L2 and L5 FL-FR and EX-FR ratios for the three phases at the initial visit.

than for the Chronic group. The Recurrent group did not significantly differ from the other two groups, but for all comparisons correlations were intermediate to the other two groups. No significant differences were observed for either flexion or extension ratios at the L2 level.

The groupings based on pain resolution produced similar trends among the correlation coefficients as did the pain history analysis.

Table 2. Mean (s.d.) Spearman correlation coefficients between pain scores and EMG ratings, and function ratings and EMG ratings, grouped by pain history and pain resolution criteria.

	FL-FR$_{L2}$	FL-FR$_{L5}$	EX-FR$_{L2}$	EX-FR$_{L5}$
Correlation of Pain Score to sEMG ratio:				
Pain History				
Transient	−0.35 (0.54)	−0.32 (0.50)^A	−0.15(0.67)	−0.41 (0.40)^A
Chronic	0.03 (0.28)	0.26 (0.37)^B	−0.04 (0.23)	0.09 (0.33)^B
Recurrent	−0.09 (0.45)	−0.16 (0.34)	−0.16 (0.37)	−0.18 (0.34)
Resolution of Pain				
Resolved	−0.24 (0.54)	−0.36 (0.45)^A	−0.10 (0.57)	−0.38 (0.37)
Partial	−0.16(0.35)	0.06 (0.27)	−0.23 (0.24)	−0.08 (0.23)
No Res	−0.02 (0.44)	−0.06 (0.40)^B	−0.11 (0.38)	0.01 (0.40)
Correlation of Function Rating to sEMG ratio:				
Pain History				
Transient	0.28 (0.62)	0.43 (0.42)^A	0.01 (0.69)	0.50 (0.34)^A
Chronic	−0.04 (0.36)	−0.12 (0.45)^B	0.04 (0.37)	0.00 (0.46)^B
Recurrent	0.06 (0.40)	0.15 (0.35)	0.08 (0.33)	0.15 (0.40)
Resolution of Pain				
Resolved	0.27 (0.60)	0.42 (0.41)^A	0.18 (0.62)	0.49 (0.32)^A
Partial	0.16 (0.19)	0.08 (0.33)	0.20 (0.09)	0.19 (0.35)
No Res	0.02 (0.34)	0.02 (0.37)^B	−0.02 (0.29)	−0.01 (0.41)^B

A and B designations indicate significant differences in correlation coefficients between groupings.

The MANOVA indicated significant differences in correlation to pain score for FL-FR$_{L5}$. However, though the tendency was similar, the correlation to EX-FR$_{L5}$ was not significant (p = 0.058). The correlation to function rating was significant for both FL-FR$_{L5}$ and EX-FR$_{L5}$. The Tukey's post hoc analysis showed significantly greater correlations for the Resolved group than for the Unresolved group. The correlations of the Partial resolution group were not significantly different than for either other group. No significant between-group differences were observed at the L2 level.

Discussion

Significantly greater L5 sEMG amplitude was observed in the LBP group than the Control group at the time of the initial visit. This finding supports the observation generally reported throughout the literature of elevated sEMG amplitudes at full static flexion for those experiencing back pain [19–25,27,28,30]. Disturbances of flexion relaxation response and how it changes over time may bear some relationship to reports of differing activation patterns of the lumbar musculature in individuals with nonspecific LBP. Different motor strategies in response to postural challenges in those with chronic LBP as compared to those without pain have been attributed to disturbances in sensory integration [35]. Other research suggests that those with chronic, nonspecifc LBP were less efficient and thus used more energy in controlling postural sway than healthy individuals [36]. Further research into how these motor behaviors might relate to the potential for developing chronicity could have implications for clinical management.

There were no significant between-group differences in the sEMG ratios between at the time of the first study session. This finding is contrary to a meta-analysis finding that FR ratios were often associated with lower FR ratios at full static flexion [18]. This may be due in large part to differences in study populations. The cohort of the present study had a varied pain experience as compared to the populations of the studies in the meta-analytic review, which generally had greater chronicity and functional disability. In addition to severity, other factors may explain differences between results of the present study and the reports of recovery of FR following rigorous functional restoration [29,30] and exercise [29] interventions that involve strengthening of the back extensors. It is likely that training effects within the ES could be in part responsible for changes in activation patterns. Participants in the present study were not enrolled in any such programs.

A unique feature of the present study was the ability, by virtue of the repeated measures, to observe the interplay between a physiologic measure, and self-reported measures of pain and function over the course of the low back pain episode in a high functioning population. Comparing the strength of these correlations between participant groupings based on their pain history has allowed us to draw some inferences as to how an individual's perception or physiologic response to pain may vary relative to the activation patterns of the erector spinae. The post hoc tests showed that FL-FR_{L5} and EX-FR_{L5} ratios to both pain scores and functional rating were significantly greater for the Transient pain group than for those classified as having and chronic pain. The correlations between the ratios of flexion relaxation to both the forward bending and extension phases demonstrated a significantly stronger inverse relationship to pain report, and positive correlation with function, in the group experiencing transient symptoms than those with more chronic pain. In the Transient group, as pain decreased over the reporting period there was more often an increase in relative amplitude of both the flexion and extension phases relative to FR, reflecting a more "normal" behavior. This was generally not the case for the Chronic group. One explanation might be that because of either physiologic or perceptual changes, pain fear or avoidance behaviors can result in changes to lumbar movement patterns [37] that may not allow for as great a relative degree of relaxation of the trunk extensor musculature during full flexion, when ligamentous structures would normally bear the tissue loads. This speculation is strengthened by the fact that the correlations for the Recurrent group, who by definition are intermediate to the other groups, were also intermediate in response. The groupings based on the relative resolution of LBP over the reporting period produced similar trends. Here again, those who experienced a resolution of pain symptoms had a significantly stronger relationship between both pain and function to the flexion relaxation ratios than their cohort in whom LBP persisted to the end of the study. The speculations made above could apply as well to these results.

There was a trend worth noting in the strength of relationship between the sEMG ratios and the subjective reports dependent upon the level of erector spinae at which the sEMG was recorded. In general, correlations were weaker for the sEMG recorded at the L2 than the L5 level for both the Transient group in the pain history analysis, and in the Resolved group in the pain resolution analysis. Though the reason for this is not known, it has been reported that flexion relaxation occurs less consistently in progression in a cephalad (towards the head) direction [3]. This was particularly pronounced when comparing the correlations of the EX-FR_{L2} and EX-FR_{L5} ratios to both pain and function ratings in both group analyses.

The groupings based on degree of resolution of LBP during the course of the study suggest that in retrospect those whose symptoms resolved had a significantly stronger relationship between changes in the erector spinae activation patterns and their reports of pain and function changes. Participants who ultimately got better were, on some conscious or unconscious level, better able to relax their back extensors as their pain and function improved. One might speculate that as their muscle physiology returned to a more "normal" status, their perceived pain and reported functional status responded accordingly. Conversely,

those whose symptoms and functional deficits persisted throughout the course of the study had significantly weaker relationships with muscle activation patterns, being unable to alter those patterns when at full trunk flexion in response to changes in pain, and ultimately function. This would lead to speculation that for those individuals, other psychosocial factors such as pain beliefs or anxiety [38] may be modulating their perceptions, if flexion relaxation is robust phenomenon. A similar logic can be applied to analysis based on grouping by pain history. This significant relationship, though not providing as strong a correlation between measures, also makes sense in that light. Those experiencing a first episode of LBP of less than six months duration were better able to relax the lower lumbar erector spinae as their pain resolved and function improved. In those facing more prolonged experience with low back pain a dissociation seems to develop between physical behaviors and perception of pain as well as function in daily living.

One limitation of the present study was that though the sample size was sufficient to observe statistically significant differences between participant groupings in some of the measures, power may not have been sufficient to observe others effects. Another potential limitation was the possibility of confounding with the treatment some participants were receiving. This risk was mitigated by having participants complete their ratings, and perform the experimental protocol prior to any treatment. Whether changes were secondary to the natural history, or secondary to treatment or other factors should not be of significant concern as the study investigated correlation of pain or function to EMG- derived variables, independent of potential cause.

The analysis of the relation of pain and function to the FR measures over time suggest that these relationships may have some utility in identifying those likely to progress to resolution of pain over a short period (eight weeks or less) from those who whose pain symptoms, and functional deficits persist. An important consideration in interpreting the results was that the participants more closely represented a cross-section of LBP in the community, as opposed to other studies with populations characterized by greater severity or functional deficits, making direct comparison of results difficult. Further study of the changes in the relationship of physiologic responses to LBP and function over time in such a cohort might help improve our understanding of the complex interplay of psychosocial factors and physical responses to back pain behaviors. Though it is not possible to draw conclusions about factors that may perpetuate back pain, improved understanding of this EMG phenomenon, and its relation to pain and function could ultimately provide measures useful in guiding clinical management.

Acknowledgments

The authors would like to acknowledge Glenn Pransky, MD for his contribution during the participant recruitment process and for his clinical insights, and William Shaw, Ph.D., for his consultations during the preparation of the manuscript. Both researchers are from the Center for Disability Research at the Liberty Mutual Research Institute for Safety.

Author Contributions

Conceived and designed the experiments: RM. Performed the experiments: RM. Analyzed the data: RM JHL. Contributed reagents/materials/analysis tools: RM JHL. Wrote the paper: RM JHL.

References

1. Floyd WF, Silver PHS (1955) The function of erectores spinae muscles in certain movements and postures in man. J Physiol (London) 129: 184–203.
2. Kippers V, Parker AW (1984) Posture related to myoelectric silence of erector spinae during trunk flexion. Spine 9: 740–745.
3. McGill SM, Kippers V (1994) Transfer of loads between lumbar tissues during the flexion-relaxation phenomenon. Spine 19: 2190–2196.
4. Adams MA, Hutton WC, Stott JR (1980) The resistance to flexion of the lumbar intervertebral joint. Spine 5: 245–253.
5. Shirado O, Ito T, Kaneda K, Strax TE (1995) Flexion-relaxation phenomenon in the back muscles. A comparative study between healthy participants and patients with chronic low back pain. Am J Phys Med Rehabil 74: 139–144.
6. Schultz AB, Haderspeck-Grib K, Sinkora G, Warwick DN (1985) Quantitative studies of the flexion-relaxation phenomenon in the back muscles. J Orthop Res 3: 189–197.
7. Sihvonen T, Partanen J, Hanninen O (1991) Electric behavior of low back muscles during lumbar pelvic rhythm in low back pain patients and healthy controls. Arch Phys Med Rehab 72: 1080–1087.
8. Ambroz C, Scott A, Ambroz A, Talbott EO (2000) Chronic low back pain assessment using surface electromyography. J Occup Environ Med. 42: 660–669.
9. Sarti MA, Lison JF, Monfort M, Fuster MA (2001) Response of the flexion-relaxation phenomenon relative to the lumbar motion to load and speed. Spine 26: E421–426.
10. Solomonow M, Baratta RV, Banks A, Freudenberger C, Zhou BH (2003) Flexion-relaxation response to static lumbar flexion in males and females. Clin Biomech 18: 273–279.
11. Paquet N, Malouin F, Richards CL (1994) Hip-spine movement interaction and muscle activation patterns during sagittal trunk movements in low back pain patients. Spine 19: 596–603.
12. Holleran K, Pope M, Haugh L, Absher R (1995) The response of the flexion-relaxation phenomenon in the low back to loading. Iowa Orthop J 15: 24–28.
13. Olson MW, Li L, Solomonow M (2004) Flexion-relaxation response to cyclic lumbar flexion. Clin Biomech 19: 769–776.
14. Descarreau M, Lafond D, Jeffrey-Gauthier R, Centomo H, Cantin V (2008) Changes in the flexion relaxation response induced by lumbar muscle fatigue. BMC Musculoskelet Disord 24; 9:10.
15. Tanii K, Masuda T (1985) A kinesiologic study of erectores spinae activity during trunk flexion and extension. Ergonomics 28: 883–893.
16. Watson PJ, Booker CK, Main CJ, Chen AC (1997) Surface electromyography in the identification of chronic low back pain patients: the development of the flexion relaxation ratio. Clin Biomech 12: 165–171.
17. Kaigle AM, Wessberg P, Hansson TH (1998) Muscular and kinematic behavior of the lumbar spine during flexion-extension. J Spinal Disord 11: 163–174.
18. Geisser ME, Ranavaya M, Haig AJ, Roth RS, Zucker R, et al. (2005) A meta-analytic review of surface electromyography among persons with low back pain and normal, healthy controls. J Pain 6: 711–726.
19. Marshall P, Murphy B (2006) Changes in the flexion relaxation response following an exercise intervention. Spine 31: E877–E883.
20. Wallbom AS, Geisser ME, Koch J, Haig AJ, Guido C, et al. (2009) Lumbar flexion and dynamic EMG among persons with single level disk herniation pre-
and post-surgery with radicular low-back pain. Am J Phys Med Rehabil. 88: 302–307.
21. Mayer TG, Neblett R, Brede E, Gatchel RJ (2009) The quantified lumbar flexion-relaxation phenomenon is a useful measurement of improvement in a functional restoration program. Spine 34: 2458–65.
22. Alschuler KN, Neblett R, Wiggert E, Haig AJ, Geisser ME (2009) Flexion-relaxation and clinical features associated with chronic low back pain: A comparison of different methods of quantifying flexion-relaxation. Clin J Pain 25: 760–766.
23. Ahern DK, Follick MJ, Council JR, Laser-Wolston N, Litchman H (1988) Comparison of lumbar paravertebral EMG patterns in chronic low back pain patients and non-patient controls. Pain 34: 153–160.
24. Ahern DK, Hannon DJ, Goreczny AJ, Follick MJ, Parziale JR (1990) Correlation of chronic low-back pain behavior and muscle function examination of the flexion-relaxation response. Spine 15: 92–95.
25. Haig AJ, Weismann G, Haugh LD, Pope M, Grobler LJ (1993) Prospective evidence for change in paraspinal muscle activity after herniated nucleus pulposus. Spine 18: 926–930.
26. Hides JA, Richardson CA, Jull GA (1996) Multifidus muscle recovery is not automatic after resolution of acute, first-episode low back pain. Spine 21: 2763–2769.
27. Mannion AF, Taimela S, Müntener M, Dvorak J (2001) Active therapy for chronic low back pain part 1. Effects on back muscle activation, fatigability, and strength. Spine 26: 897–908.
28. Neblett R, Mayer TG, Gatchel RJ, Keeley J, Proctor T, et al. (2003) Quantifying the lumbar flexion-relaxation phenomenon: theory, normative data, and clinical applications. Spine 28:1435–1446.
29. Murphy BA, Marshall PW, Taylor HH (2010) The cervical flexion-relaxation ratio: reproducibility and comparison between chronic neck pain patients and controls. Spine 35: 2103–2108.
30. Neblett R, Mayer TG, Brede E, Gatchel RJ (2010) Correcting abnormal flexion-relaxation in chronic lumbar pain: responsiveness to a new biofeedback training protocol. Clin J Pain 26: 403–409.
31. Triano JJ, Schultz AB (1987) Correlation of objective measure of trunk motion and muscle function with low-back disability ratings. Spine 12: 561–565.
32. Jensen MP, Karoly P (1992) Pain-specific beliefs, perceived symptom severity, and adjustment to chronic pain. Clin J Pain 8: 123–130.
33. Stratford PW, Binkley JM, Riddle DL (2000) Development and initial validation of the back pain functional scale. Spine 25: 2095–2102.
34. Von Korff M (1994) Studying the natural history of back pain. Spine 19: 2041S–2046S.
35. Popa T, Bonifazi M, Della Volpe R, Rossi A, Mazzocchio R (2007) Adaptive changes in postural strategy selection in chronic low back pain. Exp Brain Res. 177: 411–418.
36. Matheron E, Kapoula Z. (2011) Vertical heterophoria and postural control in nonspecific chronic low back pain. PLoS One 6: e18110.
37. Thomas JS, France CR (2008) The relationship between pain-related fear and lumbar flexion during natural recovery from low back pain. Eur Spine J 17: 97–103.
38. Linton SJ, Shaw WS (2011) Impact of psychological factors in the experience of pain. Phys Ther 91: 700–711.

15

Predictors for Half-Year Outcome of Impairment in Daily Life for Back Pain Patients Referred for Physiotherapy: A Prospective Observational Study

Sven Karstens[1,2]*, Katja Hermann[2], Ingo Froböse[1], Stephan W. Weiler[3,4]

1 Institute of Health Promotion and Clinical Movement Science, German Sport University Cologne, Cologne, Germany, 2 Department of General Practice and Health Services Research, University Hospital Heidelberg, Heidelberg, Germany, 3 Audi Medical Services, Audi, Ingolstadt, Germany, 4 Department of Occupational Medicine, University Medical Center Schleswig-Holstein, Campus Luebeck, Luebeck, Germany

Abstract

Background and Objective: From observational studies, there is only sparse information available on the predictors of development of impairment in daily life for patients receiving physiotherapy. Therefore, our aim was to identify factors which predict impairment in daily life for patients with back pain 6 months after receiving physiotherapy.

Methods: We conducted a prospective cohort study with 6-month follow-up. Patients were enrolled for treatment in private physiotherapy practices. Patients with a first physiotherapy referral because of thoracic or low back pain, aged 18 to 65 years were included. Primary outcome impairment was measured utilising the 16-item version of the Musculoskeletal Function Assessment Questionnaire. Therapy was documented on a standardized form. Baseline scores for impairment in daily life, symptom characteristics, sociodemographic and psychosocial factors, physical activity, nicotine consumption, intake of analgesics, comorbidity and delivered primary therapy approach were investigated as possible predictors. Univariate and multiple linear regression analyses were performed.

Results: A total of 792 patients participated in the study (59% female, mean age 44.4 (SD 11.4), with 6-month follow-up results available from 391 patients. In univariate analysis 17 variables reached significance. In multiple linear regression identified predictors were: impairment in daily life before therapy, mental disorders, duration of the complaints, self-prognosis on work ability, rheumatoid arthritis, age, form of stress at work and physical activity. The variables explain 34% of variance (adjusted R^2, $p<0.001$).

Conclusions: With minimal information available from observational studies on the predictors of development of back problems for physiotherapy patients, this study adds new knowledge for forming appropriate referral guidelines. Impairment in daily life before therapy, mental disorder as comorbidity and the duration of the complaints can be named as outstanding factors. The results of this study can be used to facilitate comparison of patient therapy goals with the prognosis in everyday practice.

Editor: Steve Milanese, University of South Australia, Australia

Funding: This work was supported by the German Association of Physiotherapy (ZVK) e.V., ZVK Nordverbund (www.zvk-nordverbund.de); payment for printing of questionnaires and assistance in recruitment of research-centers. The chosen assessment-instruments were discussed in a working group "assessment". The Association had no role in data collection and analysis, decision to publish, or preparation of the manuscript.

Competing Interests: Dr SW Weiler is currently employed at Audi Medical Services as an Occupational Health physician and was working for the University of Luebeck when the study was performed. All data were collected on behalf of Institute of Occupational Medicine, University of Luebeck, Germany. To our best knowledge, none of the participants worked for Audi. Audi had in no way influence on the results nor took economical benefit from this study.

* E-mail: sven.karstens@med.uni-heidelberg.de

Introduction

Back pain frequently leads to a limitation in quality of life and working ability [1]. Patients with chronic complaints may suffer from distinct restrictions in their social life [2,3]. Sets of factors useful for prediction of the transition from acute to chronic status include both biomedical and psychosocial aspects [4]. Physiotherapy referrals for treatment are often made, and therapists can positively influence the various factors [5,6,7]. On average, in 2008, every seventh person insured with a major German health insurance company received physical therapy [8]. In about 40 percent of cases, the diagnoses related to low back pain [9]. Commonly in therapy utilized approaches include exercise as active and manual therapy, or physical strategies like electrotherapy as passive approaches. Effectivity for these approaches differs: largest effect sizes were shown for exercise, which reaches a level comparable to acupuncture or behavioral therapy [10].

Various studies have been performed to investigate whether referrals for rehabilitation have been appropriate. In this context, Jensen et al. criticize decision-making on the need for rehabilitation as generally being based on expert opinion and thus being non-transparent [11]. They demonstrated that neither physicians among themselves nor physicians and physiotherapists come to corresponding results. Similar results are provided by Archer et al. and Wagemakers et al. [12,13]. Important information for the referral process is the therapy prognosis. Consequently, models to determine whether the issued referrals have been adequate, regard this factor as essential [14]. However, determining the prognosis is particularly difficult in the case of low back pain patients. Whilst there is extensive information on the natural course of the complaints, only sparse information is available from observational studies on the predictors of development of impairment in daily life specifically under physiotherapy [4,15]. In a recently published systematic review, Verkerk et al. identified some relevant studies. They have shown that for back pain patients different predictors for impairment in daily life exist, but only in a few studies interactions between predictors and physiotherapy were examined and the predictors were mainly investigated only once [16]. Exceptions in which conservative approaches were taken are those conducted by Underwood et al. and Bekkering et al. [17,18]. An additional value of these large trials (n≥500) is the setting, since patient samples were from primary health care, which occurs rather seldom. Harms et al. accomplished a cohort study at a multidisciplinary back pain clinic, in which among others physiotherapists were practicing [19].

For patients undergoing spine surgery, Mannion and Elfering give an overview for predictors [20], but therapy-related predictors are only poorly considered and in the private practice sector these patients are only a minority of the patients.

The objective of this study was to identify factors which predict impairment in daily life for patients with back pain 6 months after receiving physiotherapy.

Methods

Data were collected in a prospective, multicenter cohort study with six-month catamnesis. Patients with thoracic or low-back pain related diagnosis that were referred for physiotherapy by a physician were consecutively admitted to the physiotherapy-centres under consideration of the inclusion and exclusion criteria depicted in **Table 1**. Assignment was based on the standardised referral code "WS" meaning back, as marked on the corresponding form by the physician [21]. The criterion specific back pain meant that patients with serious traumatic conditions or inflammatory rheumatic diseases as referral diagnosis were excluded. Patients with nerve root irritation were included.

Outcomes were measured using the German 16-item-version of the Musculoskeletal Function Assessment Questionnaire [22]. The well known 46-item instrument (SMFA) has been implemented in many countries around the world [23,24]. The questionnaire comprises two subscales with the underlying constructs impairment (BI) and dysfunction (FI). The instrument is scaled from 0–

100 with 0 signifying no and 100 maximal limitation. The result is indicated as "percent"-value. Wollmerstedt et al. have shown good psychometric properties for the questionnaire in various patient groups. Internal consistency for functioning is $\alpha \geq 0.86$ and $\alpha \geq 0.78$ for impairment respectively. Construct validity was determined by correlation with the corresponding SMFA-subscales, resulting in $r \geq 0.93$ for the FI and $r \geq 0.87$ for the BI [22,24].

Potential prognostic factors comprised sociodemographics, diagnosis and symptoms, behavioural aspects, comorbidities and psychosocial factors.

All independent variables including coding are presented in **Table 2**. Sociodemographics were assessed referring to standards set by an epidemiological expert panel [25]. The diagnostic subgroups were determined in a qualitative assessment, using information given on the referral form. Examples for diagnosis assigned to the different groups are depicted in **Table 3**. Pain intensity was measured using an 11-point box scale [26]. Nicotine consumption and physical activity were assessed using self-developed questions. Comorbidities and psychosocial factors were assessed using the Work Ability Index Questionnaire (WAI) [27,28]. Comorbidities were identified with the WAI sickness list. Mental resources were determined via a subscale of the WAI, which encompasses 3 questions concerning enjoyment of regular daily activities, being active and alert and being hopeful about the future. Self-prognosis on work ability was assessed through a single item WAI-dimension.

Treatment was not influenced by the investigators. It was documented on a standardized form by the therapists after the final session. They had to select from the options depicted in **Table 4**. One option was to mark as primary approach, as many as useful as secondary approaches.

The patients were enrolled between May 2007 and August 2008. Questioning took place immediately before the first therapy session (t1) and 6 months after treatment (t2). The latter was accomplished via mail.

Ethical approval was granted by the Ethics Committee of the University of Luebeck, Germany (registration ID: 07-019). All patients gave their written informed consent for participation, before entering the study in the participating practice.

Statistics

A multiple linear regression model was calculated [29]. As dependent variable the impairment subscale of the Musculoskeletal Function Assessment Questionnaire 6 months after therapy was set [22]. Before the selection procedure, the independent variables of each case were checked for extremes. Cases were eliminated as outliers, if their value exceeded or presented a shortfall of the arithmetic average by 3 standard deviations. To enable inclusion of treatment into the analyses, the primary approaches were assigned to two variables: active (see **Table 4**,

Table 1. Inclusion and exclusion criteria.

Inclusion criteria	Thoracic- or low-back-related diagnosis
	First prescription* of physical therapy (according to form)
	Age between 18 and 65
Exclusion criteria	Specific back pain (e.g. Bechterew disease or fracture)
	Not capable of reading, writing and/or understanding German language
	Prescription for massage or lymph drainage as primary therapy

*"First prescription" according to German regulations means no therapy for at least 12 weeks.

Table 2. Independent variables.

Independent Variables		Characteristic/value label
Sociodemographic details	Age	scale
	Gender	1 = female, 2 = male
Diagnosis and Symptoms	Subgroup nonspecific, subgroup thoracic, subgroup disc/root irritation, post surgery	1 = yes, 0 = no
	Impairment/pain intensity prior to treatment	scale
	Duration of complaints ≥ ½ year, radiation into lower extremity, multifocal complaints	1 = yes, 0 = no
Behavioural factors	Physically active, smoker, intake of analgesics	1 = yes, 0 = no
	Body mass index,	scale
Comorbidities	Rheumatoid arthritis, mental disorder, neurological-sensory disease, genitourinary or digestive disease, tumours, diabetes	1 = yes, 0 = no
Psychosocial Factors	Employed, white collar worker, good self-prognosis on work ability in 2 years	1 = yes, 0 = no
	Mental resources	scale
Primary therapy	Active, passive	1 = yes, 0 = no

treatment 1–6) and passive treatment (treatment 7–13). Patient education, active assisted exercises and "other therapy" were not ascribed as not being clearly active or passive and were therefore considered only indirectly as a counterpart of the two variables.

To ensure a basic correlation between the dependent and the independent variables, statistical selection was done in two steps. For all potential variables a univariate regression analysis was calculated. First, all variables whose coefficients exceeded p = 0.25 were eliminated [30]. After that, the multiple linear regression model was calculated backwards stepwise entering all remaining variables. Missing values were excluded casewise as threshold for variable exclusion in the multivariate procedure p≥0.1 was set.

Following the recommendations given by Schendera for identification of outliers, the standardized residuals, the standardized Difference in Fit (DfFit) and Cook-distance were saved [29]. Cases were excluded if standardized residuals exceeded ±3 and if in addition results showed DfFit >2*sqrt(p/n) [sqrt = square root, p = amount of independent variables, n = number of cases] or Cook-distance >1 [29,31]. The procedure was repeated until no more outliers could be identified.

For testing the significance of the final regression model an ANOVA was carried out. Data were analyzed using SPSS version 19.0.

Results

84 practices participated with the mean number of therapists in each being 3.4 (SD 2.2). After checking for inclusion and exclusion criteria, results from 792 patients were available for analysis; for catamnesis, data from 391 patients was available (median per practice 4, IQR 2 to 6.5, range 1 to 63). Baseline characteristics

are presented in **Table 5**. The mean impairment six months after treatment was 25.3 (SD 22.4).

There were no significant baseline differences between responders and dropouts by age and impairment, but dropouts were more likely to be men (p<0.05). The treatment provided is shown in **Figure 1**.

Predictors of outcome

Three patients with an extremely high body mass index (>44) were excluded as outliers before final model formulation.

24 variables were adopted in the multivariate regression calculation after univariate analyses because their p-values satisfied the set threshold of 0.25 (see **Table 6**). Differentiated information regarding the unstandardized coefficient B are given in **Table 7**.

After first regression calculation, two additional outliers were eliminated, since leverage-values exceeded the specified threshold. There were 9 variables identified to have an influence on impairment six months after therapy (**Table 8**). With p>0.05 the body mass index must be regarded as a moderating variable.

The sign of the unstandardized regression coefficient B (**Table 8**) shows in which direction the variable influences the prognosis of impairment in daily life half a year after therapy. Metrically scaled predictors "Impairment prior to treatment" and "age" are signed positive. The prognosis thus worsens with higher impairment prior to treatment and/or higher age. Also the dichotomous predictors "mental disorder", "rheumatoid arthritis" and "duration of complaints ≥ ½ year" are signed positive. The prognosis thus worsens if the patient suffers from one of the mentioned illnesses and/or has a long history of complaints. The dichotomous predictors "good self-prognosis on work ability in 2 years", "white collar worker" and "physically active" show a

Table 3. Diagnostic Subgroups; examples for assigned referral-diagnosis.

Subgroup	Examples for assigned referral-diagnosis
- nonspecific	Back pain, low back pain, sacroiliac joint pain, sacroiliac joint dysfunction, lumbar spine blockage
- disc/root irritation	Lumbar intervertebral disc displacement, radiculopathy segment L4, lumbosacral disc displacement, slipped disc L3
- thoracic	thoracic spine pain, thoracic spine blockage

Table 4. Documentation categories therapy.

1. Therapeutic exercises	7. Manual therapy	13. Ultrasound
2. Stretching exercises	8. Traction	14. Patient education
3. Proprioception	9. Massage	15. Active assisted exercises
4. Strength training (including machines)	10. Cold therapy	16. Other therapy (free text)
5. Home exercises	11. Heat therapy	
6. Activities of daily life	12. Electrotherapy	

negative sign. If the patient is confident before therapy, is a white collar worker or physically active the prognosis improves.

ANOVA for the final regression model resulted in p<0.001. Our baseline variables predicted 34% of the variance in impairment in daily life 6 months after therapy (adjusted R^2).

Discussion

We developed a model for prognosis of disability in back patients half a year after receiving physiotherapy. Outstanding predictors are restrictions in daily life before therapy, mental disorder as secondary diagnosis and duration of complaints; of further relevance are self-prognosed work ability in 2 years, rheumatoid arthritis, age, workplace demands and physical activity. To our knowledge a variable set comparable to ours has not been previously investigated.

At this stage, the comparison of the predictor set as a whole with other studies is not feasible because of the limited number of comparable studies and the diverging sets used. Possibilities for comparison for the variables "age", "Impairment prior to treatment" and "duration of the complaints" are provided by secondary analysis of two large randomized controlled trials [17,18]. The strength of the comparison lies within the therapy-specific approach of the trials. In our study, age was a significant factor, as was the case for Underwood et al. However, Bekkering et al. found no such association [17,18]. Consensus can be found for the significant variable "duration of the complaints" [17,18]. If the variable "Impairment prior to treatment" is compared with

functioning or pain and disability there also can be shown a homogeneous result underlining relevance [17,18]. A connected predictor was found to be of relevance by another group of researchers, who adopted a follow-up similar to ours. Harms et al. found an episodic pain character to be advantageous [19].

The systematic review by van der Hulst et al. facilitates evaluation for similarities for the variables "physical activity", "white collar worker" and "self-prognosis" [15]. They also investigated a therapy-specific approach with referral to multidisciplinary rehabilitation or back school. Whether the variable was of importance differed depending on the specific therapy for physical activity. Unlike our results, van der Hulst et al. were not able to describe relevance for the aspect white versus blue collar worker [15]. Reflection on the significant predictors "self-prognosis on work ability" and "mental disorder" is difficult, because many different constructs were investigated in the trials adopted by van der Hulst et al. [15]. An association for the latter may be seen in the Symptom Checklist-90 and the Distress scale, but once more the comparison results in an inconsistency. Findings vary depending on therapy and outcome measure.

Table 5. Baseline characteristics.

Measure	Overall
	(n = 792)
Mean Age in years (SD)	44.4 (11.4)
Gender female (%)	58.8
Subgroup (%)	
- non-specific low back pain	73.4
- disc/root irritation	17.3
- thoracic spine	9.3
Duration of complaints >1/2 year (%)	56.8
Pain radiation lower extremity (%)	58.4
Mean Impairment prior to treatment (SD)	46.4 (22.4)
Mean pain intensity prior to treatment (SD)	6.0 (2.1)
Mean body mass index in kg/m² (SD)	26.3 (5.3)
Not employed (%)	18.8

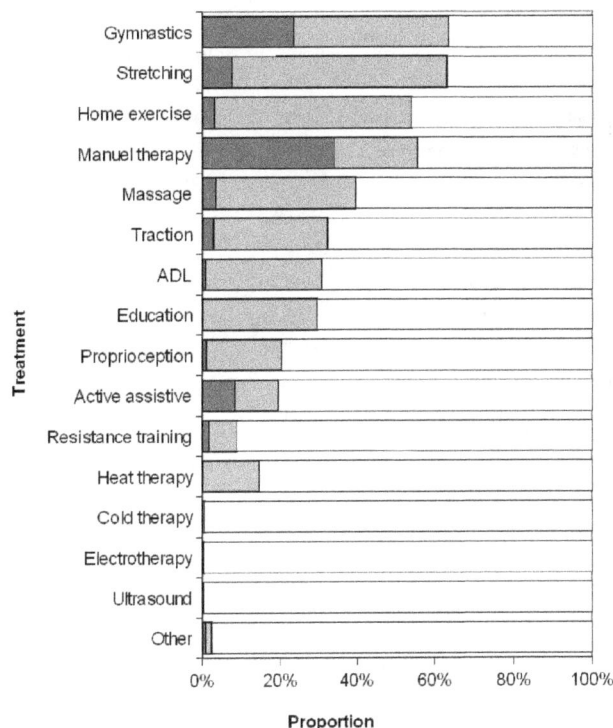

Figure 1. Treatment. Dark grey: primary treatment approach, light grey: secondary. ADL: Activities of daily living.

Table 6. Variables adopted in the multivariate regression analysis.

1. Good self-prognosis on work ability in 2 years	9. Multifocal complaints	17. Subgroup thoracic spine
2. Mental disorder	10. White collar worker	18. Primary therapy passive
3. Impairment prior to treatment	11. Analgesics intake	19. Genitourinary or digestive disease
4. Rheumatoid arthritis	12. Neurological-sensory disease	20. Tumours
5. Mental resources	13. Employed	21. Smoker
6. Duration of complaints $\geq \frac{1}{2}$ year	14. Pain radiation lower extremity	22. Diabetes or metabolic disease
7. Pain intensity at t1	15. Physically active	23. Subgroup low back non-specific
8. Age	16. Body mass index	24. Primary therapy active

The influence of the predictor rheumatoid arthritis can be easily explained by the destructive character of the underlying autoimmune disease [32,33].

In our study, different subgroups of back pain patients were included. From the relating variables, only the subgroup thoracic spine reached significance and this only in univariate analysis. This

Table 7. Predictors for impairment at 6 Month: Results of univariate Regression Analysis.

Prognostic factor	B	Lower CI	Upper CI
Age	0.47*	0.28	0.66
Gender	0.45	−4.22	5.13
Subgroup non-specific	3.49	−1.48	8.45
Subgroup disc/root irritation	1.12	−4.68	6.92
Subgroup thoracic spine	−10.19*	−17.76	−2.61
Therapy post surgery	−1.93	−26.59	22.72
Impairment prior to treatment	0.34*	0.25	0.44
Pain prior to treatment	2.85*	1.77	3.93
Duration $\geq \frac{1}{2}$ year	12.30*	7.96	16.65
Radiation into lower extremity	7.48*	2.97	11.99
Multifocal complaints	14.16*	8.34	19.98
Physically active	−7.43*	−12.05	−2.82
Smoker	4.99	−0.58	10.55
Intake of analgesics	8.84*	4.35	13.32
Body mass index	0.68*	0.23	1.14
Employed	−9.88*	−15.49	−4.28
Mental resources	−7.12*	−9.57	−4.68
Good self-prognosis on work ability in 2 years	−19.69*	−24.53	−14.84
White collar worker	−9.57*	−14.06	−5.07
Rheumatoid arthritis	19.87*	13.47	26.28
Diabetes	9.21	−1.74	20.17
Tumours	11.91	−1.20	25.02
Mental disorder	18.92*	13.64	24.21
Neurological-sensory disease	9.20*	4.18	14.21
Genitourinary or digestive disease	5.49	−0.03	11.02
Primary therapy active	−3.02	−7.58	1.55
Primary therapy passiv	1.94	−2.58	6.45

B = unstandardized Coefficients B, CI: confidence interval,
*P<0.05.

result may be partly attributed to the source of the diagnoses, which were taken from the referral-forms and issued by the physician for therapeutic and not for research purposes. According to Thomas et al. pain radiation into the lower extremity may have influence on the persistence of back pain [34]. Also, for our corresponding variable this could have been confirmed only in univariate analysis.

The mean impairment at baseline given for our study is comparable to the results of other research groups [24]. During therapy it was reduced considerably. In a meta-analysis, it was shown for non-specific low back pain patients with chronic complaints that exercise therapy is effective [35]. Therefore, regarding the conducted therapy approaches (**Figure 1**) one may conclude that these had an influence. For passive approaches, results are controversial [36,37]. However, since some patients had acute complaints the shown reduction could partly be explained by the natural course.

The primary therapy approach was utilized via two variables in our study: Primary therapy approach active or Primary therapy approach passive. Both variables did not reach significance and correspondingly our results do not reinforce the assumption that active approaches show a superior effect. A different allocation of the therapy approaches may have led to different results, moreover in future trials the duration and frequency of therapy may be included as additional factors.

Implications for practice

For assessment of the need for physiotherapy, the results allow comparison of the patients' therapy odds with the prognosis before treatment starts. Raspe et al. regard this as an essential aspect in needs assessment [14]. In addition, the results add information for compiling more homogeneous cohorts in future experimental studies. Different examinations point to the fact that studies on the efficiency of therapeutic services – seen from a biopsychosocial perspective – are currently carried out with heterogeneous groups of patients. Selected therapy approaches specifically compiled or selected for specified groups of patients could lead to an increase of efficiency in the measures [5,38,39].

Three of the four most often used treatment approaches were different types of exercise. This is in accordance with the National Disease Management Guideline for Low Back Pain, in which such approaches are strongly recommended [40]. Manual therapy, the fourth approach is declared as an option. Evidence indicates, that for chronic back pain it may especially be of use in combination with exercise [37], as it was normally conducted by the participating therapists. Particularly the frequent application of traction should be reconsidered. For acute as well as for chronic patients, it is strongly recommended in the guideline not to use it.

Table 8. Result of multivariate Regression Analysis.

Independent Variables	Unstandardized Coefficients		Standardized Coefficients	T	p	VIF
	B	SE	Beta			
(Constant)	−3.837	8.066		−0.476	0.635	
Good self-prognosis on work ability	−5.675	2.662	−0.116	−2.132	0.034	1.353
Mental disorder	11.002	2.756	0.202	3.991	0.000	1.181
Impairment prior to treatment	0.205	0.048	0.213	4.251	0.000	1.151
Rheumatoid arthritis	9.368	3.343	0.141	2.802	0.005	1.158
Duration of complaints ≥ ½ year	8.378	2.213	0.192	3.786	0.000	1.177
Age	0.218	0.097	0.111	2.256	0.025	1.117
White collar worker	−6.233	2.112	−0.141	−2.951	0.003	1.048
Physically active	−4.733	2.126	−0.107	−2.226	0.027	1.064
Body mass index	0.379	0.218	0.086	1.743	0.082	1.123

Dependent variable: Impairment 6 months after therapy.

Particularly when considering the question about changes of health status after therapy, the developed study design has the advantage that it embodied "usual therapy", as treatment was not influenced experimentally. The multicentered structure additionally increases the external validity in comparison to a mono-centered design [41]. Moreover, the large sample size can be seen as a strength.

Study Limitations

For observational studies, the dropout rate for follow-up is a classical challenge [41]. To counteract this, trial-conductance was carefully planned and tested; beyond that the material to be used during the study was developed as user-friendly as possible [42]. In this trial, a response rate of about 50% was obtained; this result is comparable with other prospective studies on musculoskeletal problems [38,43,44]. Furthermore, the number of cases made it possible to include all variables, which arose from univariate analyses into final analysis. The higher dropout rate for men may be regarded as a limiting factor for validity.

Multiple linear regression modeling is a complex procedure, which is commonly applied as an iterative process [29,45]. Correspondingly, in this investigation more than one course of analysis was necessary. Three patients had to be excluded from the analysis before first calculation due to an extremely high body mass index. The values for these patients show a difference of more than three standard deviations from the group average. Thus, the inclusion of them could have led to a distortion of the regression coefficient. Graphical analyses reinforced this hypothesis. Considering recommended thresholds, two additional patients had to be excluded because of their leverage-values [29,31]. A subsequently performed comparison showed that variables determined as significant before exclusion did not differ from that after exclusion. Correspondingly the coefficients also only differed slightly.

Only exceptionally a regression model leads to a nearby 100% prognosis. However, the level of explained variance with 34% is comparable to that of similarly analysed trials [17,18].

Conclusions

In summary, we identified prognostic factors for back patients' impairment in daily life half a year after receiving physiotherapy. Outstanding predictive factors are impairment in daily life before therapy, mental disorder as comorbidity and the duration of the complaints. Our results indicate that prognosis for the individual patient can be estimated and aligned with his or her therapy odds. This may be realistically and simply estimated using a short questionnaire at initial assessment.

Author Contributions

Acquisition of data: SK SWW. Critical revision of the article: IF. Conceived and designed the experiments: SK IF SWW. Analyzed the data: SK KH IF SWW. Wrote the paper: SK KH SWW.

References

1. EU (2009) The Status of Health in the European Union: Towards a healthier Europe; extended Summary. Available: http://euglorehcd.eulogos.it/IXT/_EXT-SUMM/_INDEX.HTM. Accessed 2012 Aug 20.

2. Leeuw M, Goossens ME, Linton SJ, Crombez G, Boersma K, et al. (2007) The fear-avoidance model of musculoskeletal pain: current state of scientific evidence. J Behav Med 30: 77–94.

3. Osborn M, Smith JA (1998) The personal experience of chronic benign lower back pain: An interpretative phenomenological analysis. British Journal of Health Psychology 3: 65–83.

4. Hayden JA, Chou R, Hogg-Johnson S, Bombardier C (2009) Systematic reviews of low back pain prognosis had variable methods and results: guidance for future prognosis reviews. J Clin Epidemiol 62: 781–796.

5. Hill JC, Whitehurst DG, Lewis M, Bryan S, Dunn KM, et al. (2011) Comparison of stratified primary care management for low back pain with current best practice (STarT Back): a randomised controlled trial. Lancet 378: 1560–1571.

6. Klaber Moffett JA, Carr J, Howarth E (2004) High fear-avoiders of physical activity benefit from an exercise program for patients with back pain. Spine (Phila Pa 1976) 29: 1167–1172; discussion 1173.

7. Smeets RJ, Vlaeyen JW, Hidding A, Kester AD, van der Heijden GJ, et al. (2006) Active rehabilitation for chronic low back pain: cognitive-behavioral, physical, or both? First direct post-treatment results from a randomized controlled trial [ISRCTN22714229]. BMC Musculoskelet Disord 7: 5.

8. Kemper C, Sauer K, Glaeske G (2009) GEK-Heil- und Hilfsmittel-Report 2009; Auswertungsergebnisse der GEK-Heil- und Hilfsmitteldaten aus den Jahren 2007 und 2008.Schwäbisch Gmünd : GEK - Gmünder Ersatzkasse. 226 p.

9. WIdO (2010) Wissenschaftliches Institut der AOK: Heilmittelbericht 2010. Berlin: AOK-Bundesverband GbR. 58 p.

10. Keller A, Hayden J, Bombardier C, van Tulder M (2007) Effect sizes of non-surgical treatments of non-specific low-back pain. Eur Spine J 16: 1776–1788.

11. Jensen IB, Bodin L, Ljungqvist T, Gunnar Bergstrom K, Nygren A (2000) Assessing the needs of patients in pain: a matter of opinion? Spine (Phila Pa 1976) 25: 2816–2823.

12. Archer KR, Mackenzie EJ, Castillo RC, Bosse MJ (2009) Orthopedic surgeons and physical therapists differ in assessment of need for physical therapy after traumatic lower-extremity injury. Phys Ther 89: 1337–1349.

13. Wagemakers HP, Luijsterburg PA, Heintjes EM, Berger MY, Verhaar J, et al. (2010) Outcome of knee injuries in general practice: 1-year follow-up. Br J Gen Pract 60: 56–63.

14. Raspe H, Ekkernkamp M, Matthis C, Raspe A, Mittag O (2005) Being in Need of Rehabilitation Services: Concept and Data. Rehabilitation (Stuttg) 44: 325–334.

15. van der Hulst M, Vollenbroek-Hutten MM, Ijzerman MJ (2005) A systematic review of sociodemographic, physical, and psychological predictors of multidisciplinary rehabilitation-or, back school treatment outcome in patients with chronic low back pain. Spine (Phila Pa 1976) 30: 813–825.

16. Verkerk K, Luijsterburg PA, Miedema HS, Pool-Goudzwaard A, Koes BW (2012) Prognostic factors for recovery in chronic nonspecific low back pain: a systematic review. Phys Ther 92: 1093–1108.

17. Bekkering GE, Hendriks HJ, van Tulder MW, Knol DL, Simmonds MJ, et al. (2005) Prognostic factors for low back pain in patients referred for physiotherapy: comparing outcomes and varying modeling techniques. Spine (Phila Pa 1976) 30: 1881–1886.

18. Underwood MR, Morton V, Farrin A (2007) Do baseline characteristics predict response to treatment for low back pain? Secondary analysis of the UK BEAM dataset Rheumatology (Oxford) 46: 1297–1302.

19. Harms MC, Peers CE, Chase D (2010) Low back pain: what determines functional outcome at six months? An observational study. BMC Musculoskelet Disord 11: 236.

20. Mannion AF, Elfering A (2006) Predictors of surgical outcome and their assessment. Eur Spine J 15 Suppl 1: S93–108.

21. GBA (2004) Richtlinien des Gemeinsamen Bundesausschusses über die Verordnung von Heilmitteln in der vertragsärztlichen Versorgung; Zweiter Teil - Zuordnung der Heilmittel zu Indikationen (Heilmittel-Katalog). Available: www.g-ba.de/downloads/17-98-1085/RL-Heilmittel-Katalog-04-12-21.pdf. Accessed 2013 Mar 22.

22. Wollmerstedt N, Faller H, Ackermann H, Schneider J, Glatzel M, et al. (2006) Evaluation of the Extra Short Musculoskeletal Function Assessment Questionnaire XSMFA-D in Patients with Musculoskeletal Disorders and Surgical or Medical In-Patient Treatment. Rehabilitation (Stuttg) 45: 78–87.

23. Barei DP, Agel J, Swiontkowski MF (2007) Current utilization, interpretation, and recommendations: the musculoskeletal function assessments (MFA/SMFA). J Orthop Trauma 21: 738–742.

24. Swiontkowski MF, Engelberg R, Martin DP, Agel J (1999) Short musculoskeletal function assessment questionnaire: validity, reliability, and responsiveness. J Bone Joint Surg Am 81: 1245–1260.

25. AEM (1997) Arbeitsgruppe "Epidemiologische Methoden" in der Deutschen Arbeitsgemeinschaft Epidemiologie, der Gesellschaft für Medizinische Informatik, Biometrie und Epidemiologie und der Deutschen Gesellschaft für Sozialmedizin und Prävention: Messung und Quantifizierung soziographischer Merkmale in epidemiologischen Studien. Available: http://www.gesundheitsforschung-bmbf.de/_media/Empfehlungen__Epidemiologische_Studien.pdf. Accessed 2013 Mar 22.

26. Sim J, Waterfield J (1997) Validity, reliability an responsiveness in the assessment of pain. Physiotherapy Theory and Practice 13: 23–37.

27. Tuomi K (1998) Work ability index. Helsinki: Finnish Inst. of Occupational Health. 30 p.

28. WAI-Netzwerk (2012) WAI Online Questionnaire (short version). Available: http://www.arbeitsfaehigkeit.uni-wuppertal.de/index.php?wai-online-en. Accessed 2012 Aug 20.

29. Schendera CFG (2008) Regressionsanalyse mit SPSS. München: Oldenbourg. 466 p.

30. van der Waal JM, Bot SD, Terwee CB, van der Windt DA, Scholten RJ, et al. (2005) Course and prognosis of knee complaints in general practice. Arthritis Rheum 53: 920–930.

31. Urban D, Mayerl J (2008) Regressionsanalyse: Theorie, Technik und Anwendung. Wiesbaden: VS Verlag für Sozialwissenschaften/Springer Fachmedien. 336 p.

32. Reeuwijk KG, de Rooij M, van Dijk GM, Veenhof C, Steultjens MP, et al. (2010) Osteoarthritis of the hip or knee: which coexisting disorders are disabling? Clin Rheumatol 29: 739–747.

33. Smolen JS, Aletaha D (2009) Developments in the clinical understanding of rheumatoid arthritis. Arthritis Res Ther 11: 204.

34. Thomas E, Silman AJ, Croft PR, Papageorgiou AC, Jayson MI, et al. (1999) Predicting who develops chronic low back pain in primary care: a prospective study. BMJ 318: 1662–1667.

35. Hayden JA, van Tulder MW, Tomlinson G (2005) Systematic review: strategies for using exercise therapy to improve outcomes in chronic low back pain. Ann Intern Med 142: 776–785.

36. Clarke JA, van Tulder MW, Blomberg SE, de Vet HC, van der Heijden GJ, et al. (2007) Traction for low-back pain with or without sciatica. Cochrane Database Syst Rev: CD003010.

37. Rubinstein SM, van Middelkoop M, Assendelft WJ, de Boer MR, van Tulder MW (2011) Spinal manipulative therapy for chronic low-back pain. Cochrane Database Syst Rev 2: CD008112.

38. Foster NE, Thomas E, Bishop A, Dunn KM, Main CJ (2010) Distinctiveness of psychological obstacles to recovery in low back pain patients in primary care. Pain 148: 398–406.

39. Kent P, Mjosund HL, Petersen DH (2010) Does targeting manual therapy and/ or exercise improve patient outcomes in nonspecific low back pain? A systematic review. BMC Med 8: 22.

40. Chenot J-F, Becker A (2011) The National Disease Management Guideline for Low Back Pain: A Summary for Family Medicine. ZFA 87: 14–21.

41. Röhrig B, du Prel J-B, Blettner M (2009) Study Design in Medical Research: Part 2 of a Series on the Evaluation of Scientific Publications. Dtsch Arztebl International 106: 184–189.

42. Edwards P, Roberts I, Clarke M, DiGuiseppi C, Pratap S, et al. (2002) Increasing response rates to postal questionnaires: systematic review. BMJ 324: 1183.

43. Rutten GM, Degen S, Hendriks EJ, Braspenning JC, Harting J, et al. (2010) Adherence to clinical practice guidelines for low back pain in physical therapy: do patients benefit? Phys Ther 90: 1111–1122.

44. van den Hoogen HJ, Koes BW, van Eijk JT, Bouter LM, Deville W (1998) On the course of low back pain in general practice: a one year follow up study. Ann Rheum Dis 57: 13–19.

45. Backhaus K (2006) Multivariate Analysemethoden: eine anwendungsorientierte Einführung. Berlin, Heidelberg: Springer. 583 p.

Threshold of Musculoskeletal Pain Intensity for Increased Risk of Long-Term Sickness Absence among Female Healthcare Workers in Eldercare

Lars L. Andersen[1]*, Thomas Clausen[1], Hermann Burr[2], Andreas Holtermann[1]

1 National Research Centre for the Working Environment, Copenhagen Ø, Denmark, **2** Federal Institute for Occupational Safety and Health (BAuA), Berlin, Germany

Abstract

Purpose: Musculoskeletal disorders increase the risk for absenteeism and work disability. However, the threshold when musculoskeletal pain intensity significantly increases the risk of sickness absence among different occupations is unknown. This study estimates the risk for long-term sickness absence (LTSA) from different pain intensities in the low back, neck/shoulder and knees among female healthcare workers in eldercare.

Methods: Prospective cohort study among 8,732 Danish female healthcare workers responding to a questionnaire in 2004–2005, and subsequently followed for one year in a national register of social transfer payments (DREAM). Using Cox regression hazard ratio (HR) analysis we modeled risk estimates of pain intensities on a scale from 0–9 (reference 0, where 0 is no pain and 9 is worst imaginable pain) in the low back, neck/shoulders and knees during the last three months for onset of LTSA (receiving sickness absence compensation for at least eight consecutive weeks) during one-year follow-up.

Results: During follow-up, the 12-month prevalence of LTSA was 6.3%. With adjustment for age, BMI, smoking and leisure physical activity, the thresholds of pain intensities significantly increasing risk of LTSA for the low back (HR 1.44 [95%CI 1.07–1.93]), neck/shoulders (HR 1.47 [95%CI 1.10–1.96]) and knees (HR 1.43 [95%CI 1.06–1.93]) were 5, 4 and 3 (scale 0–9), respectively, referencing pain intensity of 0.

Conclusion: The threshold of pain intensity significantly increasing the risk for LTSA among female healthcare workers varies across body regions, with knee pain having the lowest threshold. This knowledge may be used in the prevention of LTSA among health care workers.

Editor: Sam Eldabe, The James Cook University Hospital, United Kingdom

Funding: The study was supported by a grant from the Danish Parliament (SATS 2004). The funder had no role in study design, data collection and analysis, decision to publish, or preparation of the manuscript.

Competing Interests: The authors have declared that no competing interests exist.

* E-mail: LLA@NRCWE.DK

Introduction

Sickness absence from work is considered a global health indicator [1]. Long-term sickness absence (LTSA) is especially relevant, because workers being absent for several consecutive weeks have increased risk for not returning to the labor market [2]. Because being gainfully employed plays an important role in well-being and societal identity [3] prevention of LTSA should have high priority. Knowledge of prognostic factors for LTSA is important for optimally targeting preventive efforts.

More than 100 million European citizens suffer from chronic musculoskeletal pain [4], and musculoskeletal disorders are the most common causes of work disability and consequent absence from work [5]. Low back pain and neck/shoulder pain are associated with both short-term sickness absence and LTSA in several occupations [6–11]. However, the consequence of pain from different body regions and severities of pain may vary between occupations with different physical demands. For example, whereas knee pain did not predict LTSA in the general working population [12], knee pain was a strong risk factor for

LTSA among healthcare workers in eldercare [13]. However, previous studies have used different definitions and cut-points of pain severity making comparisons between the types of pain and occupations difficult. Thus, the association between musculoskeletal pain and risk of sickness absence should be evaluated separately for each specific occupation, body part and thresholds of pain intensity.

The prevalence of musculoskeletal disorders and LTSA is high in occupations with physically demanding work [14]. Healthcare work is particularly physically demanding [15], and in a survey involving more than 8000 healthcare workers in eldercare 23%, 28%, and 12% reported chronic pain (>30 days last year) in the low back, neck/shoulders, and knees, respectively [13]. Thus, healthcare work in eldercare may be particularly physically demanding. In spite of preventive efforts in the healthcare sector – e.g. provision of manual handling equipment – elimination of all incidences of musculoskeletal pain is probably unrealistic. Thus, prevention of the consequences of musculoskeletal pain may be more realistic. To provide better recommendations for protecting individual healthcare workers from LTSA and consequent job loss there is a need for knowing when pain intensity reaches a critical level for increasing the risk of LTSA.

The aim of our study was to estimate the risk for long-term sickness absence (LTSA) from different pain intensities in the low back, neck/shoulder and knees among female healthcare workers in eldercare.

Methods

Population

The present study is based on survey data collected among employees in the eldercare-services merged with the Danish Register for Evaluation of Marginalization (DREAM), which is a National register on social transfer payments [16]. A survey on health and working conditions among 12,744 employees in the eldercare-sector of 36 Danish municipalities was conducted in 2004–5, yielding a response percentage of 78% (9,947 persons). All respondents of the survey were identified and followed in the DREAM register for one year after completion of the survey. Employees being engaged in management or in production of services not directly related to the provision of health-related care services (e.g. kitchen staff, janitors, administrators) were excluded from the analyses (N = 995). Further, male respondents were excluded (N = 220). Thus, the target population comprised 8,732 female employees being directly engaged in the provision of health-related care services in the Danish eldercare-sector (e.g. nurses, nurses aides).

Ethical approval

The study has been notified to and registered by Datatilsynet (the Danish Data Protection Agency). According to Danish law, questionnaire and register based studies do not need approval by ethical and scientific committees, nor informed consent [17,18]. All data was de-identified and analyzed anonymously.

Outcome variable: Long-term sickness absence

Data on sickness absence were drawn from the DREAM register [16,19], and linked to the survey data via the unique personal identification number given to all Danish citizens at birth. The DREAM register contains weekly information on granted sickness absence, education, employment, disability pension etc for all citizens in Denmark. Due to Danish law the reason for sickness absence is not registered. Sickness absence compensation is given to the employer, who can apply for a refund from the state for employees after two weeks of sickness absence. Because the employer has a strong economic incentive to report sickness absence, the validity of the sickness absence data has been found to be high [16]. Long-term sickness absence was defined as the occurrence of a period of eight or more consecutive weeks of sickness absence in a one-year follow-up period from the date of the questionnaire reply. We chose an absence period for eight or more consecutive weeks as empirical evidence indicates that employees who are absent for eight weeks or more have a substantially increased risk for not returning to work [2].

Risk factor: Intensity of musculoskeletal pain

Participants rated pain in the low back, neck/shoulders, and knees, respectively, as average pain during the last three months on a numerical rating scale from 0–9, where 0 is 'no pain' and 9 is 'worst imaginable pain'. The rating scale was horizontally oriented to represent a modified visual-analogue scale [20]. A drawing from the Nordic Questionnaire defined the three respective body

regions [21]. Respondents with pain intensities of 0 were set as reference.

To ease the discussion we term pain intensities of 0–2 as 'low', 3–5 as 'moderate' and more than 5 as 'severe'.

Confounders

Potential confounders included age, body mass index (BMI = weight/height^2), smoking status (dichotomous variable depicting current smoker/non-smoker), seniority (years working as healthcare worker; continuous variable), leisure physical activity (4-categories from low to a very high level of leisure physical activity) [13,22], physical workload based on the Hollmann Index (scale of 0–62, with 62 representing the highest degree of physical workload) questionnaire asking about body postures and weight lifted during the working day [23], and four indicators of psychosocial work conditions from the Copenhagen Psychosocial Questionnaire (COPSOQ) [24,25]: emotional demands, role conflicts, influence at work, and quality of leadership (normalized on a 0–100 scale according to the test-score manual).

Statistics

Using the Cox proportional hazards model, we estimated the risk of pain intensities from 1 to 9 for onset of LTSA, referencing pain intensity of 0. Hazard ratios (HR) and 95% confidence intervals (95% CI) were calculated separately for the three body regions. Smoking status and leisure time physical activity were treated as categorical variables in the analysis. Age, BMI, tenure, physical workload and the four indicators of psychosocial work conditions were treated as continuous variables. Respondents were followed in the DREAM-register for one year and respondents were censored after first case of LTSA. Respondents were furthermore censored in case of retirement, immigration or death. In Model 1 we adjusted for age. In Model 2 we additionally adjusted for life-style related factor (BMI, leisure physical activity and smoking status). In Model 3 we additionally adjusted for work-related factors (seniority, physical workload, and psychosocial work conditions). The data on LTSA correspond to survival times which in most cases are censored as the cohort is only followed for one year. When individuals had an onset of LTSA in the one-year follow-up period, the survival times were non-censored and referred to as event times. The estimation method was maximum likelihood and the PHREG procedure of SAS 9.2 was used. We included the TEST statement in the PHREG procedure to test the proportional hazards assumption. We used the LIFETEST procedure of SAS 9.2. to produce Kaplan-Meier curves for a visual representation of the hazards.

Results

Table 1 presents descriptive data for the main study variables. Of the 8,732 female healthcare workers 38%, 37% and 18% had moderate pain and 12%, 17% and 6% had severe pain in the low back, neck/shoulders and knees, respectively. Only 0.5% had severe pain in all three regions. Moreover, 6.3% of the respondents developed at least one period of LTSA during the follow-up year. In comparison, among non-respondent females 11.0% had at least one period of LTSA during the survey period or follow-up year.

Figure 1 shows a visual representation of the hazards. Table 2 summarizes pain intensities from 1 to 9 (reference: 0) in the different body regions for the risk of LTSA. Trend tests for the relationship between increasing pain intensities and increasing risk of LTSA was highly significant for all three body regions (P<0.001) (not shown in Table 2). With adjustment for age

Table 1. Descriptive statistics for the main study variables.

	Mean (SD) or pecentage
Long-term sickness absence (%)	6.3%
Age (years)	45 (10)
Life-style related factors	
Body Mass Index (kg·m⁻²)	25 (4)
Smoker (%)	37%
Leisure physical activity (%)	
Low	5%
Medium	42%
High	49%
Very high	5%
Work related factors	
Seniority (years)	9 (7)
Physical workload (Hollmann Index, scale 0–62)*	20 (10)
Psychosocial working conditions (0–100)§	
Emotional demands	46 (19)
Influence at work	45 (21)
Role conflicts	42 (16)
Quality of leadership	57 (22)
Musculoskeletal pain	
Low back pain (%)	
Pain intensity 0–2	50%
Pain intensity 3–5	38%
Pain intensity >5	12%
Neck/shoulder pain (%)	
Pain intensity 0–2	46%
Pain intensity 3–5	37%
Pain intensity >5	17%
Knee pain (%)	
Pain intensity 0–2	76%
Pain intensity 3–5	18%
Pain intensity >5	6%

Values are given as means (SD) or percentage of the female healthcare workers (N = 8,732).
*) Higher values indicate higher physical workloads.
§) Higher values indicate higher levels of Emotional demands, Role conflicts, Influence at work and Quality of leadership.

(Model 1), the threshold of pain intensities for significantly increased risk of LTSA was 5, 4 and 3 (scale 0–9) for the low back, neck/shoulders and knees, respectively. With additional adjustment for life-style related factors (Model 2) these findings remained. At the upper boundary of the scale, pain intensities of 8–9 for the different body regions resulted in three- to fivefold increased risk for LTSA. With additional adjustment for work-related factors (Model 3) the hazard ratios generally decreased and the thresholds for significantly increased risk of LTSA was 7, 7 and 5 (scale 0–9) for the low back, neck/shoulders and knees, respectively.

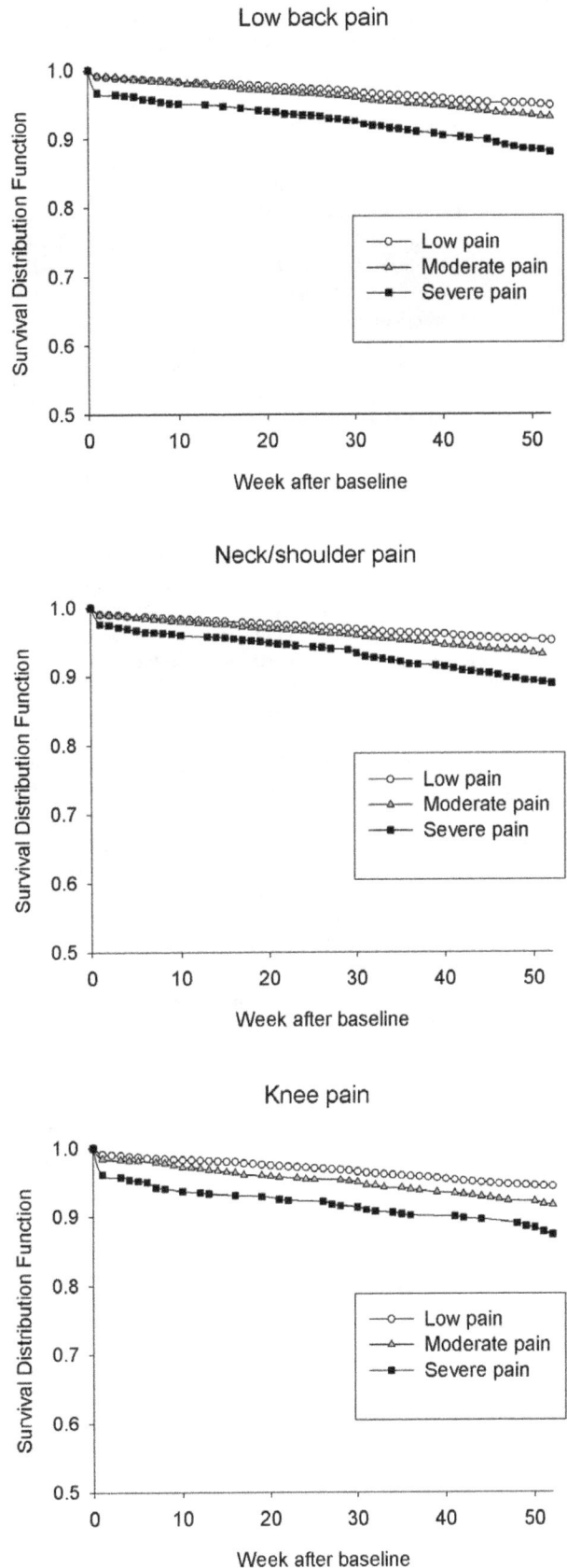

Figure 1. Visual representation of the hazards (Kaplan-Meier curves) at 0–52 weeks from baseline for low back pain, neck/shoulder pain and knee pain, respectively. The Y-axis represents

the proportion of female healthcare workers not having LTSA. Pain intensity is stratified into low (0–2), medium (3–5) and severe (>5) pain on a scale of 0–10.

Discussion

Our study showed that thresholds of pain intensity increasing the risk for LTSA vary across body regions, with knee pain having the lowest threshold. With adjustment for life-style related factors the findings remained, but the hazard ratios decreased when adjusting for work-related factors.

In our study, moderate to severe pain from the low back, neck/shoulder and knees were significant risk factors for LTSA among healthcare workers. Importantly, specific thresholds for each body region existed, with pain intensity thresholds of 5, 4 and 3 for the low back, neck/shoulders and knees, respectively, referencing pain intensity of 0 (Model 2). Prospective cohort studies have documented that pain from the back, neck and shoulders among different occupational groups increase the risk for sickness absence by a range from 30% to 390% [6–11,26]. Differences in definitions and specific cut-points of pain severity between the studies as well as inclusion of different occupational groups may explain this wide range in risk estimates. Our study elaborates on these previous findings by documenting specific thresholds of pain intensity for significantly increased risk of long-term sickness absence in female healthcare workers.

An unexpected finding is the relatively high threshold for low back pain, i.e. 5 on a scale of 0–9, compared with the thresholds of 3–4 for the other body regions. Even with minimal adjustment for other factors associated with sickness absence (Model 1) the HR's for pain intensities below 5 was close to 1. As a possible explanation, the healthcare sector has during the last decades introduced several initiatives to manage work in spite of low back pain – for example back schools and provision of manual handling equipment. Also, many countries have provided much public information about the benefits of staying active in spite of back pain [27].

The pain intensity threshold of 4 in the neck/shoulders for increased risk of LTSA among the healthcare workers in our study is roughly in line with a previous study in sewing machine operators showing that clinical findings occurred more frequently with moderate levels of self-reported complaints [28]. In that study, a summation of four complaint scores on a scale of 0–9 (i.e. range 0–36), showed a cut-point of 12 (i.e. ~3 on a scale of 0–9) for increased prevalence of myofascial pain syndrome and rotator cuff tendinitis. Further, a Danish study among the general working population showed that higher pain intensity in the neck/shoulder was related to increased risk of LTSA [29].

Knee pain intensities at 3 or above were associated with significantly increased risk for LTSA. Thus, although knee pain is less prevalent than low back and neck/shoulder pain, the consequences of individual knee pain appear to be higher among female healthcare workers. By contrast, among 5000 Danish employees from different occupations chronic knee pain, defined as at least 30 days with knee pain during the last year, was not a significant risk factor for LTSA [12]. Thus, the consequences of musculoskeletal pain in different body regions may vary across occupations and with different cut-points and definitions of pain. For example, employees in sedentary occupations may not experience the same consequences of knee pain as employees with strenuous physical labor. This stresses the importance of determining occupation-specific thresholds of pain intensity for increased risk of LTSA.

Table 2. Hazard ratios (HR) and 95% confidence intervals for onset of long-term sickness absence during 12 months follow-up for the different levels of pain intensity (scale 0–9) for the low back, neck/shoulders, and knees.

	n	Model 1 HR	Model 1 95% CI	Model 2 HR	Model 2 95% CI	Model 3 HR	Model 3 95% CI
Low back pain (scale 0–9)							
0	2811	1	-	1	-	1	-
1	472	0.64	(0.38–1.07)	0.59	(0.34–1.02)	0.53	(0.29–0.95)
2	949	0.95	(0.69–1.32)	0.93	(0.67–1.31)	0.87	(0.61–1.23)
3	1364	1.16	(0.88–1.52)	1.11	(0.84–1.46)	0.99	(0.74–1.33)
4	1047	1.19	(0.89–1.59)	1.14	(0.85–1.53)	0.97	(0.71–1.33)
5	851	1.51	(1.13–2.02)	1.44	(1.07–1.93)	1.26	(0.93–1.72)
6	532	1.55	(1.11–2.18)	1.43	(1.00–2.04)	1.19	(0.82–1.72)
7	339	2.46	(1.75–3.47)	2.37	(1.67–3.35)	2.03	(1.41–2.92)
8	86	5.23	(3.31–8.27)	4.97	(3.10–7.98)	4.17	(2.55–6.84)
9	74	3.96	(2.20–7.13)	4.28	(2.37–7.74)	3.43	(1.79–6.57)
Neck/shoulder pain (scale 0–9)							
0	2700	1	-	1	-	1	-
1	375	0.86	(0.51–1.45)	0.83	(0.48–1.44)	0.83	(0.47–1.47)
2	869	0.83	(0.58–1.21)	0.90	(0.62–1.30)	0.91	(0.63–1.34)
3	1156	1.15	(0.86–1.55)	1.17	(0.86–1.58)	1.18	(0.86–1.62)
4	1042	1.50	(1.14–1.99)	1.47	(1.10–1.96)	1.32	(0.97–1.79)
5	946	1.38	(1.03–1.87)	1.42	(1.04–1.92)	1.26	(0.91–1.74)
6	652	1.55	(1.12–2.15)	1.54	(1.10–2.16)	1.21	(0.84–1.75)
7	522	2.28	(1.67–3.12)	2.25	(1.64–3.10)	1.95	(1.39–2.72)
8	218	3.58	(2.46–5.19)	3.44	(2.35–5.03)	2.74	(1.82–4.13)
9	98	4.03	(2.43–6.68)	4.25	(2.52–7.15)	3.86	(2.27–6.56)
Knee pain (scale 0–9)							
0	5637	1	-	1	-	1	-
1	296	1.17	(0.74–1.86)	1.30	(0.82–2.08)	1.42	(0.89–2.26)
2	584	0.97	(0.67–1.40)	0.92	(0.63–1.36)	0.86	(0.57–1.29)
3	689	1.39	(1.03–1.87)	1.43	(1.06–1.93)	1.32	(0.96–1.81)
4	456	1.52	(1.08–2.15)	1.44	(1.01–2.06)	1.39	(0.96–2.01)
5	354	1.82	(1.27–2.61)	1.85	(1.28–2.67)	1.72	(1.17–2.51)
6	224	1.35	(0.82–2.23)	1.18	(0.69–2.02)	1.16	(0.67–1.99)
7	172	3.16	(2.13–4.70)	3.16	(2.12–4.70)	3.22	(2.14–4.84)
8	93	2.93	(1.68–5.10)	2.99	(1.71–5.21)	2.84	(1.62–4.97)
9	54	3.77	(2.00–7.09)	3.27	(1.61–6.63)	2.90	(1.42–5.96)

Model 1: Adjusted for age.
Model 2: Adjusted for age, BMI, smoking, and leisure physical activity.
Model 3: Adjusted for age, BMI, smoking, leisure physical activity, seniority, physical workload, and psychosocial work environment.

The hazard ratios decreased when adjusting for work-related factors, resulting in higher thresholds of pain intensity for increased risk of LTSA (Model 3). With adjustment for seniority, physical workload and psychosocial work conditions the thresholds for LTSA were 7, 7 and 5 for pain intensities in the low back, neck/shoulder and knees. We adjusted for these factors because physical as well as psychosocial working conditions are shown to be related to both the predictor (musculoskeletal pain) and the outcome (LTSA) [30–34]. In this regard, a good working environment may be viewed as a potential resource protecting workers from LTSA in spite of relatively high intensities of musculoskeletal pain. By contrast, if musculoskeletal pain simply mediates the relation between work exposures and LTSA then adjusting for these work related factors is not meaningful. Thus, asking only a single-item question about pain intensity, the thresholds of 5, 4 and 3 determined from Model 1 and 2 are likely more relevant for guidelines aiming to prevent the consequences of musculoskeletal pain.

Our study has both strengths and limitations. The large sample size of female healthcare workers from several different municipalities strengthens the validity of the estimates for this specific occupational group. However, the sample size of the reference groups as well as the sample size of each pain-intensity group also influences the range of the confidence intervals. Thus, statistically significant thresholds may have been found at lower pain intensities had the sample size been larger. Therefore, the practical relevance of our findings should also be considered. The 43% to 47% increased risk for LTSA from pain intensities of 5, 4, and 3 in the low back, neck/shoulder and knees (Model 2), respectively, seems highly relevant. By contrast, one level below the statistically significant thresholds the hazard ratios were near 1 ranging from 0.92 to 1.17 and may therefore not be relevant even if statistically significant with a larger sample size. Thus, the practical relevant thresholds are likely very near the statistically significant thresholds of 5, 4 and 3 determined in the present study. Due to the rather homogeneous group of female healthcare workers we did not control for socioeconomic factors. The inclusion criteria limit the generalizability of our findings to female healthcare workers in eldercare. As another limitation, recall bias regarding a three-month recall for musculoskeletal pain

may exist. Also, due to the study design no causal relations can be established. Further, among the total target population of female healthcare workers 11.0% and 6.3% of the non-respondents and respondents, respectively, had LTSA during follow-up. Thus, response bias may exist, i.e. non-respondents may have poorer health than respondents. Because the present questionnaire survey was conducted at the workplace, employees on sick leave during the survey period did not have the opportunity to reply. Future studies should consider mailing questionnaire surveys to employees on sick leave during the study period. Furthermore, we had no information regarding co-morbitidies, e.g. osteoarthritis or fibromyalgia, which may also influence the thresholds, and could be a target for future research.

In conclusion, the threshold of pain intensity increasing the risk for LTSA among female healthcare workers varies across body regions, being 5, 4 and 3 (scale 0–9) for the low back, neck/shoulders and knees, respectively. This knowledge may be used to better protect individual healthcare workers from LTSA by initiating preventive actions when reporting pain intensities at or above the respective thresholds.

Acknowledgments

The authors thank the co-workers from the DHCWC-2004 study group for their contribution to data collection.

Author Contributions

Conceived and designed the experiments: LLA TC HB AH. Performed the experiments: TC. Analyzed the data: LLA. Wrote the paper: LLA TC HB AH.

References

1. Kivimaki M, Head J, Ferrie JE, Shipley MJ, Vahtera J, et al. (2003) Sickness absence as a global measure of health: evidence from mortality in the Whitehall II prospective cohort study. BMJ 327: 364. 10.1136/bmj.327.7411.364 [doi];327/7411/364 [pii].
2. Høgelund J, Filges T, Jensen S (2003) Long-term sickness absence – what happens and how does it go? The Danish National Institute of Social Research, Copenhagen. Report 03:20.
3. Waddell G, Burton K (2006) Is Work Good for Your Health and Well-being? London: The Stationary Office.
4. Veale DJ, Woolf AD, Carr AJ (2008) Chronic musculoskeletal pain and arthritis: impact, attitudes and perceptions. Ir Med J 101: 208–210.
5. Bevan S, Quadrello T, McGee R, Mahdon M, Vovrovsky A, et al. (2009) Fit For Work – Musculoskeletal disorders in the European workforce. 1–143.
6. Bergstrom G, Bodin L, Bertilsson H, Jensen IB (2007) Risk factors for new episodes of sick leave due to neck or back pain in a working population. A prospective study with an 18-month and a three-year follow-up. Occup Environ Med 64: 279–287.
7. Holmberg SA, Thelin AG (2006) Primary care consultation, hospital admission, sick leave and disability pension owing to neck and low back pain: a 12-year prospective cohort study in a rural population. BMC Musculoskelet Disord 7: 66.
8. Morken T, Riise T, Moen B, Hauge SH, Holien S, et al. (2003) Low back pain and widespread pain predict sickness absence among industrial workers. BMC Musculoskelet Disord 4: 21.
9. Natvig B, Eriksen W, Bruusgaard D (2002) Low back pain as a predictor of long-term work disability. Scand J Public Health 30: 288–292.
10. Nyman T, Grooten WJ, Wiktorin C, Liwing J, Norrman L (2007) Sickness absence and concurrent low back and neck-shoulder pain: results from the MUSIC-Norrtalje study. Eur Spine J 16: 631–638.
11. van den Heuvel SG, Ariens GA, Boshuizen HC, Hoogendoorn WE, Bongers PM (2004) Prognostic factors related to recurrent low-back pain and sickness absence. Scand J Work Environ Health 30: 459–467.
12. Andersen LL, Mortensen OS, Hansen JV, Burr H (2011) A prospective cohort study on severe pain as a risk factor for long-term sickness absence in blue- and white-collar workers. Occup Environ Med 68: 590–592.
13. Andersen LL, Clausen T, Mortensen OS, Burr H, Holtermann A (2011) A prospective cohort study on musculoskeletal risk factors for long-term sickness absence among healthcare workers in eldercare. Int Arch Occup Environ Health DOI: 10.1007/s00420-011-0709-5.
14. Holtermann A, Jorgensen MB, Gram B, Christensen JR, Faber A, et al. (2010) Worksite interventions for preventing physical deterioration among employees in job-groups with high physical work demands: background, design and conceptual model of FINALE. BMC Public Health 10: 120.
15. Waters T, Collins J, Galinsky T, Caruso C (2006) NIOSH research efforts to prevent musculoskeletal disorders in the healthcare industry. Orthop Nurs 25: 380–389.
16. Hjollund NH, Larsen FB, Andersen JH (2007) Register-based follow-up of social benefits and other transfer payments: accuracy and degree of completeness in a Danish interdepartmental administrative database compared with a population-based survey. Scand J Public Health 35: 497–502.
17. Committee System on Biomedical Research Ethics (2011) Guidelines about Notification. http://www.dnvk.dk/English/guidelinesaboutnotification.aspx.
18. The Danish Data Protection Agency (2008) Standard terms for research projects – AUTHORISATION to process personal data. http://www.datatilsynet.dk/erhverv/forskere-og-medicinalfirmaer/standard-terms-for-research-projects/.
19. Lund T, Labriola M, Christensen KB, Bultmann U, Villadsen E, et al. (2005) Psychosocial work environment exposures as risk factors for long-term sickness absence among Danish employees: results from DWECS/DREAM. J Occup Environ Med 47: 1141–1147. 00043764-200511000-00007 [pii].
20. Pincus T, Bergman M, Sokka T, Roth J, Swearingen C, et al. (2008) Visual analog scales in formats other than a 10 centimeter horizontal line to assess pain and other clinical data. J Rheumatol 35: 1550–1558.
21. Kuorinka I, Jonsson B, Kilbom Å, Vinterberg H, Biering-Sørensen F, et al. (1987) Standardised Nordic questionnaires for the analysis of musculoskeletal symptoms. Appl Ergo 18: 233–237.
22. Saltin B, Grimby G (1968) Physiological analysis of middle-aged and old former athletes. Comparison with still active athletes of the same ages. Circulation 38: 1104–1115.
23. Hollmann S, Klimmer F, Schmidt KH, Kylian H (1999) Validation of a questionnaire for assessing physical work load. Scand J Work Environ Health 25: 105–114.
24. Clausen T, Nielsen K, Carneiro IG, Borg V (2012) Job demands, job resources and long-term sickness absence in the Danish eldercare services: a prospective analysis of register-based outcomes. J Adv Nurs 68: 127–36.
25. Pejtersen JH, Kristensen TS, Borg V, Bjorner JB (2010) The second version of the Copenhagen Psychosocial Questionnaire. Scand J Public Health 38: 8–24.
26. Tubach F, Leclerc A, Landre MF, Pietri-Taleb F (2002) Risk factors for sick leave due to low back pain: a prospective study. J Occup Environ Med 44: 451–458.
27. Buchbinder R, Jolley D, Wyatt M (2001) Population based intervention to change back pain beliefs and disability: three part evaluation. BMJ 322: 1516–1520.

28. Kaergaard A, Andersen JH, Rasmussen K, Mikkelsen S (2000) Identification of neck-shoulder disorders in a 1 year follow-up study. Validation Of a questionnaire-based method. Pain 86: 305–310.

29. Holtermann A, Hansen JV, Burr H, Sogaard K (2010) Prognostic factors for long-term sickness absence among employees with neck-shoulder and low-back pain. Scand J Work Environ Health 36: 34–41.

30. Kuiper JI, Burdorf A, Verbeek JH, Frings-Dresen M, van der Beek A, et al. (1999) Epidemiological evidence on manual material handling as a risk factor for back disorders: a systematic review. Int J Ind Erg 24: 389–404.

31. Hoogendoorn WE, van Poppel MNM, Bongers PM, Koes BW, Bouter LM (1999) Physical load during work and leisure time as risk factors for back pain. Scand J Work Environ Health 25: 387–403.

32. Lotters F, Burdorf A, Kuiper J, Miedema H (2003) Model for the work-relatedness of low-back pain. Scand J Work Environ Health 29: 431–440.

33. Eriksen W, Bruusgaard D, Knardahl S (2004) Work factors as predictors of intense or disabling low back pain; a prospective study of nurses' aides. Occup Environ Med 61: 398–404.

34. Herin F, Paris C, Levant A, Vignaud MC, Sobaszek A, et al. (2011) Links between nurses' organisational work environment and upper limb musculoskeletal symptoms: independently of effort-reward imbalance! The ORSOSA study. Pain 152: 2006–2015.

Assessing Sleep Disturbance in Low Back Pain: The Validity of Portable Instruments

Saad M. Alsaadi[1]*, James H. McAuley[2], Julia M. Hush[3], Delwyn J. Bartlett[4], Zoe M. McKeough[5], Ronald R. Grunstein[4,6], George C. Dungan II[4], Chris G. Maher[2]

1 Department of physiotherapy, King Fahd Hospital of the University, The University of Dammam, Khobar, Saudi Arabia, 2 The George Institute for Global Health, Faculty of Medicine, The University of Sydney, Sydney, Australia, 3 Department of Health Professions, Faculty of Human Sciences, Australian School of Advanced Medicine, Macquarie University, Sydney, Australia, 4 The Woolcock Institute of Medical Research, The University of Sydney, Sydney, Australia, 5 Clinical and Rehabilitation Sciences, The University of Sydney, Sydney, New South Wales, Australia, 6 Department of Respiratory and Sleep Medicine, Royal Prince Alfred Hospital, Sydney, Australia

Abstract

Although portable instruments have been used in the assessment of sleep disturbance for patients with low back pain (LBP), the accuracy of the instruments in detecting sleep/wake episodes for this population is unknown. This study investigated the criterion validity of two portable instruments (Armband and Actiwatch) for assessing sleep disturbance in patients with LBP. 50 patients with LBP performed simultaneous overnight sleep recordings in a university sleep laboratory. All 50 participants were assessed by Polysomnography (PSG) and the Armband and a subgroup of 33 participants wore an Actiwatch. Criterion validity was determined by calculating epoch-by-epoch agreement, sensitivity, specificity and prevalence and bias- adjusted kappa (PABAK) for sleep versus wake between each instrument and PSG. The relationship between PSG and the two instruments was assessed using intraclass correlation coefficients (ICC 2, 1). The study participants showed symptoms of sub-threshold insomnia (mean ISI = 13.2, 95% CI = 6.36) and poor sleep quality (mean PSQI = 9.20, 95% CI = 4.27). Observed agreement with PSG was 85% and 88% for the Armband and Actiwatch. Sensitivity was 0.90 for both instruments and specificity was 0.54 and 0.67 and PABAK of 0.69 and 0.77 for the Armband and Actiwatch respectively. The ICC (95%CI) was 0.76 (0.61 to 0.86) and 0.80 (0.46 to 0.92) for total sleep time, 0.52 (0.29 to 0.70) and 0.55 (0.14 to 0.77) for sleep efficiency, 0.64 (0.45 to 0.78) and 0.52 (0.23 to 0.73) for wake after sleep onset and 0.13 (−0.15 to 0.39) and 0.33 (−0.05 to 0.63) for sleep onset latency, for the Armband and Actiwatch, respectively. The findings showed that both instruments have varied criterion validity across the sleep parameters from excellent validity for measures of total sleep time, good validity for measures of sleep efficiency and wake after onset to poor validity for sleep onset latency.

Editor: Berthold Langguth, University of Regensburg, Germany

Funding: This research was supported by a grant from the University of Sydney, Sydney Medical School, Sydney, Australia. Prof. Maher's fellowship is funded by the Australian Research Council. Dr. Alsaadi was supported by the University of Dammam, Kingdom of Saudi Arabia during the study. The funders had no role in study design, data collection and analysis, decision to publish, or preparation of the manuscript.

Competing Interests: The authors have declared that no competing interests exist.

* E-mail: alsaadis@gmail.com

Introduction

Low back pain (LBP) is a common health condition; it has a lifetime prevalence of 40%, and a point prevalence (at any point in time) of 20% [1]. LBP is associated with both physical and psychological consequences, for example disability, depression and anxiety [2]. Studies have also found that between 50–60% of patients with LBP report sleep disturbance [3,4]. A recent systematic review found that people with chronic LBP report increased duration to sleep onset, reduced total sleep time, and lower sleep efficiency [5].

Sleep disturbance in patients with LBP is associated with psychological distress, physical disability [6], fatigue and day-time sleepiness [7]. Patients with LBP who complain of sleep disturbance have been found to experience more severe pain [4] and are more likely to be hospitalized for their LBP than those without sleep problems [8]. The literature suggests that there is a bidirectional relationship between disturbed sleep and intensity of pain. (i.e. pain may lead to the reporting sleep disturbance and poor sleep may cause or exacerbate the pain) [9]. It is plausible

therefore that disturbed sleep is likely to adversely impact LBP management. Moreover, the consequences of sleep disturbance can hinder treatment effectiveness. For example, exercise therapy, used to reduce pain, improve function and enhance return to work [10], is a critical component of LBP management. Clinicians prescribe exercise therapy for approximately half of their patients with LBP [11]. The effects of sleep disturbance such as fatigue are likely to hinder exercise performance and consequently lead to poorer treatment outcomes. For these reasons the assessment of sleep disturbance in patients with LBP is an important clinical and research question.

The gold standard for assessing sleep quality is Polysomnography (PSG). However, due to its complexity and expense it is infrequently used in research on sleep quality in patients with LBP. Most studies reporting on sleep quality and LBP have used data from self-report questionnaires [5]. Self-report measures however correlate poorly with PSG and therefore estimates of sleep parameters in patients with LBP may not be accurate [12]. Newly developed portable instruments provide a less expensive, objective alternative to PSG and are a potentially more accurate method of measuring sleep quality in a free-living environment than self-report measures [13]. A commonly used portable method is actigraphy, in which a small device containing an accelerometer to detect limb movement is worn on the wrist or ankle. A mathematical algorithm is used to estimate sleep/wake episodes. The accuracy of actigraphy to evaluate sleep parameters has been investigated by comparison with PSG in several medical conditions and for some sleep disorders, but not for the LBP population [14–16].

In addition to accelerometry, the BodyMedia SenseWear Armband, acquires other physiological signals including skin temperature, galvanic skin response and heat flux which are thought to be important in determining sleep/wake cycles [17]. This instrument may therefore provide a more accurate assessment of sleep quality than actigraphy alone [18]. Further, because the Armband is worn on the upper arm interference from fine limb movement associated with limb dominance is minimised. Despite the potential superiority of the Armband, only 4 studies have investigated its accuracy in detecting sleep/wake episodes measured by polysomnography. These studies were performed in healthy children and adolescents [19], healthy volunteers placed on hypnotics or placebo [20] and sleep apnea [21,22]. There was variability in findings across the studies with the Armand able to detect patients' sleep with more accuracy than detecting wake episodes. Only one study examined a different actigraphy device in parallel with the Armband [20].

Although a number of studies [6,23–25] have employed actigraphy for the assessment of sleep disturbance in patients with LBP, the accuracy of the instrument for this population is uncertain. In particular, there is some evidence that patients with LBP exhibit higher body activity during sleep than those without LBP [26], which might adversely affect the accuracy of the actigraphy in detection of an individual's sleep/wake episodes. This casts some doubt on whether findings of previous validity studies in other conditions generalise for the LBP population. Therefore, the aim of the current study was to determine the criterion validity of the actigraph and the BodyMedia SenseWear Armband for measuring sleep parameters in a sample of patients with LBP by comparing the instruments' recordings of sleep/wake to those of the PSG. A secondary aim was to investigate whether the additional physiological measures provided by the Armband increase the accuracy of sleep parameters compared with accelerometry alone (i.e. actigraph).

Materials and Methods

This was a cross-sectional study conducted between March 2010 and June 2011. The study protocol was approved by the University of Sydney Human Research Ethics Committee, Australia (09-2009/12100). All participants signed informed consent forms before participation in the study. Participants were compensated for their time and transportation expenses.

Participants

Participants with non-specific LBP were recruited from physiotherapy clinics in the Sydney metropolitan area and from the community through advertising. The inclusion criteria were: patients aged between 18 and 79 years with a primary complaint of LBP (pain between the 12th rib and buttock crease) with or without leg pain (pain radiating to the lower limb "sciatica") and possessing sufficient fluency in the English language to understand and respond to instructions. Exclusion criteria were: LBP caused by a serious spinal pathology, according to medical/physiotherapy evaluation or patient report; nerve root compromise (evidenced by

at least two of myotomal weakness, dermatomal sensory loss, or hypo-reflexia of the lower limb reflexes); spinal surgery within the preceding 6 months; previously diagnosed with a sleep disorder for which they were receiving care; and patients receiving care for a mental health condition.

Procedures

Participating physiotherapists informed patients about the study. If a patient indicated an interest in participating, the physiotherapist provided them with comprehensive information about the study procedures and then passed on their contact details to the study researcher. The researcher contacted the patient, screened the patient for eligibility, and arranged a time to meet eligible patients at the sleep laboratory. Potential participants from the community were provided with comprehensive information about the study through the post or electronic mail. Those who showed an interest in participating were then contacted and screened for inclusion by the study researcher. All who met the eligibility criteria met the study researcher at the sleep laboratory.

The sleep assessments were conducted at the sleep laboratory of the Woolcock Institute of Medical Research, the University of Sydney, Australia. The study researcher, who was a trained physiotherapist, met the participants to screen for neurological signs, obtain informed consent, collect basic demographic information (including age; gender; body mass index; nationality; level of education; whether currently seeking care) and participant's clinical condition (including pain intensity; pain duration; disability; psychological distress; fatigue –see Table S1). Although participant's clinical profiles were not included in the analysis, they were assessed to describe the study sample. At the end of the interview the researcher fitted the Armband and the Actiwatch and provided instructions on how to avoid getting the Armband and Actiwatch wet during bathing/showering. A sleep laboratory technician then carried out the overnight PSG study.

Sleep measurement

Each participant had measures of sleep parameters taken with the Armband and Actiwatch and also with PSG, which is considered the criterion measure, while sleeping overnight in the sleep laboratory. The assessed sleep parameters were: total sleep time (TST); sleep onset latency (SOL); sleep efficiency (SE) and wake after sleep onset (WASO). These parameters were calculated as below:

TST: the total number of minutes scored as sleep from lights out to lights on.

SOL: the total number of minutes scored as awake beyond lights out prior to sleep onset.

SE: the ratio of minutes spent asleep to total minutes in bed, X 100 (expressed as percentage).

WASO: the total minutes scored as wake after sleep onset before lights on.

The evaluation of these sleep parameters (TST, SOL, SE and WASO) was based on "lights off" and "lights on" time according to the PSG recording. Lights off was the time that the patient started trying to sleep (start of PSG) and lights on was the time that the patient was awakened (end of PSG), as recorded by the sleep laboratory technician.

Armband

An Armband (SenseWear-Pro3, BodyMedia Monitoring System, Pittsburgh PA, USA) was attached on the right upper arm during testing according to the manufacturer's instructions. The software (SenseWear Professional Software version 6.1) used average variations in body movements, differential and proportional changes in heat-flux and skin temperature and the galvanic skin response to score each 60 second time epoch as either sleep or awake [18].

Actiwatch

Following the manufacturer's instructions the Actiwatch (Actiwatch 2; Philips Respironics, Murrysville PA, USA) was attached to the non-dominant wrist during testing. Epoch length was set at 30 secs to match the PSG setting. The data were downloaded and analysed using ActiWare (R) software version 5.52.0003 (Philips Respironics, Murrysville, PA, USA). The standard factory-default algorithm was used for sleep interval detection. The parameters were: wake threshold set as "medium" and the sleep interval detection algorithm set as "immobile minutes." Immobile minutes for sleep onset and end of sleep were set at 10 minutes.

The software scored each epoch as either asleep or awake by evaluating the level of activity compared to the immediate prior and subsequent epochs of activity (± 2 min). The threshold value was set to medium (wake threshold value = 40). The medium threshold value has been validated in a previous technical report [27]. If the number of activity movements (count) exceeded the threshold, the epoch was scored as wake. If activity counts fell below or were equal to the threshold, the epoch was scored as sleep [28].

Polysomnography (PSG)

Overnight attendance in-laboratory polysomnography (PSG) was performed in a university-based research sleep laboratory. The contemporary standard technique was used for the recording and included measurements obtained from the following: electro-encephalogram (EEG) central channels (C3-M2, C4-M1) and occipital channels (O1-M2, O2-M1), bilateral electrooculogram (EOG), chin electromyogram (EMG), bilateral tibialis anterior EMG, Lead II electrocardiogram (ECG), nasal air-flow (pressure derived), fingertip pulse oxygen saturation (SpO2), snoring using a PTAF lite pressure transducer sensor, and body position using a body position sensor. The PSG study was performed using the Sandman system (Tyco Healthcare, Colorado, USA). Sleep staging was scored using current American Academy of Sleep Medicine criteria AASM [29]. Each epoch was assigned a stage of sleep or wake on the basis of the EEG, EOG and EMG channels. Respiratory events and arousals were scored according to standard AASM (alternative hypopnoea definition) and the American Sleep Disorders Association criteria ASDA [30], respectively. The Apnea-Hypopnea index (AHI) was calculated by dividing the total number of apneas and hypopneas by the total sleep time (hours).

As synchronisation of time is critical to accurately compare the device and PSG epochs optimal matching between the "lights off" and "lights on" time agreement was tested a number of times within a ± 2 min time range. The peak agreement value was used in the final analysis [31].

Data Analysis and Statistical Methods

Epoch by epoch sleep/wake agreement. We evaluated the criterion validity of the Armband and Actiwatch by comparing sleep/wake episodes reported by these devices to the sleep/wake episodes reported by PSG. For each participant we calculated epoch by epoch sleep/wake agreement using the Prevalence and Bias-Adjusted Kappa (PABAK) [32], sensitivity and specificity. Agreement, sensitivity and specificity calculations were based on results of 2×2 table, where PSG is considered the reference standard and the two portable sleep instruments are considered as index tests.

The PSG and the Actiwatch evaluate individual's sleep in 30 seconds intervals, whereas the Armband evaluates sleep in 60 seconds intervals, called sleep epochs. The Armband's epoch length is calibrated by the manufacturer and could not be altered. Therefore, to compare the 60-second epochs of the Armband to the 30-second epochs of the PSG each Armband's epoch score was harmonised to 60 seconds before the analysis.

Evaluation of sleep parameters. Sleep parameters (total sleep time TST, sleep onset latency SOL, sleep efficiency SE, wake after sleep onset WASO) estimated by the Armband and Actiwatch described above, were compared to sleep parameters estimated by the PSG (the reference standard measure) in a parallel form of reliability using the intraclass correlation coefficients (ICC 2, 1) with two-way model using single measure and absolute agreement, (reported with 95% confidence intervals (CIs). In addition, scatter plots, regression analyses and Bland and Altman plots were used for comparison purposes. We chose this approach because it is generally agreed that there is no single statistical procedure that adequately covers this issue [33,34]. To describe the criterion validity of the continuous sleep parameters we compared the obtained ICC values to the benchmarks proposed by Fleiss for excellent reliability (>0.75), fair to good reliability (0.4 to 0.75) and poor reliability (<0.4) [35]. Finally, to compare the criterion validity of the Armband to that of the Actiwatch we compared the 95% CI of the obtained statistics.

Statistical analyses were conducted using SPSS version 17 (SPSS Inc., Chicago, IL) and MedCalc for Windows, version 9.5.0.0 (MedCalc Software, Mariakerke, Belgium).

Results

Characteristics of study participants

Fifty patients with non-specific LBP participated in the study. The sample's demographic information and clinical description are shown in Table 1. The majority (92%) of the sample had chronic LBP with a mean (SD) pain intensity of 4.12 (1.9) on a 0–10 scale. Twenty-eight participants (56%) were seeking care for their LBP. The sample's mean (SD) weight was 76.7 (20.9) kg, with a body mass index of 25.7 (5.2) kg/m^2.

The psychological distress assessment, using the DASS-21, indicated that the majority of participants were within normal level of depression, anxiety and stress. Thirty two (64%) participants scored within normal levels for depression (total DAAS-21 depression subscale <9), 28 (56%) participants scored within normal levels for anxiety (total DAAS-21 anxiety subscale <7) and 27 (54%) participants scored within normal levels for stress (total DAAS-21 stress subscale <14). Likewise, the fatigue assessment showed that 27 (54%) participants had fatigue scores within the normal levels (i.e. total FSS <36). After completing the PSG testing a sleep physician diagnosed 4 (8%) participants with severe obstructive sleep apnea (OSA), 3 (6%) participants with moderate OSA, and 18 (36%) participants with mild OSA. Self-reported sleep measurement showed that 37 (74%) participants had poor sleep quality according to the Pittsburgh Sleep Quality Index PSQI (i.e. >5) [36,37], and 32 (64%) participants had symptoms of clinical insomnia according to the Insomnia Severity Index ISI (i.e. >14), [38,39]. Similarly, 38 (76%) participants showed evidence of excessive day-time sleepiness as measured by the ESS (i.e. <10). Two patients used escitalopram, an oral drug used for treating depression and/or generalized anxiety disorder.

For the duration of the PSG recording, all 50 participants wore the Armband, while only 33 participants wore the Actiwatch, due to limited Actiwatch availability. The mean (SD) time spent in bed during the PSG recording was 7.13 (1.2) hrs, with mean (SD) total

Table 1. Characteristics of study participants.

	Mean (SD)
Age (years)	42.7 (15.15)
BMI (kg/m²)‡	25.7 (5.21)
Pain intensity NRS (0–10)*	4.2 (1.90)
Low back symptoms duration (year)	10.6 (9.92)
Disability (RMDQ) (0–24)#	8.48 (5.49)
Depression (DASS-21) (0–21)$	10.1 (10.1)
Anxiety (DASS-21) (0–21)	8.8 (7.90)
Stress (DASS-21) (0–21)	14.8 (9.74)
Fatigue (FSS) (0–63)†	35.3 (12.63)
Sleep quality (PSQI) (0–21)**	9.2 (4.27)
Insomnia severity (ISI) (0–28)⌀	13.2 (6.36)
Day-time sleepiness (ESS) (0–24)α	8.2 (5.55)
	N (%)
Female gender	24 (48)
Seeking care	28 (56)
University degree holder	25 (50)

‡BMI, body mass index;
*NRS, numerical rating scale (pain right now);
#RMDQ-24, Roland and Morris disability questionnaire: 24-item version;
$DASS-21, depression, anxiety and stress scale: 21-item version;
†FSS, fatigue severity scale.
**PSQI, Pittsburgh sleep quality index;
⌀ISI, insomnia severity index;
αESS, Epworth sleepiness scale.

sleep time of 6.02 (1.0) hrs, mean (SD) sleep onset latency 15.19 (14.2) mins, mean (SD) wake after sleep onset of 47.30 (35.7) mins and overall sleep efficiency of 84.5%.

Epoch by epoch sleep/wake agreement

Table 2 shows the sensitivity, specificity, PABAK, and agreement (proportion and 95% CI) results derived from epoch by epoch comparison between the Armband, Actiwatch and PSG.

The Armband and Actiwatch both had sensitivity (i.e. detecting sleep) of 0.90. Specificity (i.e. detecting being awake) for the Armband and the Actiwatch was 0.54 and 0.67 respectively. Both instruments demonstrated a high level of observed agreement (i.e. detecting both sleep and being awake), 85% for the Armband and 88% for the Actiwatch. The prevalence-and bias-adjusted kappa

(PABAK) measurement showed that both instruments have high level of agreement with the PSG in detection of sleep and wake, 0.69 and 0.77 for the Armband and for the Actiwatch, respectively.

Continuous measures of sleep

Descriptive statistics for the continuous measures of sleep parameters derived from the PSG, Armband and Actiwatch, and the ICC values are presented in Table 3. The criterion validity, as reflected in the ICC values, are similar for the Armband and Actiwatch but varied across the sleep parameters from excellent validity for measures of total sleep time, good validity for measures of sleep efficiency and wake after onset to poor validity for sleep onset latency. With exception of a few extreme scores, the scatter

Table 2. Epoch-by-Epoch Sleep/Wake Agreement between Armband, Actiwatch and PSG.

Measure	Armband n = 50	Actiwatch n = 33
	Mean (95% CI)	Mean (95% CI)
Sensitivity	0.90 (0.88 to 0.93)	0.90 (0.88 to 0.93)
Specificity	0.54 (0.46 to 0.62)	0.67 (0.60 to 0.74)
Agreement	0.85 (0.81 to 0.88)	0.88 (0.86 to 0.90)
PABAK	0.69 (0.63 to 0.75)	0.77 (0.73 to 0.81)

Sensitivity is the proportion of "sleep" epochs as defined by PSG that were judged as "sleep" by Armband/Actiwatch. Specificity is the proportion of the "wake" epochs as defined by PSG that were judged as "wake" by Armband/Actiwatch. Agreement is proportion of epochs where there was agreement between PSG and instrument. PABAK is the prevalence and bias adjusted kappa.

Armband vs. PSG

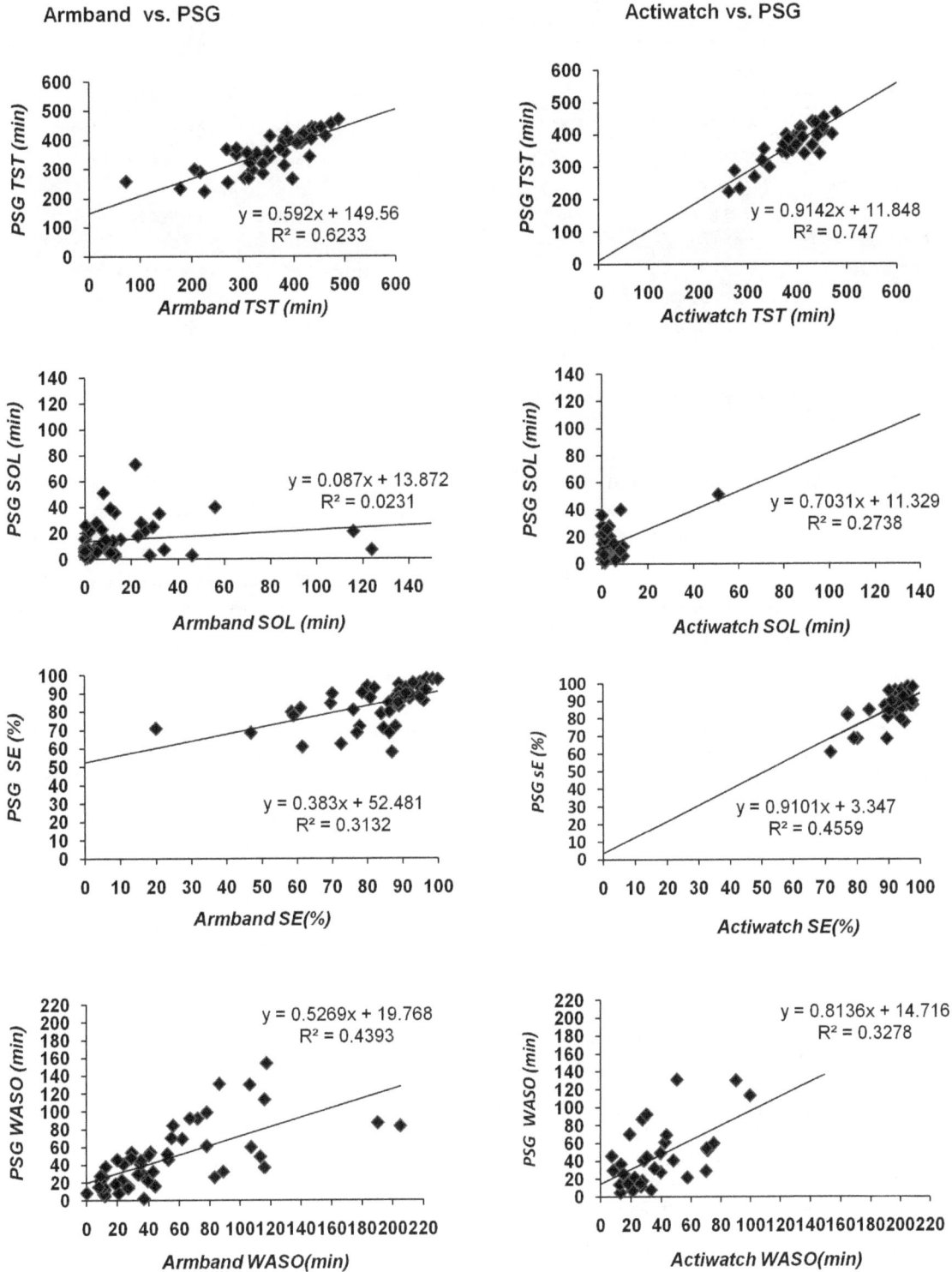

Actiwatch vs. PSG

Figure 1. Scatter plots for sleep parameters association evaluated by Armband and Actiwatch compared to PSG. The horizontal axis represents instrument's estimation of sleep parameters: TST, total sleep time; SOL, sleep onset latency; SE, sleep efficiency and WASO, wake after sleep onset. The vertical axis represents these sleep parameters estimated by the reference standard, the PSG. Each square represents data from each participant.

Table 3. Sleep parameters' comparison between the Armband, Actiwatch and PSG.

Distribution of scores: Mean (SD) & [Range]				Parallel forms' reliability ICC (2,1) with (95% CI)	
Sleep parameter	PSG	Armband	Actiwatch	Armband vs. PSG	Actiwatch vs. PSG
TST (mins)	361.60 (62.21)	358.37 (83.04)	395.31 (56.65)	0.76 (0.61 to 0.86)	0.80 (0.46 to 0.92)
	[223.00–468.30]	[72.00–488.00]	[261.30–479.30]		
SOL (mins)	15.19 (14.23)	15.23 (24.98)	4.46 (8.80)	0.13 (−0.15 to 0.39)	0.33 (−0.05 to 0.63)
	[2.00–73.00]	[0.00–124.00]	[0.00–51]		
SE (%)	84.49 (10.28)	83.59 (15.02)	90.54 (6.67)	0.52 (0.29 to 0.70)	0.55 (0.14 to 0.77)
	[58.00–98.00]	[20.00–100.00]	[71.70–97.60]		
WASO (mins)	47.30 (35.76)	52.26 (44.99)	37.06 (24.05)	0.64 (0.45 to 0.78)	0.52 (0.23 to 0.73)
	[2.00–154.00]	[0.00–205.00]	[7.30–99.30]		

ICC, intraclass correlation coefficient: two-way model using single measure and absolute agreement; CI: confidence interval; mins, minutes; TST, total sleep time; SOL, sleep onset latency; SE, sleep efficiency; WASO, wake after sleep onset.

plots and regression analyses in Figure 1 are consistent with the ICC analyses; again showing that the two instruments have a similar relationship with PSG, but the strength of the relationship varied substantially across the four continuous sleep measures.

Comparative performance of the two measures

There was no evidence that the Armband had greater criterion validity than the Actiwatch with the 95% CIs for the PABAK and ICC statistics overlapping.

Results from the Bland and Altman plots can be found in the supporting information section (Figure S1). These plots show the agreement between the instruments and the PSG for each sleep parameter by assessing the difference between a PSG sleep parameter and the instrument sleep parameter against the PSG sleep parameter. These plots show similar performance for the two measures.

Discussion

Both the Armband and actigraph provided valid measures of total sleep time, sleep efficiency and wake after sleep onset but not sleep onset latency. As the Armband does not appear to have superior criterion validity to the actigraph we conclude that the parameters sampled by the Armband do not provide additional accuracy in identifying sleep/wake epochs in the way that they are measured by this device.

To our knowledge, this is the first study to evaluate the validity of actigraphy in detecting sleep/wake in patients with LBP. The study findings are consistent with results from recent systematic reviews that investigated the role of actigraphy in sleep/wake detection for other health conditions [15,16]. These reviews have reported that actigraphy is sensitive in detecting sleep episodes, however, wakefulness detection remains somewhat problematic. Additionally, we have confirmed that the estimation of sleep onset latency is a limitation of actigraphy. This limitation may be attributed to the nature of the accelerometry which is based on body mobility detection rather than body physiological changes, as in the case of PSG [40]. Nevertheless, investigation of different types of sleep algorithms with different activity sensitivity may overcome these limitations. For example, a recent study found that lowering the actigraphy threshold to 5 minutes of immobility, rather than the standard 10 minutes, improved the detection of sleep onset latency [41].

Our study findings suggest that the Armband and the Actiwatch are useful objective tools to assess sleep parameters in patients with LBP (total sleep time, sleep efficiency, and wake after sleep onset). As these instruments are portable we conclude that they are likely to be useful for assessing sleep in a naturalistic setting. If the accurate assessment of sleep onset latency is of primary importance, researchers or clinicians could consider other devices such as the "Sleep Switch" [42], which has been found to be very strongly associated with sleep onset latency of PSG [43].

This study had several strengths. It is the first evaluation of the validity of the Armband to assess sleep parameters and the first to evaluate actigraphy in a group of patients with LBP by comparing the instruments to the widely accepted gold standard of sleep/wake detection, PSG. The study sample was recruited from both the community and primary care clinics and therefore forms a sample representative of those seeking care as well as those not currently seeking care for their LBP. Finally, we followed current recommended methods for conducting and analysing portable instruments validation against PSG [15,34].

This study also had some limitations. First, our data were collected in a sleep laboratory setting, and therefore, may not generalize to a home environment. Further research to validate these instruments using a home portable PSG are potentially worthwhile. Second, PSG data and Actiwatch data were collected in 30-sec epochs and the Armband data were collected in 60-sec epochs. This difference may have reduced the potential for agreement for the Armband with the PSG. Third, inspection of the plots (Figure 1) identified several outliers in the data. As these cases may exert undue influence on the results, we conducted a post-hoc sensitivity analysis by removing them and re-running the statistical analyses. However, since this did not change the results, we retained these cases in the analysis. In addition, the analysis showed the 95% confidence intervals are often wide and should also be taken into consideration when interpreting the study findings. For example, the point estimate for the ICC for total sleep time by Actiwatch is 0.80, which is relatively strong (Table 3). However, the lower bound of the 95% CI is 0.46 which is only moderate and reflects some uncertainty with the results. Finally, there are a variety of sleep/wake algorithm modes with different activity sensitivities (i.e. low, medium and high). In this study we used the medium threshold setting, the commonly used threshold [44]. However, we acknowledge that other settings might improve the accuracy of the device. Thus, future research is needed to identify the optimal threshold setting to detect sleep/wake in this group of patients. Further investigation is also needed to assess the accuracy of actigraphy in detecting change (responsiveness) in sleep quality in patients with LBP that might occur following intervention.

Supporting Information

Figure S1 Bland and Altman Plots of Difference vs. PSG Score for Sleep Parameters Evaluated by Armband/ Actiwatch against PSG. TST, total sleep time; SOL, sleep onset latency; SE, sleep efficiency; WASO, wake after sleep onset.

References

1. Hoy DG, Bain C, Williams G, March L, Brooks P, et al. (2012) A systematic review of the global prevalence of low back pain. Arthritis Rheum 64: 2028–2037.
2. Manchikanti L, Singh V, Datta S, Cohen SP, Hirsch JA, et al. (2009) Comprehensive review of epidemiology, scope, and impact of spinal pain. Pain Physician 12: E35–70.
3. Marin R, Cyhan T, Miklos W (2006) Sleep disturbance in patients with chronic low back pain. Am J Phys Med Rehab 85: 430–435.
4. Alsaadi SM, McAuley JH, Hush JM, Maher CG (2012) Erratum to: Prevalence of sleep disturbance in patients with low back pain. Eur Spine J 21: 554–560.
5. Kelly GA, Blake C, Power CK, O'Keeffe D, Fullen BM (2011) The association between chronic low back pain and sleep: a systematic review. Clin J Pain 27: 169–181.
6. van de Water AT, Eadie J, Hurley DA (2011) Investigation of sleep disturbance in chronic low back pain: an age- and gender-matched case-control study over a 7-night period. Man Ther 16: 550–556.
7. McCracken LM, Iverson GL (2002) Disrupted sleep patterns and daily functioning in patients with chronic pain. Pain Res Manag 7: 75–79.
8. Kaila-Kangas L, Kivimaki M, Harma M, Riihimaki H, Luukkonen R, et al. (2006) Sleep disturbances as predictors of hospitalization for back disorders-A 28-year follow-up of industrial employees. Spine 31: 51–56.
9. O'Brien EM, Waxenberg LB, Atchison JW, Gremillion HA, Staud RM, et al. (2011) Intraindividual variability in daily sleep and pain ratings among chronic pain patients: bidirectional association and the role of negative mood. Clin J Pain 27: 425–433.
10. Hayden JA, van Tulder MW, Tomlinson G (2005) Systematic review: strategies for using exercise therapy to improve outcomes in chronic low back pain. Ann Intern Med 142: 776–785.
11. Freburger JK, Carey TS, Holmes GM, Wallace AS, Castel LD, et al. (2009) Exercise prescription for chronic back or neck pain: who prescribes it? who gets it? What is prescribed? Arthritis Rheum 61: 192–200.
12. Silva GE, Goodwin JL, Sherrill DL, Arnold JL, Bootzin RR, et al. (2007) Relationship between reported and measured sleep times: the sleep heart health study (SHHS). J Clin Sleep Med 3: 622–630.
13. Ancoli-Israel S, Cole R, Alessi C, Chambers M, Moorcroft W, et al. (2003) The role of actigraphy in the study of sleep and circadian rhythms. Sleep 26: 342–392.
14. van de Water ATM, Holmes A, Hurley DA (2011) Objective measurements of sleep for non-laboratory settings as alternatives to polysomnography–a systematic review. J Sleep Res 20: 183–200.
15. Sadeh A (2011) The role and validity of actigraphy in sleep medicine: an update. Sleep Med Rev 15: 259–267.
16. Martin J, Hakim A (2011) Wrist actigraphy. Chest 139: 1514–1527.
17. Germain A, Buysse D, Kupfer D (2006) Preliminary validation of a new device for studying sleep. "SLEEP 2006"-20th Anniversary Meeting of the Associated Professional Sleep Societies (AOSS). Salt Lake City, Utah USA.
18. Sunseri M, Liden C, Farringdon J, Pelletier R, Safier S, et al. (2009) The Sensewear Armband as a sleep detection device, BodyMedia internal white paper.
19. Soric M, Turkalj M, Kucic D, Marusic I, Plavec D, et al. (2013) Validation of a multi-sensor activity monitor for assessing sleep in children and adolescents. Sleep Med 14: 201–205.
20. Peterson B, Chiao P, Pickering E, Freeman J, Zammit G, et al. (2012) Comparison of actigraphy and polysomnography to assess effects of zolpidem in a clinical research unit. Sleep Med 13: 419–424.
21. Sharif MM, BaHammam AS (2013) Sleep estimation using BodyMedia's SenseWear(TM) armband in patients with obstructive sleep apnea. Ann Thorac Med 8: 53–57.
22. O'Driscoll D, Turton A, Copland J, Strauss B, Hamilton G (2013) Energy expenditure in obstructive sleep apnea: validation of a multiple physiological sensor for determination of sleep and wake. Sleep Breath 17: 139–146.
23. O'Donoghue GM, Fox N, Heneghan C, Hurley DA (2009) Objective and subjective assessment of sleep in chronic low back pain patients compared with healthy age and gender matched controls: a pilot study. BMC Musculoskelet Disord 10: 122.
24. Harman K, Pivik RT, D'Eon JL, Wilson KG, Swenson JR, et al. (2002) Sleep in depressed and nondepressed participants with chronic low back pain: electroencephalographic and behaviour findings. Sleep 25: 775–783.
25. Lavie P, Epstein R, Tzischinsky O, Gilad D, Nahir M, et al. (1992) Actigraphic measurements of sleep in rheumatoid arthritis: comparison of patients with low back pain and healthy controls. J Rheumatol 19: 362–365.
26. Bulthuis Y, Vollenbroek-Hutten M, Hermens H, Vendrig L, van Lummel R (2004) Psychological distress, disturbed sleep and physical activity during the night in chronic low-back pain patients. J Back Musculoskelet Rehabil 17: 69–76.
27. Oakley N (1997) Validation with polysomnography of the sleepwatch sleep/wake scoring algorithm used by the actiwatch activity monitoring system. Technical Report to Mini Mitter Co, Inc,.
28. Mini Mitter Company IAR, Inc. Company (2005) Actiware Software: Actiwatch Instruction Manual Software version 5.0 ed. Oregon, USA: Respironics,.
29. Iber C, Ancoli-Israel S, Chesson A, Quan S (2007) The AASM manual for the scoring of sleep and associated events: rules, terminology and technical specifications. Wenchester, IL USA: American Academy of Sleep Medicine. 59 p.
30. American Sleep Disorders Association (1992) EEG arousals: scoring rules and examples: a preliminary report from the Sleep Disorders Atlas Task Force of the American Sleep Disorders Association. Sleep 15: 173–184.
31. Wang D, Wong KK, Dungan GC, 2nd, Buchanan PR, Yee BJ, et al. (2008) The validity of wrist actimetry assessment of sleep with and without sleep apnea. J Clin Sleep Med 4: 450–455.
32. Byrt T, Bishop J, Carlin JB (1993) Bias, prevalence and kappa. J Clin Epidemiol 46: 423–429.
33. Bland JM, Altman DG (1986) Statistical methods for assessing agreement between two methods of clinical measurement. Lancet 1: 307–310.
34. Terwee CB, Bot SDM, de Boer MR, van der Windt DAWM, Knol DL, et al. (2007) Quality criteria were proposed for measurement properties of health status questionnaires. Jo Clin Epidemiol 60: 34–42.
35. Fleiss J (1986) The design and analysis of clinical experiments. New York: John Wiley and Sons.
36. Buysse DJ, Reynolds CF, 3rd, Monk TH, Berman SR, Kupfer DJ (1989) The Pittsburgh Sleep Quality Index: a new instrument for psychiatric practice and research. Psychiatry Res 28: 193–213.
37. Backhaus J, Junghanns K, Broocks A, Riemann D, Hohagen F (2002) Test-retest reliability and validity of the Pittsburgh Sleep Quality Index in primary insomnia. J Psychosom Res 53: 737–740.
38. Bastien CH, Vallières A, Morin CM (2001) Validation of the Insomnia Severity Index as an outcome measure for insomnia research. Sleep Med 2: 297–307.
39. Smith S, Trinder J (2001) Detecting insomnia: comparison of four self-report measures of sleep in a young adult population. J Sleep Res 10: 229–235.
40. Lichstein KL, Stone KC, Donaldson J, Nau SD, Soeffing JP, et al. (2006) Actigraphy validation with insomnia. Sleep 29: 232–239.
41. Chae KY, Kripke DF, Poceta JS, Shadan F, Jamil SM, et al. (2009) Evaluation of immobility time for sleep latency in actigraphy. Sleep Med 10: 621–625.
42. Tryon WW (2004) Issues of validity in actigraphic sleep assessment. Sleep 27: 158–165.
43. Hauri PJ (1999) Evaluation of a sleep switch device. Sleep 22: 1110–1117.
44. Chae KY, Kripke DF, Poceta JS, Shadan F, Jamil SM, et al. (2009) Evaluation of immobility time for sleep latency in actigraphy. Sleep Med 10: 621–625.

Table S1 Construct and description of clinical assessment measures.

Author Contributions

Conceived and designed the experiments: JM JH SA. Performed the experiments: SA GD RG DB JM. Analyzed the data: SA JM ZM CM GD. Contributed reagents/materials/analysis tools: SA GD JM. Wrote the paper: SA JH JM CM. Obtained funds for the study: JM. Obtained Ethics approval: SM.

Evaluation of the Validity of Job Exposure Matrix for Psychosocial Factors at Work

Svetlana Solovieva[1,2]*, **Tiina Pensola**[1], **Johanna Kausto**[1,2], **Rahman Shiri**[1,2], **Markku Heliövaara**[3],
Alex Burdorf[4], **Kirsti Husgafvel-Pursiainen**[1,2], **Eira Viikari-Juntura**[2]

1 Centre of Expertise for Health and Work Ability, Finnish Institute of Occupational Health, Helsinki, Finland, 2 Disability Prevention Centre, Finnish Institute of Occupational Health, Helsinki, Finland, 3 National Institute for Health and Welfare, Helsinki, Finland, 4 Erasmus MC, University Medical Center Rotterdam, Rotterdam, The Netherlands

Abstract

Objective: To study the performance of a developed job exposure matrix (JEM) for the assessment of psychosocial factors at work in terms of accuracy, possible misclassification bias and predictive ability to detect known associations with depression and low back pain (LBP).

Materials and Methods: We utilized two large population surveys (the Health 2000 Study and the Finnish Work and Health Surveys), one to construct the JEM and another to test matrix performance. In the first study, information on job demands, job control, monotonous work and social support at work was collected via face-to-face interviews. Job strain was operationalized based on job demands and job control using quadrant approach. In the second study, the sensitivity and specificity were estimated applying a Bayesian approach. The magnitude of misclassification error was examined by calculating the biased odds ratios as a function of the sensitivity and specificity of the JEM and fixed true prevalence and odds ratios. Finally, we adjusted for misclassification error the observed associations between JEM measures and selected health outcomes.

Results: The matrix showed a good accuracy for job control and job strain, while its performance for other exposures was relatively low. Without correction for exposure misclassification, the JEM was able to detect the association between job strain and depression in men and between monotonous work and LBP in both genders.

Conclusions: Our results suggest that JEM more accurately identifies occupations with low control and high strain than those with high demands or low social support. Overall, the present JEM is a useful source of job-level psychosocial exposures in epidemiological studies lacking individual-level exposure information. Furthermore, we showed the applicability of a Bayesian approach in the evaluation of the performance of the JEM in a situation where, in practice, no gold standard of exposure assessment exists.

Editor: James Coyne, University of Pennsylvania, United States of America

Funding: The study was financially supported by the Finnish Work Environment Fund (project no 109364). The funders had no role in study design, data collection and analysis, decision to publish, or preparation of the manuscript.

Competing Interests: The authors have declared that no competing interests exist.

* Email: svetlana.solovieva@ttl.fi

Introduction

During the past three decades, the effects of psychosocial factors at work on health have received considerable attention in research. Psychosocial factors at work are numerous, with psychological job demands, job control (decision latitude), efforts and rewards [1,2] comprising the key dimensions. Another factor of importance is social support at work [3].

The job strain model, introduced by Karasek in 1979 [4], is one of the most studied occupational stress models. According to the model, workers with a combination of high psychosocial job demands and low control over a job (high job strain) have a higher risk of developing an illness as compared to workers with low psychosocial job demands and high job control (low job strain) [1]. The job strain model has been successfully used to predict the risk of cardiovascular disease [5,6], major mental disorders [7], type II

diabetes [8] and musculoskeletal diseases [9]. The effects of the individual components of the job strain model on health have also been evaluated, although the results have often been inconsistent across the studies and health outcomes [7,9].

The interpretation of the observed associations between psychosocial factors at work and health mainly depends on the validity of the assessment methods of the risk factors. Self-reported questionnaires are widely used to measure psychosocial factors at work [10]. Self-reports provide subjective information representing a worker's perception of occupational stress and are therefore susceptible to reporting bias. The subjective assessment of psychosocial factors at work has been the largest concern in the debate on the interpretation of associations and on the possible causal role of these factors for illness. It has been suggested that common source bias due to subjective measures of psychosocial factors at work increases the likelihood of false positive findings, particularly in cross-sectional studies with the self-reported health outcomes [11–13]. Workers having health problems are more likely to report certain psychosocial exposures than healthy workers. Such tendency might lead to differential misclassification, which results either in an overestimation or underestimation of the true effect [14], particularly, when exposures and outcome are measured simultaneously.

The assessment of psychosocial factors at work with a job exposure matrix (JEM), where exposure level is assigned based on the job-specific average of exposure, is not prone to information bias and may therefore guarantee some degree of objectivity. The major advantage of the JEM in epidemiological studies is that it can be applied to the populations with lacking exposure information. However, such method of exposure assessment induces Berkson type error, which may not cause notable bias on the effect estimates but weakens the precision of the estimates [15]. A JEM neglects both within worker (over time variation) and between worker (variation in tasks, activities and work processes) variation in a job [16] and therefore may result in false positive and negative exposure assignments for a considerable proportion of the subjects. A non-differential misclassification bias induced by JEM will attenuate the observed associations towards null [15,17,18]. Knowing the magnitude of measurement error (e.g. sensitivity and specificity) and exposure prevalence, the extent of non-differential bias can be estimated [15,19].

Several psychosocial job exposure matrices have been developed and used in epidemiological studies [20–26]. Even though the JEM measures are more objective than self-reported ones, they cannot be seen as a gold standard in the context of psychosocial factors at work [13]. Therefore, the question of the reliability of the associations between JEM-based exposures and health outcomes is always warranted. The validity of psychosocial JEM measures in the absence of a gold standard method is challenging to evaluate and, as a result, has rarely been examined and reported [24–28]. Furthermore, the magnitude of misclassification bias of psychosocial JEM measures on effect estimates has not been examined so far.

The aims of the study were 1) to examine the accuracy of a developed gender-specific job exposure matrix in the assessment of psychosocial factors at work applying the Bayesian approach, 2) to evaluate the theoretical impact of exposure misclassification on exposure-outcome associations and 3) to examine the ability of the matrix to detect known associations between psychosocial factors at work and health outcomes.

Materials and Methods

Study population

We utilized two large Finnish population samples. The Health 2000 (H2000) Study was used to construct the JEM and to examine the inter-method agreement, and the national Finnish Work and Health (FWH) Surveys were used to test the performance of the matrix. The study populations consisted of 18–64 year-old individuals, who had been working during the preceding 12 months.

The Health 2000 Study is a large Finnish population-based study carried out in 2000–01. The main objective of the study was to obtain representative information on the current health status of the whole non-institutional adult population in Finland. The survey consisted of several questionnaires, a home interview, and a health examination. A nationally representative sample of the population was obtained using a two-stage stratified cluster sampling design. The original samples consisted of 8028 subjects

aged 30 years or over and 1894 subjects aged 18–29. The participation rates were 87% and 90%, respectively. A detailed comprehensive description of the methods and processes has been published elsewhere [29,30]. The sample of this study comprised 4619 persons aged 18–64 who were working during the preceding 12 months and for whom information on occupational titles and exposures were available. The age and gender distribution of the study population matched those of the employed persons in Finland in the year 2000.

The national Finnish National Work and Health Surveys have been conducted every third year since 1997 to collect information on perceived working conditions and the health of the working-age population. For the 1997–2003 Surveys, random samples of subjects aged 25–64 years independent of their working status (e.g., working, unemployed, retired or student) were drawn from the Finnish population register. For the 2009 Survey a random sample of subjects aged 20–64 years was drawn from Finnish employment statistics. The sample size has varied between 2031 and 2355 persons from year to year with a response rate of 58–72% [31]. At each survey, a phone number was not found for about 10–16% of subjects. The proportion of non-participants in each survey was slightly higher among men than women and among subjects aged 24–34 years than among the older subjects. Age, gender, education, socioeconomic status and occupational sector of the respondents were compared with the Census data. No major differences were found. Thus, the respondents to the FWH Surveys represent rather well the targeted population. The data from all five surveys were combined. Hence, the total number of the interviewed persons with information on occupation during 1997–2009 was 11326.

The H2000 Study and the FWH Surveys have all obtained ethical approval from the appropriate ethics committees.

Classification of occupations

Occupations in both surveys were classified on the 4-digit level (including few occupations coded with 5 digits) according to the Classification of Occupations 2001 by Statistics Finland, which is based on the International Standard Classification of Occupations (ISCO-88). The classification is based on ten categories of professional skills. In total, the classification includes 444 job titles.

Psychosocial exposures

Psychosocial exposures in the H2000 Study were measured with a Finnish version of the Job Content Questionnaire (JCQ) [32]. The JCQ has been shown to be a valid and reliable instrument to assess job stress and social support in many occupational settings worldwide [10,13]. Responses were given on a five point Likert-scale from 1 (fully agree) to 5 (fully disagree).

Psychological *job demands* scale is the sum of the following five items: "work fast", "work hard", "excessive work", "not enough time", and "hectic job". In the current study, Cronbach's alpha for the scale was 0.76 for men and 0.81 for women. *Job control* scale is the sum of two subscales. Decision authority was measured with three items: "allows own decisions", "decision freedom", and "a lot of say on the job"), and skill discretion was measured with five items: "learn new things", "requires creativity", "high skill level", "variety", and "develop own abilities". Cronbach's alpha for the scale was 0.85 for men and 0.86 for women. Since *monotonous (repetitive) work* was weakly correlated with the other five items of the skill discretion scale we treated it as a separate exposure. Job demands, job control and monotonous work were dichotomized using gender-specific median cut-off points.

Job strain was operationalized using the quadrant approach proposed by Karasek and Theorell [1]. It defines workers who are above the median on job demands and below the median on job control as having a high strain job. Other categories are: low strain (low demands and high control), passive (low demands and low control) and active (high demands and high control). Low strain job was used as the reference category in the analyses.

Social *support* at work was measured with four items: "support from supervisor", "supervisor appreciates", "support from co-workers", "discussion on work". Cronbach's alpha for the scale was 0.80 for men and 0.82 for women. Social support was dichotomized at a gender-specific median in order to define low and high support.

Development of the job exposure matrix (JEM)

We constructed a gender-specific matrix with exposure estimates at each intersection between rows (occupational groups) and columns (psychosocial exposures). The exposure axis of the matrix included the above mentioned five psychosocial risk factors at work. The occupation axis of the matrix was based on the original job titles or occupational groups.

Previous studies showed that ten individuals with the same job title will be sufficient for a reliable estimation of exposures [33,34]. The exposure estimates for job demands, job control, monotonous work and social support at work were calculated as a median score of exposures in each occupation which included at least 10 subjects in order to obtain reasonably precise estimates. The exposure estimates for job strain were calculated as the proportion of exposed to passive, active and high strain work. The job titles with a small number (<10) of respondents were grouped based on the similarities of these job titles with regard to work tasks (including supervising), work environment, and required educational level. The gender differences in the exposures were also considered. If there was no reasonable way to merge the occupation with other occupations within the gender (such as female frontier guards), the exposure estimates of both genders in that occupation/occupational group were combined.

The sample size of the H2000 Study was large enough to enable us to develop a gender-specific job exposure matrix and to keep several job titles unmerged. Out of 444 possible job titles, altogether 363 (300 among men and 267 among women) were available in the Health 2000 Study. There were 61 job titles among men and 58 among women with at least 10 subjects. These job titles covered 69% of the study sample. After merging the smaller groups the number of job titles or occupational groups reduced to 110 among men and 101 among women.

The exposure estimates for job demands, job control, monotonous work and social support at work were dichotomized using gender-specific median as a cut-off point. The categories of job strain were obtained based on the dichotomized JEM-based job demands and job control.

Health outcomes

Based on the current evidence we chose two health outcomes that are known to be associated with psychosocial factors at work. Both cross-sectional and longitudinal studies have shown that high level of psychological demands and job strain are associated with major mental disorders [7,35–37]. Suggestive evidence for a relationship of job demands, job control and monotonous work with low back pain has also been reported [9,38,39].

Depressive symptoms. In both studies, depressive symptoms were assessed with the following question: "Have you had melancholy or depression during the last month (30 days)?". The response categories ranged from 1 = not at all to 5 = very often. The occurrence of depressive symptoms was dichotomized as no (categories 1 and 2) or yes (categories from 3 to 5).

Low back pain. In the H2000 Study information on low back pain was inquired with the following question: "Have you had pain in your back during the past month (30 days)?" (yes/no). In the FWH Surveys, data on low back pain were collected with an interview using the question: "Have you during the past month (30 days) had long-lasting or recurrent pain in the lumbar spine?" (yes/no).

Data analyses

In the H2000 Study, the inter-method agreement between self-reported and JEM measures was examined using intra-class correlation (ICC). Two-way mixed total ICC agreements were computed. In the FWH Surveys, the performance of the matrix was evaluated by examining the accuracy of the matrix in the identification of exposed/non-exposed individuals, estimating exposure misclassification error, and looking at the ability of the matrix to detect associations of psychosocial factors at work with one-month prevalence of depression or low back pain (predictive validity) [40]. The accuracy of the JEM was evaluated using five indicators: sensitivity (Se), specificity (Sp), Youden's J index, likelihood ratio positive (LR+) and likelihood ratio negative (LR−).

Sensitivity (ability of the test to identify positive results) and specificity (ability of the test to identify negative results) are usually determined against a reference standard test (gold standard). Errors in measuring the sensitivity and specificity of a test will arise if the reference test itself does not have 100% sensitivity and 100% specificity. Since there is no gold standard measure for psychosocial factors at work, we estimated sensitivity and specificity using a Bayesian approach, proposed by Joseph et al. [41]. As the first step, the posterior distribution of sensitivity and specificity of the JEM measures was calculated using self-reported and JEM measures of exposures from H2000 Study. For these analyses, the prior distribution of the parameters was derived based on the assumption that the self-reported measures have almost perfect sensitivity and specificity and no prior information on sensitivity and specificity of JEM measures is available. As the second step, the posterior distribution of sensitivity and specificity of the JEM measures was calculated using data from FWH Surveys. For these analyses the prior distributions of the parameters were derived based on the posterior distributions obtained in the first step. At each step, the posterior medians and their 95% Bayesian credible intervals were estimated using Gibbs sampler algorithm with WinBUGS software version 1.4.3.

The estimated sensitivity and specificity were used to calculate Youden's J index as well as LR+ and LR−. The Youden's J index (J = Se+Sp−1) has been used as a measure of the effectiveness of the JEM to discriminate between exposed and non-exposed individuals. The possible range of the Youden's J index value is between 0 (totally useless) and 1 (perfect). Likelihood ratio positive is the probability of an exposed person to be classified as exposed divided by the probability of a non-exposed person to be classified as exposed. Likelihood ratio negative is the probability of an exposed person to be classified as non-exposed divided by the probability of a non-exposed person to be classified as non-exposed. A likelihood ratio equal to 1 will indicate that the JEM measure is unable to distinguish between exposed and non-exposed. A LR>1 will indicate that the JEM is likely to identify exposed and LR<1 will indicate that the JEM is likely to identify non-exposed. The higher LR+ value and lower the LR− value, the better is the JEM performance.

To estimate the theoretical magnitude of exposure misclassification, biased odds ratios (OR′) were calculated based on the obtained estimates of sensitivity (Se) and specificity (Sp) and assumed "true prevalence" (Pr) and "true odds ratios" (OR) using

Table 1. Prevalence of self-reported and JEM-based psychosocial exposures.

Exposures	Men				Women		
	H2000 Study			FWH Surveys	H2000 Study		FWH Surveys
	Self-reported	JEM		JEM	Self-reported	JEM	JEM
	Prev. (95% CI)	Prev. (95% CI)		Prev. (95% CI)	Prev. (95% CI)	Prev. (95% CI)	Prev. (95% CI)
High job demands	43.1 (41.1, 45.0)	33.1 (29.4, 33.3)		32.2 (31.0, 33.4)	44.2 (42.2, 46.3)	35.3 (33.4, 37.3)	36.0 (34.7, 37.3)
Low job control	52.6 (50.5, 54.7)	49.8 (47.8, 51.9)		49.8 (48.5, 51.1)	56.1 (54.1, 58.1)	56.5 (54.5, 58.5)	55.4 (54.1, 56.7)
Job strain							
Low strain job	26.2 (24.4, 28.1)	36.3 (34.3, 38.3)		36.3 (34.1, 36.6)	23.8 (22.1, 25.6)	24.6 (22.9, 26.4)	25.6 (24.4, 26.3)
Passive job	30.7 (28.8, 32.7)	32.4 (30.5, 34.4)		32.5 (31.3, 33.8)	32.0 (30.1, 33.9)	40.0 (38.1, 42.1)	38.4 (37.2, 39.7)
Active job	21.2 (19.5, 22.9)	13.9 (12.5, 15.4)		14.9 (14.0, 15.8)	20.0 (18.4, 21.7)	18.9 (17.3, 20.5)	19.0 (18.0, 20.1)
High strain job	21.9 (20.2, 23.6)	17.4 (15.9, 19.1)		17.3 (16.3, 18.3)	24.2 (22.5, 26.0)	16.4 (15.0, 18.0)	16.9 (16.0, 18.0)
Low social support	47.3 (45.3, 49.4)	48.5 (46.4, 50.1)		48.4 (47.1, 49.7)	44.2 (42.2, 46.2)	37.1 (35.2, 39.1)	37.5 (36.2, 38.7)
Monotonous work	28.5 (26.6, 30.4)	17.2 (15.7, 18.8)		17.1 (16.1, 18.1)	31.8 (29.9, 33.7)	24.0 (22.3, 25.8)	22.1 (21.0, 23.2)

H2000 Study- the Health 2000 Study; FWH Surveys- the Finnish Work and Health Surveys.

the following formula [19]:

$$OR' = \frac{((Se*OR*Pr+(1-Sp)*(1-Pr))*((1-Se)*Pr+Sp*(1-Pr))}{((Se*Pr+(1-Sp)*(1-Pr))*((1-Se)*OR*Pr+Sp*(1-Pr))}$$

The true prevalence was fixed at 0.50 for high job demands, low job control and low social support, at 0.33 for monotonous work and at 0.25 for high strain job. The true odds ratios were fixed at three values OR = 1.5, OR = 2 and OR = 3. The relative difference between biased and true estimates was calculated ((OR'-OR)/OR) and used as quantitative measure for the magnitude of exposure misclassification.

Logistic regression analyses with age, education and year of survey (the FWH Surveys) adjusted odds ratios (OR) and 95% confidence intervals (CIs) were carried out to study the associations between the JEM measures and one-month prevalence of depression or low back pain. These analyses were performed using SAS version 9.1. The effect estimates were adjusted for misclassification error using WINPEPI COMPARE2 program, version 3.08 [42].

All analyses were performed separately for men and women.

Results

In both genders, the prevalence of high job demands, high job strain and monotonous work measured by job exposure matrix was statistically significantly lower than that assessed by self-reports (Table 1). In women, the prevalence of low social support was lower for JEM measures than for self-reported measures. There were no differences in the distribution of exposures assessed by JEM between the two study populations, reflecting a similar job distribution in both surveys. In general, total agreement between self-reported and JEM measures assessed by ICC was slightly better among women than men, with the largest ICC values observed for job control followed by monotonous work (Table 2).

Bayesian estimates of sensitivity and specificity and magnitude of exposure misclassification error

The Bayesian estimates of sensitivity and specificity were calculated based on the data from the Health 2000 Study and

The Finnish Work and Health Surveys and are shown in the form of posterior medians and 95% Bayesian intervals (Table 3). The posterior estimates were very similar in both study populations. The specificity of JEM measures was higher than sensitivity for all exposures except job control among women. Specificity ranged from 0.62 to 0.90 in men, and from 0.68 to 0.86 in women. Sensitivity was the lowest for high strain job (0.46) in men and for low social support (0.52) in women. The best matrix performance assessed by Youden's J index and likelihood ratios was found for high strain job, particularly in women. The JEM was least effective in identification of men exposed to high demands (J = 0.17) and women exposed to low social support (J = 0.15).

The theoretical effect of exposure misclassification error on estimated ORs is shown in Table 4. In both genders, the smallest misclassification error was observed for high job strain, followed by that for low job control. The largest misclassification error was found for low social support (both genders) and high job demands (men). In general, when the true OR is equal to 1.5, the effect of misclassification error on point estimates is relatively small, though there is a high likelihood of false negative findings. A statistically significant association can be detected only for low job control and high job strain in women. With the increase of true OR, there is a larger reduction in the biased odds ratios, but at the same time the likelihood of false negative findings is lowered.

Table 2. Intra-class correlation (ICC) between individual-based and group-based measures of psychosocial exposures for men and women in the H2000 Study.

	Men	Women
Job demands	0.31	0.40
Job control	0.53	0.60
Monotonous work	0.45	0.51
Social support	0.36	0.33
Job strain	0.21	0.29

H2000 Study- the Health 2000 Study.

Table 3. Posterior medians and lower and upper limits of the posterior equally tailed 95% credible intervals (Bayesian confidence interval).

	H2000 Study		FWH Surveys				
	Sensitivity	Specificity	Sensitivity	Specificity	J[1]	LR+[2]	LR−[3]
High demands							
Men	0.41 (0.38–0.44)	0.76 (0.74–0.78)	0.41 (0.39–0.44)	0.76 (0.74–0.78)	0.17	1.71 (1.53–1.91)	0.78 (0.73–0.82)
Women	0.49 (0.46–0.52)	0.75 (0.73–0.78)	0.49 (0.46–0.52)	0.75 (0.73–0.78)	0.24	2.00 (1.77–2.25)	0.68 (0.63–0.72)
Low control							
Men	0.67 (0.64–0.70)	0.69 (0.67–0.72)	0.67 (0.64–0.69)	0.70 (0.67–0.72)	0.37	2.20 (2.01–2.42)	0.48 (0.43–0.52)
Women	0.75 (0.73–0.78)	0.68 (0.65–0.71)	0.76 (0.73–0.78)	0.68 (0.65–0.71)	0.44	2.35 (2.14–2.59)	0.36 (0.32–0.40)
High strain job							
Men	0.58 (0.52–0.64)	0.87 (0.84–0.91)	0.60 (0.55–0.65)	0.82 (0.77–0.86)	0.42	3.34 (2.52–4.45)	0.49 (0.42–0.57)
Women	0.77 (0.71–0.82)	0.88 (0.84–0.92)	0.78 (0.73–0.83)	0.86 (0.81–0.90)	0.64	5.75 (4.13–8.03)	0.25 (0.19–0.31)
Low social support							
Men	0.60 (0.57–0.63)	0.62 (0.59–0.65)	0.60 (0.57–0.63)	0.62 (0.59–0.65)	0.22	1.59 (1.45–1.74)	0.65 (0.59–0.71)
Women	0.48 (0.45–0.51)	0.72 (0.70–0.74)	0.44 (0.42–0.46)	0.71 (0.69–0.73)	0.15	1.52 (1.40–1.65)	0.79 (0.75–0.83)
Monotonous work							
Men	0.35 (0.32–0.39)	0.90 (0.88–0.91)	0.36 (0.32–0.39)	0.90 (0.88–0.91)	0.26	3.39 (2.84–4.01)	0.72 (0.68–0.76)
Women	0.46 (0.42–0.50)	0.86 (0.84–0.88)	0.46 (0.42–0.50)	0.86 (0.84–0.88)	0.32	3.31 (2.79–3.91)	0.63 (0.58–0.68)

The sensitivity and specificity of JEM-based measures for men and women in the H2000 Study and the FWH Surveys.
H2000 Study- the Health 2000 Study; FWH Surveys- the Finnish Work and Health Surveys;
[1] J - Youden's index = sensitivity+specificity−1.
[2] LR+ likelihood ratio positive.
[3] LR− likelihood ratio negative.

Table 4. Biased odds (OR′) ratios according to sensitivity and specificity of the job exposure matrix when the true odds ratios (OR) were assumed to equal 1.5, 2 or 3.

	OR = 1.5		OR = 2.0		OR = 3.0	
	Men	Women	Men	Women	Men	Women
High job demands[1]	1.08	1.11	1.13	1.18*	1.21*	1.28*
Low job control[1]	1.16	1.20*	1.28*	1.35*	1.45*	1.58*
Monotonous work[2]	1.17	1.17	1.30*	1.31*	1.50*	1.52*
Low social support[1]	1.09	1.07	1.16	1.11	1.25*	1.17*
High job strain[3]	1.18	1.27*	1.34*	1.53*	1.60*	1.99*

[1]Prevalence of exposure is assumed to equal 0.50.
[2]Prevalence of exposure is assumed to equal 0.33.
[3]Prevalence of exposure is assumed to equal 0.25.
*Statistical significance at the 5% level (two-sided test) of the biased odds ratios is calculated for a study population of 5000 men and 5000 women.

Predictive validity of the JEM measures

The one-month prevalence of depression was statistically significantly higher in the H2000 Study as compared with the FWH Surveys, while the prevalence of low back pain during the preceding 30 days was similar (Table 5). In both study populations, women tended to report depression and LBP more frequently than men.

In the H2000 Study, associations between all self-reported psychosocial factors at work and depression were statistically significant in both genders (Table 5). In the FWH Surveys, the point estimates of associations between the JEM-based exposures and depression were reduced by 22–65% as compared with those for self-reported exposures in the H2000 Study, particularly in women. The smallest drop was found for low job control (men) and monotonous work (women), while the largest reduction in estimates was observed for low social support in women. After correction for exposure misclassification, the odds ratios obtained with JEM regained their statistical significance for low job control (both genders), monotonous work (women), and high job demands, low social support and high strain job (men). However, women with high job demands or low social support assessed by JEM had reduced odds of depression. Similarly, monotonous work seemed to be associated with lower risk of depression in men.

All self-reported psychosocial factors at work, except monotonous work, were statistically significantly associated with LBP in women (Table 5). In men, high job demands, low job control and low social support tended to increase the odds of LBP, although the association was statistically significant for high job strain only. The estimated odds for JEM-based exposures were reduced by 6–21% in men and by 12–32% in women as compared with those for self-reported exposures. Unexpectedly, for monotonous work, the odds ratios obtained with JEM were increased by 21% as compared to odds ratios obtained with self-reports. After correction for exposure misclassification error, all JEM-based exposures in men and all except high job demands in women were statistically significantly associated with LBP. Women with low social support had a low prevalence of LBP.

Discussion

We comprehensively validated a gender-specific job exposure matrix that we constructed for the assessment of psychosocial factors at work. The matrix showed a good accuracy in identification of individuals exposed to low job control and high job strain, while its performance for job demands and social support was relatively low. The largest misclassification error was found for low social support (women) and high job demands (men). The difference between the odds ratios based on self-reports and JEM was larger for depression than for low back pain, especially in women. Without correction for exposure misclassification, the JEM was able to detect the association between job strain and depression in men and that between monotonous work and low back pain in both genders. The predictive ability of the matrix substantially improved after correction for possible misclassification bias.

Although several psychosocial JEMs exist, their validity is poorly explored. Most of the previous studies on the validation of JEMs examined their ability to detect known associations between JEM measures and health outcomes (predictive validity) [24–28]. Few studies evaluated inter-method agreement between JEM and self-reported measures [24,43]. There are several parameters that can be used to evaluate the performance of an exposure assessment method, of which sensitivity, specificity, Youden's J index and likelihood ratios are the most commonly applied. Considering all performance indicators, the performance of our JEM was good for job control and job strain and was rather low for job demands and social support. These findings are in line with the results of the previous studies that reported higher validity of the JEM measures for job control and job strain than for job demands and social support [13,43,44]. The relatively low validity of job demands may suggest that variation of this factor between occupations is smaller than that within occupation [20,21]. However, the poor performance for social support may alternatively reflect that some psychosocial factors are highly individually oriented in that a particular job may be perceived as very strenuous for some whereas not for others.

Among performance indicators, sensitivity and specificity are the key ones, because all others are calculated based on them. Theoretically, sensitivity and specificity should be determined against a reference test (gold standard). In practice, the sensitivity and specificity of the JEMs are usually evaluated against self-reports, even if it is well known that the self-reported exposures may be subject to information bias. In the current study, we used the Bayesian approach to estimate sensitivity and specificity of JEM measures. The similarity of estimates obtained in both of our study samples suggests their robustness. The sensitivity of the JEM-based estimates for job control and high strain job was acceptable, while it was reduced for job demands, monotonous work and social support. The specificity of all our JEM-based estimates varied from good to very good and was substantially higher,

Table 5. The association of psychosocial exposures measured at individual (ind) level and at group level (job exposure matrix (JEM)) with one-month prevalence of depression and low back pain among men and women.

	Prevalence (95% CI)	High demands		Low control		Monotonous work		Low social support		High strain job	
		OR	95% CI	OR	95% CI	OR	95% CI	OR	95% CI	OR	95% CI
Men											
Depressive symptoms											
H2000 (ind)[1]	13.9 (12.3–15.5)	1.98	1.51–2.59	1.52	1.16–2.01	1.45	1.07–1.95	2.07	1.59–2.74	3.07	2.05–4.62
FWH (JEM)[2]	10.6 (9.8–11.5)	1.15	0.96–1.37	1.19	0.98–1.43	0.95	0.75–1.21	1.11	0.93–1.31	1.34	1.04–1.72
FWH (JEM)[3]		2.08	1.74–2.48	1.33	1.12–1.59	0.81	0.67–0.99	1.54	1.30–1.72	1.70	1.34–2.15
Low back pain											
H2000 (ind)[1]	26.8 (25.0–28.7)	1.19	0.99–1.44	1.13	0.93–1.37	1.01	0.81–1.26	1.16	0.96–1.41	1.37	1.04–1.80
FWH (JEM)[2]	29.8 (28.6–31.0)	1.04	0.92–1.18	1.06	0.94–1.21	1.22	1.05–1.42	1.06	0.94–1.19	1.10	0.92–1.30
FWH (JEM)[3]		1.20	1.07–1.34	1.73	1.54–1.95	2.38	2.10–2.69	1.50	1.33–1.68	1.77	1.51–2.09
Women											
Depressive symptoms											
H2000 (ind)[1]	18.7 (17.0–20.5)	1.55	1.22–1.95	1.49	1.17–1.90	1.29	1.00–1.67	2.75	2.16–3.50	2.38	1.68–3.37
FWH (JEM)[2]	15.9 (14.9–16.9)	0.99	0.85–1.15	1.07	0.91–1.28	1.01	0.84–1.22	0.97	0.83–1.13	1.09	0.87–1.37
FWH (JEM)[3]		0.88	0.76–1.01	1.33	1.15–1.54	1.24	1.05–1.45	0.79	0.69–0.92	1.20	0.96–1.50
Low back pain											
H2000 (ind)[1]	29.7 (27.8–31.6)	1.29	1.08–1.55	1.27	1.05–1.54	1.16	0.95–1.43	1.28	1.07–1.54	1.68	1.28–2.20
FWH (JEM)[2]	31.4 (30.2–32.)	1.00	0.89–1.13	1.12	0.99–1.27	1.19	1.03–1.38	1.00	0.89–1.12	1.14	0.95–1.38
FWH (JEM)[3]		0.92	0.82–1.03	1.76	1.56–1.97	2.38	2.10–2.71	0.83	0.74–0.94	1.52	1.27–1.81

Odds ratios (OR) and their 95% confidence intervals (95% CI).
H2000 – the Health 2000 Study; FWH– the Finnish Work and Health Surveys;
[1] ORs calculated based on self-reports and adjusted for age and education.
[2] ORs calculated based on JEM and adjusted for age, education and year of survey.
[3] ORs calculated based on JEM adjusted for exposure misclassification bias.

especially in women, as compared to those found in a French study [24].

The studies that examined the predictive validity of the psychosocial JEM measures have consistently reported weaker associations between JEM measures and health outcomes than what has been found for the corresponding self-reported factors [24–28]. In general, the associations of JEM measures for job strain and job control with health outcomes were better reproducible than the associations for job demands. However, even unexpected results of a protective effect of high job demands assessed by JEM on anxiety disorders [25] and self-rated health [24] have been reported.

When JEM is used to study the association between an exposure and a health outcome, there is always some loss of information because the individual values are replaced with the group-based (job title) ones. Both self-reported exposures and JEM are prone to classification errors whose consequences on effect estimates need to be considered when interpreting the association between the exposure and the outcome. The measurement error in exposures assessed by JEM is always of a Berkson type, while the error of self-reported measures is of a classical type. The group-specific average of exposures used in our JEM was obtained based on nationally representative self-reported exposure data; therefore, the measurement error of our JEM has both classical and Berkson component, with the latter being dominant. The classical and Berkson errors bias the effect estimates differently [15]. The Berkson error has almost no effect on the point estimate, while it severely affects the estimate's precision. In case of classical error, the direction and magnitude of bias are more difficult to assess. We observed a larger difference between the self-reported and JEM-based exposures in the ORs for depressive symptoms than for LBP. This may suggest the presence of a higher common source bias in self-reported exposure measures among those reporting depressive symptoms than among those reporting LBP. As a result, for depressive symptoms, the risk estimates based on JEM measures may be closer to the true risk than the risk estimates based on self-reports. These benefits support the use of the JEM in epidemiological studies.

The ability of the JEM to detect known associations between risk factors and health outcomes primarily depends on the magnitude of misclassification error. Even though studies have examined the predictive validity of psychosocial JEM measures, none of them examined the effect of exposure misclassification on observed associations. Our results suggest that, due to misclassification error, we were not able to observe associations between job demands, job control and social support assessed by JEM with either depression or low back pain. However, after correction for misclassification bias, the ability of the matrix to detect the expected associations improved substantially. Furthermore, the bias-adjusted effect estimates for low job control and high job strain in our study were about the same as those reported in previous meta-analyses [7,9].

Conclusions

Our results suggest that JEM more accurately identifies occupations with low control and high strain than those with high demands or low social support. Although the JEM is a rather crude exposure assessment method, it can be a useful source of job-level psychosocial exposures in epidemiological studies lacking individual-level exposure. Furthermore, we showed the applicability of a Bayesian approach in the evaluation of the performance of the JEM in a situation where, in practice, no gold standard of exposure assessment exists.

Acknowledgments

We would like to thank Dr. Timo Kauppinen for his expertise in the development of the job exposure matrix.

Author Contributions

Conceived and designed the experiments: SS TP JK RS AB KH-P EV-J. Performed the experiments: SS TP JK RS AB KH-P EV-J. Analyzed the data: SS. Contributed reagents/materials/analysis tools: MH EV-J. Wrote the paper: SS TP EV-J KH-P. Contributed substantially to the interpretation of the findings and critically revised the manuscript: SS TP JK RS MH AB KH-P EV-J.

References

1. Karasek RA, Theorell T (1990) Healthy Work: Stress, Productivity, and the Reconstruction of Working Life. New York: Basic Books.
2. Siegrist J (1996) Adverse health effects of high-effort/low-reward conditions. J Occup Health Psychol 1:27–41.
3. Johnson JV, Hall EM (1988) Job strain, work place social support, and cardiovascular disease: a cross-sectional study of a random sample of the Swedish working population. Am J Public Health 78: 1336–42.
4. Karasek RA (1979) Job demands, job decision latitude, and mental strain: Implications for job redesign. Adm Sci Q 24:285–308.
5. Diène E, Fouquet A, Esquirol Y (2012) Cardiovascular diseases and psychosocial factors at work. Arch Cardiovasc Dis 105:33–9.
6. Kivimäki M, Nyberg ST, Batty GD, Fransson EI, Heikkilä K, et al. (2012) Job strain as a risk factor for coronary heart disease: a collaborative meta-analysis of individual participant data. Lancet 380(9852):1491–7.
7. Stansfeld S, Candy B (2006) Psychosocial work environment and mental health–a meta-analytic review. Scand J Work Environ Health 32:443–62.
8. Cosgrove MP, Sargeant LA, Caleyachetty R, Griffin SJ (2012) Work-related stress and Type 2 diabetes: systematic review and meta-analysis. Occup Med (Lond) 62:167–73.
9. Lang J, Ochsmann E, Kraus T, Lang JW (2012) Psychosocial work stressors as antecedents of musculoskeletal problems: a systematic review and meta-analysis of stability-adjusted longitudinal studies. Soc Sci Med 75:1163–74.
10. Tabanelli MC, Depolo M, Cooke RM, Sarchielli G, Bonfiglioli R, et al. (2008) Available instruments for measurement of psychosocial factors in the work environment. Int Arch Occup Environ Health 82:1–12.
11. Landsbergis P, Theorell T, Schwartz J, Greiner BA, Krause N (2000) Measurement of psychosocial workplace exposure variables. Occup Med 15:163–88.
12. Macleod J, Davey Smith G (2003) Psychosocial factors and public health: a suitable case for treatment? J Epidemiol Community Health 57:565–70.

13. Theorell T, Hasselhorn HM (2005) On cross-sectional questionnaire studies of relationships between psychosocial conditions at work and health–are they reliable? Int Arch Occup Environ Health 78:517–22.
14. Blair A, Stewart P, Lubin JH, Forastiere F (2007) Methodological issues regarding confounding and exposure misclassification in epidemiological studies of occupational exposures. Am J Ind Med 50:199–207.
15. Armstrong BG (1998) Effect of measurement error on epidemiological studies of environmental and occupational exposures. Occup Environ Med 55:651–6.
16. Tielemans E, Heederik D, Burdorf A, Vermeulen R, Veulemans H, et al. (1999) Assessment of occupational exposures in a general population: comparison of different methods. Occup Environ Med 56:145–151.
17. Siemiatycki J, Dewar R, Richardson L (1989) Costs and statistical power associated with five methods of collecting occupation exposure information for population-based case-control studies. Am J Epidemiol 130:1236–46.
18. Bouyer J, Dardenne J, Hémon D (1995) Performance of odds ratios obtained with a job-exposure matrix and individual exposure assessment with special reference to misclassification errors. Scand J Work Environ Health 21:265–71.
19. Flegal KM, Brownie C, Haas JD (1986) The effects of exposure misclassification on estimates of relative risk. Am J Epidemiol 123:736–51.
20. Schwartz JE, Pieper CF, Karasek RA (1988) A procedure for linking psychosocial job characteristics data to health surveys. Am J Public Health 78:904–9.
21. Johnson JV, Stewart WF (1993) Measuring work organization exposure over the life course with a job-exposure matrix. Scand J Work Environ Health 19:21–8.
22. Mariani M (1999) Replace with a database: O*NET replaces the Dictionary of Occupational Titles. Occup Outlook Quarterly 43:3–9.
23. Kauppinen T, Toikkanen J, Pukkala E (1998) From cross-tabulations to multipurpose exposure information systems: a new job-exposure matrix. Am J Ind Med 33:409–17.
24. Niedhammer I, Chastang JF, Levy D, David S, Degioanni S, et al. (2008) Study of the validity of a job-exposure matrix for psychosocial work factors: results

from the national French SUMER survey. Int Arch Occup Environ Health 82:87–97.

25. Wieclaw J, Agerbo E, Mortensen PB, Burr H, Tuchsen F, et al. (2008) Psychosocial working conditions and the risk of depression and anxiety disorders in the Danish workforce. BMC Public Health 8:280.

26. Rijs KJ, van der Pas S, Geuskens GA, Cozijnsen R, Koppes LL, et al. (2013) Development and Validation of a Physical and Psychosocial Job-Exposure Matrix in Older and Retired Workers. Ann Occup Hyg 2013 Dec 11. [Epub ahead of print], doi:10.1093/annhyg/met052.

27. Theorell T, Tsutsumi A, Hallquist J, Reuterwall C, Hogstedt C, et al. (1998) Decision latitude, job strain, and myocardial infarction: a study of working men in Stockholm. The SHEEP Study Group. Stockholm Heart epidemiology Program. Am J Public Health 88:382–8.

28. Cohidon C, Santin G, Chastang JF, Imbernon E, Niedhammer I (2012) Psychosocial exposures at work and mental health: potential utility of a job-exposure matrix. Occup Environ Med 54:184–91.

29. Aromaa A, Koskinen S (2004) Population and methods. Health and functional capacity in Finland. In: Aromaa A. and Koskinen S, editors. Baseline result of the Health 2000 Helath Examination Survey. Helsinki: The National Public Health Institute pp. 11–23.

30. Laiho J, Djerf K, Lehtonen R (2006) Sampling design. In: Heistaro S, editor. Methodology report Health 2000 Survey. Helsinki: the National Public Health Institute B26: 13–5.

31. Perkiö-Mäkelä M, Hirvonen M, Elo A-L, Kauppinen K, Kauppinen T, et al. (2010) Työ ja terveys -haastattelututkimus. 2009; Helsinki: Työterveyslaitos (in Finnish).

32. Karasek R, Brisson C, Kawakami N, Houtman I, Bongers P, et al. (1998) The Job Content Questionnaire (JCQ): an instrument for internationally comparative assessments of psychosocial job characteristics. J Occup Health Psychol 3:322–55.

33. Le Moual N, Bakke P, Orlowski E, Heederik D, Kromhout H, et al. (2000) Performance of population specific job exposure matrices (JEMs): European collaborative analyses on occupational risk factors for chronic obstructive pulmonary disease with job exposure matrices (ECOJEM). Occup Environ Med 57:126–32.

34. Solovieva S, Pehkonen I, Kausto J, Miranda H, Shiri R, et al. (2012) Development and validation of a job exposure matrix for physical risk factors in low back pain. PLoS One 7(11):e48680.

35. Bonde JP (2008) Psychosocial factors at work and risk of depression: a systematic review of the epidemiological evidence. Occup Environ Medicine 65:438–45.

36. Netterstrøm B, Conrad N, Bech P, Fink P, Olsen O, et al. (2008) The relation between work-related psychosocial factors and the development of depression. Epidemiologic reviews 30:118–32.

37. Niedhammer I, Sultan-Taïeb H, Chastang JF, Vermeylen G, Parent-Thirion A (2013). Fractions of cardiovascular diseases and mental disorders attributable to psychosocial work factors in 31 countries in Europe. Int Arch Occup Environ Health 2013 Apr 27. [Epub ahead of print], doi 10.1007/s00420-013-0879-4

38. Hartvigsen J, Lings S, Leboeuf-Yde C, Bakketeig L (2004). Psychosocial factors at work in relation to low back pain and consequences of low back pain; a systematic, critical review of prospective cohort studies. Occup Environ Med 61:e2.

39. Macfarlane GJ, Pallewatte N, Paudyal P, Blyth FM, Coggon D, et al. (2009) Evaluation of work-related psychosocial factors and regional musculoskeletal pain: results from a EULAR Task Force. Ann Rheum Dis 68:885–91.

40. Bouyer J, Hémon D (1993) Studying the performance of a job exposure matrix. Int J Epidemiol 22 (Suppl 2):S65–71.

41. Joseph L, Gyorkos TW, Coupal L (1995) Bayesian estimation of disease prevalence and the parameters of diagnostic tests in the absence of a gold standard. Am J Epidemiol 141:263–72.

42. Abramson JH (2011) WINPEPI updated: computer programs for epidemiologists, and their teaching potential. Epidemiol Perspect Innov 8:1.

43. Cifuentes M, Boyer J, Gore R, d'Errico A, Tessler J, et al. (2007) Inter-method agreement between O*NET and survey measures of psychosocial exposure among healthcare industry employees. Am J Ind Med 50:545–53.

44. Ostry AS, Marion SA, Demers PA, Hershler R, Kelly S, et al. (2001) Measuring psychosocial job strain with the job content questionnaire using experienced job evaluators. Am J Ind Med 39:397–401.

Disrupted TH17/Treg Balance in Patients with Chronic Low Back Pain

Benjamin Luchting*, Banafscheh Rachinger-Adam, Julia Zeitler, Lisa Egenberger, Patrick Möhnle, Simone Kreth, Shahnaz Christina Azad

Department of Anesthesiology and Pain Medicine, Ludwig-Maximilians University Munich, Munich, Germany

Abstract

Chronic low back pain (CLBP) is a leading cause of disability and costs in health care systems worldwide. Despite extensive research, the exact pathogenesis of CLBP, particularly the individual risk of chronification remains unclear. To investigate a possible role of the adaptive immune system in the pathophysiology of CLBP, we analyzed T cell related cytokine profiles, T cell related mRNA expression patterns and the distribution of T cell subsets in 37 patients suffering from nonspecific CLBP before and after multimodal therapy in comparison to 25 healthy controls. Serum patterns of marker cytokines were analyzed by Luminex technology, mRNA expression of cytokines and specific transcription factors was measured by real-time PCR, and distribution of TH1-, TH2-, TH17- and regulatory T cell (Tregs) subsets was determined by multicolor flow cytometry. We found that CLBP patients exhibit an increased number of anti-inflammatory Tregs, while pro-inflammatory TH17 cells are decreased, resulting in an altered TH17/Treg ratio. Accordingly, FoxP3 and TGF-β-mRNA expression was elevated, while expression of IL-23 was reduced. Serum cytokine analyses proved to be unsuitable to monitor the adaptive immune response in CLBP patients. We further show that even after successful therapy with lasting reduction of pain, T cell subset patterns remained altered after a follow-up period of 6 months. These findings suggest an involvement of TH17/Treg cells in the pathogenesis of CLBP and emphasize the importance of these cells in the crosstalk of pain and immune response.

Trial Registration: German Clinical Trial Register: Registration Trial DRKS00005954.

Editor: Mohammed Shamji, Toronto Western Hospital, Canada

Funding: This work was supported by grants from the Hella-Langer-Stiftung, Germany. The funders had no role in study design, data collection and analysis, decision to publish, or preparation of the manuscript.

Competing Interests: The authors have declared that no competing interests exist.

* Email: benjamin.luchting@med.uni-muenchen.de

Introduction

Low back pain (LBP) is a common condition with a lifetime prevalence of nearly 84%. Although most patients recover completely within 4–8 weeks, a subset of patients is prone to develop chronic low back pain (CLBP). CLBP has become a major challenge for public health care systems worldwide [1]. The prevalence of CLBP is about 23%; around 12% of the afflicted patients are severely disabled [2,3]. Still, mechanisms driving the chronification of low back pain syndromes remain largely elusive. Pathological physical conditions such as microtraumata, incorrect posture and degenerative processes as well as psychological factors such as overtaxing, emotional distress and inadequate coping have been described to contribute to the pathogenesis of CLBP [4,5]. Increasing evidence indicates a pivotal role of the immune system in acute and chronic pain [6].

Recent studies have reported enhanced serum levels of pro-inflammatory cytokines in various pain syndromes [7,8,9,10]. In the pathogenesis of CLBP, a possible impact of TNF-α was suggested [11]. Moreover, an increased expression of Il-17 in herniated and degenerated lumbar intervertebral discs has been reported, indicating a possible role of this cytokine in the chronification of pain [9].

While the innate immune system has been found to play an important role in acute pain [12], T-Lymphocytes as key players of the adaptive immune system are supposed to be of major importance [13,14] in the pathogenesis of chronic pain. In patients with complex regional pain syndrome (CRPS) and in those suffering from abacterial chronic pelvic pain [15,16], a TH1/TH2 imbalance with increased numbers of TH1 cells has been shown. In recent years, TH1/TH2 dichotomy has been expanded by two further CD4[+] T cell lineages, Th17 and regulatory T cells (Tregs). These two T-cell subsets play prominent roles in immune functions: Th17 cells exerting pro-inflammatory effects are key players in the pathogenesis of autoimmune diseases and protection against bacterial infections, while Tregs function to restrain excessive effector T-cell responses. The role of both T cell subsets has extensively been analyzed in tumor growth and in the development of inflammatory and autoimmune diseases [17,18,19,20,21]. Recently published data also indicate an involvement of both T cell subsets in the development of chronic pain [22,23,24,25]. For example, in patients with postherpetic neuralgia (PHN), increased Treg numbers have been found [26]. In addition, there is evidence that these cells play a central role in endogenous recovery from neuropathic pain [27]. Due to the antagonistic functions of TH17 and Treg cells, and in analogy to the well-known TH1/TH2 paradigm, the ratio between TH17 and Tregs is increasingly used to characterize immune responses.

In CLBP, however, specific alterations in the adaptive immune system have not conclusively been analyzed, yet.

In the current study, we investigated cytokine profiles and T helper cell subset compositions in CLBP patients and healthy controls. Our results indicate that CLBP is associated with characteristic alterations of T helper cell subsets: The TH17/Treg ratio was significantly decreased. We further provide evidence that these alterations persist even in those patients exhibiting significant pain reduction after participation in a standardized multimodal therapy program.

Materials and Methods

Ethics statement

The study followed the principles of the Declaration of Helsinki and was approved by the Ethics Committee of the LMU Munich.

Subjects

During a prospective recruitment period of two years (September 2011 until September 2013), all patients seeking treatment for nonspecific CLBP at our pain clinic were assessed for study specific inclusion and exclusion criteria. Inclusion criteria were CLBP defined as low back pain persisting longer than two month, not attributable to a recognized specific pathological condition (e.g., disc herniation, any type of radiculopathy or other neuropathic pain, infection, tumor, osteoporosis, trauma, structural deformity or inflammatory disorders) and planned participation in a specific 4 week multimodal outpatient program (see Therapy). Exclusion criteria were concomitant autoimmune, chronic, inflammatory, neoplastic-, and psychiatric diseases, drug abuse and pregnancy as well as any preexisting long-term medication with opioids, non-opioid analgesics or co-analgesics. Healthy pain free volunteers without any signs or history of CLBP and concomitant diseases were asked for their participation in the study as controls. In total, 37 patients and 25 healthy controls matching the criteria listed above provided written informed consent and were enrolled in the study. None of the enrolled individuals had been treated with corticosteroids or had received immunomodulatory agents currently or in the past. Acute inflammatory diseases at the time of blood sampling were ruled out by measurement of body temperature and laboratory assessment of C-reactive-Protein (CRP) as wells as total- and differential leucocyte count. This study is registered on German Clinical Trial Register (Registration Trial DRKS00005954), but was not registered before enrollment of participants since all patients received only standard treatment and no further study-related interventions. The authors confirm that all ongoing and related trials for this drug/intervention are registered.

Therapy

The multimodal outpatient program (MRIP, "Muenchner Ruecken Intensiv Programm") performed at the University of Munich is a clinically established outpatient program for patients with chronic low back pain. In line with specific recommendations for the treatment of chronic disabling low back pain [2,3,28], the program follows a bio-psycho-social approach and comprises medical (examination, education), physical (exercise), work-related and behavioral therapy components. The program is conducted by specialists from at least four professional groups with different backgrounds (e.g. physicians, physiotherapists, psychotherapists, occupational therapists). The group size is limited to 10 patients.

The duration of the program is 4 weeks, 5 days a week and 8 hours a day.

Outcome assessment

Pain and stress levels were routinely evaluated by standardized questionnaires before treatment, at the end of the program and six months after completion of the program (follow-up). Patients were asked to rate their recalled average pain intensity using an 11-point numerical rating scale (NRS): 0 means "no pain" and 10 means "worst pain imaginable". Self-perceived stress was evaluated using the Short Questionnaire on Current Burden (KAB, "Kurzfragebogen zur aktuellen Beanspruchung"). The KAB is able to repeatedly determine an individual's psychological state under the conditions of acute or chronic stress and is highly sensitive to short-term or situational changes during a stressful experience [29]. The rating is based on a 6-point scale ranging from 1 to 6 for all six matched adjectives. Higher KAB values indicate increased perceived stress levels. Responders were defined as patients with improvements in NRS by $\geq 50\%$ due to the treatment program. Healthy controls were asked to fill out questionnaires once.

Blood sampling

Blood samples were taken from all patients before treatment, at the end of the program and at the follow-up six months after completion of the program. Blood samples from healthy volunteers were taken once at enrollment.

Cytokine Assessment. Blood samples were collected, centrifuged and stored in polypropylene aliquot tubes at $-80°C$. Samples were then assessed for levels of T cell related cytokines using a human cytokine multiplex immunoassay by Myriad Rules-Based Medicine Inc., Austin, Texas, USA. The multiplex microbead assay is based on Luminex technology and measures proteins in a similar manner to standard sandwich ELISA, with comparable sensitivity and range. Regarding the detection limits, the LLOQ (Lower Limit of Quantitation) for the cytokines were: TNF-α: 23.0 pg/ml, IFN-γ: 1.5 pg/ml, IL-4: 29.0 pg/ml, IL-6: 11.0 pg/ml, IL-10: 6.9 pg/ml, IL-17: 4.0 pg/ml, IL-23: 0.59 pg/ml. The LLOQ is the lowest concentration of an analyte in a sample that can be reliably detected and at which the total error meets the laboratory's requirements for accuracy [30].

Flow cytometric staining and analysis

After collection of heparinized venous blood samples, peripheral blood mononuclear cells (PBMCs) were separated by density gradient preparation over Ficoll-Uropoline (Sigma Aldrich, Taufkirchen, Germany). Hereupon, PBMCs were cryopreserved in RPMI freezing media containing 10% FCS and 10% DMSO [31] and stored at $-30°C$ for 24 h and then at $-196°C$ until measurement. After storage, samples were thawed rapidly in a water bath at $37°C$ and washed twice to eliminate DMSO. For TH1, TH2 and TH17 analysis, cells were stimulated 5 h with cell stimulation cocktail including protein transport inhibitors (Phorbol 12-myristate 13-acetate (PMA), ionomycin, brefeldin A and monensin, eBioscience, San Diego, CA, USA) according to the manufacturer's protocol. Subsequently, cells were extracellulary stained with anti-human CD4 antibody and consecutively fixed and permeabilized (Fix-Perm-Solutions A and B, Life Technologies, Darmstadt, Germany) for intracellular staining with anti-human INF-γ (detection of TH1 cells), IL-4 (detection of TH2 cells) and IL-17 antibody (detection of TH17 cells, all Biolegend, San Diego, CA, USA). T cell distribution was measured by FACS analysis with the Attune Acoustic Focusing Cytometer (Life Technologies, Carlsbad, USA). Tregs were identified and quantified using multicolor flow cytometry after surface staining of PBMCs with mAbs specific for anti-human CD4, CD25 and CD127 and intracellular staining with an anti-human FoxP3 antibody. The frequencies of $CD4^+CD25^{high}$ and $CD4^+CD25^{high}CD127^{low}FoxP3^+$ T cells were expressed as percentage of total $CD4^+$ T cells by sequential gating on lymphocytes. Isotype controls (Biolegend, San Diego, CA, USA) were given for compensation and confirmation of antibody specificity.

RNA isolation and synthesis of cDNA

$CD4^+$ cells were isolated from PBMCs by magnetic separation with Whole Blood CD4 MicroBeads (MACS Miltenyi Biotec, Auburn, CA, USA). Subsequently, total RNA was isolated using the mirVana miRNA Isolation Kit followed by a DNase-digest with Turbo DNA-free Kit (Ambion). Quantity and purity of the isolated RNA were measured using a NanoDrop ND-1000 spectrophotometer (Peqlab). After amplification of total RNA using TargetAmp 1-Round aRNA Amplification Kit (Epicentre Biotechnologies, Madison, WI, USA) and purification using RNeasy Mini Kit (Qiagen), cDNA synthesis was performed with SuperScript III First Strand Synthesis System (Invitrogen) and random hexamers (Qiagen).

Quantitative real-time PCR (qPCR)

Quantitative RT-PCR was performed in duplicates with the LightCycler 480 instrument (Roche Diagnostics, Mannheim, Germany) using LightCycler 480 Probes Master and RealTime ready single assays (Roche Diagnostics) and UPL probes. The RealTime ready single assays contain target specific primers and a Universal ProbeLibrary LNA probe. Primer sequences and qPCR characteristics are given in Table 1. The cycling conditions comprised an initial denaturation phase at 95°C for 10 min, followed by 45 cycles at 95°C for 10 s, 60°C for 30 s and 72°C for 1 s. Relative mRNA expression was calculated by Relative Quantification Software (Roche Diagnostics) using an efficiency-corrected algorithm with standard curves and reference gene normalization against the reference genes succinate dehydrogenase complex subunit A (SDHA) and TATA box binding protein (TBP) as described in [32].

Statistical analyses

All statistical analyses were performed using SigmaStat 12.0 (Systat Software, Chicago, USA). Every statistical analysis was started with testing for normal distribution using the Shapiro Wilk Test. Testing for differences between groups was accomplished by the T-Test for all data with normal distribution (IL-17, IL-23, TGF-β-mRNA, $CD25^+CD25^{high}$) and the nonparametric Mann-Whitney Rank Sum Test for all data without normal distribution (IL-6, IL-10, IL-23-mRNA, IFN-γ-mRNA, FoxP3-mRNA, RORγT-mRNA, Tregs, TH17 cells, TH17/Treg Ratio, TH1/TH2 Ratio). Values are expressed as mean ± standard deviation (SD) in the text and figures and p-values≤0.05 were considered statistically significant.

Results

Subjects and treatment variables

23 female and 14 male patients were enrolled. The median age of the patients at inclusion was 44.5 (range 21–73) years. The control group consisted of 25 (13 female/12 male) healthy pain free individuals aged 43.0 (range 24–54) years.

At inclusion, the average pain intensity of the patients was NRS 3.37 (±2.4) at rest and NRS 4.18 (±2.5) during movement. The average pain duration was 70.1 (±78.3) months. Using the KAB to evaluate the intensity of self-perceived stress, patients rated average KAB values at inclusion with 3.31 (±0.83). The average KAB of healthy controls was 1.80 (±0.64).

Upon therapy, 13 of 37 patients (35%) showed a significant reduction of pain scores (NRS) within 4 weeks, as defined by a decrease of pain ratings of ≥50%. They were therefore defined as therapy responders. Follow-up responders were defined as patients with persisting favorable effects according to the aforementioned criteria after 6 months.

Serum cytokine profiles

Serum protein levels of TNF-α, IFN-γ and IL-4 were neither detectable in the peripheral blood of CLBP patients nor in blood samples of healthy controls. Generally, for both CLBP patients and healthy controls, the serum levels of IL-6, IL-10, Il-17 and IL-23 were found to be just marginally above the detection thresholds. No differences were found for IL-6, IL-10 and IL-17 (Figs. 1A, 1B, 1C). However, only levels of the pro-inflammatory cytokine IL-23 were found to be significantly higher in patients with CLBP before initiation of therapy as compared to healthy controls. (IL-23: 0.94±0.29 pg/ml in healthy controls vs. 1.21±0.43 pg/ml in CLBP patients; p = 0.009; Fig. 1D).

mRNA expression of T cell cytokines

As measurements of specific cytokine profiles in serum turned out to be not conclusive, we determined the mRNA expression of cytokines and T cell specific transcription factors directly in the compartment of $CD4^+$ cells of CLBP patients and healthy volunteers. By means of qPCR, we evaluated the mRNA expression of the TH1 cytokines TNF-α and IFN-γ, the TH2 cytokines IL-4 and IL-10, FoxP3 and TGF-β indicative for Tregs, and IL-6, IL-17, IL 23 and the transcription factor RORγT specific for TH17 cells.

The expression of the TH1 specific cytokine IFN-γ did not exhibit significant differences in CLBP patients as compared to healthy controls (IFN-γ: 4.19±3.54 in CLBP patients vs. 3.60±2.20 in healthy controls, n.s., Fig. 2A). Expression levels of TNF-α, IL-4 and IL-10 were neither detectable in $CD4^+$ T cells of CLBP patients nor in healthy controls. As shown in Fig. 2B, the expression of IL-23 in $CD4^+$ T cell samples of CLBP patients was found to be significantly decreased compared to healthy controls (IL-23: 4.88±2.44 in CLBP patients vs. 7.73±3.77 in healthy controls, p = 0.006). The expression of both TGF-β and the transcription factor FoxP3 was significantly increased in $CD4^+$ cells of CLBP patients compared to healthy controls, thereby implying an increased Treg abundance (TGF-β: 0.21±0.07 in CLBP patients vs. 0.14±0.05 in healthy controls, p = 0.014, Fig. 3A, FoxP3: 0.21±0.14 in CLBP patients vs. 0.14±0.06 in healthy controls, p = 0.009, Fig. 3B). Regarding factors specific for TH17 cells, the expression of IL-6 and IL-17 was neither detectable in $CD4^+$ samples of CLBP patients nor in healthy controls. Expression levels of RORγT did not differ in CLBP patients and healthy controls (RORγT: 0.028±0.02 in CLBP patients vs. 0.025±0.01 in healthy controls, n.s., Fig. 3C). Taken together, qPCR results promoted the hypothesis that CLBP patients may exhibit altered distribution patterns of Treg and TH17 subsets whereas TH1/TH2 balance appeared to be unchanged.

Table 1. RT-PCR Assay Characteristics and Primer Sequences.

Gene	Primer Sequence
SDHA	Roche RealTime Ready Single Assay ID 102136
TBP	Roche RealTime Ready Single Assay ID 101145
FoxP3	Roche RealTime Ready Single Assay ID 113503
IL-4	for 5'TGCCTCACATTGTCACTGC 3'
	rev 5'GCACATGCTAGCAGGAAGAAC 3', UPL probe #38
IL-6	for 5'GATGAGTACAAAAGTCCTGATCCA 3'
	rev 5'CTGCAGCCACTGGTTCTGT 3', UPL probe #40
IL-10	for 5'TGCCTTCAGCAGAGTGAAGA 3'
	rev 5'GCAACCCAGGTAACCCTTAAA 3', UPL probe #67
IL-17	for 5'TGGGAAGACCTCATTGGTGT 3'
	rev 5'GGATTTCGTGGGATTGTGAT 3', UPL probe #8
IL-23	for 5'CAGCTTCATGCCTCCCTACT 3'
	rev 5'GACTGAGGCTTGGAATCTGC 3', UPL probe #14
TGF-β	for 5'ACTACTACGCCAAGGAGGTCAC 3'
	rev 5'TGCTTGAACTTGTCATAGATTTCG 3', UPL probe #31
TNF-α	for 5'CAGCCTCTTCTCCTTCCTGAT 3'
	rev 5'GCCAGAGGGCTGATTAGAGA 3', UPL probe #29
IFN-γ	for 5'GGCATTTTGAAGAATTGGAAAG 3'
	rev 5'TTTGGATGCTCTGGTCATCTT 3', UPL probe #21
RoRγT	for 5'CAGCGCTCCAACATCTTCT 3'
	rev 5'CCACATCTCCCACATGGAC 3', UPL probe #69

CLBP patients exhibit an increased Treg frequency while the TH17 frequency is decreased

To test this hypothesis, we next evaluated the distribution of T cell subsets in blood samples of patients and healthy volunteers by flow cytometric analyses. The relative number of Tregs was assessed by using two different staining protocols: First, with antibodies specific for CD4$^+$CD25^{high} cells and second, specific for CD4$^+$CD25^{high}CD127^{low}FoxP3$^+$ cells (Gating strategy is displayed on Fig. 4). TH17 cells were identified by intracellular staining with anti-human IL-17 antibody (gating strategy is displayed on Fig. 5).

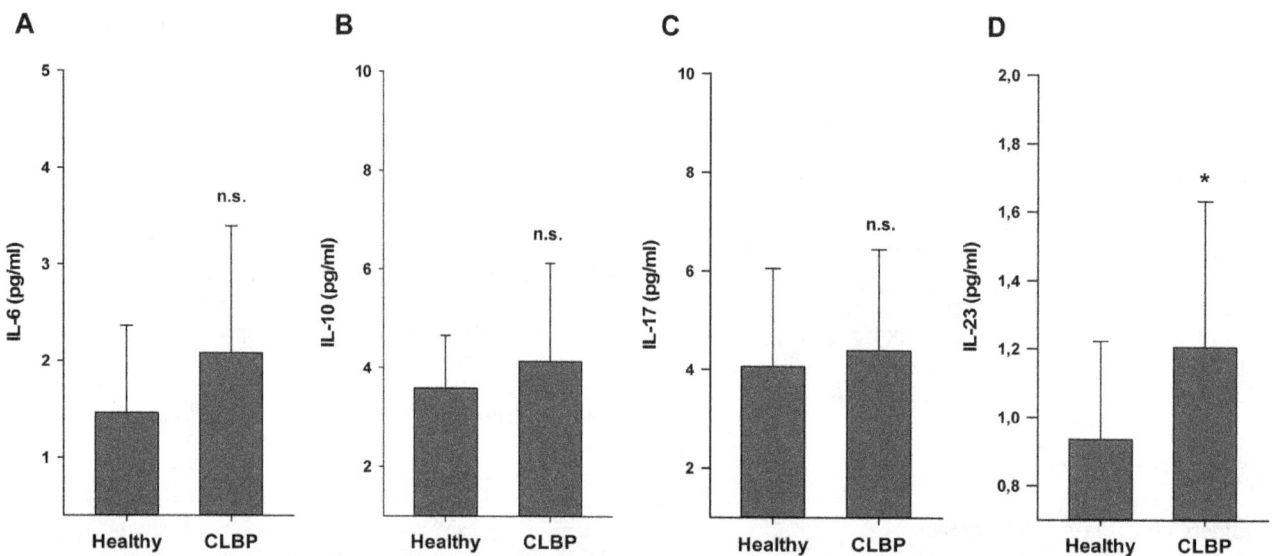

Figure 1. **Concentrations of serum cytokines, determined by using a Human Cytokine multiplex immunoassay.** No differences are found analyzing serum protein levels of IL-6, IL-10 and IL-17 between patients and healthy controls (Fig. 1A, 1B, 1C). Protein levels of pro-inflammatory cytokine IL-23 are significantly higher in the peripheral blood of patients with CLBP compared to healthy controls. Values are expressed as mean ± standard deviation. (IL-23: 0.94±0.29 pg/ml in healthy controls vs. 1.21±0.43 pg/ml in CLBP patients; p=0.009; Fig. 1D).

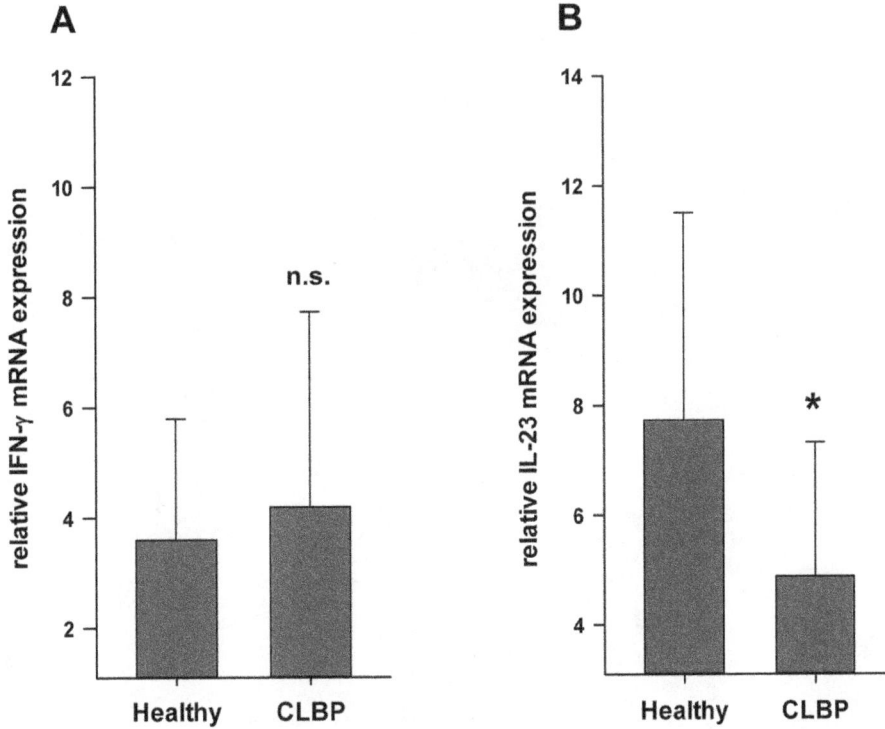

Figure 2. Expression levels of T cell related cytokine mRNA measured by qPCR. TNF-α, IL-4 and IL-10 were neither detectable in CD4$^+$ T cells of CLBP patients nor in healthy controls. The expression of IFN-γ did not exhibit significant differences in CLBP patients as compared to healthy controls (IFN-γ: 4.19±3.54 in CLBP patients vs. 3.60±2.20 in healthy controls, n.s.; Fig. 2A) whereas IL-23 expression of in CD4$^+$ T cell samples of CLBP patients was found to be significantly decreased (4.88±2.44 in CLBP patients vs. 7.73±3.77 in healthy controls, p=0.006; Fig. 2B).

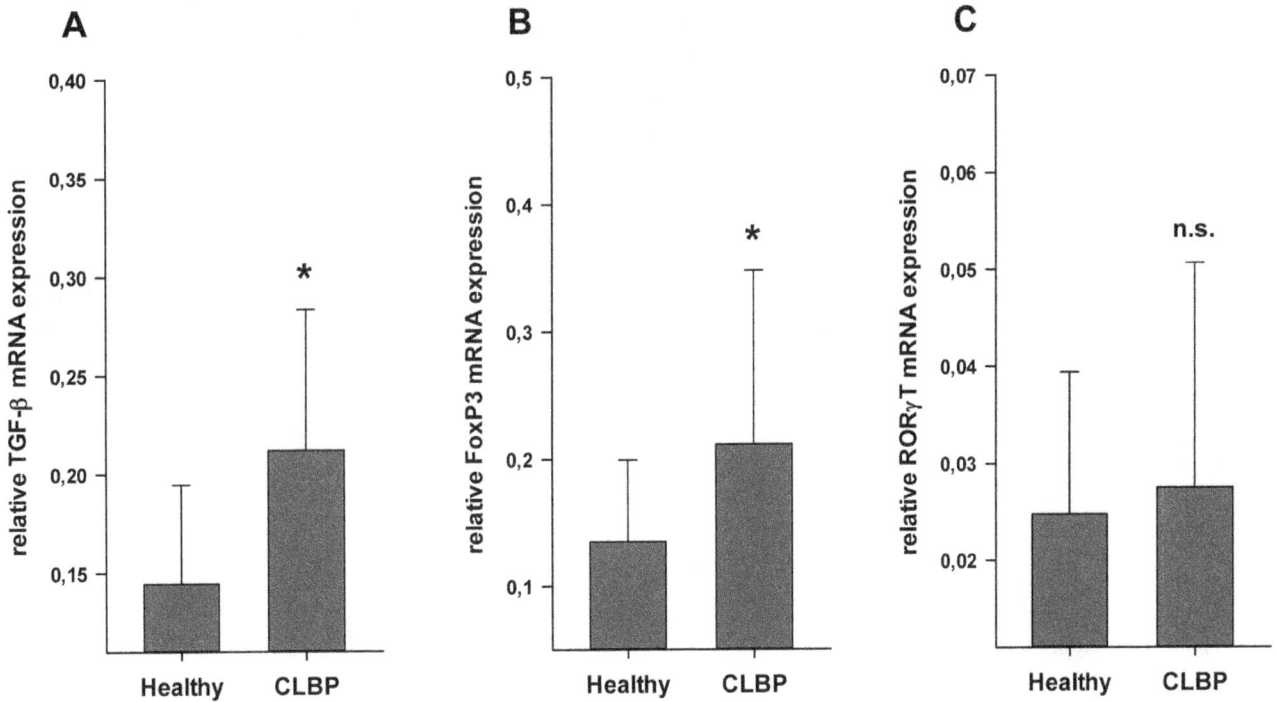

Figure 3. Expression levels of T cell subset related mRNA measured by qPCR. TGF-β and FoxP3 mRNA expression, specific for Tregs, was significantly higher in patients with CLBP than in healthy controls (TGF-β: 0.21±0.07 in CLBP patients vs. 0.14±0.05 in healthy controls, p=0.014; Fig. 3A), (FoxP3: 0.21±0.14 in CLBP patients vs. 0.14±0.06 in healthy controls, p=0.009; Fig. 3B). TH17 specific expression of IL-17 was neither detectable in CD4$^+$ samples of CLBP patients nor in healthy controls. Expression levels of RORγT did not differ in CLBP patients and healthy controls (RORγT: 0.028±0.02 in CLBP patients vs. 0.025±0.01 in healthy controls, p=n.s.; Fig. 3C).

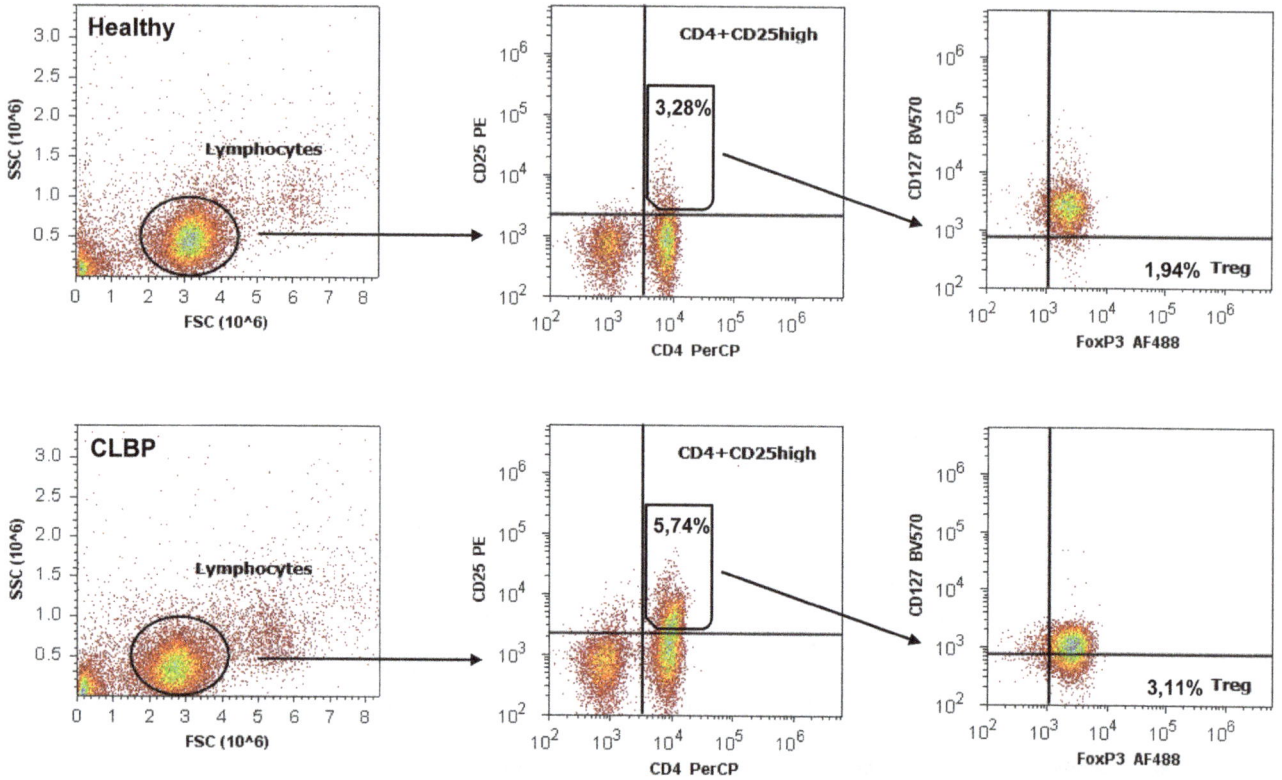

Figure 4. Gating strategy for the detection of Tregs. PBMCs extracellular stained with PerCP labeled anti-human CD4-antibody, PE labeled anti CD25-antibody, Brilliant Violet (BV570) labeled anti CD127-antibody and intracellular stained with Alexa Fluor (AF488) labeled anti-human FoxP3-antibody. Lymphocyte population was gated from PBMCs according to forward scatter (FSC) characteristics and side scatter (SSC) characteristics (left). Gated lymphocytes were then separated in CD4+CD25^{high} cells/T cells (middle) and CD4+CD25^{high}CD127^{low}FOXP3$^+$ cells/CD4+T cells (right, named Treg). Upper row represents the result of a healthy control with less CD4+CD25^{high} T cells (3.28%) and less CD4+CD25^{high}CD127^{low}FoxP3$^+$ T cells (1.94%) compared to a patient with CLBP (lower row, 5.74% and 3.11%).

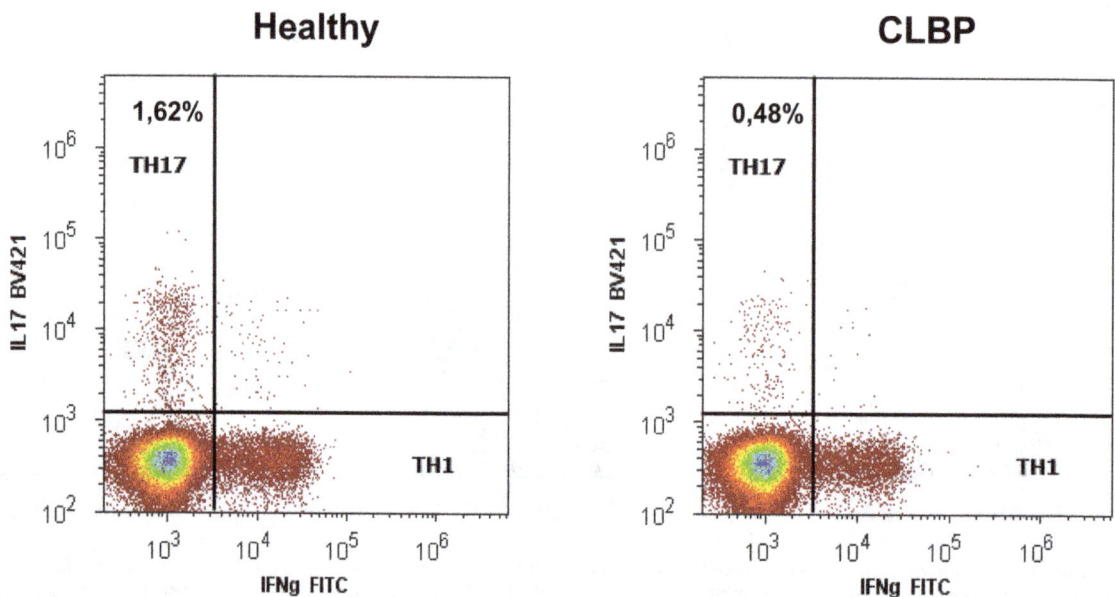

Figure 5. Gating strategy for the detection of TH1 and TH17 cells. PBMCs stimulated with cell stimulation cocktail for 5 h followed by intracellular staining with Brilliant Violet (BV421) labeled anti-human IL-17 antibody and FITC labeled anti-human IFN-γ antibody.

With both Treg staining protocols, a significantly increased frequency of Tregs was seen in CLBP patients as compared to healthy controls. FACS analysis applying the $CD4^+CD25^{high}$ staining protocol resulted in $4.45\pm0.88\%$ $CD4^+CD25^{high}$ cells in CLBP patients vs. $3.49\pm0.5\%$, $CD4^+CD25^{high}$ cells in healthy controls ($p<0.001$, Figure 6A). $CD4^+CD25^{high}CD127^{low}FoxP3^+$ staining as a more specific staining protocol for Tregs revealed similar results with $2.89\pm1.07\%$ Tregs in CLBP patients vs. $1.93\pm0.66\%$ Tregs in healthy controls ($p=0.001$, Figure 6B). The frequency of TH17 cells, however, was found to be significantly decreased in CLBP patients as compared to healthy volunteers (TH17: $0.46\pm0.24\%$ in CLBP patients vs. $1.14\pm0.73\%$ in healthy controls, $p=<0.001$, Figure 6C). Conclusively, ratios of Th17/$CD4^+CD25^{high}$ resp. Th17/$CD4^+CD25^{high}CD127^{low}FoxP3^+$ were significantly decreased in CLBP patients as compared to healthy controls (Th17/$CD4^+CD25^{high}$: 0.12 ± 0.08 in CLBP patients vs. 0.33 ± 0.23 in healthy controls, $p<0.001$, Fig. 7A; Th17/$CD4^+CD25^{high}CD127^{low}FoxP3^+$: 0.23 ± 0.17 in CLBP patients vs. 0.64 ± 0.79 in healthy controls, $p<0.001$, Fig. 7B).

TH1/TH2 balance is not altered in CLBP patients

As depicted in Fig. 7C, TH1/TH2 balance did not reveal significant differences between CLBP patients and healthy controls; however, a trend towards a decreased TH1/TH2 ratio was observed (TH1/TH2: 9.76 ± 7.27 in CLBP patients vs. 14.72 ± 12.81 in healthy controls, $p=$ n.s.).

T cell ratios remain altered in CLBP patients after multimodal therapy

To evaluate the impact of therapeutic interventions on the observed T cell subset alterations in CLBP patients, the distribution of TH cells subsets (TH1, TH2, TH17 and Tregs) was analyzed in the group of therapy responders before, immediately after therapy and 6 months later. As depicted in Fig. 8A, these patients showed an ongoing decrease of NRS by $\geq$ 50% due to the treatment program. The pain reduction was also accompanied by a decrease of the KAB values. However, as shown in Figure 8B, this therapeutic effect was not reflected in any respective adaptation of the T cell subsets.

Discussion

Pathomechanisms driving the chronification of low back pain still remain largely elusive. While a growing body of evidence suggests a pivotal role of adaptive immune responses in the pathogenesis of chronic pain, these issues have not conclusively been analyzed for CLBP, yet.

Our results indicate that CLBP is associated with characteristic alterations of T helper cell subsets: The ratio between regulatory T cells, playing a vital role in controlling adaptive immune responses, and TH17 cells, one of the key effector T cells mediating autoimmunity [33], was significantly decreased. We further provide evidence that these alterations persist even in these patients exhibiting significant pain reduction after participation in a standardized multimodal therapy program [3].

Assuming that cytokines as central mediators of cellular immunity may mirror immune cell functions, we first analyzed seven T cell related cytokines (TNF-α, IFN-γ, IL-4, IL-6, IL-10, IL-17, IL-23) in serum samples of CLBP patients and healthy controls. TNF-α, IFN-γ and IL-4 were below the detection limits in patients as well as in healthy controls, and the results of the remaining four analytes were only slightly above the detectable limit. Values for the proinflammatory cytokines IL-6 and IL-17 in

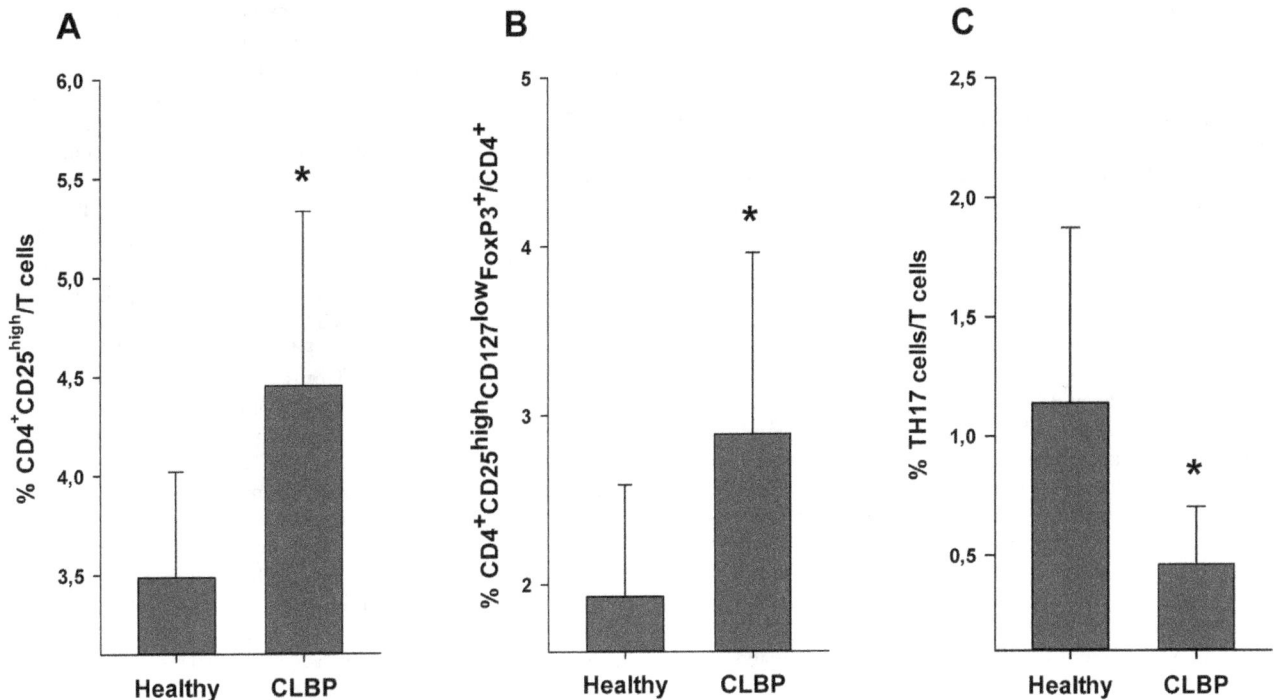

Figure 6. Flow cytometric quantification of Tregs and TH17 cells. Results show significantly higher percentage of anti-inflammatory Tregs in patients with CLBP in both staining protocols ($CD4^+CD25^{high}$ cells: $4.45\pm0.88\%$ in CLBP patients vs. $3.49\pm0.53\%$ in healthy controls, $p<0.001$; Fig. 6A), ($CD4^+CD25^{high}CD127^{low}FoxP3^+$ cells: $2.89\pm1.07\%$ in CLBP patients vs. $1.93\pm0.66\%$ in healthy controls, $p=0.001$; Fig. 6B). Number of TH17 cells as percentage of T cells in peripheral blood show significantly lower percentage of pro-inflammatory TH17 cells in patients with CLBP (TH17 cells: $0.46\pm0.24\%$ in CLBP patients vs. $1.14\pm0.73\%$ in healthy controls, $p<0.001$; Fig. 6C).

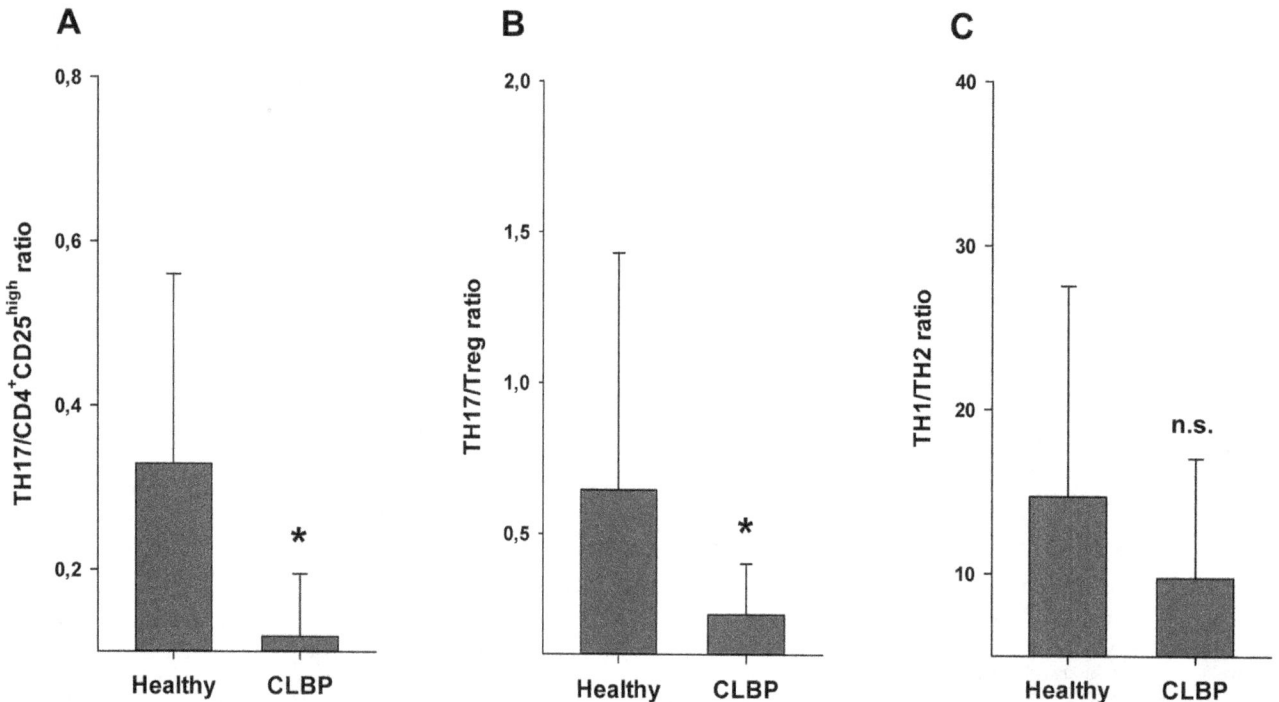

Figure 7. Ratios of TH17/CD4⁺CD25ʰⁱᵍʰ, TH17/Tregs and TH1/TH2 cells. Ratios of Th17/CD4⁺CD25^high and Th17/CD4⁺CD25^highCD127^low-FoxP3⁺ were significantly decreased in CLBP patients as compared to healthy controls (Th17/CD4⁺CD25^high: 0.12±0.08 in CLBP patients vs. 0.33±0.23% in healthy controls, p<0.001; Fig. 7A), (Th17/CD4⁺CD25^highCD127^lowFoxP3⁺: 0.23±0.17 in CLBP patients vs. 0.64±0.79 in healthy controls, p<0.001; Fig. 7B). Ratio of TH1/TH2 cells in peripheral blood of patients with CLBP and healthy controls were tendencially decreased in patients with CLBP, but did not reach significance (9.76±7.27 in CLBP patients vs. 14.72±12.81 in healthy controls, p=0.19, Fig. 7C).

blood samples of CLPB patients were slightly elevated as compared to controls. However, this finding may be of limited clinical relevance as normal plasma concentrations for IL-6 of healthy controls are about 1 pg/ml with immense increases in situations of severe systemic infection ranging up to 10.000-fold. Our results demonstrate only an 1.5-fold increase in IL-6 levels in patients with CLBP, which could even occur after physical activity or in obesity [34]. However, the relevance of cytokine measurements should generally be regarded with caution as serum levels of most cytokines are influenced by a complex interplay of macrophages/monocytes, fibroblasts, endothelial−/epithelial cells and dendritic cells thus complicating the extrapolation from plasma cytokines to immune cell functions. Moreover, ranges of detection exhibits considerable variances between the different assays used [35]. Even different types of Luminex-based platforms exhibit differences in their ability to measure serum levels of cytokines and thus, may be more useful in studies in which relative rather than absolute changes in cytokines are of interest [36,37].

Overall, these data suggest that serum levels of cytokines are not suitable to monitor the adaptive immune response in CLBP and prompted us to analyze the expression of cytokines directly in the compartment of CD4⁺ cells as central players of the T cell response. While no differences in the expression of TH1 and TH2 cytokines were observed, qPCR results clearly pointed to an increased abundance of Tregs in CLBP patients, as expression of both TGF-β and the transcription factor FoxP3 were significantly increased. Moreover, expression of IL-23 was clearly decreased supporting the assumption that TH17 frequency may be reduced. IL-17 and RORγT, however, did not differ significantly between CLBP and controls which may be due to the fact that the subset of TH17 cells per se is only less than 2% of CD4+ cells. Thus,

resolving differences of cytokine expression without prior cell sorting may be difficult. The opposite results of increased IL-23 protein levels and decreased IL23-mRNA-expression is in line with a wide body of literature showing a big discrepancy between mRNA expression and protein levels as a result of control mechanisms. These can affect post-transcriptional, translational and protein degrading processes [38,39].

Our findings encouraged us to investigate T cell subset compositions by flow cytometric analyzes. We used standard staining procedures to identify TH1, TH2, and TH17 cells, whereas for identification of anti-inflammatory Tregs, both classic extracellular staining of CD4⁺CD25^high and a more specific extra- and intracellular staining of CD4⁺CD25^highCD127^lowFoxP3⁺ was applied. As activated human T cells can transiently express FoxP3 and CD25, differentiation of Tregs from activated effector T cells by only using these two markers may suffer from inaccuracies. CD127 is a newly described surface marker that allows distinguishing regulatory T cells from other CD25⁺ cells [40]. For TH17 identification, we chose two experimental approaches: determination the mRNA expression of the TH17 specific transcription factor RORγT by qPCR, and FACS analyses of IL-17 production, which has revealed as a very reliable method to identify TH17 cells [41]. However, flow cytometry staining protocols combining IL-17 with further markers, e.g. CD161 or CCR6, may further refine these measurements and thus may be implemented in future studies.

Flow cytometry clearly proved the assumed alterations of the TH17/Treg balance, as a significantly increased frequency of Tregs and decreased frequency of TH17 cells was observed in our CLBP patients. Even in flow cytometric analyzes, no differences in the TH1/TH2 ratio were detectable. There are several investi-

A

B

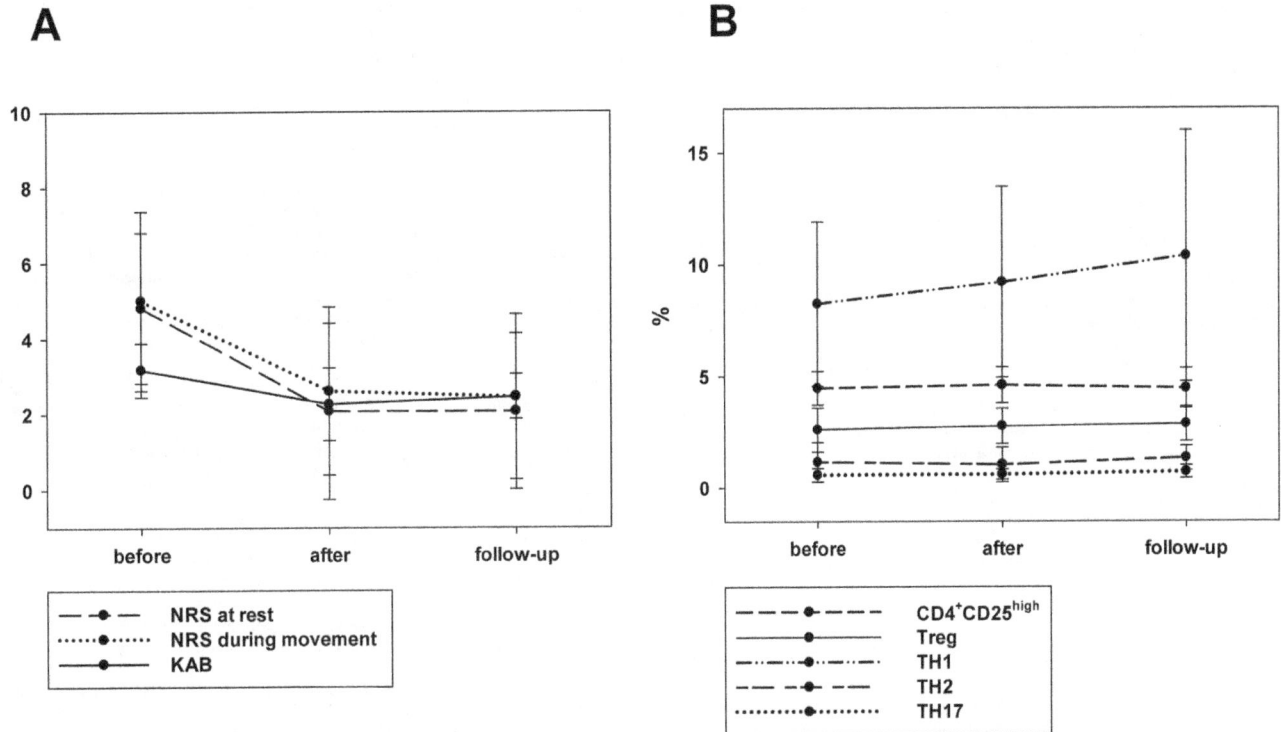

Figure 8. NRS pain scores, KAB stress scores and T cell subsets before and after treatment. 35% [n = 13] of all patients benefited by the 4 weeks intensive multimodal therapy with long lasting pain- and stress reduction (Fig. 8A). Even all responders showed a significant pain- and stress reduction of ≥50%, no transformation were observed regarding T cell subsets. None of our analyzed T cell subsets (TH1, TH2, TH17, Tregs) normalized after successful therapy (Fig. 8B). (NRS at rest before/after: p = 0.025, NRS at rest before/follow up: p = 0.003, NRS during movement before/after: p = 0.046, NRS during movement before/follow up: p = 0.012, KAB before/after: p = 0.024, KAB before/follow up: p = 0.019).

gations which point to a beneficial role of anti-inflammatory cells and cytokines together with a detrimental function of a pro-inflammatory immune response in pain patients [6,7,8,9]. In contrast to these findings, our results showing an anti-inflammatory shift on cellular level are in accordance with other chronic diseases like mild depression or chronic fatigue syndrome [42,43]. A potential explanation for our findings on TH17/Treg balance may therefore be that pain-related, long lasting chronic stress and fatigue induces an ongoing dysregulation of immune cells towards an anti-inflammatory phenotype [44,45,46]. On the other hand, it may also be discussed that dysregulation of the TH17/Treg balance may exist first, thus predisposing the affected individuals to experience chronification of pain symptoms. The latter theory may be supported by our surprising findings that the observed TH17/Treg imbalance persisted despite clinical improvement after multimodal therapy even after a follow-up period of 6 months.

In summary, we found a persisting TH17/Treg imbalance with an increased count of anti-inflammatory Tregs and a decreased number of pro-inflammatory TH17 cells in peripheral blood of CLBP patients pointing to a strong association between chronic

pain and immune suppression rather than immune activation. Importantly, these findings are not reflected by serum cytokine concentration, indicating a major role of specific T cell subset measurements in the analysis of pain-related immune responses.

Taken together, the results of the current study suggest an involvement of TH17/Treg in the pathogenesis of CLBP and emphasize the importance of these cells in the crosstalk of pain and immune response.

Acknowledgments

The authors are grateful to G. Groeger and J. Rink for excellent technical assistance.

The results of the present study are a part of the dissertation of J.Z.

Author Contributions

Conceived and designed the experiments: BL BR SCA. Performed the experiments: BL BR JZ LE. Analyzed the data: BL JZ LE SCA. Contributed reagents/materials/analysis tools: BL JZ LE SCA. Wrote the paper: BL SK SCA. Interpretation of data, making intellectual contributions to the manuscript: PM.

References

1. Becker A, Held H, Redaelli M, Strauch K, Chenot JF, et al. (2010) Low back pain in primary care: costs of care and prediction of future health care utilization. Spine (Phila Pa 1976) 35: 1714–1720.
2. Balague F, Mannion AF, Pellise F, Cedraschi C (2012) Non-specific low back pain. Lancet 379: 482–491.
3. Airaksinen O, Brox JI, Cedraschi C, Hildebrandt J, Klaber-Moffett J, et al. (2006) Chapter 4. European guidelines for the management of chronic nonspecific low back pain. Eur Spine J 15 Suppl 2: 192–300.
4. Sullivan MJ, Reesor K, Mikail S, Fisher R (1992) The treatment of depression in chronic low back pain: review and recommendations. Pain 50: 5–13.
5. Edit V, Eva S, Maria K, Istvan R, Agnes C, et al. (2013) Psychosocial, educational, and somatic factors in chronic nonspecific low back pain. Rheumatol Int 33: 587–592.
6. Austin PJ, Moalem-Taylor G (2010) The neuro-immune balance in neuropathic pain: involvement of inflammatory immune cells, immune-like glial cells and cytokines. J Neuroimmunol 229: 26–50.

7. Koch A, Zacharowski K, Boehm O, Stevens M, Lipfert P, et al. (2007) Nitric oxide and pro-inflammatory cytokines correlate with pain intensity in chronic pain patients. Inflamm Res 56: 32–37.

8. Lenz M, Uceyler N, Frettloh J, Hoffken O, Krumova EK, et al. (2013) Local cytokine changes in complex regional pain syndrome type I (CRPS I) resolve after 6 months. Pain 154: 2142–2149.

9. Shamji MF, Setton LA, Jarvis W, So S, Chen J, et al. (2010) Proinflammatory cytokine expression profile in degenerated and herniated human intervertebral disc tissues. Arthritis Rheum 62: 1974–1982.

10. DeLeo JA, Yezierski RP (2001) The role of neuroinflammation and neuroimmune activation in persistent pain. Pain 90: 1–6.

11. Wang H, Schiltenwolf M, Buchner M (2008) The role of TNF-alpha in patients with chronic low back pain-a prospective comparative longitudinal study. Clin J Pain 24: 273–278.

12. Perkins NM, Tracey DJ (2000) Hyperalgesia due to nerve injury: role of neutrophils. Neuroscience 101: 745–757.

13. Hu P, Bembrick AL, Keay KA, McLachlan EM (2007) Immune cell involvement in dorsal root ganglia and spinal cord after chronic constriction or transection of the rat sciatic nerve. Brain Behav Immun 21: 599–616.

14. Costigan M, Moss A, Latremoliere A, Johnston C, Verma-Gandhu M, et al. (2009) T-cell infiltration and signaling in the adult dorsal spinal cord is a major contributor to neuropathic pain-like hypersensitivity. J Neurosci 29: 14415–14422.

15. Liu HH, Xia XY, Wu YM, Pan LJ, Jin BF, et al. (2006) [Detection of peripheral blood Th1/Th2 cell ratio in patients with chronic abacterial prostatitis/chronic pelvic pain syndrome]. Zhonghua Nan Ke Xue 12: 330–332, 336.

16. Schinkel C, Gaertner A, Zaspel J, Zedler S, Faist E, et al. (2006) Inflammatory mediators are altered in the acute phase of posttraumatic complex regional pain syndrome. Clin J Pain 22: 235–239.

17. Homey B (2006) [After TH1/TH2 now comes Treg/TH17: significance of T helper cells in immune response organization]. Hautarzt 57: 730–732.

18. Whiteside TL (2012) Disarming suppressor cells to improve immunotherapy. Cancer Immunol Immunother 61: 283–288.

19. Baecher-Allan C, Brown JA, Freeman GJ, Hafler DA (2001) CD4+CD25high regulatory cells in human peripheral blood. J Immunol 167: 1245–1253.

20. Sakaguchi S (2004) Naturally arising CD4+ regulatory t cells for immunologic self-tolerance and negative control of immune responses. Annu Rev Immunol 22: 531–562.

21. Sakaguchi S, Ono M, Setoguchi R, Yagi H, Hori S, et al. (2006) Foxp3+ CD25+ CD4+ natural regulatory T cells in dominant self-tolerance and autoimmune disease. Immunol Rev 212: 8–27.

22. Kleinschnitz C, Hofstetter HH, Meuth SG, Braeuninger S, Sommer C, et al. (2006) T cell infiltration after chronic constriction injury of mouse sciatic nerve is associated with interleukin-17 expression. Exp Neurol 200: 480–485.

23. Hirota K, Hashimoto M, Yoshitomi H, Tanaka S, Nomura T, et al. (2007) T cell self-reactivity forms a cytokine milieu for spontaneous development of IL-17(+) Th cells that cause autoimmune arthritis. Journal of Experimental Medicine 204: 41–47.

24. Tian P, Ma XL, Wang T, Ma JX, Yang X (2009) Correlation between radiculalgia and counts of T lymphocyte subsets in the peripheral blood of patients with lumbar disc herniation. Orthop Surg 1: 317–321.

25. Cheng L, Fan W, Liu B, Wang X, Nie L (2013) Th17 lymphocyte levels are higher in patients with ruptured than non-ruptured lumbar discs, and are correlated with pain intensity. Injury 44: 1805–1810.

26. Xing Q, Hu D, Shi F, Chen F (2013) Role of regulatory T cells in patients with acute herpes zoster and relationship to postherpetic neuralgia. Arch Dermatol Res 305: 715–722.

27. Austin PJ, Kim CF, Perera CJ, Moalem-Taylor G (2012) Regulatory T cells attenuate neuropathic pain following peripheral nerve injury and experimental autoimmune neuritis. Pain 153: 1916–1931.

28. Becker A, Held H, Redaelli M, Chenot JF, Leonhardt C, et al. (2012) Implementation of a guideline for low back pain management in primary care: a cost-effectiveness analysis. Spine (Phila Pa 1976) 37: 701–710.

29. Chouker A, Kaufmann I, Kreth S, Hauer D, Feuerecker M, et al. (2010) Motion sickness, stress and the endocannabinoid system. PLoS One 5: e10752.

30. Chowdhury F, Williams A, Johnson P (2009) Validation and comparison of two multiplex technologies, Luminex and Mesoscale Discovery, for human cytokine profiling. J Immunol Methods 340: 55–64.

31. Venet F, Malcus C, Ferry T, Poitevin F, Monneret G (2010) Percentage of regulatory T cells CD4+CD25+CD127- in HIV-infected patients is not reduced after cryopreservation. J Immunol Methods 357: 55–58.

32. Ledderose C, Heyn J, Limbeck E, Kreth S (2011) Selection of reliable reference genes for quantitative real-time PCR in human T cells and neutrophils. BMC Res Notes 4: 427.

33. Afzali B, Lombardi G, Lechler RI, Lord GM (2007) The role of T helper 17 (Th17) and regulatory T cells (Treg) in human organ transplantation and autoimmune disease. Clin Exp Immunol 148: 32–46.

34. Fischer CP, Berntsen A, Perstrup LB, Eskildsen P, Pedersen BK (2007) Plasma levels of interleukin-6 and C-reactive protein are associated with physical inactivity independent of obesity. Scand J Med Sci Sports 17: 580–587.

35. Breen EC, Reynolds SM, Cox C, Jacobson LP, Magpantay L, et al. (2011) Multisite comparison of high-sensitivity multiplex cytokine assays. Clin Vaccine Immunol 18: 1229–1242.

36. Huckans M, Fuller BE, Olavarria H, Sasaki AW, Chang M, et al. (2014) Multi-analyte profile analysis of plasma immune proteins: altered expression of peripheral immune factors is associated with neuropsychiatric symptom severity in adults with and without chronic hepatitis C virus infection. Brain Behav 4: 123–142.

37. Bozza FA, Salluh JI, Japiassu AM, Soares M, Assis EF, et al. (2007) Cytokine profiles as markers of disease severity in sepsis: a multiplex analysis. Crit Care 11: R49.

38. Maier T, Guell M, Serrano L (2009) Correlation of mRNA and protein in complex biological samples. FEBS Lett 583: 3966–3973.

39. Vogel C, Marcotte EM (2012) Insights into the regulation of protein abundance from proteomic and transcriptomic analyses. Nat Rev Genet 13: 227–232.

40. Hartigan-O'Connor DJ, Poon C, Sinclair E, McCune JM (2007) Human CD4+ regulatory T cells express lower levels of the IL-7 receptor alpha chain (CD127), allowing consistent identification and sorting of live cells. J Immunol Methods 319: 41–52.

41. Brucklacher-Waldert V, Steinbach K, Lioznov M, Kolster M, Holscher C, et al. (2009) Phenotypical characterization of human Th17 cells unambiguously identified by surface IL-17A expression. J Immunol 183: 5494–5501.

42. Hong M, Zheng J, Ding ZY, Chen JH, Yu L, et al. (2013) Imbalance between Th17 and Treg cells may play an important role in the development of chronic unpredictable mild stress-induced depression in mice. Neuroimmunomodulation 20: 39–50.

43. Torres-Harding S, Sorenson M, Jason LA, Maher K, Fletcher MA (2008) Evidence for T-helper 2 shift and association with illness parameters in chronic fatigue syndrome (CFS). Bull IACFS ME 16: 19–33.

44. Raison CL, Miller AH (2011) Is depression an inflammatory disorder? Curr Psychiatry Rep 13: 467–475.

45. Licciardone JC, Gatchel RJ, Kearns CM, Minotti DE (2012) Depression, somatization, and somatic dysfunction in patients with nonspecific chronic low back pain: results from the OSTEOPATHIC Trial. J Am Osteopath Assoc 112: 783–791.

46. Miller AH (2010) Depression and immunity: a role for T cells? Brain Behav Immun 24: 1–8.

Preoperative MRI Findings Predict Two-Year Postoperative Clinical Outcome in Lumbar Spinal Stenosis

Pekka Kuittinen[1]*, **Petri Sipola**[2], **Ville Leinonen**[3], **Tapani Saari**[4], **Sanna Sinikallio**[5], **Sakari Savolainen**[6], **Heikki Kröger**[7], **Veli Turunen**[8], **Olavi Airaksinen**[9], **Timo Aalto**[10]

1 Department of Neurosurgery, Kuopio University Hospital, Kuopio, Finland and Institute of Clinical Medicine, University of Eastern Finland, Kuopio, Finland, 2 Department of Clinical Radiology, Kuopio University Hospital, Kuopio, Finland and Unit of Radiology, Institute of Clinical Medicine, University of Eastern Finland, Kuopio, Finland, 3 Department of Neurosurgery, Kuopio University Hospital, Kuopio, Finland and Unit of Neurosurgery, Institute of Clinical Medicine, University of Eastern Finland, Kuopio, Finland, 4 Department of Clinical Radiology, Kuopio University Hospital, Kuopio, Finland, 5 Institute of Public Health and Clinical Nutrition, University of Eastern Finland, Kuopio, Finland, 6 Department of Neurosurgery, Kuopio University Hospital, Kuopio, Finland, 7 Department of Orthopaedics and Traumatology, Kuopio University Hospital and Bone and Cartilage Research Unit, University of Eastern Finland, Kuopio, Finland, 8 Department of Orthopaedics and Traumatology, Kuopio University Hospital, Kuopio, Finland, 9 Department of Physical and Rehabilitation Medicine, Kuopio University Hospital, Kuopio, Finland, 10 Health Center Ikioma OY, Mikkeli, Finland

Abstract

Purpose: To study the predictive value of preoperative magnetic resonance imaging (MRI) findings for the two-year postoperative clinical outcome in lumbar spinal stenosis (LSS).

Methods: 84 patients (mean age 63 ± 11 years, male 43%) with symptoms severe enough to indicate LSS surgery were included in this prospective observational single-center study. Preoperative MRI of the lumbar spine was performed with a 1.5-T unit. The imaging protocol conformed to the requirements of the American College of Radiology for the performance of MRI of the adult spine. Visual and quantitative assessment of MRI was performed by one experienced neuroradiologist. At the two-year postoperative follow-up, functional ability was assessed with the Oswestry Disability Index (ODI 0–100%) and treadmill test (0–1000 m), pain symptoms with the overall Visual Analogue Scale (VAS 0–100 mm), and specific low back pain (LBP) and specific leg pain (LP) separately with a numeric rating scale from 0–10 (NRS-11). Satisfaction with the surgical outcome was also assessed.

Results: Preoperative severe central stenosis predicted postoperatively lower LP, LBP, and VAS when compared in patients with moderate central stenosis ($p<0.05$). Moreover, severe stenosis predicted higher postoperative satisfaction ($p=0.029$). Preoperative scoliosis predicted an impaired outcome in the ODI ($p=0.031$) and lowered the walking distance in the treadmill test ($p=0.001$). The preoperative finding of only one stenotic level in visual assessment predicted less postoperative LBP when compared with patients having 2 or more stenotic levels ($p=0.026$). No significant differences were detected between quantitative measurements and the patient outcome.

Conclusions: Routine preoperative lumbar spine MRI can predict the patient outcome in a two-year follow up in patients with LSS surgery. Severe central stenosis and one-level central stenosis are predictors of good outcome. Preoperative finding of scoliosis may indicate worse functional ability.

Editor: Paul Arnold, University of Kansas, United States of America

Funding: This study was supported by the Kuopio University Hospital (grant number 596013 - URL: http://www.psshp.fi/). The funder had no role in study design, data collection and analysis, decision to publish, or preparation of the manuscript.

Competing Interests: The authors have declared that no competing interests exist.

* Email: pekkaku@student.uef.fi

Introduction

Lumbar spinal stenosis (LSS) is defined as "buttock or lower extremity pain, which may occur with or without low back pain (LBP), associated with diminished space available for the neural and vascular elements in the lumbar spine" [1,2]. LSS is the most common indication for lumbar spinal surgery in people aged over 65 years. Incidence of lumbar spinal stenosis is increasing due to the aging population, which increase also the frequency of more

complex lumbar spine procedures, which in turn is associated with the more demand for the healthcare [3]. The aim of surgery is to improve functional ability and relieve symptoms with adequate decompression of the neural elements. However, the long-term results of surgery are good to excellent only in two-thirds of patients [3,4]. Accordingly, preoperative patient selection is considered critical [5–8]. Clinically, routine magnetic resonance imaging (MRI) is the standard method in the diagnostic workup of patients with suspected LSS [9–10]. However, impacts of the MRI findings to the patients' symptoms have been also questioned [11].

We have earlier reported that depressive symptoms are a strong predictor for a worse short-term outcome [12,13] and for the two-year outcome in LSS surgery [7]. Depression and disability were also clearly associated in a cross-sectional setting [14].

There are several a cross-sectional studies on preoperative radiological findings and preoperative patient's symptoms, but only few with prospective setting. A clear association in a cross-sectional setting has been reported between the minimum dural sac cross-sectional (DSCA) area in lumbar MRI and several outcome measures (walking ability, symptom severity, quality of life) with the 82 and 88 LSS patient groups [15,16]. In another study with 50 patients population a smaller central anterior–posterior (AP) canal have reported greater perceived disability, but no other group differences emerged [17]. In contrast, a lack of association has been reported between the ODI and DSCA, qualitative evaluation of the lateral recess, and foraminal stenosis with the 63 LSS patients [18]. Thus there is discrepancy in the previous literature.

Yukawa et al reported in their prospective study with the 62 LSS patients that multilevel central stenosis were, on average, older and walked a shorter distance preoperatively and postoperatively, although the improvement in their postoperative self-assessment scores was similar to that of patients with single-level stenosis [19]. Sigmundsson et al. investigated the predictive value of MRI findings among a study population consisting of 109 LSS patients undergoing surgery with a one-year follow-up. They found in their prospective study that a smaller dural sac area predicted less leg pain postoperatively and more pain relief in low LBP [20]. None of these studies have, however, investigated the predictive value of visual and quantitative findings from preoperative lumbar spine MR images for both subjective and objective clinical outcome measures with a two-year follow-up [19,20].

The use of the standardized Oswestry Disability Index (ODI) [21,22], visual analogue scale for pain (VAS) [23], Beck Depression Inventory (BDI) [24], and specific back pain and leg pain assessment with a numeric rating scale (NRS-11) [25] has improved the accuracy and reproducibility in reliably grading functional disability, pain and depressive symptoms in patients. Keeping in mind the strong association of depressive symptoms and outcome measures of LSS, depressive symptoms should be adjusted. As far as we are aware, there have been no earlier LSS studies on MRI predictors that have adjusted the clinical outcome for depressive symptoms.

The purpose of the current study was to investigate the predictive value of preoperative MRI findings for the postoperative clinical outcome by comparing the preoperative imaging findings with the postoperative symptoms and function measured using standardized methods in a prospective study setting in LSS.

Materials and Methods

Patients

This prospective single-center study was approved by the Ethics Committee of Kuopio University Hospital, and the patients provided written informed consent to participate this study which was also documented. Ethics committee approved this procedure. The original study population consisted of 102 LSS patients, including 84 patients with central stenosis and lateral stenosis, and 18 patients having only lateral stenosis (5, 7, 13, 26). In the current study we included only these 84 central stenosis patients (mean age 63 ± 11 years, male 43%) with both clinically and radiologically defined LSS who had been selected for surgical treatment.

Selection for surgery was made by an orthopedist or neurosurgeon at Kuopio University Hospital, Kuopio, Finland. The inclusion criteria were: 1) the presence of severe back, buttock, and/or lower extremity pain, with radiographic evidence (computed tomography, magnetic resonance imaging, myelography) of compression of the cauda equina or exiting nerve roots by degenerative changes (ligamentum flavum, facet joints, osteophytes, and/or disc material), and 2) the surgeon's judgment in clinical and radiological evaluation that the patient had degenerative LSS requiring operative treatment. In addition, all patients had a history of ineffective response to conservative treatment.

The exclusion criteria for this current study were: pure lateral stenosis; emergency or urgent spinal surgery precluding recruitment and protocol investigations; cognitive impairment prohibiting completion of the questionnaires or other failures in co-operation, and the presence of metallic particles in the body preventing the magnetic resonance imaging investigation. A previous spine operation or coexisting disc herniation were not exclusion criteria, but the main diagnosis of the study patients had to be LSS. The surgeons sent the information on eligible patients to the Department of Physical and Rehabilitation Medicine, which organized the study [26].

MRI was performed preoperatively for all patients, and functional ability, clinical symptoms, and patient satisfaction were assessed at the two-year follow-up.

Magnetic resonance imaging

MR imaging of the lumbar spine was performed with a 1.5-T imager (Vision; Siemens Medical Solutions, Erlangen, Germany) and a dedicated receive-only spine coil. All patients were imaged prospectively with the same study protocol for study purposes. The imaging protocol conformed to the requirements of the American College of Radiology for the performance of MRI of the adult spine [27]. The following sequences were used: (a) sagittal T1-weighted spin-echo (repetition time/echo time (TR/TE) 600/12 ms; flip angle, 150°; 4-mm sections; intersection gap, 0.4 mm; field of view (FOV), 290 mm; rectangular FOV, 80%; three signals acquired per data line; matrix 288×512); (b) sagittal T2-weighted fast spin-echo (3500/120; flip angle, 180°; echo train length of five; 4-mm sections; intersection gap, 0.4 mm; FOV 290 mm; rectangular FOV, 63%; two signals acquired; matrix 180×512); (c) transverse T1-weighted spin-echo (700/15; flip angle, 90°; 4-mm sections; intersection gap, 0.4 mm; FOV, 250 mm; rectangular FOV, 80%; two signals acquired per data line; matrix 288×512); and (d) transverse T2-weighted fast spin-echo (5000/120; flip angle, 180°; echo train length of 15; 4-mm sections; intersection gap, 0.4 mm; FOV, 250 mm; rectangular FOV, 100%; three signals acquired per data line; matrix 330×512).

The entire lumbar spine was studied from the sagittal images (T12-S1), including parasagittal imaging of all the neural foramina bilaterally. Transverse images were obtained from the inferior aspect of L1 to the inferior aspect of S1, and the orientation of the sections was planned parallel to the major axis of each disc. In all sequences, a saturation band was placed over abdominal vessels.

MRI predictors

Image evaluation was performed with Numaris software (Siemens Medical Systems) by a neuroradiologist with 15 years of experience of spinal MRI (T.S.). Image analysis was performed independently without knowledge of the patients' clinical symptoms and data. Each level from the inferior aspect of L1 to the inferior aspect of S1 was analyzed separately. The central spinal canal was evaluated both visually and quantitatively. The lateral recess, lateral foramen, scoliosis, stenotic levels and spondylolisthesis were evaluated visually. The central canal was visually classified into three grades: 0 = normal or mild changes (ligamentum flavum hypertrophy and/or osteophytes and/or or disk bulging without narrowing in the central spinal canal); 1 = moderate stenosis (central spinal canal is narrowed but spinal fluid is still clearly visible between the nerve roots in the dural sac); 2 = severe stenosis (central spinal canal is narrowed and there is only a faint amount of spinal fluid or no fluid between the nerve roots in the dural sac). In quantitative image evaluation, each level was first assessed visually. On the image with the visually smallest cross-sectional area of the dural sac (mm^2), this area was manually traced. The number of stenotic levels was graded as: 1 = 1 stenotic level, 2 = two stenotic levels, 3 = three stenotic levels, 4 = four stenotic levels. The number of stenotic levels was also dichotomously classified as 1 (one-level stenosis) or 2 (two or more stenotic levels).

The lateral canal of the lumbar spine was divided into subarticular (entrance) and foraminal (mid) zones. The subarticular zone (lateral recess) was the most cephalad part of the lateral lumbar canal and located medial to or underneath the superior articular process. The foraminal zone was located below the pedicle. Each subarticular zone and foraminal zone was evaluated separately and bilaterally. In visual analysis, the grading system classified the lumbar nerve root canals into three grades: 0 = normal, 1 = narrowing without root compression and 2 = nerve root compression [28].

Scoliosis was evaluated visually and categorized into: 0 = no scoliosis, 1 = mild scoliosis, 2 = severe scoliosis. Spondylolisthesis was visually analyzed and categorized as 0 = no spondylolisthesis or 1 = spondylolisthesis.

Assessment of postoperative symptoms, functional disability and satisfaction with surgical outcome

The overall current low back and leg pain intensity was assessed using a self-administered VAS (range 0–100 mm) in a sitting position during study visits. This has been demonstrated to be a valid index of experimental, clinical, and chronic pain [23].

Back pain at rest (during last week) and leg pain on walking (during last week) were measured separately with a numerical rating scale from 0–10 (NRS-11) [25]. The questions about pain were anchored on the left (0) with the descriptor "no pain" and on the right (10) with the descriptor "intolerable pain".

Subjective disability was measured using the validated Finnish version of the ODI, where 0% represents no disability and 100% extreme debilitating disability [21–22,29].

The treadmill test (0–1000 m) was supervised by a physiotherapist. The patient was asked to keep a straight upright position during walking (on a zero-degree ramp). The starting speed was 0.67 m/s for the first 10 min (400 m), then 1 m/s for the next 10 min (600 m), and the maximum result was thus 1000 m in 20 min. If the patient was unable to start with a speed of 0.67 m/s, another test with a starting speed of 0.5 m/s was applied.

Satisfaction with the surgical outcome was assessed using a seven-category scale as follows: −3 = surgery was a total failure; −2 = condition is now considerably worse; −1 = condition is now slightly worse; 0 = no change; 1 = condition has slightly improved; 2 = condition has considerably improved; and 3 = totally cured. With respect to satisfaction, a "good outcome" consisted of those patients who were either "totally cured" or reported "condition considerably improved", whereas a "worse outcome" consisted of the other responses [26].

Statistical analyses

Analysis was performed using a general linear univariate model, and for patient satisfaction using a generalized linear model. Adjusting factors in the analysis were the age at operation (years), spondylodesis (yes/no) at operation (with or without instrumentation), and depressive symptoms (Beck Depression Inventory as a continuous scale, 0–63) [24] at two-year follow-up.

The predictive value of the radiological factors was assessed as follows: all the MRI predictors and adjusting factors were included together in the model, and tested together against each outcome measure. We applied a backward stepwise method in the analysis, using SPSS for Windows (version 19.0; SPSS, IBM, Chicago IL, USA). Statistical significance was set at p<0.05.

Results

Preoperative clinical characteristics and surgical outcome

Patient characteristics are summarized in Table 1. The mean age of the study patients (n = 84) at the time of surgery was 63 years (range 33–83), and 36 (43%) of the subjects were male. Twelve patients (14%) had undergone a previous spine operation.

All the pre- and postoperatively evaluated outcome measures displayed a statistically significant improvement after surgery (p<0.001; Table 1). Postoperative satisfaction was as follows: 9 (11.1%) "totally cured"; 39 (48.1%) "considerable improvement"; 25 (30.9%) "slight improvement"; 2 (2.5%) "no change"; 3 (3.7%) "condition is now slightly worse"; and 3 (3.7%) patients "considerably worse outcome".

Radiological findings

In visual analysis, none of the patients had a normal central canal. The central canal was moderately and severely stenosed in 40 (47.6%) and 44 (52.4%) patients, respectively. In quantitative analysis, the mean minimal DSCA was 55.2±20.9 mm2 (range 12–120). The lateral spinal canal recess was moderately and severely stenosed in 60 (71.1%) and 24 (28.9%) patients, respectively. The lateral spinal foramina was normal, moderately, and severely stenosed in 47 (55.4%), 30 (36.1%), and 7 (8.4%) patients, respectively. One-, two-, three-, and four-level central stenosis was observed in 29 (34.5%), 34 (40.5%), 13 (15.5%), and 8 (9.5%) patients, respectively. In dichotomous classification, one-level stenosis was recorded in 29 (34.5%) and stenosis of two or more levels in 55 (65.5%) patients. Scoliosis was severe in 3 (3.6%), mild in 19 (22.9%) and normal in 61 (73.5%) patients. One-level spondylolisthesis was found in 2 (2.4%) patients.

Predictive value of imaging findings for 2-year postoperative outcome

In parentheses below, the means and standard deviations of the study groups are presented, in addition to p-values and statistical tests of subgroups not mentioned in the methods.

Severe stenosis predicted less postoperative LP compared to moderate stenosis (2.75±2.6 vs 4.25±3.1; p = 0.028). Nevertheless, the improvement in LP was statistically also significant among patients in the moderate stenosis group (p<0.001; paired t-test).

Similarly, severe stenosis predicted less postoperative LBP compared to moderate stenosis (1.6±2.3 vs 2.4±2.5; p = 0.046). The improvement in LBP was also statistically significant among patients in the moderate stenosis group (p<0.001; paired t-test).

Moreover, severe stenosis predicted a lower postoperative overall VAS score compared to moderate stenosis (7.8±13.2 vs 17.8±20.9; p = 0.010) (Figure 1). The improvement in the VAS score was also statistically significant among patients with moderate stenosis (p<0.001; paired t-test).

Table 1. Clinical characteristics of the study subjects (n = 84).

Phase	Preoperative phase	2-year post-operative	P-value
Male/Female	36/48 (43/57)		
Marital status married or co-habiting	54 (64)		
Current smoker	17 (20)		
Previous lumbar operation	12 (14)		
Age	63 (11.0)		
BMI (kg/m²)	29.6 (4.0)		
Number of somatic diseases	5.2 (3.0)		
BDI score	10.4 (6.1)	7.6 (5.7)	<0.001
ODI	44.8 (16.1)	27.1 (19.8)	<0.001
VAS overall	32.8 (24.5)	12.6 (17.7)	<0.001
NRS LBP	4.1 (2.6)	1.9 (2.3)	<0.001
NRS LP on walking	6.4 (2.6)	3.2 (2.7)	<0.001
Walking distance (m)	551 (446)	729 (384)	<0.001

Note: Except where indicated, the data are numbers of patients, with percentages or means ± standard deviations in parentheses.
P-values: Paired T-test was used.
ODI = Oswestry Disability Index scale (0–100), VAS overall = Visual analogue pain scale (0–100), VAS LBP = specific back pain scale (0–10), VAS LP = specific leg pain scale (0–10), BDI = Beck Depression Inventory (0–63).

Finally, severe stenosis predicted better postoperative satisfaction with the surgical outcome compared to moderate stenosis (OR 0.297; 95% CI 0.100–0.880; p = 0.029).

Mild scoliosis predicted a worse 2-year outcome with the ODI compared to patients who had no scoliosis (34.3±21.5 vs 24.6±18.5; p = 0.031). The improvement in the ODI was also statistically significant among patients with scoliosis (p = 0.003; paired t-test).

In addition, scoliosis predicted a shorter postoperative treadmill test result compared to patients who had no preoperative scoliosis (547 m ± 464 m vs 820 m ± 315 m; p = 0.001). The improvement in walking ability in the treadmill test was not statistically significant among patients with scoliosis (p = 0.397; paired t-test).

One-level central stenosis predicted lower postoperative LBP compared to patients who had two or more stenotic levels (1.55±2.1 vs 2.22±2.5; p = 0.026).

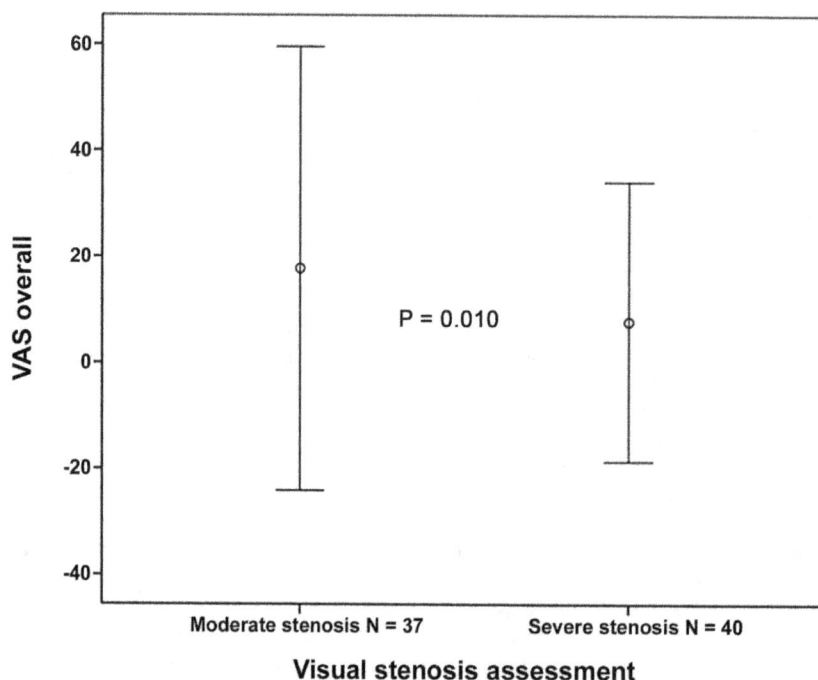

Figure 1. Visual analogue pain (mean ± SD) on two-year follow-up in patients with moderate and severe central spinal stenosis in visual analysis of lumbar spine magnetic resonance images.

We did not find any predictive value for quantitative evaluation of the central spinal canal or visual evaluation of spondylolisthesis, the lateral spinal canal recess and foramina.

Discussion

Our main finding was that the visually evaluated severity of lumbar spinal stenosis correlated with the postoperative clinical outcome. Interestingly, in the visual classification of the central spinal canal, the LP, LBP, and overall VAS were postoperatively higher in patients with moderate than with severe central canal stenosis. In addition, more severe stenosis also associated with better postoperative satisfaction with the surgical outcome. However, according to subgroup analysis, patients with only moderate stenosis also displayed a statistically significant improvement in LP, LBP, and overall VAS. Thus, patients with only moderate stenosis still appear to experience significant pain relief following surgical treatment for LSS.

Mild scoliosis predicted a worse postoperative ODI and walking distance in the treadmill test compared with patients who had no scoliosis. However, despite the scoliosis, subgroup analysis revealed that patients had a significant improvement in the ODI but not in the walking distance in the treadmill test. Consistently with this, Frazier et al. observed that greater preoperative scoliosis predicted more postoperative back pain. However, their radiological evaluation was based on plain X-ray images [30]. In our study, scoliosis also predicted a worse postoperative outcome in the ODI and treadmill test, but not worse LBP. Thus, patients who have scoliosis still benefit from surgical treatment for LSS in terms of their overall functional ability, but the effect on walking ability appears to be non-significant.

Patients who preoperatively had only one stenotic level reported lower postoperative LBP than patients who had two or more stenotic levels. This could be expected, since the degenerative changes are then also often more severe. In contrast, Sigmundsson et al. found that multilevel stenosis patients had less leg pain postoperatively than patients with single-level stenosis [20]. Amundsen et al. did not find any association between the number of stenotic levels and the surgical outcome in their study [31].

In the literature, there are only a few earlier prospective studies on the predictive value of preoperative MRI findings for an adequately determined postoperative clinical outcome on two-year follow-up. Yukawa et al. observed a correlation between better postoperative ODI scores in patients who had a DSCA under 70 mm2 in preoperative MRI [19]. However, the authors did not visually evaluate the severity of stenosis, which we found an elementary part of image analysis, especially in patients with stenosis in the upper part of the lumbar spine. Sigmundsson et al. found in their prospective study that a smaller dural sac area predicted less leg pain postoperatively and more pain relief for LBP. However, they did not visually evaluate the severity of LSS, and walking distance was only subjectively estimated by the patient, depressive symptoms were not adjusted, and the clinical outcome was only evaluated with a one-year follow-up [20]. Our results are generally in line with these studies, i.e. more severe visually determined preoperative central canal stenosis predicted less pain and better satisfaction postoperatively.

Studies on visually analyzed spinal canal stenosis of the whole lumbar spine are rare. In our study, we found a clear correlation between visually assessed central spinal canal stenosis and the patient outcome, but no correlation in quantitative preoperative measurements. How can this discrepancy be explained? The amount of neural tissue at the L1–2 and L2–3 levels is significantly greater than at the L4–5 or presacral levels. Thus by measuring only the cross-sectional area of the dural sac, subjects with reduced space for neural tissue may not be correctly recognized. According to our findings, quantitative evaluation with the used methods cannot replace visual interpretation performed by an experienced radiologist. To the best of our knowledge, there have been no previous prospective studies in which the predictive value of lateral spinal stenosis has been examined. Despite the visually evaluated lateral spinal recess and foraminal stenosis not predicting any postoperative outcome in our study, it may have clinical relevance. Lateral stenosis, if not decompressed properly, might be associated with a poor outcome. All our patients had central canal stenosis, which is always associated with a stenotic lateral recess but only few had foraminal stenosis, which may explain our results.

The strengths of this study are the prospective, observational study setting, carefully characterized study population. The study included clinically relevant subjective and validated outcome measures together with objectively measured walking distance, and the analyses were adjusted for depressive symptoms, age, and fusion. A two-year follow-up is considered as a "golden standard" in spine surgery studies. The standardized MRI protocol was planned and carefully performed for the study purposes, and the evaluation was performed with visually and quantitatively by an experienced neuroradiologist.

The limitation of this study are relatively small number of the patients, however number of the patients in the previous prospective studies are less than in this study expect in the study by Sigmundsson et al where was several shortages compared to this study as pointed out earlier (20). In our study number of patients was sufficient for detecting clinically relevant associations.

The results of the current study relate to routine clinical MRI with patients lying in the supine position. Imaging patients in the supine position is also a limitation, because the symptoms may worsen in the upright position, and the upright position may also alter the anatomy of the neural canal. Accordingly, an upright position would be the most appropriate image acquisition position to link image findings to the patient's symptoms [32,33]. Hiwatashi et al. found in their study that axial loading with imaging can even influence treatment decisions [34].

The incidence of lumbar spinal stenosis is increasing due to the aging of population [35]. This also increase the number of LSS operations. However, the selection of patients for surgical treatment still remains challenging. Our results strengthen the classical conception that the diagnosis of this syndrome depends on the clinical history and radiographic evidence of a demonstrable stenosis [36,37]. This study shows that pre-operative lumbar spine MRI imaging can predict the two-year clinical outcome in LSS surgery patients. The results of our study can be used to improve patient information and selection of patients for surgery.

Conclusions

Routine preoperative lumbar spine MRI can predict the two-year clinical outcome in LSS surgery. Severe central stenosis, compared with moderate stenosis, predicted better postoperative satisfaction and less pain. One-level stenosis, compared to patients who had two or more stenotic levels, predicted less low back pain. Preoperative scoliosis may indicate a worse functional outcome.

Author Contributions

Conceived and designed the experiments: PK TJA PS VL OA HK VT S. Sinikallio TS S. Savolainen. Performed the experiments: PK TJA PS VL OA HK VT S. Sinikallio TS S. Savolainen. Analyzed the data: PK TJA PS VL. Contributed reagents/materials/analysis tools: PK TJA PS VL OA HK VT S. Sinikallio TS S. Savolainen. Wrote the paper: PK TJA PS VL.

References

1. North American Spine Society (NASS) (2011) Diagnosis and treatment of degenerative lumbar spinal stenosis. Burr Ridge (IL): North American Spine Society (NASS).

2. Wunschmann BW, Sigl T, Ewert T, Schwarzkopf SR, Stucki G (2003) Physical therapy to treat spinal stenosis. Orthopade 32: 865–868.

3. Deyo RA, Mirza SK, Martin BI, Kreuter W, Goodman DC, et al (2010) Trends, major medical complications, and charges associated with surgery for lumbar spinal stenosis in older adults. JAMA 303: 1259–1265.

4. Atlas SJ, Keller RB, Wu YA, Deyo RA, Singer DE (2005) Long-term outcomes of surgical and nonsurgical management of lumbar spinal stenosis: 8 to 10 year results from the maine lumbar spine study. Spine (Phila Pa 1976) 30: 936–943.

5. Aalto T, Sinikallio S, Kroger H, Viinamaki H, Herno A, et al (2012) Preoperative predictors for good postoperative satisfaction and functional outcome in lumbar spinal stenosis surgery - a prospective observational study with a two-year follow-up. Scand J Surg 101: 255–260.

6. Sinikallio S, Aalto T, Airaksinen O, Herno A, Kroger H (2007) Depression is associated with poorer outcome of lumbar spinal stenosis surgery. Eur Spine J 16: 905–912.

7. Sinikallio S, Aalto T, Airaksinen O, Lehto SM, Kroger H, et al (2011) Depression is associated with a poorer outcome of lumbar spinal stenosis surgery: a two-year prospective follow-up study. Spine (Phila Pa 1976) 36: 677–682.

8. Mannion AF, Elfering A (2006) Predictors of surgical outcome and their assessment. Eur Spine J 1: S93–108.

9. Geisser ME, Haig AJ, Tong HC, Yamakawa KS, Quint DJ, et al (2007) Spinal canal size and clinical symptoms among persons diagnosed with lumbar spinal stenosis. Clin J Pain 23: 780–785.

10. Jonsson B, Annertz M, Sjoberg C, Stromqvist B (1997) A prospective and consecutive study of surgically treated lumbar spinal stenosis. Part I: Clinical features related to radiographic findings. Spine (Phila Pa 1976) 22: 2932–2937.

11. Haig AJ, Geisser ME, Tong HC, Yamakawa KS, Quint DJ, et al (2007) Electromyographic and magnetic resonance imaging to predict lumbar stenosis, low-back pain, and no back symptoms. J Bone Joint Surg Am 89: 358–366.

12. Sinikallio S, Aalto T, Airaksinen O, Herno A, Kroger H, et al (2007) Depression is associated with poorer outcome of lumbar spinal stenosis surgery. Eur Spine J 16: 905–912.

13. Sinikallio S, Aalto T, Airaksinen O, Herno A, Kroger H, et al (2009) Depressive burden in the preoperative and early recovery phase predicts poorer surgery outcome among lumbar spinal stenosis patients: a one-year prospective follow-up study. Spine (Phila Pa 1976) 34: 2573–2578.

14. Sinikallio S, Aalto T, Airaksinen O, Herno A, Kroger H, et al (2006) Depression and associated factors in patients with lumbar spinal stenosis. Disabil Rehabil 28: 415–422.

15. Kanno H, Ozawa H, Koizumi Y, Morozumi N, Aizawa T, et al (2012) Dynamic change of dural sac cross-sectional area in axial loaded magnetic resonance imaging correlates with the severity of clinical symptoms in patients with lumbar spinal canal stenosis. Spine (Phila Pa 1976) 37: 207–213.

16. Ogikubo O, Forsberg L, Hansson T (2007) The relationship between the cross-sectional area of the cauda equina and the preoperative symptoms in central lumbar spinal stenosis. Spine (Phila Pa 1976) 32: 1423–8.

17. Geisser ME, Haig AJ, Tong HC, Yamakawa KS, Quint DJ, et al (2007) Spinal canal size and clinical symptoms among persons diagnosed with lumbar spinal stenosis. Clin J Pain 23: 780–785.

18. Sirvanci M, Bhatia M, Ganiyusufoglu KA, Duran C, Tezer M, et al (2008) Degenerative lumbar spinal stenosis: correlation with Oswestry Disability Index and MR imaging. Eur Spine J 17: 679–685.

19. Yukawa Y, Lenke LG, Tenhula J, Bridwell KH, Riew KD, et al (2002) A comprehensive study of patients with surgically treated lumbar spinal stenosis with neurogenic claudication. J Bone Joint Surg Am 84-A: 1954–1959.

20. Sigmundsson FG, Kang XP, Jonsson B, Stromqvist B (2012) Prognostic factors in lumbar spinal stenosis surgery. Acta Orthop 83: 536–542.

21. Fairbank JC, Couper J, Davies JB, O'Brien JP (1980) The Oswestry low back pain disability questionnaire. Physiotherapy 66: 271–273.

22. Fairbank JC, Pynsent PB (2000) The Oswestry Disability Index. Spine (Phila Pa 1976) 25: 2940–52.

23. Price DD, McGrath PA, Rafii A, Buckingham B (1983) The validation of visual analogue scales as ratio scale measures for chronic and experimental pain. Pain 17: 45–56.

24. Beck AT (1961) An inventory for measuring depression. Arch Gen Psychiatry 4: 561–571.

25. Breivik EK, Bjornsson GA, Skovlund E (2000) A comparison of pain rating scales by sampling from clinical trial data. Clin J Pain 16: 22–28.

26. Kuittinen P, Aalto TJ, Heikkila T, Leinonen V, Savolainen, etal (2012) Accuracy and reproducibility of a retrospective outcome assessment for lumbar spinal stenosis surgery. BMC Musculoskelet Disord 29: 83.

27. (ACR) TACoR: Practice guideline for the performance of magnetic resonance imaging (MRI) of the adult spine. http://www.acr.org/~/media/5B165A70F9E342D4B77F0680A573C7ED.pdf.

28. Sipola P, Leinonen V, Niemelainen R, Aalto T, Vanninen R, et al (2011) Visual and quantitative assessment of lateral lumbar spinal canal stenosis with magnetic resonance imaging. Acta Radiol 52: 1024–31.

29. Pekkanen L, Kautiainen H, Ylinen J, Salo P, Hakkinen A (2011) Reliability and Validity Study of the Finnish Version 2.0 of the Oswestry Disability Index. Spine (Phila Pa 1976) 36: 332–8.

30. Frazier DD, Lipson SJ, Fossel AH, Katz JN (1997) Associations between spinal deformity and outcomes after decompression for spinal stenosis. Spine (Phila Pa 1976) 22: 2025–2029.

31. Amundsen T, Weber H, Nordal HJ, Magnaes B, Abdelnoor M, et al (2000) Lumbar spinal stenosis: conservative or surgical management?: A prospective 10-year study. Spine (Phila Pa 1976) 25: 1424–35.

32. Kanno H, Endo T, Ozawa H, Koizumi Y, Morozumi N, et al (2012) Axial Loading During Magnetic Resonance Imaging in Patients with Lumbar Spinal Canal Stenosis: Does It Reproduce the Positional Change of the Dural Sac Detected by Upright Myelography? Spine (Phila Pa 1976) 37: E985–92.

33. Kanno H, Ozawa H, Koizumi Y, Morozumi N, Aizawa T, et al (2012) Dynamic change of dural sac cross-sectional area in axial loaded MRI correlates with the severity of clinical symptoms in patients with lumbar spinal canal stenosis. Spine (Phila Pa 1976) 37: 207–13.

34. Hiwatashi A, Danielson B, Moritani T, Bakos RS, Rodenhause TG, et al (2004) Axial loading during MR imaging can influence treatment decision for symptomatic spinal stenosis. AJNR Am J Neuroradiol 25: 170–174.

35. Lurie JD, Birkmeyer NJ, Weinstein JN (2003) Rates of advanced spinal imaging and spine surgery. Spine (Phila Pa 1976) 28: 616–620.

36. Katz JN, Dalgas M, Stucki G, Katz NP, Bayley J, et al (1995) Degenerative lumbar spinal stenosis. Diagnostic value of the history and physical examination. Arthritis Rheum 38: 1236–1241.

37. Spengler DM (1987) Degenerative stenosis of the lumbar spine. J Bone Joint Surg Am 69: 305–308.

21

Do Abnormal Serum Lipid Levels Increase the Risk of Chronic Low Back Pain? The Nord-Trøndelag Health Study

Ingrid Heuch[1]*, Ivar Heuch[2], Knut Hagen[3], John-Anker Zwart[1,4]

1 Department of Neurology and FORMI, Oslo University Hospital, Oslo, Norway, 2 Department of Mathematics, University of Bergen, Bergen, Norway, 3 Department of Neuroscience, Norwegian University of Science and Technology, and Norwegian National Headache Centre, Department of Neurology, St. Olavs Hospital, Trondheim, Norway, 4 Faculty of Medicine, University of Oslo, Oslo, Norway

Abstract

Background: Cross-sectional studies suggest associations between abnormal lipid levels and prevalence of low back pain (LBP), but it is not known if there is any causal relationship.

Objective: The objective was to determine, in a population-based prospective cohort study, whether there is any relation between levels of total cholesterol, high density lipoprotein (HDL) cholesterol and triglycerides and the probability of experiencing subsequent chronic (LBP), both among individuals with and without LBP at baseline.

Methods: Information was collected in the community-based HUNT 2 (1995–1997) and HUNT 3 (2006–2008) surveys of an entire Norwegian county. Participants were 10,151 women and 8731 men aged 30–69 years, not affected by chronic LBP at baseline, and 3902 women and 2666 men with LBP at baseline. Eleven years later the participants indicated whether they currently suffered from chronic LBP.

Results: Among women without LBP at baseline, HDL cholesterol levels were inversely associated and triglyceride levels positively associated with the risk of chronic LBP at end of follow-up in analyses adjusted for age only. Adjustment for the baseline factors education, work status, physical activity, smoking, blood pressure and in particular BMI largely removed these associations (RR: 0.96, 95% CI: 0.85–1.07 per mmol/l of HDL cholesterol; RR: 1.16, 95% CI: 0.94–1.42 per unit of lg(triglycerides)). Total cholesterol levels showed no associations. In women with LBP at baseline and men without LBP at baseline weaker relationships were observed. In men with LBP at baseline, an inverse association with HDL cholesterol remained after complete adjustment (RR: 0.83, 95% CI: 0.72–0.95 per mmol/l).

Conclusion: Crude associations between lipid levels and risk of subsequent LBP in individuals without current LBP are mainly caused by confounding with body mass. However, an association with low HDL levels may still remain in men who are already affected and possibly experience a higher pain intensity.

Editor: Sam Eldabe, The James Cook University Hospital, United Kingdom

Funding: This study was supported in part by grants from Olav Raagholt and Gerd Meidel Raagholt's Legacy and the Legacy of Trygve Gythfeldt and Wife. The funders had no role in study design, data collection and analysis, decision to publish, or preparation of the manuscript.

Competing Interests: The authors have declared that no competing interests exist.

* Email: ingrid.heuch@ous-hf.no

Introduction

Low back pain (LBP) is a common disabling disorder, representing a substantial economic burden to society [1]. Only in about 15% of the patients suffering from LBP is it possible to give a precise underlying pathoanatomical diagnosis [2]. It is therefore important to clarify general theories about causal relationships.

It has been suggested that LBP may be related to lumbar artery disease, with atherosclerosis in the feeding arteries producing reduced blood supply and disc degeneration [3]. LBP has been found more frequently in individuals with missing or narrow lumbar or middle sacral arteries [4] or with calcification in the abdominal aorta [5,6]. In this way, LBP can possibly be compared to chest pain arising on the basis of atherosclerosis or to intermittent claudication with leg pain caused by impaired blood flow [7].

If the risk of LBP is affected by lesions in the arteries, risk factors for atherosclerosis should also be related to LBP, but results of epidemiological studies are equivocal [8,9]. Only few studies [8–15] have dealt with associations between LBP and abnormal serum lipid levels, representing established risk factors for atherosclerosis [16]. In particular, large prospective studies of potential relationships between lipid levels and risk of LBP are needed.

The purpose of the present study was to investigate associations between serum lipid levels and occurrence of LBP using a prospective design, considering data from two large health surveys,

Back Pain: Assessment and Treatment

carried out in a Norwegian county 11 years apart. As the course of LBP is often recurrent, with patients moving between acute and more chronic stages [17], risk factors may also be associated with subsequent occurrence in those already experiencing LBP. Thus one section of this study dealt with risk of LBP in participants not suffering from the disorder at baseline, while another part dealt with subsequent occurrence in participants with LBP at baseline.

Previous work based on the same cohort has shown positive associations between body mass index (BMI) and risk of LBP in both women and men [18]. High values of systolic and pulse pressure were also found to be related to a lower risk of LBP among women [19]. The present work includes adjustment for BMI and blood pressure, in addition to other potential confounders.

Materials and Methods

Participants

From 1995 to 1997, a large health survey, HUNT 2, was carried out in Nord-Trøndelag County in Norway. The entire population aged 20 years or more received a health questionnaire in which they indicated whether they had experienced LBP lasting for at least three months consecutively during the last year, which was regarded as chronic LBP. The participants underwent a clinical examination, including blood samples, with measurement of serum lipid levels [20]. In the HUNT 3 survey, carried out in 2006 to 2008 in the same county with a corresponding target population, similar questionnaires were distributed [21].

The present follow-up study was based on individual background information from HUNT 2 linked to information about chronic LBP collected in the subsequent HUNT 3 survey. The study aimed at the cohort consisting of 44,923 individuals who were 30 to 69 years old when they participated in the HUNT 2 survey and had information available on total cholesterol, high density lipoprotein (HDL) cholesterol, triglycerides and presence or absence of chronic LBP. Participants outside this age interval in HUNT 2 were excluded due to relatively low participation rates in the subsequent HUNT 3 survey [22]. During the period of follow-up, from HUNT 2 to HUNT 3, 2663 persons in this cohort died, 1686 persons left the county of Nord-Trøndelag, and one person disappeared. Furthermore, 15,123 members of the cohort residing in Nord-Trøndelag at the time of HUNT 3 did not participate or did not supply information about LBP. Thus a total of 25,450 persons, 14,053 women and 11,397 men, were available for analysis after follow-up, representing 62.7% of the remaining individuals resident in the county and 56.7% of the original cohort.

Definitions

Participants in HUNT 2 had levels of total cholesterol, HDL cholesterol and triglycerides measured in non-fasting blood. Total cholesterol was measured applying an enzymatic colorimetric cholesterolesterase method, and HDL cholesterol was measured after precipitation with phosphortungsten and magnesium ions [20]. Triglycerides were also measured by an enzymatic colorimetric method. All lipid levels were categorized in five groups by quintiles, determined in the overall HUNT 2 population [13].

Systolic blood pressure was categorized in intervals less than 120, 120–139, 140–159 and 160 mm Hg or more, and diastolic blood pressure in intervals less than 80, 80–89, 90–99 and 100 mm Hg or more. BMI, defined as weight/height^2, was subdivided into three groups, less than 25, 25–29.9, and 30 kg/m^2 or more.

For work status, one category comprised those who were employed or carried out professional work. This category was further subdivided according to the level of physical activity at work, in four subcategories. The second category of work status included individuals temporarily unemployed, students and those in military service. The third category included pensioners and people receiving social security support, and the fourth category included women occupied full time with housework.

Leisure-time physical activity was categorized in 3 groups, as light activity only or hard activity less than 1 hour per week, hard activity 1–2 hours per week, and hard activity 3 hours per week or more. Hard activity was defined as activity leading to participants sweating or being out of breath. Physical activity in leisure time included moving to and from work.

Duration of education was considered in 3 groups, 9 years or less, 10–12 years, and 13 years or more. Categories of cigarette smoking represented current daily smoking, previous daily smoking, and never daily smoking. Age was categorized in 10-year intervals within the range 30–69 years.

Statistical analyses

The percentage of chronic LBP at end of follow-up was computed within categories of total cholesterol, HDL cholesterol and triglycerides, separately for those without and with chronic LBP at baseline, to assess crude associations with lipid levels.

Associations adjusted for potential confounders were evaluated by generalized linear modeling for binomially distributed data with a log link. This procedure produced estimates of the risk ratio for any particular category of lipid levels relative to a reference category defined as the lowest category considered. As LBP is a relatively common disorder, this approach was preferred to logistic regression producing estimates of odds ratios which are poor approximations to risk ratios. In addition to categorical analyses involving quintiles of lipid levels, linear analyses were conducted with lipid levels considered as continuous variables. All such analyses were based on the actual recorded values of the lipid levels, not the quintiles. Likelihood tests were performed to test for trend. Triglyceride levels showed strongly skewed distributions and were logarithmically transformed (with base 10) before analysis.

One set of analyses included adjustment for age only. Further analyses were adjusted additionally for other factors potentially associated both with LBP and lipid levels, as education [23,24], work status [25,26], physical activity [27,28], cigarette smoking [29,30], BMI [18,31] and systolic and diastolic blood pressure [19,32]. All such factors were entered as categorical variables in the analyses. Because lipid measurements were performed on non-fasting blood, adjustment was made also for time between last meal and blood sampling. The main statistical strategy included tests for interaction between lipid levels and all variables adjusted for in the situations when a significant association was observed with a lipid level after full adjustment. In these tests, lipid levels were considered as continuous variables. Additional separate checks were made of the adequacy of the statistical model (Appendix S1), including tests for linearity in the effects of lipid levels and interaction terms for lipids showing no significant main effect.

Information was missing on some confounders in a minor fraction of the data set, and analyses with complete adjustment were based on a somewhat lower number of individuals than the basic age-adjusted analyses. All statistical analyses were carried out using IBM SPSS version 19 (IBM Corp, Armonk, NY).

Ethics

Each participant in the HUNT 2 and HUNT 3 surveys signed a written informed consent regarding the collection and use of data for research purposes. This procedure was approved by the Norwegian Data Inspectorate and by the Regional Committee for Ethics in Medical Research. The analysis was approved by the Regional Committee for Ethics in Medical Research.

Results

Associations among participants without LBP at baseline

A total of 10,151 women and 8731 men reported not having chronic LBP at baseline. In this group, 2028 women (20.0%) and 1226 men (14.0%) reported chronic LBP at end of follow-up. No definite association was seen between crude risk of chronic LBP and total cholesterol in either sex among the participants free of LBP at baseline (Table 1), but moderate inverse associations were suggested with levels of HDL in both women and men. The crude risk of LBP showed a weak tendency to increase with increasing levels of triglycerides among these participants.

Generalized linear modeling revealed no associations with total cholesterol (Table 2). Analyses adjusted for age only showed inverse associations with HDL levels and positive associations with triglyceride levels, although statistical significance was not reached for HDL in men (Table 2). However, after complete adjustment for other potential risk factors, these associations were substantially weakened and were no longer significant. Separate analyses carried out on participants with known values for all factors adjusted for, but with age adjustment only, gave very similar risk estimates to the age adjusted values shown in Table 2.

To determine which factor contributed most to the effect of the adjustment, analyses were also carried out with adjustment for each separate factor in addition to age. Adjustment for education, smoking, physical activity, work status and blood pressure had relatively little influence on associations between triglyceride levels and chronic LBP (Table 3), whereas adjustment for BMI led to substantial weakening of the associations. A similar tendency was seen for associations with HDL levels (Table 3), except that adjustment for smoking had an effect on the association in women of about the same magnitude as that for BMI. As total cholesterol levels showed no associations with LBP, neither with adjustment for age nor with complete adjustment, results are not shown for this variable in Table 3. No significant interaction was observed between lipid levels and BMI.

Associations among participants with LBP at baseline

In the group who reported chronic LBP at baseline, including 3902 women and 2666 men, a total of 2327 women (59.6%) and 1270 men (47.6%) also experienced chronic LBP at end of follow-up. Crude percentages did not indicate any relation between occurrence of chronic LBP in this group and total cholesterol (Table 1), while only weak inverse associations with HDL and positive associations with triglycerides were suggested.

Associations indicated with triglyceride levels largely disappeared after complete adjustment for other risk factors (Table 4). This was also the case with the inverse association with HDL levels in women, but in men the association persisted after complete adjustment. Separate risk ratios relative to levels ≤1.0 mmol/l were 0.92 (95% confidence interval [CI] 0.83–1.02), 0.90 (95% CI 0.80–1.01), 0.85 (95% CI 0.74–0.97) and 0.89 (95% CI 0.75–1.07) for HDL levels in the 1.1–1.2, 1.3–1.4, 1.5–1.7 and ≥1.8 mmol/l intervals, respectively. No significant interaction was found between levels of HDL in this case and age or any other variable adjusted for.

Discussion

In initial age-adjusted analyses of this prospective data set, the risk of chronic LBP was inversely associated with HDL levels and positively associated with triglyceride levels. However, further adjustment indicated that these associations were, at least to some extent, a product of confounding by other risk factors, in particular BMI. Yet in men who were already affected by chronic LBP at baseline, the inverse association between HDL and subsequent occurrence of chronic LBP remained after complete adjustment.

An important strength of this study was the opportunity to take into account relevant potential confounders, although information on such factors was missing in 8.7% of the subjects without LBP at baseline and 11.2% of those with LBP at that time. However, as the results with age adjustment only were very similar regardless of whether these subjects were included or not, missing values probably had little influence on the estimates concerned. Laboratory measurements were carried out by standardized procedures and the period between assessment of risk factors and final reporting of back pain was relatively long. Yet information on LBP was only available at baseline and end of follow-up, and other changes in back pain status during the intervening period were not recorded. Moreover, information on LBP was based on self-reported data and did not rely on a specific clinical examination.

Unfortunately no information was available on pain intensity or on cholesterol lowering medication. If abnormal lipid levels form part of a causal pathway to LBP, it is not obvious that use of such medication constitutes a potential confounder, but with sufficient information it might have been reasonable to analyse data separately for users and non-users. Furthermore, lipid measurements made on non-fasting blood may not represent the correct average over time for each participant. An attempt was made to compensate to some extent for this problem by adjusting for time since last meal. Finally, despite a relatively high response rate in the first survey, the response was lower at the second survey. There is no particular reason, however, why this should have introduced a noticable bias in the risk estimates.

Many patients who are affected by back pain recover after a certain period but are later prone to recurrent episodes [33]. In our study, chronic LBP was defined in the conventional manner requiring a continuous duration of at least 3 months [34], but if additional information had been available on pain intensity over an extended period, a more precise definition [35] could have made it easier to select those who were genuinely suffering from long-lasting LBP. However, even with a stricter definition of chronic LBP, some patients will later recover [35], so the percentage of chronic LBP observed at follow-up in our data among those with LBP at baseline is not surprising. Under these conditions it is not easy to distinguish between risk factors among subjects without LBP and factors affecting recurrence or persistence in those already experiencing LBP. This was the motivation in our study for considering assocations with lipid levels also among subjects with LBP at baseline.

To maintain the temporal relation between potential risk factors and the outcome variable representing LBP at follow-up, no other individual information collected at follow-up was included as predictors in our analyses. It is thus unlikely that the final disease status has influenced the values recorded for risk factors. Previous prospective epidemiological studies of relationships between lipid levels and occurrence of back pain have been based on follow-up of occupational cohorts. A long-term Finnish study of employees in an engineering company [9,36] showed positive associations with tryglyceride levels for both local and radiating LBP, and

Table 1. Proportion of individuals with chronic LBP at end of follow-up, by lipid levels and LBP status at baseline.

	Among individuals without LBP at baseline				Among individuals with LBP at Baseline			
	Women		Men		Women		Men	
	Total	With LBP at end of follow-up (%)	Total	With LBP at end of follow-up (%)	Total	With LBP at end of follow-up (%)	Total	With LBP at end of follow-up (%)
Total cholesterol (mmol/l)								
≤4.8	2173	442 (20.3)	1421	200 (14.1)	643	341 (53.0)	400	192 (48.0)
4.9–5.5	2316	441 (19.0)	2015	288 (14.3)	791	452 (57.1)	572	269 (47.0)
5.6–6.1	1957	419 (21.4)	1947	286 (14.7)	788	507 (64.3)	595	287 (48.2)
6.2–6.9	1873	364 (19.4)	1932	236 (12.2)	836	502 (60.0)	601	296 (49.3)
≥7	1832	362 (19.8)	1416	216 (15.3)	844	525 (62.2)	498	226 (45.4)
HDL cholesterol (mmol/l)								
≤1.0	847	190 (22.4)	2520	389 (15.4)	410	265 (64.6)	806	420 (52.1)
1.1–1.2	1497	340 (22.7)	2300	315 (13.7)	636	383 (60.2)	698	328 (47.0)
1.3–1.4	2169	442 (20.4)	1856	249 (13.4)	863	528 (61.2)	519	239 (46.1)
1.5–1.7	2966	542 (18.3)	1447	198 (13.7)	1113	631 (56.7)	436	188 (43.1)
≥1.8	2672	514 (19.2)	608	75 (12.3)	880	520 (59.1)	207	95 (45.9)
Triglycerides (mmol/l)								
≤0.94	3155	599 (19.0)	1129	137 (12.1)	969	533 (55.0)	336	152 (45.2)
0.95–1.29	2481	466 (18.8)	1541	214 (13.9)	845	510 (60.4)	470	220 (46.8)
1.30–1.70	1872	393 (21.0)	1768	244 (13.8)	797	476 (59.7)	529	253 (47.8)
1.71–2.38	1537	346 (22.5)	2008	267 (13.3)	712	422 (59.3)	595	262 (44.0)
≥2.38	1106	224 (20.3)	2285	364 (15.9)	579	386 (66.7)	736	383 (52.0)

LBP, low back pain.

Table 2. Associations between lipid levels and risk of chronic LBP among individuals without chronic LBP at baseline.

	Women		Men	
	Adjustment for age only	Complete adjustment*	Adjustment for age only	Complete adjustment*
	Risk ratio (95% CI)	Risk ratio (95% CI)	Risk ratio (95% CI)	Risk ratio (95% CI)
Number of individuals	10151	9159	8731	8078
Total cholesterol (mmol/l)				
≤4.8	1.00 (reference)	1.00 (reference)	1.00 (reference)	1.00 (reference)
4.9–5.5	0.93 (0.82–1.05)	0.90 (0.79–1.02)	1.02 (0.86–1.21)	0.99 (0.83–1.18)
5.6–6.1	1.04 (0.92–1.18)	1.04 (0.91–1.18)	1.06 (0.89–1.25)	1.00 (0.84–1.19)
6.2–6.9	0.95 (0.83–1.08)	0.91 (0.79–1.05)	0.88 (0.74–1.06)	0.83 (0.69–1.00)
≥7	0.97 (0.84–1.12)	0.93 (0.80–1.08)	1.11 (0.92–1.33)	1.00 (0.83–1.21)
Continuous results				
Per mmol/l	0.99 (0.95–1.02)	0.98 (0.94–1.02)	1.00 (0.96–1.06)	0.97 (0.92–1.02)
P for log-linear association	0.46	0.27	0.87	0.29
HDL cholesterol (mmol/l)				
≤1.0	1.00 (reference)	1.00 (reference)	1.00 (reference)	1.00 (reference)
1.1–1.2	1.02 (0.87–1.18)	1.05 (0.88–1.24)	0.89 (0.78–1.02)	0.96 (0.83–1.11)
1.3–1.4	0.91 (0.78–1.06)	0.98 (0.83–1.15)	0.88 (0.76–1.01)	0.95 (0.82–1.11)
1.5–1.7	0.81 (0.70–0.94)	0.89 (0.76–1.04)	0.90 (0.77–1.05)	0.94 (0.79–1.11)
≥1.8	0.86 (0.74–0.99)	0.96 (0.82–1.13)	0.81 (0.64–1.02)	0.86 (0.67–1.11)
Continuous results				
Per mmol/l	0.87 (0.78–0.97)	0.96 (0.85–1.07)	0.86 (0.73–1.01)	0.91 (0.77–1.08)
P for log-linear association	0.008	0.45	0.07	0.29
Triglycerides (mmol/l)				
≤0.94	1.00 (reference)	1.00 (reference)	1.00 (reference)	1.00 (reference)
0.95–1.29	1.00 (0.89–1.11)	0.95 (0.85–1.07)	1.15 (0.94–1.40)	1.09 (0.88–1.34)
1.30–1.70	1.12 (0.99–1.25)	1.06 (0.93–1.20)	1.15 (0.94–1.40)	1.10 (0.90–1.36)
1.71–2.38	1.20 (1.07–1.35)	1.12 (0.99–1.28)	1.10 (0.91–1.34)	1.05 (0.85–1.29)
≥2.38	1.08 (0.94–1.25)	0.99 (0.84–1.16)	1.31 (1.09–1.58)	1.20 (0.98–1.47)
Continuous results				
Per unit of lg(triglycerides)	1.32 (1.10–1.58)	1.16 (0.94–1.42)	1.40 (1.12–1.74)	1.24 (0.96–1.58)
P for log-linear association	0.003	0.18	0.003	0.10

LBP, low back pain; CI confidence interval.
*Adjustment for age, education, work status, physical activity, smoking, BMI, blood pressure and time between last meal and blood sampling.

associations persisted after adjustment for BMI. Results for total cholesterol were more ambiguous. A prospective study of British civil servants [8] revealed a positive relationship between sick-leave due to back pain and triglyceride levels, and the relation was essentially retained after adjustment for BMI and other relevant factors. No clear association emerged with total cholesterol. Finally, an American study of a cohort involved in petroleum-manufacturing [14] produced a positive assocation with triglycerides which largely disappeared after adjustment for obesity and other risk factors.

A cross-sectional study of the HUNT 2 population [13] showed an inverse association with HDL and a positive association with triglyceride levels, which was still significant in women after adjustment for BMI and other potential confounders. No definite associations were found between back pain and lipid levels in other cross-sectional studies [10–12,15], but in many cases results were not adjusted for other risk factors. However, in a Finnish study [37] associations were observed in men between prevalence of sciatica and levels of total and low density lipoprotein (LDL)

cholesterol and triglycerides but not HDL cholesterol, in analyses adjusted for BMI and other confounders. In our study, we did not consider the LDL level as a potential risk factor for LBP as no separate measurements of LDL were available, but to a large extent total cholesterol levels reflect LDL.

The notion that LBP may be related to lumbar artery disease [3] was partly based on a comparison of postmortem angiograms showing more missing or narrow lumbar or middle sacral arteries in subjects with LBP [4]. The hypothesis was supported by subsequent studies showing an association between LBP and occluded or narrowed lumbar arteries [38,39] or presence of atherosclerotic calcifications [5,6]. Calcification of the abdominal aorta has also been associated with intervertebral disc degeneration in several studies [5,39–41]. The relationship with LBP is presumably mediated by reduced blood supply [3,42], and an association has been indicated between lumbar arterial status and diffusion in the discs [43,44]. A recent study, however, found an increased blood flow in the lumbar arteries in LBP patients [45]. Regarding lipid levels, one study found no major differences

Table 3. Log-linear associations between HDL and triglyceride levels and risk of chronic LBP among individuals without chronic LBP at baseline, with adjustment for different variables.

	Women		Men	
	Risk ratio per mmol/l of HDL cholesterol* (95% CI)	Risk ratio per unit of lg(triglycerides)* (95% CI)	Risk ratio per mmol/l of HDL cholesterol* (95% CI)	Risk ratio per unit of lg(triglycerides)* (95% CI)
Adjustment for age only	0.87 (0.78–0.97)	1.32 (1.10–1.58)	0.86 (0.73–1.01)	1.40 (1.12–1.74)
Additional adjustment[†]				
Education	0.88 (0.79–0.98)	1.27 (1.06–1.52)	0.86 (0.73–1.01)	1.34 (1.08–1.68)
Smoking	0.91 (0.82–1.01)	1.28 (1.07–1.54)	0.88 (0.75–1.03)	1.36 (1.09–1.70)
Leisure time physical activity	0.88 (0.79–0.97)	1.29 (1.07–1.55)	0.86 (0.73–1.02)	1.42 (1.13–1.77)
Work status, including physical activity at work	0.87 (0.78–0.97)	1.29 (1.08–1.55)	0.83 (0.71–0.98)	1.40 (1.12–1.75)
BMI	0.91 (0.82–1.01)	1.19 (0.99–1.45)	0.94 (0.80–1.11)	1.21 (0.95–1.52)
Blood pressure	0.87 (0.78–0.96)	1.37 (1.14–1.64)	0.87 (0.74–1.03)	1.37 (1.09–1.71)
Complete adjustment[‡]	0.96 (0.85–1.07)	1.16 (0.94–1.42)	0.91 (0.77–1.08)	1.24 (0.96–1.58)

LBP, low back pain; CI confidence interval.
*Considered as a continuous variable.
[†]Adjustment for age and factor indicated in each case.
[‡]Adjustment for age, education, work status, physical activity, smoking, BMI, blood pressure and time between last meal and blood sampling.

between patients with lumbar spinal stenosis and controls [46], although associations have been observed between levels of LDL cholesterol and disc degeneration [47] and total cholesterol and disc herniation [48]. It has also been suggested that statin use may retard the process of disc degeneration [49].

Thus although there are many indications that arterial status may be related to pain arising in the lumbar region, no firm link has been established between lipid levels, intermediate factors and back pain mechanisms. Abnormal levels of triglycerides and total and HDL cholesterol have been regarded as established independent risk factors for atherosclerosis and cardiovascular disease [50]. In view of the hypothesis that atherosclerosis may cause LBP, it may seem peculiar that no relation was indicated at all with total

cholesterol in our data set. For stroke, however, total cholesterol levels do not seem to be associated with risk at the population level [50], in contrast to associations with HDL and triglycerides, so this is not a unique finding.

It is possible that lipid levels can influence the risk of LBP by other mechanisms. Thus dyslipidemia is related to inflammation [51], which may be linked to LBP in other ways [9]. Moreover, lipid levels may be associated with lumbar spine bone mineral density [52], which could play a role in the development of LBP.

Several other variables are associated with lipid levels at the population level and also constitute potential risk factors for LBP. BMI occupies a special position in this regard, as it is a relatively strong risk factor for LBP [18] and at the same time shows

Table 4. Log-linear associations between lipid levels and probability of chronic LBP among individuals with chronic LBP at baseline.

	Women		Men	
	Adjustment for age only	Complete adjustment*	Adjustment for age only	Complete adjustment*
	Risk ratio (95% CI)	Risk ratio (95% CI)	Risk ratio (95% CI)	Risk ratio (95% CI)
Number of individuals	3902	3418	2666	2414
Total cholesterol				
Per mmol/l[†]	1.02 (0.99–1.04)	1.00 (0.98–1.03)	0.99 (0.96–1.03)	0.98 (0.94–1.01)
p[†]	0.20	0.93	0.66	0.19
HDL cholesterol				
Per mmol/l[†]	0.94 (0.88–1.00)	0.99 (0.92–1.07)	0.84 (0.74–0.96)	0.83 (0.72–0.95)
p[†]	0.06	0.81	0.007	0.007
Triglycerides				
Per unit of lg(triglycerides)[†]	1.24 (1.10–1.40)	1.08 (0.94–1.24)	1.17 (0.99–1.38)	1.07 (0.88–1.29)
p[†]	<0.001	0.27	0.07	0.51

LBP, low back pain; CI confidence interval.
*Adjustment for age, education, work status, physical activity, smoking, BMI, blood pressure and time between last meal and blood sampling.
[†]Lipid levels considered as continuous variables.

substantial associations with lipid levels over long periods of life [31]. In our study, adjustment for BMI had a major effect on the triglyceride and HDL associations with chronic LBP. Some other studies have shown similar effects of adjustment for BMI [13,14], although this is not a consistent finding [8,9]. If lipid levels influence BMI, it is possible that this to some extent represents an overadjustment, so that the true relations between risk of LBP and lipid levels are somewhere between those shown here with age adjustment only and complete adjustment.

The particular association with HDL remaining after complete adjustment, among men with chronic LBP at baseline, may represent a chance finding among many statistical tests. It is still reasonable that low HDL cholesterol levels may have an effect different from high triglyceride levels on predisposing factors for LBP. The contrast between men and women in this regard may reflect general sex differences for LBP, as the prevalence is higher in women and women may have a different pain threshold [53]. In the group of men who reported chronic LBP at baseline, subsequent LBP could represent a somewhat different, more permanent condition, possibly with higher pain intensity. Underlying associations with lipid levels may be more pronounced for particularly severe back pain, as suggested for LDL by one study [39]. General high-intensity chronic pain has also been found to be related to low HDL levels [54].

Unfortunately the present study does not provide any definite answer concerning associations between lipid levels and risk of LBP. If the LBP related to atherosclerosis of abdominal arteries represents a relatively small proportion of all LBP cases, a better classification of this heterogeneous medical condition may be important in future studies. Information on intensity and more precise duration of pain may be essential. A detailed medical classification may also help in delineating other specific causal mechanisms, although this may be difficult to achieve in large population-based studies.

Acknowledgments

The Nord-Trøndelag Health Study (the HUNT study) is a collaboration between the HUNT Research Centre, Faculty of Medicine, the Norwegian University of Science and Technology (NTNU); Norwegian Institute of Public Health; and the Nord-Trøndelag County Council. Laboratory measurements were carried out at facilities owned by the Nord-Trøndelag Hospital Trust.

Author Contributions

Conceived and designed the experiments: Ingrid Heuch JAZ. Performed the experiments: Ingrid Heuch. Analyzed the data: Ingrid Heuch Ivar Heuch. Contributed reagents/materials/analysis tools: KH JAZ. Wrote the paper: Ingrid Heuch. Revised the manuscript critically for important intellectual content: Ivar Heuch KH JAZ.

References

1. Hong J, Reed C, Novick D, Happich M (2013) Costs associated with treatment of chronic low back pain: an analysis of the UK General Practice Research Database. Spine (Phila Pa 1976) 38: 75–82.
2. Deyo RA, Weinstein JN (2001) Low back pain. N Engl J Med 344: 363–370.
3. Kauppila LI (1995) Can low-back pain be due to lumbar-artery disease? Lancet 346: 888–889.
4. Kauppila LI, Tallroth K (1993) Postmortem angiographic findings for arteries supplying the lumbar spine: their relationship to low-back symptoms. J Spinal Disord 6: 124–129.
5. Kauppila LI, McAlindon T, Evans S, Wilson PW, Kiel D, et al. (1997) Disc degeneration/back pain and calcification of the abdominal aorta: a 25-year follow-up study in Framingham. Spine (Phila Pa 1976) 22: 1642–1647.
6. Kurunlahti M, Tervonen O, Vanharanta H, Ilkko E, Suramo I (1999) Association of atherosclerosis with low back pain and the degree of disc degeneration. Spine (Phila Pa 1976) 24: 2080–2084.
7. Bøggild H (2006) Ischemia and low-back pain-is it time to include lumbar angina as a cardiovascular disease? Scand J Work Environ Health 2006; 32: 20–21.
8. Hemingway H, Shipley M, Stansfeld S, Shannon H, Frank J, et al. (1999) Are risk factors for atherothrombotic disease associated with back pain sickness absence? The Whitehall II study. J Epidemiol Community Health 53: 197–203.
9. Leino-Arjas P, Solovieva S, Kirjonen J, Reunanen A, Riihimäki H, et al. (2006) Cardiovascular risk factors and low-back pain in a long-term follow-up of industrial employees. Scand J Work Environ Health 32: 12–19.
10. Welin L, Larsson B, Svärdsudd K, Tibblin G (1978) Serum lipids, lipoproteins and musculoskeletal disorders among 50- and 60-year-old men. An epidemiologic study. Scand J Rheumatol 7: 7–12.
11. Svensson HO, Vedin A, Wilhelmsson C, Andersson GB (1983) Low-back pain in relation to other diseases and cardiovascular risk factors. Spine (Phila Pa 1976) 8: 277–285.
12. Kostova V, Koleva M (2001) Back disorders (low back pain, cervicobrachial and lumbosacral radicular syndromes) and some related risk factors. J Neurol Sci 192: 17–25.
13. Heuch I, Heuch I, Hagen K, Zwart JA (2010) Associations between serum lipid levels and chronic low back pain. Epidemiology 21: 837–841.
14. Tsai SP, Bhojani FA, Wendt JK (2011) Risk factors for illness absence due to musculoskeletal disorders in a 4-year prospective study of a petroleum-manufacturing population. Occup Environ Med 53: 434–440.
15. Ha IH, Lee J, Kim MR, Kim H, Shin JS (2014) The association between the history of cardiovascular diseases and chronic low back pain in South Koreans: a cross-sectional study. PLoS One 9: e93671.
16. Lusis AJ (2000) Atherosclerosis. Nature 407: 233–241.
17. Von Korff M, Saunders K (1996) The course of back pain in primary care. Spine (Phila Pa 1976) 21: 2833–2837.
18. Heuch I, Heuch I, Hagen K, Zwart JA (2013) Body mass index as a risk factor for developing chronic low back pain: a follow-up in the Nord-Trøndelag Health Study. Spine (Phila Pa 1976) 38: 133–139.
19. Heuch I, Heuch I, Hagen K, Zwart JA (2014) Does high blood pressure reduce the risk of chronic low back pain? The Nord-Trøndelag Health Study. Eur J Pain 18: 590–598.
20. Holmen J, Midthjell K, Krüger Ø, Langhammer A, Holmen TL, et al. (2003) The Nord-Trøndelag Health Study 1995–97 (HUNT 2): objectives, contents, methods and participation. Nor Epidemiol 13: 19–32.
21. Krokstad S, Langhammer A, Hveem K, Holmen TL, Midthjell K, et al. (2013) Cohort Profile: The HUNT Study, Norway. Int J Epidemiol 42: 968–977.
22. Langhammer A, Krokstad S, Romundstad P, Heggland J, Holmen J, et al. (2012) The HUNT study: participation is associated with survival and depends on socioeconomic status, diseases and symptoms. BMC Med Res Methodol 12: 143.
23. Dionne CE, Von Korff M, Koepsell TD, Deyo RA, Barlow WE, et al. (2001) Formal education and back pain: a review. J Epidemiol Community Health 55: 455–468.
24. Wamala SP, Wolk A, Schenck-Gustafsson K, Orth-Gomér K (1997) Lipid profile and socioeconomic status in healthy middle aged women in Sweden. J Epidemiol Community Health 51: 400–407.
25. Osti OL, Cullum DE (1994) Occupational low back pain and intervertebral disc degeneration: epidemiology, imaging, and pathology. Clin J Pain 10: 331–334.
26. Kang MG, Koh SB, Cha BS, Park JK, Baik SK, et al. (2005) Job stress and cardiovascular risk factors in male workers. Prev Med 40: 583–588.
27. Björk-van Dijken C, Fjellman-Wiklund A, Hildingsson C (2008) Low back pain, lifestyle factors and physical activity: a population based-study. J Rehabil Med 40: 864–869.
28. Monda KL, Ballantyne CM, North KE (2009) Longitudinal impact of physical activity on lipid profiles in middle-aged adults: the Atherosclerosis Risk in Communities Study. J Lipid Res 50: 1685–1691.
29. Leboeuf-Yde C (1999) Smoking and low back pain. A systematic literature review of 41 journal articles reporting 47 epidemiologic studies. Spine (Phila Pa 1976) 24: 1463–1470.
30. Craig WY, Palomaki GE, Haddow JE (1989) Cigarette smoking and serum lipid and lipoprotein concentrations: an analysis of published data. BMJ 298: 784–788.
31. Pinto Pereira SM, Power C (2013) Life course body mass index, birthweight and lipid levels in mid-adulthood: a nationwide birth cohort study. Eur Heart J 34: 1215–1224.
32. Bønaa KH, Thelle DS (1991) Association between blood pressure and serum lipids in a population. The Tromsø Study. Circulation 83: 1305–1314.
33. Hayden JA, Dunn KM, van der Windt DA, Shaw WS (2010) What is the prognosis of back pain? Best Pract Res Clin Rheumatol 24: 167–179.

34. Merskey H, Bogduk N (1994) Classification of chronic pain. Descriptions of chronic pain syndromes and definitions of pain terms. 2nd edn. Seattle: IASP Press.
35. Von Korff M, Dunn KM (2008) Chronic pain reconsidered. Pain 138: 267–276.
36. Leino-Arjas P, Kaila-Kangas L, Solovieva S, Riihimäki H, Kirjonen J, et al. (2006) Serum lipids and low back pain: an association? A follow-up study of a working population sample. Spine (Phila Pa 1976) 31: 1032–1037.
37. Leino-Arjas P, Kauppila L, Kaila-Kangas L, Shiri R, Heistaro S, et al. (2008) Serum lipids in relation to sciatica among Finns. Atherosclerosis 197: 43–49.
38. Kauppila LI (1997) Prevalence of stenotic changes in arteries supplying the lumbar spine. A postmortem angiographic study on 140 subjects. Ann Rheum Dis 56: 591–595.
39. Kauppila LI, Mikkonen R, Mankinen P, Pelto-Vasenius K, Mäenpää I (2004) MR aortography and serum cholesterol levels in patients with long-term nonspecific lower back pain. Spine (Phila Pa 1976) 29: 2147–2152.
40. Turgut AT, Sönmez I, Cakıt BD, Koşar P, Koşar U (2008) Pineal gland calcification, lumbar intervertebral disc degeneration and abdominal aorta calcifying atherosclerosis correlate in low back pain subjects: A cross-sectional observational CT study. Pathophysiology 15: 31–39.
41. Suri P, Hunter DJ, Rainville J, Guermazi A, Katz JN (2012) Quantitative assessment of abdominal aortic calcification and associations with lumbar intervertebral disc height loss: the Framingham Study. Spine J 12: 315–323.
42. Kauppila LI (2009) Atherosclerosis and disc degeneration/low back pain–a systematic review. Eur J Vasc Endovasc Surg 37: 661–670.
43. Kurunlahti M, Kerttula L, Jauhiainen J, Karppinen J, Tervonen O (2001) Correlation of diffusion in lumbar intervertebral disks with occlusion of lumbar arteries: a study in adult volunteers. Radiology 221: 779–786.
44. Tokuda O, Okada M, Fujita T, Matsunaga N (2007) Correlation between diffusion in lumbar intervertebral disks and lumbar artery status: evaluation with fresh blood imaging technique. J Magn Reson Imaging 25: 185–191.
45. Espahbodi S, Doré CJ, Humphries KN, Hughes SP (2013) Color Doppler ultrasonography of lumbar artery blood flow in patients with low back pain. Spine (Phila Pa 1976) 38: E230–E236.
46. Uesugi K, Sekiguchi M, Kikuchi SI, Konno S (2013) Relationship between lumbar spinal stenosis and lifestyle-related disorders: a cross-sectional multi-center observational study. Spine (Phila Pa 1976) 38: E540–E545.
47. Hangai M, Kaneoka K, Kuno S, Hinotsu S, Sakane M, et al. (2008) Factors associated with lumbar intervertebral disc degeneration in the elderly. Spine J 8: 732–740.
48. Jhawar BS, Fuchs CS, Colditz GA, Stampfer MJ (2006) Cardiovascular risk factors for physician-diagnosed lumbar disc herniation. Spine J 6: 684–691.
49. Shi S, Wang C, Yuan W, Wang X, Zhou X (2011) Potential prevention: orally administered statins may retard the pathologic process of disc degeneration. Med Hypotheses 76: 125–127.
50. Prospective Studies Collaboration (2007) Blood cholesterol and vascular mortality by age, sex, and blood pressure: a meta-analysis of individual data from 61 prospective studies with 55,000 vascular deaths. Lancet 370: 1829–1839.
51. van Diepen JA, Berbée JF, Havekes LM, Rensen PC (2013) Interactions between inflammation and lipid metabolism: relevance for efficacy of anti-inflammatory drugs in the treatment of atherosclerosis. Atherosclerosis 228: 306–315.
52. Makovey J, Chen JS, Hayward C, Williams FM, Sambrook PN (2009) Association between serum cholesterol and bone mineral density. Bone 44: 208–213.
53. Keogh E (2006) Sex and gender differences in pain: a selective review of biological and psychosocial factors. J Mens Health Gend 3: 236–243.
54. Goodson NJ, Smith BH, Hocking LJ, McGilchrist MM, Dominiczak AF, et al. (2013) Cardiovascular risk factors associated with the metabolic syndrome are more prevalent in people reporting chronic pain: results from a cross-sectional general population study. Pain 154: 1595–1602.

22

Clinical Significance of Tumor Necrosis Factor-α Inhibitors in the Treatment of Sciatica

Yun Fu Wang[1], Ping You Chen[2], Wei Chang[3], Fi Qi Zhu[4], Li Li Xu[1], Song Lin Wang[1], Li Ying Chang[5], Jie Luo[1]*, Guang Jian Liu[1]*

1 Department of Neurology, Taihe Hospital Affiliated to Hubei University of Medicine, Shiyan City, Hubei Province, China, 2 Medical Imaging Center, Taihe Hospital Affiliated to Hubei University of Medicine, Shiyan City, Hubei Province, China, 3 Department of Spine Surgery, Taihe Hospital Affiliated to Hubei University of Medicine, Shiyan City, Hubei Province, China, 4 Department of Neurology, Yuebei People's Hospital Affiliated to Shantou University Medical College, Shaoguan City, Guangdong Province, China, 5 Department of Neurology, Xiangyang Center Hospital Affiliated to Hubei University of Arts and Science, Xiangyang City, Hubei Province, China

Abstract

Background and Objective: Currently, no satisfactory treatment is available for sciatica caused by herniated discs and/or spinal stenosis. The objective of this study is to assess the value of tumor necrosis factor (TNF)-α inhibitors in the treatment of sciatica.

Methods: Without language restrictions, we searched PubMed, OVID, EMBASE, the Web of Science, the Clinical Trials Registers, the Cochrane Central Register of Controlled Trials and the China Academic Library and Information System. We then performed a systematic review and meta-analysis on the enrolled trials that met the inclusion criteria.

Results: Nine prospective randomized controlled trials (RCTs) and two before-after controlled trials involving 531 patients met our inclusion criteria and were included in this study. Our systematic assessment and meta-analysis demonstrated that in terms of the natural course of the disease, compared with the control condition, TNF-α inhibitors neither significantly relieved lower back and leg pain (both $p>0.05$) nor enhanced the proportion of patients who felt overall satisfaction (global perceived effect (satisfaction)) or were able to return to work (return to work) (combined endpoint; $p>0.05$) at the short-term, medium-term and long-term follow-ups. In addition, compared with the control condition, TNF-α inhibitors could reduce the risk ratio (RR) of discectomy or radicular block (combined endpoint; $RR=0.51$, 95% CI 0.26 to 1.00, $p=0.049$) at medium-term follow-up, but did not decrease RR at the short-term ($RR=0.64$, 95% CI 0.17 to 2.40, $p=0.508$) and long-term follow-ups ($RR=0.64$, 95% CI 0.40 to 1.03, $p=0.065$).

Conclusion: The currently available evidence demonstrated that other than reducing the RR of discectomy or radicular block (combined endpoint) at medium-term follow-up, TNF-α inhibitors showed limited clinical value in the treatment of sciatica caused by herniated discs and/or spinal stenosis.

Editor: Malú G. Tansey, Emory University, United States of America

Funding: This study received financial support from the Sowers Foundation for Evidence-Based Medicine of Taihe Hospital (2013). The funders had no role in study design, data collection and analysis, decision to publish, or preparation of the manuscript.

Competing Interests: The authors have declared that no competing interests exist.

* Email: liuguangjian@aliyun.com (GJL); luojie_001@126.com (JL)

Introduction

Disk herniation-induced sciatica is one of the most common causes of lower back and leg pain among young adults. Previous studies have demonstrated that the outcomes of conservative treatment, such as medication and physical therapy, are similar to the natural course of this disease [1]. Although epidural steroid injections can relieve a portion of patients' pain, they cannot restore the patients' physical function [2]. Recently, some scholars have stated that non-opioid analgesic agents, discectomy and epidural steroid injection are effective [3]; however, the opposing opinion indicates that discectomy is only effective for acute neurodynia, and its long-term outcome is not superior to that of conservative treatment [4]. In addition, because of nerve root adhesions or epidural adhesions, epidural steroid injection cannot relieve pain in a considerable number of patients [5].

Tumor necrosis factor-alpha (TNF-α) is an inflammatory factor involved in the pathophysiological mechanism underlying disk herniation-induced sciatica [6,7]. In the past decade, some scholars have attempted to use TNF-α inhibitors to treat sciatica. Previous non-randomized controlled trials have shown that this type of agent has potential efficacy and a relatively high patient tolerance [8,9]. However, afterwards, various randomized controlled trials (RCTs) demonstrated that these agents yielded inconsistent outcomes. A newly published systematic review and meta-analysis revealed that the evidence supporting the use of TNF-α inhibitors to treat sciatica is inadequate [10]. Nevertheless, this study has some limitations: (1) four high-quality RCTs [11–14] were missed; (2) among all of the enrolled trials, a visual analogue scale (VAS) score range of 0 to 100 was adopted in a portion of trials [15–19], while a score range of 0 to 10 was applied in others [20–22]. The authors used a weighted mean difference (WMD) technique to pool all of the data together; however, this is not a standard and conventional method commonly used in meta-analysis [23]; and (3) in addition, we disagree that the authors' method of pooling together all of the data regarding the outcomes of discectomy, including the data obtained during short-term, medium-term and long-term follow-ups.

The primary purpose of this study was to evaluate the treatment value of TNF-α inhibitors compared with placebos and steroids in terms of five endpoints at short-term follow-up (≤3 months), medium-term follow-up (3 to 12 months) and long-term follow-up (≥12 months). The five endpoints that were adopted were the Oswestry Disability Index, VAS pain intensity in the leg, VAS pain intensity in the lower back, global perceived effect (satisfaction) or return to work (combined endpoint), and discectomy or radicular block (combined endpoint). The secondary purpose was to evaluate the patient tolerance of the adverse reaction of TNF-α inhibitors.

Methods

Using the "Preferred Reporting Items for Systematic reviews and Meta-Analyses (PRISMA)" [24] as a guideline, we conducted this systematic review and meta-analysis. The present study is a complement to and update of the study performed by Williams *et al.* [10].

Search Strategies

The searched database included the following: PubMed, OVID, EMBASE, the Web of Science, the Clinical Trials Registers, the Cochrane Central Register of Controlled Trials and the China Academic Library and Information System. The search terms included following: "anti-tumor necrosis factor agents OR tumor necrosis factor alpha inhibitor OR infliximab OR adalimumab

OR etanercept OR rituximab OR golimumab OR certolizumab OR efalizumab OR ustekinumab OR alefacept" AND "sciatica OR lumbosacral radiculopathy" AND "controlled trial" appearing in "title/abstract". Each database was searched from January 1, 2000 to July 1, 2013. No language restrictions were applied.

Trial Selection

The inclusion criteria were as follows: (1) Participants: all patients included were older than 18 years and were diagnosed with sciatica caused by lumbar disc herniation and/or lumbar spinal stenosis confirmed with CT/MRI, regardless of the duration of symptoms. Patients who planned to undergo discectomy soon or had comorbid liver disease, tuberculosis, spinal cord tumor, infection or trauma were excluded; (2) Intervention: any trial that used TNF-α inhibitors in the TNF-α inhibitor group and placebos or steroids in the control group and in which all drugs were locally injected or systematically administered; (3) Endpoints: any trial that used subjective parameters, such as the Oswestry Disability Index and VAS scores, to evaluate lower back and leg pain and used global perceived effect (satisfaction) or return to work (combined endpoint) to represent the proportion of patients who felt overall satisfaction or were able to return to work, and adopted an objective parameter, discectomy or radicular block (combined endpoint), to evaluate the risk ratio (RR) of discectomy or radicular block; (4) Study type: the controlled trials including randomized controlled trials (RCTs), cross-over controlled trial, non-randomized concurrent trials, before-after controlled trial, and case-control study, were included regardless of their sample size and trial results.

Data Extraction

Using a unified form, two investigators extracted the data and established the data spreadsheet independently. Finally, they confirmed the accuracy of the data together, and discrepancies were resolved via discussion until a consensus was reached. A portion of the endpoint data expressed only as a line graph or

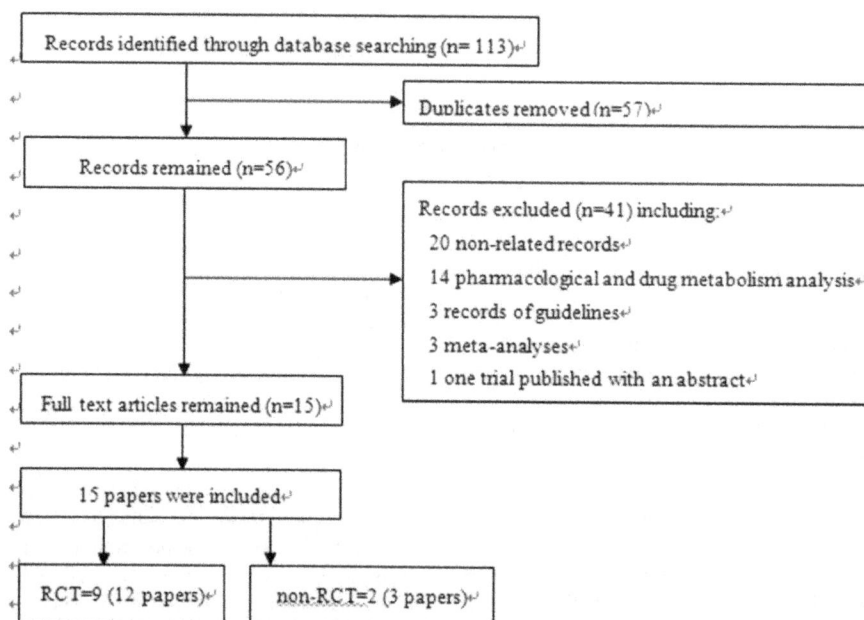

Figure 1. A flow diagram of the screening process.

Table 1. Trial characteristics.

Trial and study type	Participants	Intervention		Outcome (follow-up duration and outcome measures)
		TNF-α inhibitor group	Control group	
1 Genevay et al. [13,15], RCT	n = 61, and the average age was 49 years; males accounted for 57% of the participants; the mean duration of the symptoms was 3.6 weeks	Adalimumab 40 mg; subcutaneous injection; once a week; administered twice	Normal saline; subcutaneous injection; once a week; administered twice	Genevay et al. [15]: 6-week and 6-month follow-ups; VAS-leg pain, VAS-lower back pain, Oswestry Disability Index [28], the number of resected discs, the general health survey (12-item Short Form health survey [29]), the number of patients who returned to work, adverse reaction
				Genevay et al. [13]: 36-month follow-up; The number of resected discs, VAS-leg pain, VAS-lower back pain, Oswestry Disability Index [28], the general health survey (12-item Short Form health survey [30])
2 Cohen et al. [21], RCT	n = 84, and the average age was 42 years; males accounted for 70% of the population; the mean duration of the symptoms was 2.7 months	Etanercept 4 mg +bupivacaine 0.5 ml; foraminal injection administered twice	Normal saline + bupivacaine 0.5 ml (Group 1), or steroid methyl prednisolone 60 mg + bupivacaine 0.5 ml (Group 2); foraminal injection administered twice	1-, 3- and 6-month follow-ups; The number of patients with a positive outcome (a 50% reduction in leg pain + an overall positive feeling without any further treatment), VAS-leg pain, VAS-lower back pain, Oswestry Disability Index [28], complications
3 Ohtori et al. [12], RCT	n = 80, and the average age was 65±5.5/67±5.0[1] years; the mean duration of the symptoms was 2.5 (1 to 12)/2.3 (1 to 12)[2] months	Etanercept 10 mg; foraminal injection; administered once	Dexamethasone 3.3 mg; foraminal injection; administered once	1-month follow-up; VAS-leg pain, VAS-lower back pain, Oswestry Disability Index [28], complications
4 Okoro et al. [22], RCT	n = 15 with no indication of the average age; males accounted for 40% of the population; the duration of the symptoms was at least 24 weeks	Etanercept 25 mg; subcutaneous injection; administered once	Normal saline; subcutaneous injection; once	3-month follow-up; VAS-leg pain, VAS-lower back pain, Oswestry Disability Index [28], modified Zung Depression index, independent walking distance, the number of patients receiving discectomy or radicular block, adverse reaction
5 Cohen et al. [20], RCT	n = 24, and the median age was 41 to 46 years; males accounted for 71% of the participants; the mean duration of symptoms was 3 to 7 months	Etanercept 2 mg (Group 1), 4 mg (Group 2), 6 mg (Group 3); foraminal injection; administered once	Normal saline; foraminal injection; administered once	1-, 3- and 6-month follow-ups; VAS-leg pain, VAS-lower back pain, Oswestry Disability Index [28], the number of patients with a positive outcome (a reduction of 50% in the leg pain + an overall satisfaction), the number of resected discs
6 Karppinen et al. [17], RCT	n = 15, and the average age was 53 years; males accounted for 67% of the participants; the mean duration of symptoms was 58 days	Infliximab 5 mg/kg; intravenous injection; administered once	Normal saline; intravenous injection; administered once	3- and 6-month follow-ups; VAS-leg pain, VAS-lower back pain, Oswestry Disability Index [28], the number of patients who underwent discectomy or caudal epidural block, RAND-36-item health questionnaire, days of sick leave, adverse reaction
7 Cohen et al. [14], RCT	n = 36, and the average age was 39.3±1.9[1] years; males accounted for 78% of the participants; the mean duration of the symptoms was 5.3±0.7[1] years	Etanercept 0.1 mg (Group 1), 0.5 mg (Group 2), 0.75 mg (Group 3), 1.0 mg (Group 4), 1.5 mg (Group 5); subcutaneous injection; administered once	Normal saline; subcutaneous injection; administered once	1-, 3-and 6-month follow-ups; VAS-leg pain, VAS-lower back pain, Oswestry Disability Index [28], overall satisfaction score

Table 1. Cont.

Trial and study type	Participants	Intervention TNF-α inhibitor group	Control group	Outcome (follow-up duration and outcome measures)
8 Becker *et al.* [18], RCT	n = 84, and the average age was 54 years; males accounted for 62% of the participants; the duration of the symptoms was at least 6 weeks	Autologous conditioned serum (Group 1); epidural injections; administered three times	Triamcinolone 5 mg or 10 mg + local anesthetic 1 ml (Group 2 or Group 3); epidural injection; administered three times	6-, 10- and 22-week follow-ups; VAS-lower back pain, Oswestry Disability Index [28], adverse reaction
9 Korhonen *et al.* [11,16,19], RCT	n = 40, and the average age was 40 years; the males accounted for 60%; the mean duration of the symptoms was 61 days	Infliximab 5 mg/kg; intravenous injection; administered once	Normal saline; intravenous injection; administered once	Korhonen *et al.* [19]: 3-month follow-up; The straight leg-raising test, VAS-leg pain, VAS-lower back pain, Oswestry Disability Index [28]
				Autio *et al.* [11]: 6-month follow-up; The volume (mm³), thickness (mm) and the rim enhancement (%) of herniated nucleus pulposus, the number of resected discs, swelling of the nerve root
				Korhonen *et al.* [16]: 12-month follow-up; The straight leg-raising test, VAS-leg pain, VAS-lower back pain, Oswestry Disability Index [28], RAND-36-item health questionnaire [31], the number of resected discs, adverse reaction
10 Karppinen *et al.* [9] and Korhonen *et al.* [27], non-RCT	n = 72, and the average age was 39 years; the males accounted for 80%; the mean duration of the symptoms was 7.2 weeks	Infliximab 3 mg/kg; intravenous injection; administered once	Normal saline; Periradicular injection; administered once	Karppinen *et al* [9]: 3-month follow-up; The number of painless patients (75% decrease from baseline leg pain score), VAS-leg pain
				Korhonen *et al* [27]: 6- and 12-month follow-ups; VAS-leg pain, VAS-lower back pain, Oswestry Disability Index [28], the number of sick leave days; clinical status, adverse effects
11 Genevay *et al.* [8], non-RCT	n = 20, and the average age was 47 years; the males accounted for 50%; the mean duration of the symptoms was 3.2 weeks	Etanercept 25 mg; subcutaneous injection; every 3 days; administered three	Methylprednisolone; 250 mg, intravenous injection; administered three	6-weeks follow-up; The numbers with a good clinical result (leg pain VAS<30 or Oswestry Disability Index<20); VAS-leg pain, VAS-lower back pain, Oswestry Disability Index [28]; Roland Morris Disability Questionnaire (RMDQ) [32], the number of discectomies

RCT randomized controlled trial, non-RCT non-randomized control trial, VAS visual analogue scale.
[1]mean ± standard deviation.
[2]median (range).

histogram was obtained from the forest plots of the study conducted by Williams *et al.* [10]. The extracted data mainly included the sample size, intervention measures, the Oswestry Disability Index, VAS-leg pain, VAS-lower back pain, global perceived effect (satisfaction) or return to work (combined endpoint), and discectomy or radicular block (combined endpoint) of the experimental and control groups at various follow-up points.

Quality Evaluation

One investigator performed a methodology quality assessment of all included studies based on a 17-item quality evaluating system [25].

Statistical Analysis

Using WMD, standardized mean difference (SMD) and RR, we performed a systematic review and meta-analysis of the aforementioned five endpoints according to the follow-up time and the type of control drugs used. For global perceived effect (satisfaction) or return to work (combined endpoint), an RR>1 indicated that the outcomes of the TNF-α inhibitor group were superior to those of the control group; for discectomy or radicular block (combined endpoint), an RR<1 indicated that the outcomes of the TNF-α inhibitor group were superior to those of the control group; for Oswestry Disability Index, VAS-leg, and VAS-lower back, a negative WMD or SMD indicated that the outcomes of the TNF-α inhibitor group were superior to those of the control group. The data from reports concerning same trial were used for the analysis of the corresponding follow-up. Prior to the meta-analysis, for each

Table 2. Methodological quality scoring [25] for all trials.

Check list item	Trials										
	1 [13,15]	2 [21]	3 [12]	4 [22]	5 [20]	6 [17]	7 [14]	8 [18]	9 [11,16,19]	10 [9,27]	11 [8]
1. Is there a rationale for the study?	yes	yes	yes	yes	yes	yes	yes	yes	yes	yes	yes
2. Is a clear study objective/goal defined?	yes	yes	yes	yes	yes	yes	yes	yes	yes	no	yes
3. Are key elements of study design described (e.g. how were participants identified/recruited)?	yes	yes	yes	yes	yes	yes	yes	yes	yes	no	yes
4. Are the setting and selection criteria for the study population described?	yes	yes	yes	yes	yes	yes	yes	yes	yes	yes	yes
5. Is the follow-up period appropriate?	yes	yes	no	yes	yes	yes	yes	yes	yes	yes	no
6. Are there any strategies to avoid loss to follow-up or address missing data?	no	no	no	no	no	no	no	no	no	no	no
7. Is the sample size justified?	no	no	no	no	no	no	no	no	no	no	no
8. Is information presented about the instruments used to measure the prognostic variable(s), and does this enable replication (through the use of standardized or valid measures)?	yes	yes	yes	yes	yes	yes	yes	yes	yes	yes	yes
9. Is the outcome selected and assessed appropriately?	yes	yes	yes	yes	yes	yes	yes	yes	yes	yes	yes
10. Is the study sample described (demographic/clinical characteristics)?	yes	yes	yes	no	yes	yes	yes	no	yes	yes	yes
11. Is the final sample representative of the study's target population?	yes	yes	yes	yes	no	yes	yes	yes	yes	no	no
12. Is loss to follow-up ≤20%? (If not, are there any significant differences in baseline variables between responders and non-responders to follow-up? If yes, have the implications been considered?)	yes	yes	yes	yes	no	yes	yes	yes	yes	yes	yes
13. Are the main results reported (including the prevalence of prognostic indicator(s) and outcome, strength of association, and statistical significance)?	yes	yes	yes	yes	yes	yes	yes	yes	yes	yes	yes
14. Is the statistical analysis appropriate and described?	yes	yes	yes	no	yes	yes	yes	yes	yes	yes	yes
15. Were potential confounders and effect modifiers identified and accounted for (e.g. multivariate analysis)?	yes	yes	yes	yes	yes	yes	yes	yes	yes	no	no
16. Do the findings support the authors' interpretations?	yes	yes	yes	yes	yes	yes	yes	yes	yes	yes	yes
17. Do the authors discuss study limitations (e.g. biases/generalizability)?	no	yes	yes	no	yes	no	no	no	no	no	no
Total	14	15	14	12	13	14	14	13	14	10	11

Scoring: Total number of "yes" answers provides the overall score. 0 to 10 = poor quality, 11 to 14 = adequate quality, 15 to 17 = high quality [25].

endpoint, Cochran's Q statistic test was applied to assess the heterogeneity among the included studies. If a p-value of Cochran's Q statistic (Qp) ≥0.10, which indicated the absence of heterogeneity, a fixed-effects model was applied; otherwise, a random effects model was applied for analysis. Stata statistical software version SE 12.0 (Stata Corp LP, College Station, TX, USA) was utilized for all statistical analysis.

Results

Search Results

A total of 113 records were identified through database searches, and 16 remained [8,9,11–22,26,27] after the exclusion of unrelated and repeated studies through a careful review of the titles, abstracts and partial main text. After the exclusion of one trial that was published as an abstract without full text available [26], 15 papers were ultimately enrolled in our study [8,9,11–22,27]. These 15 papers included nine RCTs [11–22,27], two non-RCT (before-after controlled trials) [8,9,27], involving 531 patients; two of the trials were reports of the data from the 6-month and 36-month follow-up of the NCT00470509 trial [13,15], three of the trials were the reports of the data from the 3-month, 6-month and 12-month follow-ups of the FIRST II trial [11,16,19], and two records were the reports of the data from the 3-month, 6-month and 12-month follow-ups of same trial [9,27]. Among the included trials, seven used placebos as a control [9,14–17,20,22], three used steroids as a control [8,12,18], and one used placebos and steroids as a dual control [21]; eight trials involved local injection [8,12–14,18,20–22], and three involved a systematic medication [9,16,17]; the drugs were administered once in seven trials [9,12,14,16,17,22], twice in three trials [13,20,21], and three times in two trial [8,18]; six trials adopted VAS scoring in a range of 0 to100 [8,9,15–18], and five adopted VAS scoring in a range of 0 to 10 [12,14,20–22]. Figure 1 shows the screening process. The major features of the 11 trials are listed in Table 1.

Quality of all included studies

Table 2 lists the quality scores of the 11 trials, including one with high quality [21], nine with middle quality (12 records) [8,11–20,22], and one with poor quality (two records) [9,27].

Oswestry Disability Index

The trial by Cohen et al. [20] demonstrated there was no statistical difference in the Oswestry Disability Index between the two groups at post-injection Month 1 and Month 6 (p=0.11, p=0.78). Another trial by Cohen et al. [14] showed that there was no intragroup or intergroup difference in the Oswestry Disability Index at post-injection Month 1, while the Oswestry Disability Index was restored to the baseline level at post-injection Month 6. The trial conducted by Karppinen et al. [17] also indicated that there was no statistical difference in the Oswestry Disability Index between the two groups at post-injection Month 6 (p=0.52). In addition, in the FIRST II trial, there was no statistical difference in the Oswestry Disability Index between the two groups at post-injection Month 3 and Month 12 (p=0.37, p=0.79) [16,19].

The results derived from the meta-analysis showed that compared with the placebo group, the TNF-α inhibitor group had a WMD of −5.34 (−14.50 to 3.82, p=0.254, n=7) at the post-injection short-term follow-up, −8.19 (−14.53 to −1.84, p=0.011, n=5) at the medium-term follow-up (The sensitivity analysis demonstrated that after the exclusion of a low-quality trial [27], WMD=8.69, 95% CI 19.00 to 1.61, p=0.098, n=4), and −0.73 (−9.94 to 8.48, p=0.877, n=3) at the long-term follow-up; compared with the steroid group, the TNF-α inhibitor group had

a WMD of −0.82 (−5.99 to 4.36, p=0.757, n=5) at the post-injection short-term follow-up and 0.48 (−2.75 to 3.72, p=0.771, n=2) at the medium-term follow-up (Figure 2).

VAS-leg pain

The trial by Cohen et al. [20] showed no statistical difference in the reduction of VAS between the two groups at post-injection Month 1 (p=0.15). Another trial by Cohen et al. [14] indicated there was no difference in the VAS between the two groups at post-injection Month 1 [14]. The trial by Karppinen et al. [17] showed no statistical difference in the reduction of leg pain between the two groups at post-injection Month 6 (73% vs. 65%, p=0.52). In addition, in the FIRST II trial, there was no statistical difference observed in the VAS-leg pain between the two groups at post-injection Month 3 and Month 12 (p=0.82, p=0.54) [16,19]; moreover, there was no statistical difference in the percentage of patients who achieved a VAS reduction of more than 75% between the two groups at post-injection Month 12 (p=0.72) [16].

The meta-analysis showed that, compared with the placebo group, the TNF-α inhibitor group had an SMD of −0.41 (−0.85 to 0.02, p=0.061, n=7) at the post-injection short-term follow-up, −0.24 (−0.55 to 0.07, p=0.122, n=5) at the medium-term follow-up, and 0.03 (−0.54 to 0.60, p=0.928, n=3) at the long-term follow-up; compared with the steroid group, the TNF-α inhibitor group had an SMD of −1.22 (−3.27 to 0.84, p=0.246, n=3) at the post-injection short-term follow-up (Figure 3).

VAS-lower back pain

A trial by Cohen et al. [20] showed that the VAS-lower back pain of the TNF-α inhibitor group was significantly lower than that of the placebo group (p=0.01) one month after drug injection. The trial by Karppinen et al. [17] showed no statistical difference in the VAS between the two groups at post-injection Months 3 and 6 (p=0.13, p=0.25). In addition, in the FIRST II trial, there was no statistical difference observed in the VAS-lower back pain between the two groups at post-injection Month 3 and Month 12 (p=0.98, p=0.68) [16,19]. The meta-analysis demonstrated that compared with the placebo group, the TNF-α inhibitor group had an SMD of −0.34 (−0.89 to 0.22, p=0.233, n=4) at the post-injection short-term follow-up and −0.28 (−0.85 to 0.29, p=0.332, n=1) at the medium-term follow-up; compared with the steroid group, the TNF-α inhibitor group had an SMD of −0.35 (−1.38 to 0.68, p=0.503, n=3) at the post-injection short-term follow-up (Figure 4).

Global perceived effect (satisfaction) or return to work (combined endpoint)

The trial by Genevay et al. [13] demonstrated no difference in the work capability or physical condition between the two groups, and the trial by Cohen et al. [14] also indicated no intragroup and intergroup difference in the patients' global perceived effect. In the FIRST II trial, no statistical difference was observed between the two groups in the patients' days of sick leave from work because of sciatica (p=0.60) [16]. The meta-analysis indicated that compared with the placebo group, the TNF-α inhibitor group had an RR of 1.19 (0.66 to 2.16, p=0.554, n=5) for global perceived effect (satisfaction) or return to work (combined endpoint) at the post-injection short-term follow-up, 1.18 (0.76 to 1.85, p=0.465, n=5) at the medium-term follow-up and 1.40 (0.81 to 2.44, p=0.231, n=2) at the long-term follow-up; compared with the steroid group, the TNF-α inhibitor group had an RR of 1.10 (0.83 to 1.45, p=0.520, n=2) at the short-term follow-up and 1.25 (0.59 to 2.66, p=0.562, n=1) at the medium-term follow-up (Figure 5).

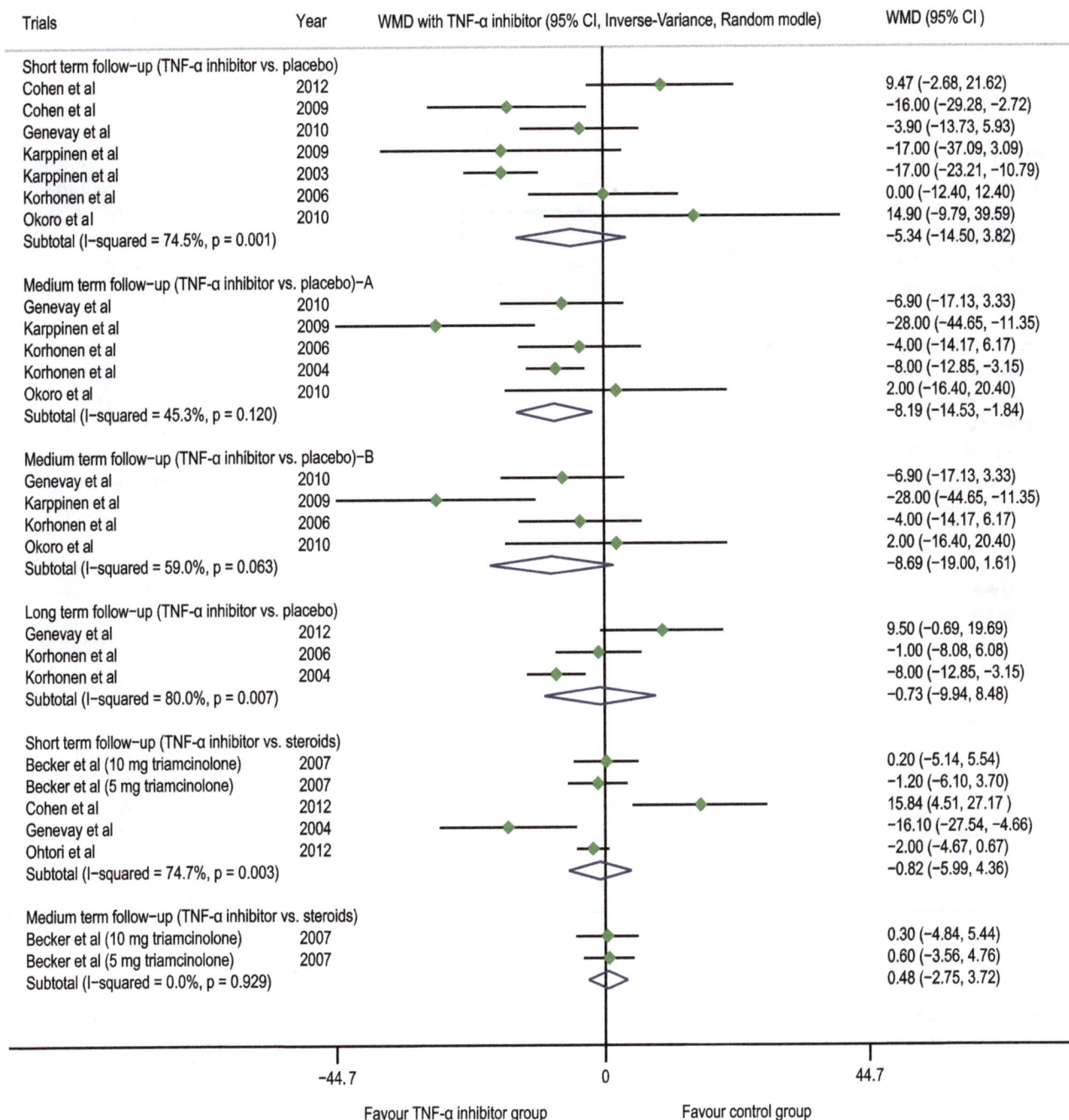

Figure 2. Forest plot of Oswestry Disability Index. The difference in the Oswestry Disability Index (WMD) at the post-injection short-term, medium-term and long-term follow-ups between the TNF-α inhibitor group and placebo group was not statistically significant (p>0.05); there was no statistically significant difference at the post-injection short-term and medium-term follow-ups between the steroid group and the TNF-α inhibitor group (p>0.05). A. Results when the trials with poor quality were included; B. Results when the trials with poor quality were excluded. TNF-α tumor necrosis factor-alpha, CI confidence interval, WMD weighted mean difference.

Discectomy or radicular block (combined endpoint)

The results derived from the meta-analysis indicated that compared with the control group, the TNF-α inhibitor group had an RR of 0.64 (0.17 to 2.40, p = 0.508, n = 4) for the discectomy or radicular block (combined endpoint) at the post-injection short-term follow-up, 0.51 (0.26 to 1.00, p = 0.049, n = 3) at the medium-term follow-up and 0.64 (0.40 to 1.03, p = 0.065, n = 4) at the long-term follow-up (Figure 6A). The sensitivity analysis

showed that after the exclusion of the trials with a systematic drug administration [11,16,27], the RR was 0.47 (0.23 to 0.96, p = 0.037, n = 2) at the medium-term follow-up and 0.52 (0.27 to 1.00, p = 0.049, n = 2) at the long-term follow-up (Figure 6B).

Adverse reaction

Four reports indicated the absence of adverse reaction [11,12,19,22], six reports did not mention adverse reaction

Trials	Year	SMD with TNF-α inhibitor (95% CI, Inverse-Variance, Random modle)	SMD (95% CI)
Short term follow–up (TNF-α inhibitor vs. placebo)			
Cohen et al	2009		−1.70 (−2.75, −0.64)
Cohen et al	2012		−0.06 (−0.58, 0.47)
Genevay et al	2010		0.08 (−0.43, 0.60)
Karppinen et al	2009		−0.56 (−1.60, 0.47)
Karppinen et al	2003		−0.95 (−1.63, −0.26)
Korhonen et al	2006		−0.46 (−1.09, 0.17)
Okoro et al	2010		0.32 (−0.70, 1.34)
Subtotal (I–squared = 60.0%, p = 0.020)			−0.41 (−0.85, 0.02)
Medium term follow–up (TNF-α inhibitor vs. placebo)			
Genevay et al	2010		−0.45 (−0.97, 0.07)
Karppinen et al	2009		−0.40 (−1.43, 0.62)
Korhonen et al	2006		−0.07 (−0.69, 0.55)
Korhonen et al	2004		−0.21 (−0.88, 0.46)
Okoro et al	2010		0.15 (−0.86, 1.17)
Subtotal (I–squared = 0.0%, p = 0.812)			−0.24 (−0.55, 0.07)
Long term follow–up (TNF-α inhibitor vs. placebo)			
Genevay et al	2012		−0.08 (−0.65, 0.48)
Korhonen et al	2006		0.59 (−0.05, 1.22)
Korhonen et al	2004		−0.44 (−1.11, 0.23)
Subtotal (I–squared = 60.0%, p = 0.082)			0.03 (−0.54, 0.60)
Short term follow–up (TNF-α inhibitor vs. steroids)			
Cohen et al	2012		0.58 (0.03, 1.12)
Genevay et al	2004		−2.02 (−3.12, −0.92)
Ohtori et al	2012		−2.26 (−2.83, −1.70)
Subtotal (I–squared = 96.3%, p = 0.000)			−1.22 (−3.27, 0.84)

-3.27   0   3.27

Favour TNF-α inhibitor group   Favour control group

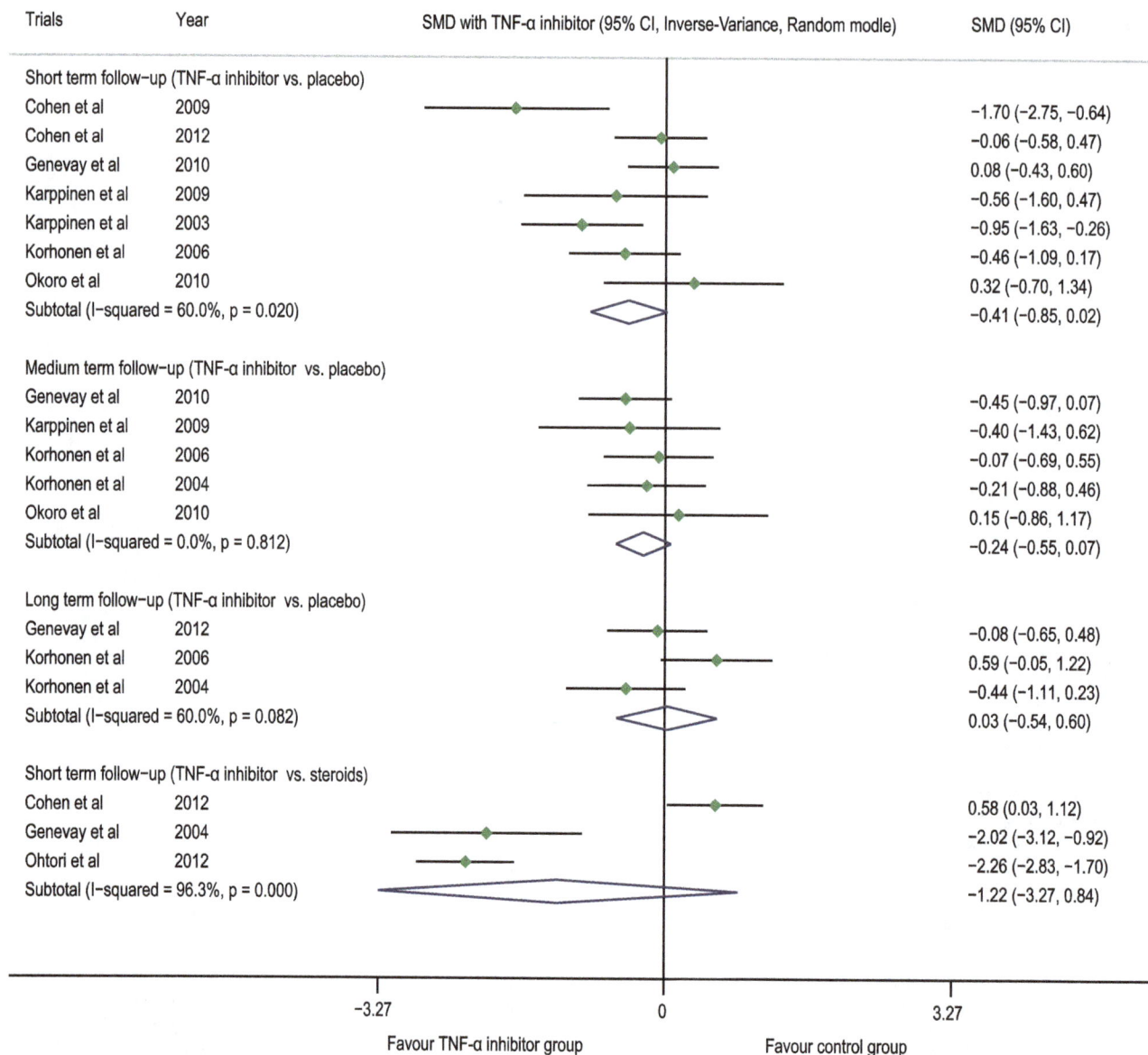

Figure 3. Forest plot of VAS-leg pain. The difference in the VAS-leg (SMD) at the post-injection short-term, medium-term and long-term follow-ups between the TNF-α inhibitor group and placebo group was not statistically significant (p>0.05); there was no statistically significant difference at the post-injection short-term follow-up between the steroid group and the TNF-α inhibitor group (p>0.05). VAS visual analogue scale, TNF-α tumor necrosis factor-alpha, CI confidence interval, SMD standardized mean difference.

[8,9,13,14,20,27], and four reported the occurrence of rhinitis, diarrhea, otitis media, maxillary sinusitis or a skin rash, but with only "mild symptoms" [15–17,21]. One patient had metastasis of cancer cells at the neck [17], and one patient had severe digestive tract bleeding after being treated with non-steroidal anti-inflammatory agents [15]. One trial reported the occurrence of puncture-associated severe headache in both groups [18]. However, there was no evidence proving the relationship between these adverse events and the use of TNF-α inhibitors.

Discussion

The major findings of this study were that TNF-α inhibitors could reduce the RR of discectomy or radicular block (combined endpoint) at medium-term follow-up, but not at short-term and

long-term follow-ups; during the natural disease course, TNF-α inhibitors neither provided additional pain relief nor improved the percentage of global perceived effect (satisfaction) or return to work (combined endpoint); the observed adverse reaction were mild and could not be proven to have any association with the use of TNF-α inhibitors.

Previous studies have found that in patients with intervertebral disc herniation, the TNF-α level on the articular surface increased [33]; the TNF-α mRNA level on the annulus fibrosus, nucleus pulposus and the yellow ligaments increased [34]; and the content of nucleus pulposus leaked to the epidural cavity, causing local acute inflammation, fiber deposition and adhesion [5]. The inflammatory reactions mediated by various biochemical and immunological factors can disturb intraradicular blood flow and disrupt the nerve-blood barrier, thus leading to swelling and

Trials	Year	SMD with TNF-α inhibitor (95% CI, Inverse-Variance, Random modle)	SMD (95% CI)
Short term follow-up (TNF-α inhibitor vs. placebo)			
Cohen et al	2012		0.29 (−0.24, 0.82)
Cohen et al	2009		−1.30 (−2.30, −0.30)
Genevay et al	2010		−0.42 (−0.95, 0.10)
Karppinen et al	2003		−0.30 (−0.97, 0.37)
Subtotal (I-squared = 65.5%, p = 0.033)			−0.34 (−0.89, 0.22)
Medium term follow-up (TNF-α inhibitor vs. placebo)			
Genevay et al	2012		−0.28 (−0.85, 0.29)
Subtotal (I-squared = .%, p = .)			−0.28 (−0.85, 0.29)
Short term follow-up (TNF-α inhibitor vs. steroids)			
Cohen et al	2012		0.53 (−0.02, 1.07)
Genevay et al	2004		−1.97 (−3.05, −0.88)
Ohtori et al	2012		0.00 (−0.44, 0.44)
Subtotal (I-squared = 87.7%, p = 0.000)			−0.35 (−1.38, 0.68)

```
        −3.05                    0                    3.05
   Favour TNF-α inhibitor group        Favour control group
```

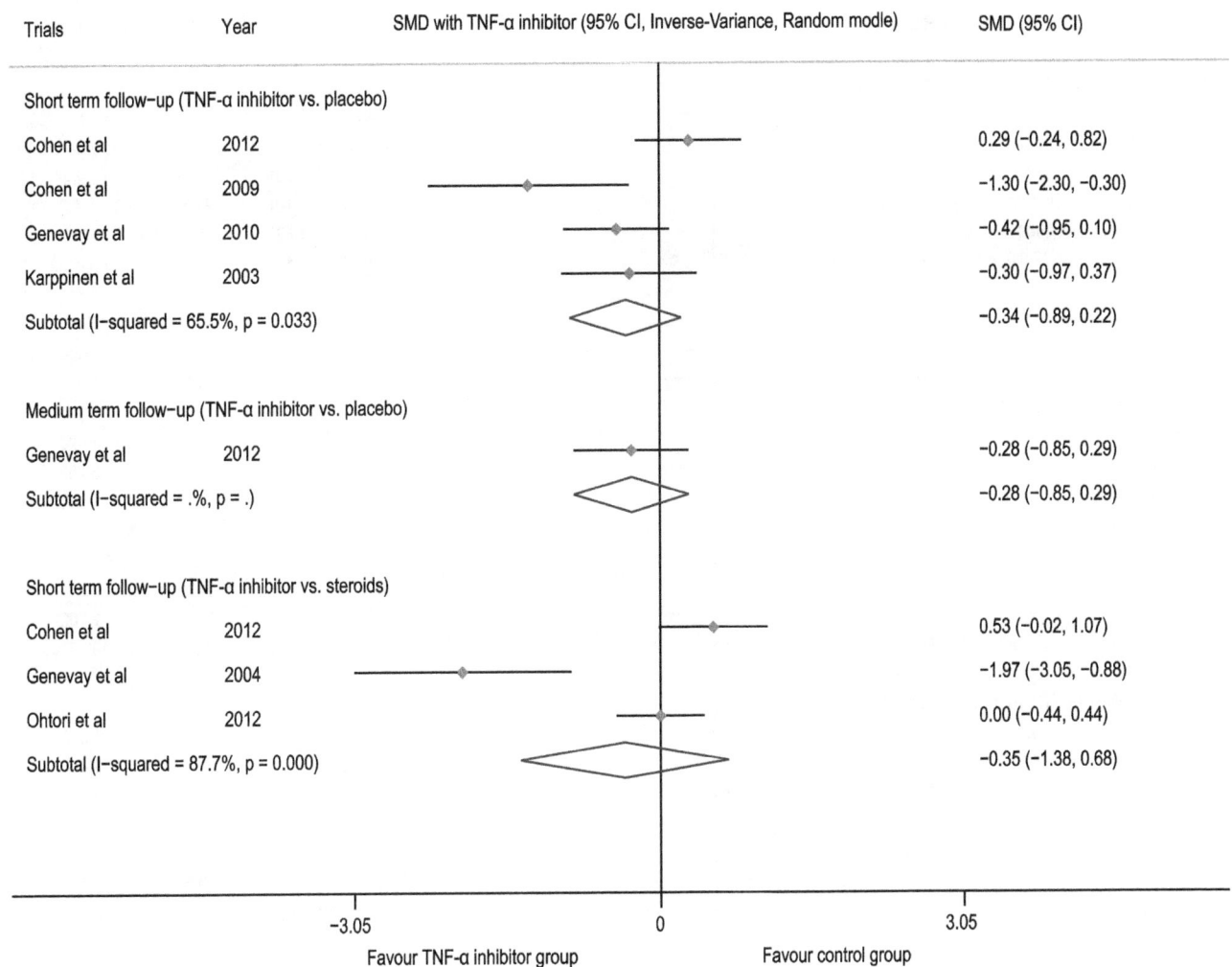

Figure 4. Forest plot of VAS-lower back pain. The difference in the VAS-lower back (SMD) at the post-injection short-term and medium-term follow-ups between the TNF-α inhibitor group and placebo group was not statistically significant (p>0.05); there was no statistically significant difference at the post-injection short-term follow-up between the steroid group and the TNF-α inhibitor group (p>0.05). VAS visual analogue scale, TNF-α tumor necrosis factor-alpha, CI confidence interval, SMD standardized mean difference.

demyelination of the nerve root [35]. TNF-α is a pleiotropic cytokine, which can induce inflammatory responses of synapses and myelin sheath [35], promote cellular apoptosis due to its cytotoxic effect [6], and induce nerve swelling and neuropathic pain [35]. Thus, this cytokine plays a pivotal role in the pathophysiology of sciatica [36]. Animal experiments and clinical studies have revealed that TNF-α inhibitors can prevent the decline of nucleus pulposus-induced neural transmission speed and neural damage and thus have a protective effect on neurodegeneration [7,37,38]. The results from clinical trials in terms of the efficacy of TNF-α inhibitors on decreasing the RR of discectomy or radicular block (combined endpoint) are inconsistent; a portion of the trials showed positive results [13,15], whereas others reported that TNF-α inhibitors had efficacy similar to that of placebos [8,9,11,12,14,16–22,27]. In this study, we found that TNF-α inhibitors could decrease the RR of discectomy or radicular block (combined endpoint) at the medium-term follow-up. We conservatively speculate that this effect might be related to their anti-inflammatory and neuroprotective functions.

Our explanations regarding the finding that TNF-α inhibitors could reduce the risk of discectomy or radicular block (combined endpoint) but could not improve the pain were as follows: (1) TNF-α inhibitors reduce the risk of discectomy or radicular block (combined endpoint) because of their neuroprotective function. Genevay et al. [13,15] believe that TNF-α inhibitors might have a "delayed mode of action on sciatica" or protective function on the nerve root, and thus the physical condition could recover better with TNF-α inhibitors; this result should be considered during the selection of discectomy. The trial by Korhonen et al. [27] showed that the recovery rate of nerve abnormalities was much higher in the TNF-α inhibitor group than in the control group (p = 0.001), indirectly indicating that TNF-α inhibitors had a protective effect on sciatic nerves. Because of this neuroprotective effect, TNF-α inhibitors can promote the recovery of physical function and reduce the risk of discectomy or radicular block (combined endpoint). (2) The anti-inflammatory effect of TNF-α inhibitors is not parallel to their pain-controlling effect. The mechanisms underlying leg pain and lower back pain remain unclear [39].

Trials	Year	RR with TNF-α inhibitor (95% CI, Mantel-Haenszel, Random modle)	RR (95% CI)	Events, TNF-α inhibitor	Events, Control
Short term follow-up (TNF-α inhibitor vs. placebo)					
Cohen et al	2009		3.89 (0.66, 22.84)	14/18	1/5
Cohen et al	2007		0.33 (0.11, 1.03)	5/30	3/6
Cohen et al	2012		0.98 (0.53, 1.79)	11/26	13/30
Genevay et al	2010		1.01 (0.73, 1.40)	22/31	21/30
Karppinen et al	2003		2.55 (1.44, 4.53)	7/10	17/62
Subtotal (I-squared = 72.8%, p = 0.005)			1.19 (0.66, 2.16)	59/115	55/133
Medium term follow-up (TNF-α inhibitor vs. placebo)					
Cohen et al	2012		0.77 (0.42, 1.41)	10/26	15/30
Cohen et al	2007		0.20 (0.01, 2.77)	1/30	1/6
Cohen et al	2009		4.33 (0.71, 26.53)	13/18	1/6
Genevay et al	2010		1.09 (0.74, 1.62)	22/31	13/20
Korhonen et al	2004		1.65 (1.11, 2.47)	8/10	30/62
Subtotal (I-squared = 53.0%, p = 0.075)			1.18 (0.76, 1.85)	54/115	60/124
Long term follow-up (TNF-α inhibitor vs. placebo)					
Korhonen et al	2006		1.06 (0.67, 1.67)	14/21	12/19
Korhonen et al	2004		1.84 (1.21, 2.80)	8/10	27/62
Subtotal (I-squared = 68.6%, p = 0.074)			1.40 (0.81, 2.44)	22/31	39/81
Short term follow-up (TNF-α inhibitor vs. steroids)					
Cohen et al	2012		0.85 (0.47, 1.51)	11/26	14/28
Ohtori et al	2012		1.17 (0.93, 1.48)	34/40	29/40
Subtotal (I-squared = 19.0%, p = 0.267)			1.10 (0.83, 1.45)	45/66	43/68
Medium term follow-up (TNF-α inhibitor vs. steroids)					
Cohen et al	2012		1.25 (0.59, 2.66)	10/26	8/26
Subtotal (I-squared = .%, p = .)			1.25 (0.59, 2.66)	10/26	8/26

0.0144   1   69.3

Favour control group   Favour TNF-α inhibitor group

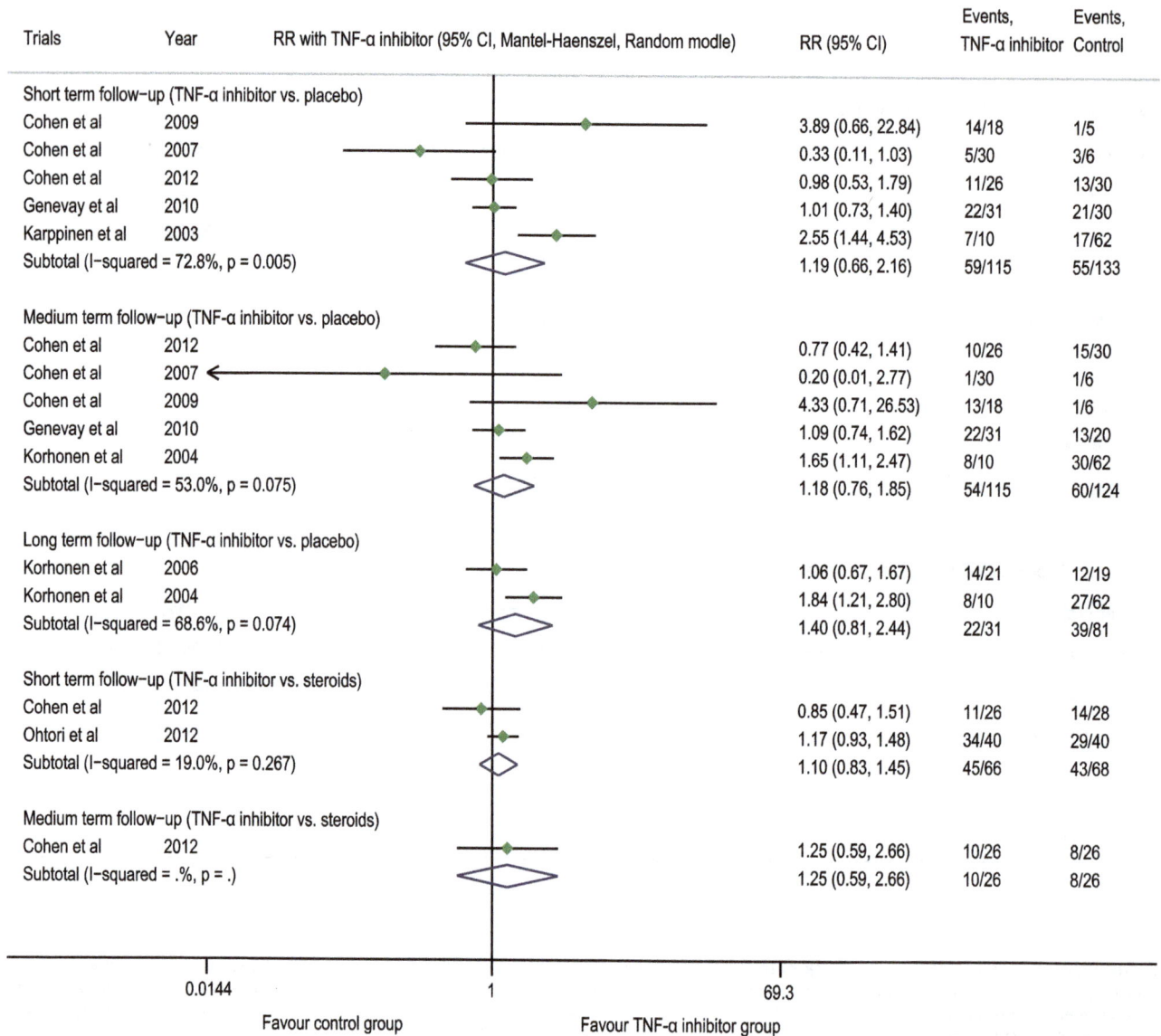

Figure 5. Forest plot of global perceived effect (satisfaction) or return to work (combined endpoint). The difference in the RR of global perceived effect (satisfaction) or return to work (combined endpoint) at the post-injection short-term, medium-term, and long-term follow-ups between the TNF-α inhibitor group and placebo group was not statistically significant (p>0.05); there was no statistically significant difference at the post-injection short-term and medium-term follow-ups between the steroid group and the TNF-α inhibitor group (p>0.05). TNF-α tumor necrosis factor-alpha, CI confidence interval, RR risk ratio.

Scholars generally believe the pain might result from the mechanical, chemical and inflammatory irritation of sinuvertebral nerves [40,41], while the pain might be associated with unstable lumbar spine or spinal stenosis in addition to inflammatory responses in a portion of patients. The trial by Andrade *et al.* [42] found that in the patients with disc herniation, the expression of TNF-α, IL-1β and IL-6 increased significantly, but the expression levels of these cytokines were unrelated to the lower back pain; therefore, the authors concluded that "these cytokines may not play a leading role in maintaining a pain generating network", indicating that TNF is not the sole inflammatory factor and TNF-mediated inflammatory response is not the leading cause responsible for the pain of disc herniation patients. Moreover, some studies demonstrated that the TNF-α expression level in the

annulus fibrosus is negatively related to VAS [34], suggesting that TNF-mediated inflammatory response is not parallel to the level of pain. Therefore, TNF-α inhibitors administered for anti-inflammation might not be sufficient to simultaneously control both leg pain and lower back pain. (3) It is difficult to relieve the pain of patients who had a long disease course. Animal experiments have revealed that treatment immediately after the nerve root injury could be effective, while drug administration 10 days after the injury is often ineffective because of the occurrence of neuropathic pain [43]. Therefore, in the trials enrolled in the present study, the pain of patients with a disease course longer than 10 days was difficult to reduce. (4) Pain is not a decisive factor for the selection of discectomy. In clinical practice, the selection of discectomy depends mainly on the functional status, particularly the degree of

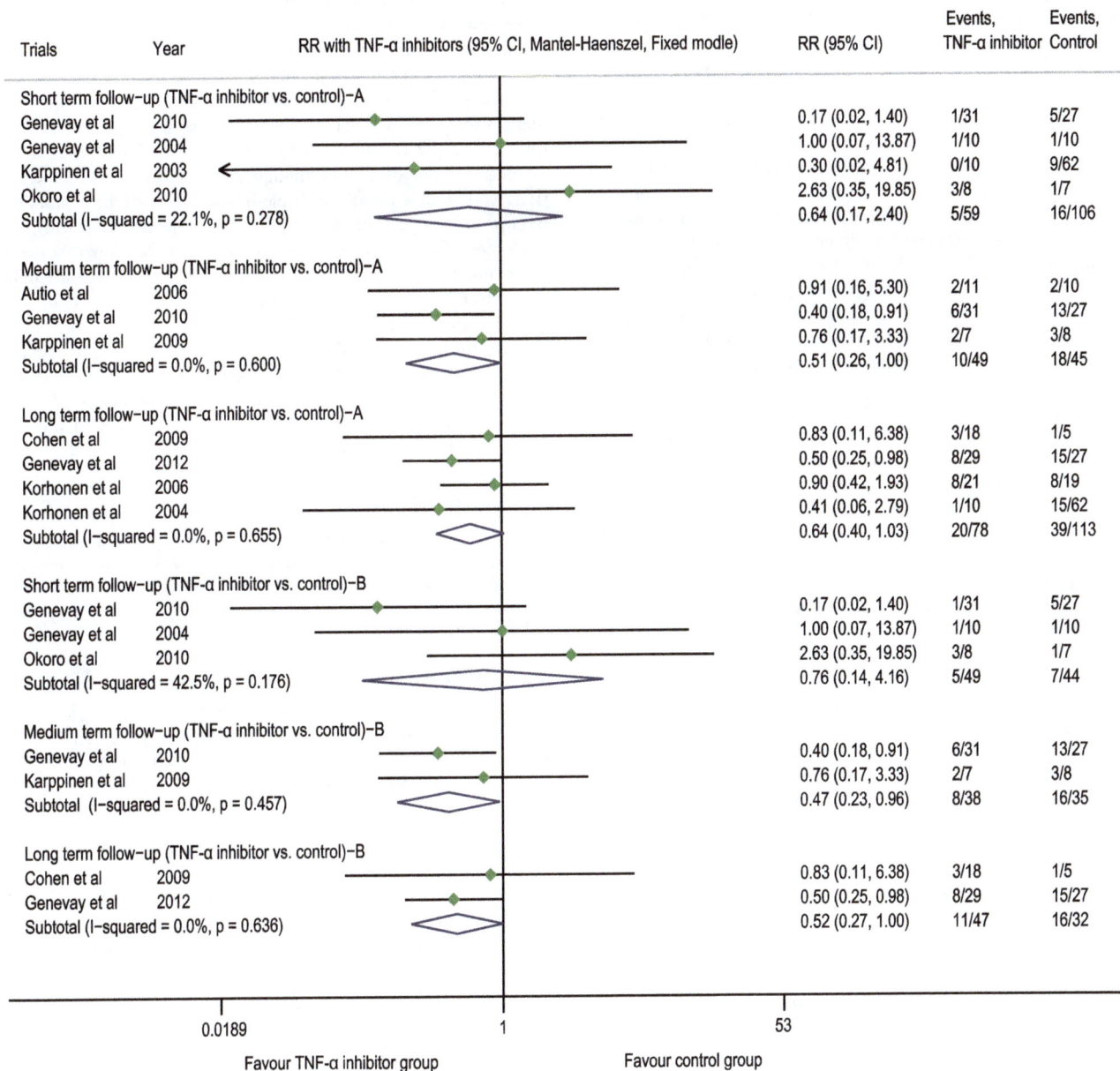

Figure 6. Forest plot of discectomy of the radicular block (combined endpoint). The difference in the RR of discectomy or the radicular block (combined endpoint) at the post-injection short-term and long-term follow-ups between the TNF-α inhibitor group and placebo group was not statistically significant (p>0.05). At the medium-term follow-up, the RR of the TNF-α inhibitor group was 66% of that of the placebo group; after the exclusion of the three trials involving a systemic medication, the RR of the TNF-α inhibitor group was 47% of that of the placebo group at the medium-term follow-up, and was 52% of that of the placebo group at the long-term follow-up. A. Results when the trials involving a systemic medication were included; B. Results when the trials involving a systemic medication were excluded. TNF-α tumor necrosis factor-alpha, CI confidence interval, RR risk ratio.

disability. Some scholars have stated that the disability level is unrelated to the acute or chronic pain [18]. Parameters such as the Oswestry Disability Index and the VAS are based on pain and thus cannot be used to assess the overall functional status of patients. In addition, Korhonen et al. [27] stated that there is no direct correlation between the selection of discectomy and the Oswestry Disability Index.

Interestingly, we found that TNF-α inhibitors could reduce the RR of discectomy or radicular block (combined endpoint) at medium-term follow-up, but not at short-term and long-term follow-up. Regarding this phenomenon, our explanations are as

follows: (1) the neuroprotective role of TNF-α inhibitors cannot been fulfilled within a short period of time; (2) we conservatively speculated that TNF-α-related inflammation and neurotoxicity are not the major pathophysiological mechanisms of sciatica; thus, TNF-α inhibitors might not exhibit clinical value at long-term follow-up; (3) the bias of drug administration approaches might be involved in this result. Although the currently available evidence is not sufficient to determine the superiority of local injection and systematic drug administration, the efficacy of intravenous injection is dubious. The sensitivity analysis demonstrated that after the exclusion of three trials in which the drugs were administered through intravenous injection [11,16,27], TNF-α inhibitors significantly decreased the risk of discectomy or radicular block (combined endpoint; p = 0.049; Figure 6B). In addition, Ohtori *et al.* [12] stated their negative opinion regarding the use of intravenous injection. Moreover, the ineffectiveness of intravenously administered steroids was also indicated in other studies [44].

Regarding the finding that TNF-α inhibitors reduced the risk of discectomy or radicular block (combined endpoint) but did not increase the percentage of global perceived effect (satisfaction) or return to work (combined endpoint), we believe a possible explanation could be as following: the endpoint, global perceived effect (satisfaction) or return to work (combined endpoint), is related to the patients' self-perceptions (such as pain), while discectomy or radicular block (combined endpoint) is related more closely to the patients' functional status, particularly in the case of discectomy.

It is worth noting that in this study, we could not draw a definitive conclusion regarding the appropriate selection of the drug dose and the frequency of drug administration based on the current available evidence. Because the endpoint data of both the treatment and control groups changed proportionately (10 times), the differences in the VAS score ranges among the enrolled trials would not affect the quantitative analysis and result interpretation in the meta-analysis using SMD.

Compared with the study by Williams *et al.* [10], the present study has the following differences: (1) This study used SMD for the meta-analysis of endpoints that had a different score range, such as VAS-leg pain and VAS-lower back pain. (2) The meta-analysis of discectomy or radicular block (combined endpoint) was conducted using the follow-up data from different time points, i.e. short-term, medium-term and long-term, to evaluate the treatment outcomes more precisely. (3) This study discovered that TNF-α inhibitors cannot provide additional pain relief at all follow-up

periods, but they can reduce the RR of discectomy or radicular block (combined endpoint) at the medium-term follow-up.

The limitations of this study are as follows: (1) the sample size was small, and the follow-up durations were inconsistent; (2) the data showed a skewed distribution, and data expressed with the mean value and without a standard deviation (e.g. the trial of Okoro *et al.* [22]) could not be included in the quantitative analysis of measurement data; (3) although the majority of the included trials were double-blinded or triple-blinded, most of the evaluating parameters adopted in these trials were subjective, and thus the outcomes of natural disease course or the medication treatment could not be distinguished; (4) most of the included trials only showed the results of the treatment analysis rather than the intention-to-treat (ITT) analysis.

Conclusion: According to the currently existing evidence, other than reducing the RR of discectomy of the radicular block (combined endpoint) at the medium-term follow-up, TNF-α inhibitors have limited clinical value in the treatment of sciatica caused by disc herniation and/or spinal stenosis.

Acknowledgments

We sincerely thank Mr. Ya Jun Li (the Library of Hubei University of Medicine) for his help with the literature search. We also greatly appreciate the help of Dr. Hui Nie. (diyahui912@gmail.com) with the translation of this paper.

Ethical approval. Not required.

Author Contributions

Conceived and designed the experiments: YFW GJL JL. Analyzed the data: YFW GJL JL. Wrote the paper: YFW GJL JL. Performed the systematic review and meta-analysis: YFW GJL JL. Data extraction and quality evaluation: PYC WC FQZ LLX SLW LYC.

References

1. Luijsterburg PA, Verhagen AP, Ostelo RW, van Os TA, Peul WC, et al. (2007) Effectiveness of conservative treatments for the lumbosacral radicular syndrome: a systematic review. Eur Spine J 16: 881–899.

2. Buenaventura RM, Datta S, Abdi S, Smith HS (2009) Systematic review of therapeutic lumbar transforaminal epidural steroid injections. Pain Physician 12: 233–251.

3. Lewis R, Williams N, Matar HE, Din N, Fitzsimmons D, et al. (2011) The clinical effectiveness and cost-effectiveness of management strategies for sciatica: systematic review and economic model. Health Technol Assess 15: 1–578.

4. Jacobs WC, van Tulder M, Arts M, Rubinstein SM, van Middelkoop M, et al. (2011) Surgery versus conservative management of sciatica due to a lumbar herniated disc: a systematic review. Eur Spine J 20: 513–522.

5. Lee JH, Lee SH (2012) Clinical effectiveness of percutaneous adhesiolysis using Navicath for the management of chronic pain due to lumbosacral disc herniation. Pain Physician 15: 213–221.

6. Kawakami M, Tamaki T, Matsumoto T, Kuribayashi K, Takenaka T, et al. (2000) Role of leukocytes in radicular pain secondary to herniated nucleus pulposus. Clin Orthop Relat Res: 268–277.

7. Chia S, Qadan M, Newton R, Ludlam CA, Fox KA, et al. (2003) Intra-arterial tumor necrosis factor-alpha impairs endothelium-dependent vasodilatation and stimulates local tissue plasminogen activator release in humans. Arterioscler Thromb Vasc Biol 23: 695–701.

8. Genevay S, Stingelin S, Gabay C (2004) Efficacy of etanercept in the treatment of acute, severe sciatica: a pilot study. Ann Rheum Dis 63: 1120–1123.

9. Karppinen J, Korhonen T, Malmivaara A, Paimela L, Kyllonen E, et al. (2003) Tumor necrosis factor-alpha monoclonal antibody, infliximab, used to manage severe sciatica. Spine (Phila Pa 1976) 28: 750–753; discussion 753–754.

10. Williams NH, Lewis R, Din NU, Matar HE, Fitzsimmons D, et al. (2013) A systematic review and meta-analysis of biological treatments targeting tumour necrosis factor alpha for sciatica. Eur Spine J.

11. Autio RA, Karppinen J, Niinimaki J, Ojala R, Veeger N, et al. (2006) The effect of infliximab, a monoclonal antibody against TNF-alpha, on disc herniation resorption: a randomized controlled study. Spine (Phila Pa 1976) 31: 2641–2645.

12. Ohtori S, Miyagi M, Eguchi Y, Inoue G, Orita S, et al. (2012) Epidural administration of spinal nerves with the tumor necrosis factor-alpha inhibitor, etanercept, compared with dexamethasone for treatment of sciatica in patients

with lumbar spinal stenosis: a prospective randomized study. Spine (Phila Pa 1976) 37: 439–444.

13. Genevay S, Finckh A, Zufferey P, Viatte S, Balague F, et al. (2012) Adalimumab in acute sciatica reduces the long-term need for surgery: a 3-year follow-up of a randomised double-blind placebo-controlled trial. Ann Rheum Dis 71: 560–562.

14. Cohen SP, Wenzell D, Hurley RW, Kurihara C, Buckenmaier CC, et al. (2007) A double-blind, placebo-controlled, dose-response pilot study evaluating intradiscal etanercept in patients with chronic discogenic low back pain or lumbosacral radiculopathy. Anesthesiology 107: 99–105.

15. Genevay S, Viatte S, Finckh A, Zufferey P, Balague F, et al. (2010) Adalimumab in severe and acute sciatica: a multicenter, randomized, double-blind, placebo-controlled trial. Arthritis Rheum 62: 2339–2346.

16. Korhonen T, Karppinen J, Paimela L, Malmivaara A, Lindgren KA, et al. (2006) The treatment of disc-herniation-induced sciatica with infliximab: one-year follow-up results of FIRST II, a randomized controlled trial. Spine (Phila Pa 1976) 31: 2759–2766.

17. Karppinen J, Korhonen T, Hammond A, Bowman C, Malmivaara A, et al. (2009) The Efficacy of Infliximab in Sciatica Induced by Disc Herniations Located at L3/4 or L4/5: A Small-Scale Randomized Controlled Trial. The Open Spine Journal 1: 9–13.

18. Becker C, Heidersdorf S, Drewlo S, de Rodriguez SZ, Kramer J, et al. (2007) Efficacy of epidural perineural injections with autologous conditioned serum for lumbar radicular compression: an investigator-initiated, prospective, double-blind, reference-controlled study. Spine (Phila Pa 1976) 32: 1803–1808.

19. Korhonen T, Karppinen J, Paimela L, Malmivaara A, Lindgren KA, et al. (2005) The treatment of disc herniation-induced sciatica with infliximab: results of a randomized, controlled, 3-month follow-up study. Spine (Phila Pa 1976) 30: 2724–2728.

20. Cohen SP, Bogduk N, Dragovich A, Buckenmaier CC, Griffith S, et al. (2009) Randomized, double-blind, placebo-controlled, dose-response, and preclinical safety study of transforaminal epidural etanercept for the treatment of sciatica. Anesthesiology 110: 1116–1126.

21. Cohen SP, White RL, Kurihara C, Larkin TM, Chang A, et al. (2012) Epidural steroids, etanercept, or saline in subacute sciatica: a multicenter, randomized trial. Ann Intern Med 156: 551–559.

22. Okoro T, TS, Longworth S, Sell PJ (2010) Tumor necrosis alpha-blocking agent (etanercept): a triple blind randomized controlled trial of its use in treatment of sciatica. J Spinal Disord Tech 23: 74–77.

23. Higgins JP, Green S (2011) Cochrane handbook for systematic reviewers of interventions version Version 5.1.0 [updated March 2011]. http://handbook. cochrane.org/(accessed July 21, 2013).

24. Liberati A, Altman DG, Tetzlaff J, Mulrow C, Gotzsche PC, et al. (2009) The PRISMA statement for reporting systematic reviews and meta-analyses of studies that evaluate health care interventions: explanation and elaboration. PLoS Med 6: e1000100.

25. Ashworth J, Konstantinou K, Dunn KM (2011) Prognostic factors in non-surgically treated sciatica: a systematic review. BMC Musculoskelet Disord 12: 208.

26. Kume K AS, Yamada S (2008) The efficacy and safety of caudal epidural injection with the TNF-alpha antagonist, etanercept, in patients with discherniation-induced sciatica. Results of a randomized, controlled, 1-month follow-up study. Ann Rheum Dis 67(Suppl II): 131.

27. Korhonen T, Karppinen J, Malmivaara A, Autio R, Niinimaki J, et al. (2004) Efficacy of infliximab for disc herniation-induced sciatica: one-year follow-up. Spine (Phila Pa 1976) 29: 2115–2119.

28. Fairbank JC, Couper J, Davies JB, O'Brien JP (1980) The Oswestry low back pain disability questionnaire. Physiotherapy 66: 271–273.

29. Ware JE Jr, Sherbourne CD (1992) The MOS 36-item short-form health survey (SF-36). I. Conceptual framework and item selection. Med Care 30: 473–483.

30. Ware J Jr, Kosinski M, Keller SD (1996) A 12-Item Short-Form Health Survey: construction of scales and preliminary tests of reliability and validity. Med Care 34: 220–233.

31. Hays RD, Morales LS (2001) The RAND-36 measure of health-related quality of life. Ann Med 33: 350–357.

32. Roland M, Morris R (1983) A study of the natural history of back pain. Part I: development of a reliable and sensitive measure of disability in low-back pain. Spine (Phila Pa 1976) 8: 141–144.

33. Igarashi A, Kikuchi S, Konno S, Olmarker K (2004) Inflammatory cytokines released from the facet joint tissue in degenerative lumbar spinal disorders. Spine (Phila Pa 1976) 29: 2091–2095.

34. Andrade P, Visser-Vandewalle V, Philippens M, Daemen MA, Steinbusch HW, et al. (2011) Tumor necrosis factor-alpha levels correlate with postoperative pain severity in lumbar disc hernia patients: opposite clinical effects between tumor necrosis factor receptor 1 and 2. Pain 152: 2645–2652.

35. Di Martino A, Merlini L, Faldini C (2013) Autoimmunity in intervertebral disc herniation: from bench to bedside. Expert Opin Ther Targets 17: 1461–1470.

36. Habtemariam A, Virri J, Gronblad M, Seitsalo S, Karaharju E (1999) The role of mast cells in disc herniation inflammation. Spine (Phila Pa 1976) 24: 1516–1520.

37. Zhou QH, Sumbria R, Hui EK, Lu JZ, Boado RJ, et al. (2011) Neuroprotection with a brain-penetrating biologic tumor necrosis factor inhibitor. J Pharmacol Exp Ther 339: 618–623.

38. Wang X, Feuerstein GZ, Xu L, Wang H, Schumacher WA, et al. (2004) Inhibition of tumor necrosis factor-alpha-converting enzyme by a selective antagonist protects brain from focal ischemic injury in rats. Mol Pharmacol 65: 890–896.

39. Liang C, Li H, Tao Y, Shen C, Li F, et al. (2013) New hypothesis of chronic back pain: low pH promotes nerve ingrowth into damaged intervertebral disks. Acta Anaesthesiol Scand 57: 271–277.

40. Ito K, Creemers L (2013) Mechanisms of Intervertebral Disk Degeneration/ Injury and Pain: A Review. Global Spine J 3: 145–152.

41. Issack PS, Cunningham ME, Pumberger M, Hughes AP, Cammisa FP Jr (2012) Degenerative lumbar spinal stenosis: evaluation and management. J Am Acad Orthop Surg 20: 527–535.

42. Andrade P, Hoogland G, Garcia MA, Steinbusch HW, Daemen MA, et al. (2013) Elevated IL-1beta and IL-6 levels in lumbar herniated discs in patients with sciatic pain. Eur Spine J 22: 714–720.

43. Xie W, Strong JA, Meij JT, Zhang JM, Yu L (2005) Neuropathic pain: early spontaneous afferent activity is the trigger. Pain 116: 243–256.

44. Roncoroni C, Baillet A, Durand M, Gaudin P, Juvin R (2011) Efficacy and tolerance of systemic steroids in sciatica: a systematic review and meta-analysis. Rheumatology (Oxford) 50: 1603–1611.

23

Percutaneous Resolution of Lumbar Facet Joint Cysts as an Alternative Treatment to Surgery

Feng Shuang[1,2], **Shu-Xun Hou**[1]*, **Jia-Liang Zhu**[1], **Dong-Feng Ren**[1], **Zheng Cao**[1], **Jia-Guang Tang**[1]*

1 Department of Orthopaedics, The First Affiliated Hospital of General Hospital of Chinese PLA, Beijing, China, 2 Department of Orthopedics, The 94th Hospital of Chinese PLA, Nanchang, China

Abstract

Purpose: A comprehensive review of the literature in order to analyze data about the success rate of percutaneous resolution of the lumbar facet joint cysts as a conservative management strategy.

Methods: A systematic search for relevant articles published during 1980 to May 2014 was performed in several electronic databases by using the specific MeSH terms and keywords. Most relevant data was captured and pooled for the meta-analysis to achieve overall effect size of treatment along with 95% confidence intervals.

Results: 29 studies were included in the meta-analysis. Follow-up duration as mean ± sd (range) was 16±10.2 (5 days to 5.7 years). Overall the satisfactory results (after short- or long-term follow-up) were achieved in 55.8 [49.5, 62.08] % (pooled mean and 95% CI) of the 544 patients subjected to percutaneous lumbar facet joint cyst resolution procedures. 38.67 [33.3, 43.95] % of this population underwent surgery subsequently to achieve durable relief. There existed no linear relationship between the increasing average duration of follow-up period of individual studies and percent satisfaction from the percutaneous resolutions procedure.

Conclusion: Results shows that the percutaneous cyst resolution procedures have potential to be an alternative to surgical interventions but identification of suitable subjects requires further research.

Editor: Sam Eldabe, The James Cook University Hospital, United Kingdom

Funding: This work was supported by the National Natural Science Foundation of China (No. 81071514). The funders had no role in study design, data collection and analysis, decision to publish, or preparation of the manuscript.

Competing Interests: The authors have declared that no competing interests exist.

* Email: jiaguangtang@yahoo.com.cn (JGT); houshuxun_2000@163.com (SXH)

Introduction

Facet joint cysts of lumbar spine (LFJCs) are benign degenerative outgrowths which are most usually associated with low back pain and radiculopathy. Two types of cysts recognized under this category are the synovial cysts and ganglion cysts [1]. The synovial cysts have vascularized lining filled with xanthochromic fluid and have communication with facet joint while the ganglion cysts are covered by fibrocartilagenous capsule filled with proteinaceous and gelatinous material and do not communicate with joint [2].

These cysts can arise because of the chronic hypermobility of the spinal segments leading to increased and more frequent loading of the zygapophyseal joint (Z-joint; a synovial joint). This causes the accumulation of fibrocartilaginous substances which provide raw material for cyst formation [3,4]. The Z-joint is thought to be involved in the genesis of cysts owing to a degenerative process, not fully understood, though herniation of synovial tissue is frequently perceived [5–7]. The LFJCs are associated with spinal stenosis, nerve root compression, neurogenic claudication and many other neurological disturbances by encroaching the local foramen [8,9].

Although, small scale studies indicate that the prevalence of LFJCs in symptomatic patients is 0.7 to 2.5% (Ayberg et al., 2008) [10], but it may be higher and even increase with increasing longevity. This neuropathological agent is strongly associated with late decades of life and females harbor more than males [1].

Diagnosis of the LFJCs utilize magnetic resonance imaging (MRI) or computed tomography (CT) and to some extent CT myelography. Seldom these cysts resolve spontaneously; mostly require treatment. Various management strategies include bed rest, non-steroidal anti-inflammatory drugs, analgesics, physical therapies, transcutaneous electrical nerve stimulation (TENS), intra-articular steroid injections/epidural steroid instillation with or without cyst rupture and CT or flouroscopy guided aspiration of the cyst materials and surgical interventions such as laminectomy, facetectomy, flavectomy, cyst excision and microsurgery.

Long term relief from the symptoms associated with the LFJCs can be achieved with surgery or percutaneous resolution procedures, however. Surgery is the most effective treatment noted so far but studies indicate that percutaneous cyst resolution procedures can be an alternative to surgery in a well-sized subgroup of patients. Moreover, older and high risk patients who are abstained from surgical interventions due to many reasons can

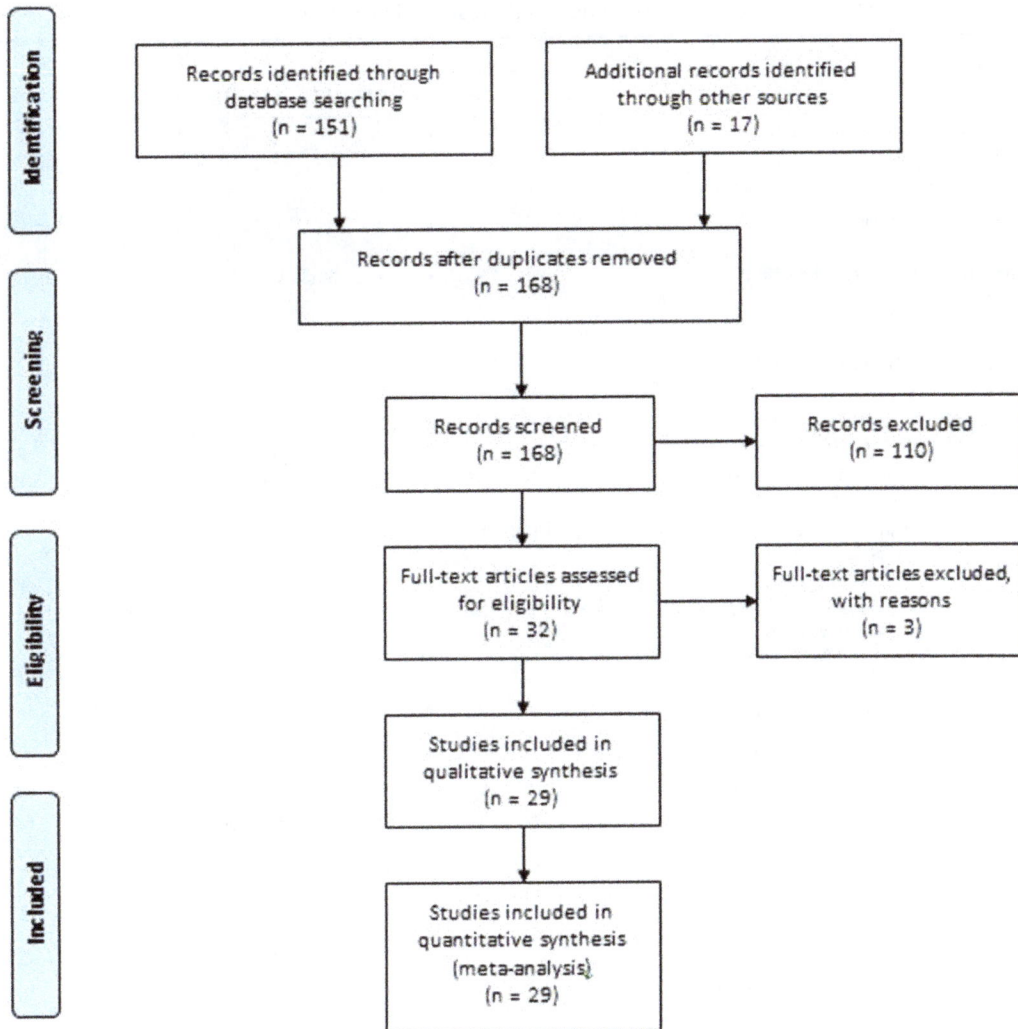

Figure 1. Flowchart of study screening and selection process.

also be benefited from later treatment regimen. In order to explore this avenue, this systematic review and meta-analysis is conducted to evaluate the success rate of percutaneous cyst resolution procedures in terms of durable relief and to attempt the identification of subgroup of patients in which chances success with this technique can be better than surgical intervention.

Materials and Methods

Study Identification

Detailed systematic search was made in several electronic databases including PubMed/Medline, Embase, EBSCO, CINAHL, Ovid SP, SCI Web of Science and Google Scholar under most relevant keywords. MeSH terms and keywords used in various logical combinations included: spinal, lumbar, cyst, synovial, ganglion, juxtafacet, facet, zygapophyseal, magnetic resonance imaging (MRI), computed tomography (CT), conservative management, percutaneous, puncture, rupture, steroid, injection, intra-articular, epidural, facet, joint, effusion. Literature search was restricted to a period from 1980 to May 2014. All retrospective analyses, prospective studies, and individual case reports were taken into consideration.

Selection criteria

The PRISMA guidelines were followed for this study. Because of the scarcity of well-designed clinical trials, selection of studies was made under a broader scope and all studies with prospective or retrospective designs and case reports were included. Inclusion criteria were: a) Studies mentioning percutaneous resolution procedures of LFJCs (synovial/ganglion) such as steroid injections, cyst rupture and cyst material aspiration by utilizing CT/fluoroscopically guided instrumentation; b) studies mentioning a short-term or long-term follow-up of the outcomes and related details, including the provision of data of the subjects who underwent surgical procedures in case of failure of the interventions. Exclusion criteria were: a) studies/case reports intervening other types of similar spinal cyst pathologies such as discal cysts, vertebroplasty etc; b) studies involving percutaneous procedures for the purpose of diagnosis only; and c) studies/case reports utilizing percutaneous procedures for the alleviation of back pain without a diagnosis of LFJC/s; d) studies/case reports which did not contain sufficient details of the outcomes of interventions of interest.

Table 1. Quality Assessment Tool for Observational Cohort and Cross-Sectional Studies.

Criteria	12	13	14	15	16	17	18	19	20	21	22	23	24	25
1. Was the research question or objective in this paper clearly stated?	Y	Y	Y	Y	Y	Y	Y	Y	Y	Y	Y	Y	Y	Y
2. Was the study population clearly specified and defined?	Y	Y	Y	Y	Y	Y	Y	Y	Y	Y	Y	Y	Y	Y
3. Was the participation rate of eligible persons at least 50%?	Y	Y	Y	Y	Y	Y	Y	Y	Y	Y	Y	Y	Y	Y
4. Were all the subjects selected or recruited from the same or similar populations (including the same time period)? Were inclusion and exclusion criteria for being in the study prespecified and applied uniformly to all participants?	Y	Y	Y	Y	Y	Y	Y	Y	Y	Y	Y	Y	Y	Y
5. Was a sample size justification, power description, or variance and effect estimates provided?	N	N	N	N	N	N	Y	N	N	N	N	Y	N	N
6. For the analyses in this paper, were the exposure(s) of interest measured prior to the outcome(s) being measured?	NA	NA	NA	NA	NA	NA	NA	NA	NA	NA	NA	NA	NA	NA
7. Was the timeframe sufficient so that one could reasonably expect to see an association between exposure and outcome if it existed?	N	N	N	Y	Y	N	N	N	Y	N	N	N	N	N
8. For exposures that can vary in amount or level, did the study examine different levels of the exposure as related to the outcome (e.g., categories of exposure, or exposure measured as continuous variable)?	Y	Y	NA	Y	Y	NA	Y	Y	Y	Y	Y	Y	Y	Y
9. Were the exposure measures (independent variables) clearly defined, valid, reliable, and implemented consistently across all study participants?	Y	Y	Y	Y	Y	Y	Y	Y	Y	Y	Y	Y	Y	Y
10. Was the exposure(s) assessed more than once over time?	Y	Y	Y	Y	Y	NR	Y	Y	Y	Y	Y	NR	Y	NR
11. Were the outcome measures (dependent variables) clearly defined, valid, reliable, and implemented consistently across all study participants?	N	N	N	Y	Y	N	Y	N	Y	N	N	N	N	N
12. Were the outcome assessors blinded to the exposure status of participants?	N	N	N	N	N	N	N	N	N	N	N	N	N	N
13. Was loss to follow-up after baseline 20% or less?	CD	CD	CD	CD	CD	CD	CD	CD	CD	CD	CD	CD	CD	CD
14. Were key potential confounding variables measured and adjusted statistically for their impact on the relationship between exposure(s) and outcome(s)?	N	N	N	N	Y	N	Y	N	N	N	N	N	N	N

Legends: CD: Cannot be determined, NA: not applicable, NR: not reported, N: no, Y: yes.

Data extraction, synthesis and analysis

Data were extracted from each research article/case report regarding the demographics of patients, clinical and pathological characteristics, diagnostic tools, procedural features, follow-up period, and outcomes. Outcome measures were the percent satisfactory response of the patient after a reasonable follow-up and the percentage of patients who subsequently underwent surgery. Pooling of dichotomous data (satisfactory outcomes vs surgery requirement) was made by calculating standard errors and 95% confidence intervals (CI) of the data from individual studies and then overall effect size of the meta-analysis was calculated. Forest graphs were plotted manually on the spreadsheets from pooled data and the overall effect size. Descriptive data are presented as mean along with either standard deviation (sd) or range. Quality of the included studies was assessed by using Quality Assessment Tool for Observational Cohort and Cross-Sectional Studies [11].

Results

Search identified 29 articles [12–40] reporting 12 retrospective studies, 2 prospective studies and 15 case reports which are included in this analytical review. Study screening and selection process has been depicted in Figure 1. Quality assessment outcomes are presented in Table 1.

Major characteristics relevant to the manifesto of the present study are present in Table 2. Overall of the 544 subjects included in this meta-analysis, age of the participants as mean $\pm$ sd (range) was 62 ± 4.2 (28–87) years and proportion of females in this population was 64%. Spinal level of the cysts was L_{2-3} in 10, L_{3-4} in 69, L_{4-5} in 384 and L_5–S_1 in 96 cases (Figure 2). Size of the cyst ranged from 6×13 to 12×18 mm. Duration of symptoms before percutaneous resolution interventions ranged from 2 weeks to 60 months. Major conditions associated with the presence of LFJCs in these patients were lower back pain and radiculopathy, especially lower extremity radiculopathy. Symptomatic features at clinical presentation are presented in Table 3.

The procedures involved cyst puncture, rupture, aspiration, intra-articular steroid injection, epidural steroid injection, and local anesthetics injections. These procedures were performed under CT/fluoroscopic guidance, though, not all studies utilized each of these interventions. Arthrography was also performed in majority of cases. Majority of the subjects were diagnosed with MRI (about 85% vs CT about 15%) for harboring one or more

Table 2. Characteristics of the included studies which utilized percutaneous resolution of lumber facet joint procedures.

Study/Design	Patients' characteristics	Pathology	Diagnosis	Intervention	Follow up	Outcome
Allen et al., 2009 [12]/ Retrospective cohort	n: 32; age: 66 (46–86) y; females: 18; Location (L$_{3-4}$/L$_{4-5}$/L$_5$–S$_1$): 2/22/8 (left 18, right 13, bilateral 1)	LBP/LER since 5 mo	MRI	FCR/ESI	12 (6–24) mo	Satisfactory: 19 (60%), Repeats: 11 (34%), Required Surgery: 6 (19%)
Amoretti et al., 2012 [13]/ prospective	n: 120; age: 68.2 (52–84) y; Location (L$_{3-4}$/L$_{4-5}$/L$_5$–S$_1$): 16/84/20; VAS change; mean ± sd: 7.2±1.2 to 2.9±1.2	Disabling LBP/radiculopathy	MRI	CTISI	12 mo	Satisfactory: 90 (75%), Repeats: 43 (36%), Required Surgery: 30 (25%)
Bjorkengren et al., 1987 [14]/ prospective	n: 3; age: 59 (44, 56 & 77) y; females: 2; Location: L$_{4-5}$ in all	LBP/LER	CT	CTISI	11 (6–14) mo	Satisfactory: 2 partially, Repeats: 1, Required surgery: 1/refused
Bureau et al., 2001 [17]/ retrospective	n: 12; age: 60 (45–79) y; females: 8; Location (L$_{3-4}$/L$_{4-5}$/L$_5$–S$_1$): 1/10/1; Cyst size: 11×13.6 (6–13×8–19)mm	LBP/radiculopathy	MRI	FCR/SI	23 (12–36) mo	Satisfactory: 9 (75%), Repeats: 7 (58%), Required Surgery: 3 (25%)
Cambron et al., 2013 [18]/ retrospective	n: 110; age: 63 (28–87) y; females: 71; Location (L$_{2-3}$/L$_{3-4}$/L$_{4-5}$/L$_5$–S$_1$): 6/17/89/22; Cyst size: 10.6 mm/intensity: H 48/L 65	LER	MRI	CT-guided FCR/SI	34 (7–93) mo	Satisfactory: 63 (57%), Repeats: 40 (36%), Required Surgery: 47 (43%)
Carrera, 1980 [19]/retrospective	n: 20; age (mean): 54 y; females: 12; Location (L$_{2-3}$/L$_{3-4}$/L$_{4-5}$/L$_5$–S$_1$): NA	LBP/symptomatic facet arthropathy	CT	IAFB	6–12 mo	Satisfactory: 6 (30%), Repeats: NA, Required Surgery: NA
Martha et al., 2009 [30]/ retrospective	n: 101; age: 59.8±1.3 y; females: 69; Location (L$_{2-3}$/L$_{3-4}$/L$_{4-5}$/L$_5$–S$_1$): 2/9/69/21	LBP/LER	MRI	FCR/SI	3.2±1.3 y (mean ± sd)	Satisfactory: 46 (46%), Repeats: 51 (51%), Required Surgery: 55 (55%)
Ortiz & Tekchandani, 2013 [32]/ retrospective	n: 20; age: 65.5 y average; females: 9; Location (L$_{2-3}$/L$_{3-4}$/L$_{4-5}$/L$_5$–S$_1$): 1/5/11/4; Cyst size: 7.3 (3–14) mm	LBP/LER	NA	CTISI/aspiration	18 (4–24)	Satisfactory: 18 (90%), Repeats: 2 (10%)
Parlier-Cuau et al., 1999 [33]/ retrospective	n: 30; age: 67 (44–82) y; females: 21; Location (L$_{2-3}$/L$_{3-4}$/L$_{4-5}$/L$_5$–S$_1$): 1/3/25/1; Symptom duration: at least 6 mo	Sciatic/femoral pain	CT: 27/MRI: 3/ arthrography	FISI	26 (8–50) mo	Satisfactory: 14 (47%), Repeats: 7 (23%), Required Surgery: 14 (47%)
Sabers et al., 2005 [35]/ retrospective	n: 23; age: 64 (28–81) y; females: 12; Location (L$_{3-4}$/L$_{4-5}$/L$_5$–S$_1$): 1/15/7; Symptom duration: 10.5 (2 wk–48 mo)	LBP/LER	MRI	FISI/aspiration	9.1 (1.5–21) mo	Satisfactory: 9 (50%), Repeats: 2 (1–4) per subject, Required Surgery: 9 (50%)
Sauvage et al., 2000 [36]/ retrospective	n: 13; age: 63 (42–87) y; females: 9; Location (L$_{3-4}$/L$_{4-5}$/L$_5$–S$_1$): 1/8/4; Cyst size: 9 (5–11) mm; largest 12×18 mm	radiculopathy	MRI	CTISI	9 (2–25) mo	Satisfactory: 6 (46%), Repeats: 6 (46%), Required Surgery: 3 (23%)
Schulz et al 2011 [37]/ prospective	n: 20; age: median 54.5 y; females: 17; Location (L$_{3-4}$/L$_{4-5}$/L$_5$–S$_1$): 1/19/0; Symptom duration: median 10.5 mo	radiculopathy	CT	CTISI	24 mo	Satisfactory: 8 (40%), Repeats: NA, Required Surgery: 12 (60%)
Shah and Lutz, 2003 [38]/ retrospective	n: 10; age: 60 (53–70) y; females: 8; Location (L$_{3-4}$/L$_{4-5}$/L$_5$–S$_1$): 0/8/2; Symptom duration: 7.9 (1–30) mo	LBP/LER	CT/MRI	FISI/aspiration/ESI	11.5 (3–30) mo	Satisfactory: 1 (10%), Repeats: 1 (10%), Required Surgery: 8 (80%)
Slipman et al., 2000 [40]/ retrospective	n: 14; age: 60.2 (39–87) y; females: 7; Location (L$_{3-4}$/L$_{4-5}$/L$_5$–S$_1$): 2/10/2; Symptom duration: 18.8 (3–60) mo	radiculopathy	CT/MRI	FISI/aspiration	1.4 (1–3) y	Satisfactory: 4 (40%), Repeats: NA, Required Surgery: 8(58%)
Case Reports						
Boissiere et al., 2013 [15]	57 y old male with cyst at L$_{4-5}$	Sciatica since 24 mo	CT	CTISI	6 mo	surgery (decompression + fusion)
Braza et al., 2005 [16]	48 y old man with cyst at L$_{4-5}$ (7 mm)	Thigh and calf pain (7 mo)	MRI	FISI/aspiration	2 mo	80% improvement in pain relief
Casselman et al 1985 [20]	65 y old woman with cyst at L$_{4-5}$	LBP/LER	CT	Intra-articular SI	3 mo	Underwent surgery

Table 2. Cont.

Study/Design	Patients' characteristics	Pathology	Diagnosis	Intervention	Follow up	Outcome
Chang et al 2009 [21]	63 y old woman with cyst at L_5-S_1 (7 mm)	Left-sided radiculopathy	MRI	CT-guided FISI	1 mo	Satisfactory relief
Foley, 2009 [22]	44 y old man with cyst at L_{4-5}	LBP	MRI	FISI/rupture	1 mo	Satisfactory relief (0/10 VAS)
Gishen & Mill., 2001 [23]	65 y old woman with cyst at L_5-S_1	Hip osteoarthris/left sciatica	MRI	CTISI/ESI	12 mo	Satisfactory (asymptomatic)
Hong et al., 1995 [24]	51 y old woman with cyst at L_{4-5}	LBP/right knee pain (6 mo)	MRI	FCA, no SI	6 mo	Satisfactory (asymptomatic)
Imai et al., 1998 [25]	77/55 y old women with cysts at L_{4-5}/L_{3-4}	LBP/LER (15 mo/10 mo)	MRI	FISI/aspiration	5 d/2 mo	surgery for durable relief (both)
Kozar & Jer. 2014 [26]	77 y old man with cyst at L_{4-5} (3×5 mm)	LBP/LER (3 y)	MRI	CTISI/rupture	1 mo	Partial relief/surgery not feasible
Lim et al., 2001 [27]	67 y old woman with cyst at L_{4-5}	LBP/right LER	MRI	CTISI	9 mo	Satisfactory (asymptomatic)
Lin et al, 2014 [28]	52 y old man with cyst at L_{4-5}	LBP/right LER since 10 mo	MRI	UISI	18 mo	Satisfactory (asymptomatic)
Lutz and Shen, 2002 [29]	48 y old woman; cyst at L_{4-5} (7×15 mm)	LBP/right LER (4 mo)	MRI	FCA, no SI	1 mo	Satisfactory (asymptomatic)
Melfi & Aprill, 2005 [31]	72 y old woman with cyst at L_{4-5}/L_5-S_1	Chronic LBP/LER (7 mo)	MRI	FISI	30 mo	Satisfactory (asymptomatic)
Rauchwerger 2011 [34]	70 y old woman with cyst at L_5-S_1	LBP/radiculopathy (1 y)	MRI	FISI	1 day	Partial relief
Shin et al., 2012 [39]	51 y old man with cyst at L_{4-5}	LBP/LER (1mo)	MRI	FISI/aspiration	6 mo	Satisfactory (asymptomatic)

Values are presented as mean (range) unless otherwise stated. Abbreviations: CTISI (CT-guided Intra-cystic/Intra-articular SI), ESI (epidural SI), FCA (fluoroscopically-guided cyst aspiration), FCR (fluoroscopically guided cyst rupture), FISI (fluoroscopic intra-articular SI), IAFB (intra-articular facet block), LBP (lower back pain), LER (lower extremity radiculopathy), mo (month/s), NA (not available), SI (steroid injection), wk (week/s), y (year/s).

LFJCs. Cyst rupture outcomes were assessed by the loss of resistance method or by the extravasation of dye.

Follow-up duration as mean ± sd (range) was 16±10.2 (5 days to 5.7 years). Overall the satisfactory results (after short- or long-term follow-up) were achieved in 55.8 [49.5, 62.08] % (pooled mean and 95% CI) of the 544 patients subjected to percutaneous lumbar cyst resolution procedures (Figure 3). Repeat procedures were performed in 115 of 323 subjects at an average duration of 4.7 (range 0.06–26.3) months after first procedure (data from 7 studies only). On the other hand, 38.67 [33.3, 43.95] % of this population underwent surgery subsequently to achieve durable relief (Figure 4). Average time from percutaneous resolution procedure to surgery was 6.7 (range 0.13–34.4) months (data from six studies only).

There was no purposeful linear relationship between the increasing average duration of follow-up period of individual studies and percent satisfaction from the percutaneous resolutions procedure (correlation coefficient: 0.13; slope: 0.057; Figure 5). However, number of studies with around 1-year follow up was highest (10), with 2-year follow-up 4 and with 3-year follow-up 2 only. For this analysis individual case reports were lumped in to three groups according to follow-up period (1, 6 and 12 months). Only one case report had a follow-up of over 2-years duration (30 months).

Discussion

Usually, the LFJCs are found as rare incidental MRI findings of elderly patients (usually in their 6th or 7th decade) presenting with low back pain and lower extremity radiculopathy. However, discovery of LFJCs remains difficult because low back pain is one of the most common presentations in a visit to physician [41]. Frequently, small cohorts of patients often develop additional bony abnormalities, including instability and spondylolisthesis.

Previously, it was difficult to pinpoint a precise existence of a cyst. Rather, the physician relied on his/her clinical acumen. For example, bilateral examinations of L_4, L_5 and S_1, supplying the knee, foot dorsiflexion and plantar flexion, respectively, could give quick insight into the functioning of these spinal nerve roots. Added to these were lumbosacral flexion-extension plain film radiographs that could provide basic information about vertebral anatomy. However, with the advent of modern imaging modalities like CT scans and MRI, primary care physicians as well as specialists started utilizing these techniques in order to obtain more reliable anatomical features leading to pathology. This has resulted in better insights of pathoanatomical diagnoses that can provide sustained and earlier relief.

The present study utilizes almost all relevant data to appraise the success rate of the percutaneous resolution of the LFJCs and finds perhaps the highest rate (56%) reviewed so far [2 e.g.]. This appears to be because of inclusion of 15 case reports which provide considerable power to analysis. Overall success rate noted in the case reports was 70%, whereas, in the pooled analysis of 14 studies the success rate was noted to about 50%. Although, follow-up period of the case reports was much less than the pooled analysis of 14 studies, yet, in the subset of 4 case reports with 9, 12, 18, and 30 months follow-up, the success rate was 100%. Overall association between the follow-up and satisfactory results was also not providing indication of declined success rate with increments in follow up period. Such a difference of success rate of percutaneous procedures in the retrospective analyses and case reports can be attributed to publication bias or scarcity of prospective studies will be clarified in future research. Nevertheless, this point is

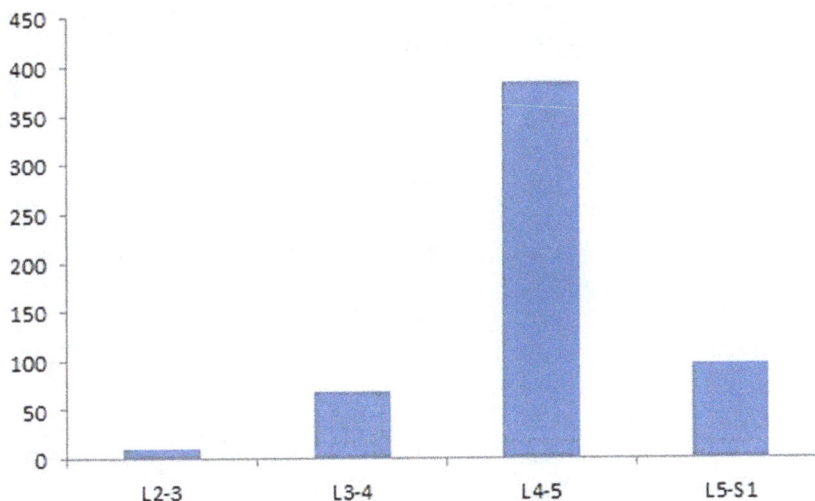

Figure 2. Spinal level of cysts diagnosed in the patients included in the meta-analysis.

encouraging enough to provide impetus for larger and longer trial/s to assess the potentials of this treatment strategy.

Natural history of the disease progression of LJFCs is not known. Frequently, patients with radicular pain may be advised for obtaining MRI scans and if there is incidental detection of LJC, detailed neurological examination is meritorious in order to seek insights into the associated pathophysiology. Patients presenting with any kind of radicular pain or associated claudication syndromes, cauda equina syndrome, or any lower extremity motor or sensory symptoms must be evaluated with advanced imaging like MRI. However, in order to avoid extra un-forecasted healthcare costs, there is sheer need of a good clinical examination at the presentation. Due to methodological issues, scarcity of categorical data and statistical power limitations, the present study could not arrive at an initiative of establishing criteria for the selection of suitable patients for percutaneous resolution procedures. Narrowing and ideally eliminating the gray areas of when to take the decision for percutaneous rupture versus the definitive strategy of cyst excision remains the hallmark of clinical research in this area. Surgical excision is precise, but is time consuming, expensive and still not risk-free. On the other hand complications may also develop following procedures such as paraplegia [42].

Because of a number of factors, the present study encounters significant limitations. Firstly, as the diagnosis of LJC remains incidental, there is only one considerable sized prospective study and all others are either retrospective analyses or case reports. Schulz et al. [37] utilized a prospective design to compare the efficacy of percutaneous resolution of LFJCs with microsurgery and noticed a clear-cut supremacy of microsurgery over percutaneous resolution attempts. Their study was not randomized but acts as a required initiative which noted satisfactory benefit of percutaneous treatment for 8 of 20 patients. Indeed, because of minimally invasiveness of this treatment, it remains a treatment of choice.

Secondly, follow-up period in the majority of studies was less than two years which makes it difficult to speculate long-term benefits of the intervention. Thirdly, data availability remained a major issue as it could be useful to apply meta-regression analyses for predicting factor by utilizing data such as age, gender cyst size, cyst type, cyst orientation/location, radiological intensity, pre-procedure duration of symptoms and previous history of treatment/s. Although, case reports were considerably detailed yet in many all relevant data was not available. Cambron et al. [18] studied the effect of low or high signal intensity of MRI on the success rate of percutaneous resolution of LFJCs and noted that patients with T2-hyperintene LFJCs can be more reliably benefited from percutaneous resolution procedures.

Table 3. Common presenting conditions of lumbar facet joint cysts.

Low back pain	Disc herniation
Unilateral or bilateral radiculopathy	Spinal stenosis
Myelopathy	Neural foraminal stenosis
Neurogenic claudication	Herniated nucleus pulposus
Caudaequina syndrome	Osteoarthritis
Intracystic or epidural hemorrhage	Arachnoiditis
Spondylolisthesis	Cauda equina compression from cyst
Trochanteric bursitis	High-intensity zone in disk
Peripheral neuropathy	

Study / Case reports	Benefitted subjects	Total	Percent benefitted subjects and 95% CI			Percent benefitted subjects and 95% CI
			Percentage	Upper limit	Lower limit	
Allen et al., 2009	19	32	59.37	32.68	86.07	
Amoretti et al., 2012	90	120	75.0	59.5	90.5	
Bjorkengren et 1987	1	3	33.33	-32.0	98.67	
Bureau et al., 2001	9	12	75.0	26.0	124.0	
Cambron et al 2013	63	110	57.27	43.13	71.42	
Carrera, 1980	6	20	30.0	5.995	54.0	
Martha et al., 2009	46	101	45.54	32.38	58.71	
Ortiz & Tekch., 2013	18	20	90.0	48.42	131.6	
Parlier-Cuau et 1999	14	30	46.66	22.22	71.11	
Sabers et al., 2005	9	23	39.13	13.57	64.7	
Sauvage et al., 2000	6	13	46.15	9.223	83.08	
Schulz et al., 2011	8	20	40.0	12.28	67.72	
Shah & Lutz, 2003	1	10	10.0	-9.6	29.6	
Slipman et al., 2000	4	14	28.57	0.571	56.57	
CR 1	4	8	50.0	1.0	99.0	
CR 2	2	3	66.66	-25.7	159.1	
CR 3	3	3	100	-13.2	213.2	
Summary	303	543	55.80	49.52	62.08	

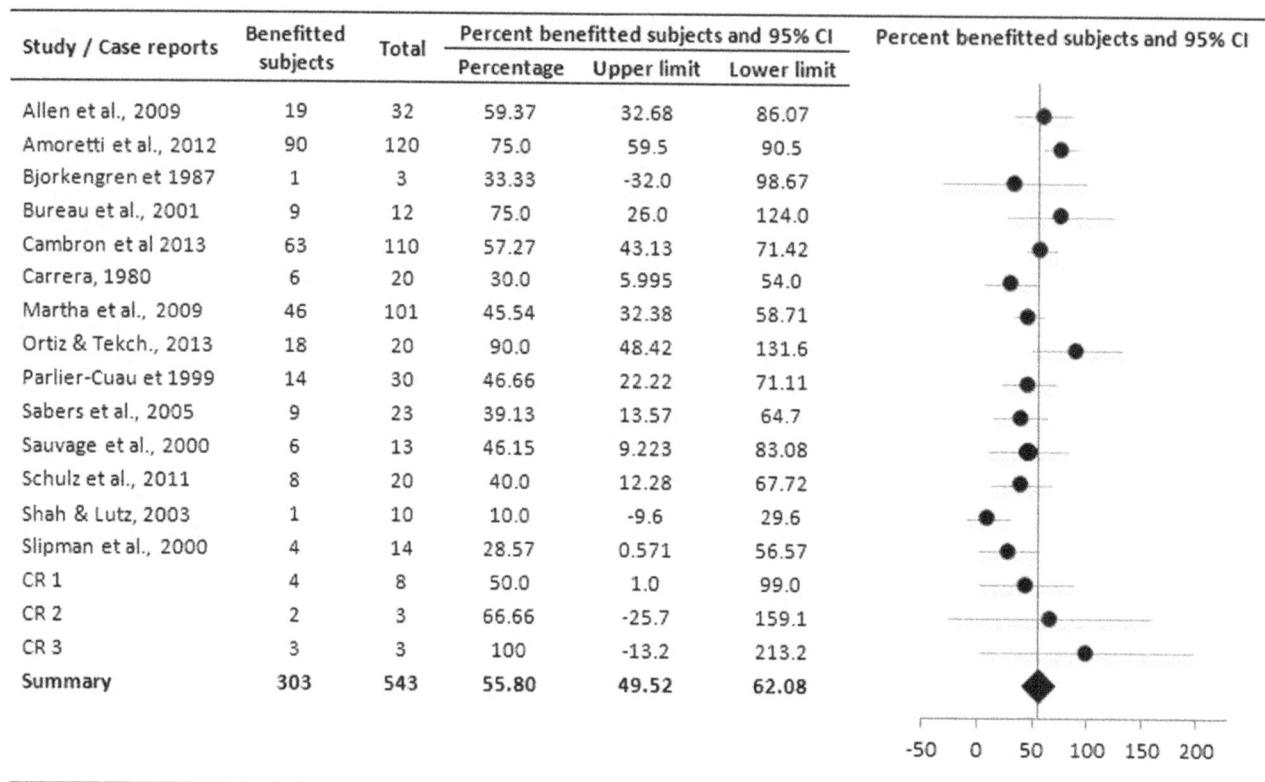

Figure 3. Forest plot showing effect sizes of satisfactory results of percutaneous treatments of the LFJCs after short- or long-term follow-up in individual studies (closed circles) and the overall effect size achieved in meta-analysis (diamond). CR 1 (follow-up 1 mo): Braza et al., 2005; Casselman et al., 1985; Chang, 2009; Foley, 2009; Imai et al., 1998; Kozar & Jeromal, 2014; Lutz and Shen, 2002; Rauchwerger et al., 2011/CR 2 (follow-up 6 month): Boissier et al., 2013; Hong et al., 1995; Shin et al., 2012/CR 3 (follow-up 1 year or more): Gishen et al., 2001; Lim et al., 2001; Lin et al., 2014; Melfi and Aprill, 2005.

Study / Case reports	Subsequent surgery	Total	Percent surgery subjects and 95% CI			Percent surgery subjects and 95% CI
			Percentage	Upper limit	Lower limit	
Allen et al., 2009	6	32	18.75	3.747	33.75	
Amoretti et al., 2012	30	120	25.0	16.05	33.95	
Bjorkengren et 1987	1	3	33.33	-32.0	98.67	
Bureau et al., 2001	3	12	25.0	-3.29	53.29	
Cambron et al 2013	47	110	42.72	30.51	54.94	
Martha et al., 2009	55	101	54.45	40.06	68.85	
Ortiz & Tekch., 2013	2	20	10.0	-3.86	23.86	
Parlier-Cuau et 1999	14	30	46.66	22.22	71.11	
Sabers et al., 2005	9	23	39.13	13.57	64.7	
Sauvage et al., 2000	3	13	23.07	-3.04	49.19	
Schulz et al., 2011	12	20	60.0	26.05	93.95	
Shah & Lutz, 2003	8	10	80.0	24.56	135.4	
Slipman et al., 2000	8	14	57.14	17.54	96.74	
CR 1	2	8	25.0	-9.65	59.65	
CR 2	1	3	33.33	-32.0	98.67	
CR 3	0	3	0	-	-	
Summary	201	523	38.62	33.30	43.95	

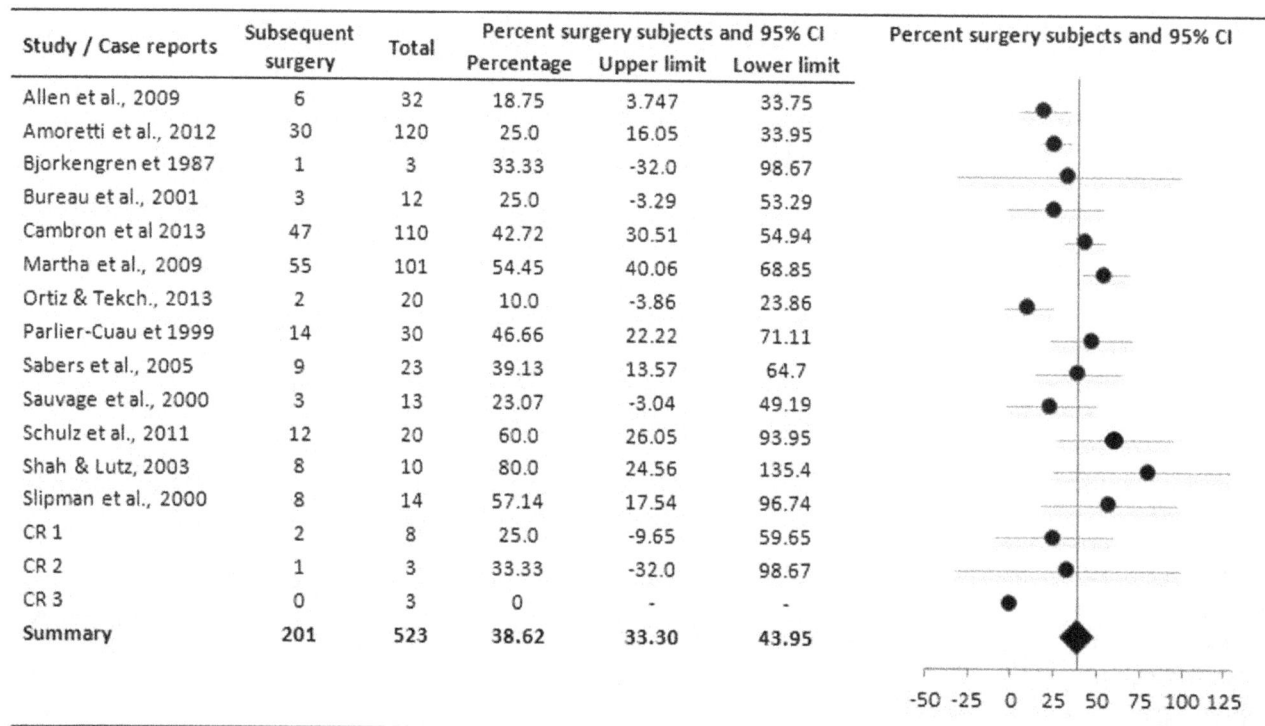

Figure 4. Forest plot showing effect sizes of subjects underwent surgical treatments subsequent to failure of percutaneous treatments of the LFJCs in individual studies (closed circles) and the overall effect size achieved in meta-analysis (diamond). CR 1/CR 2/CR 3 as given in Figure 2.

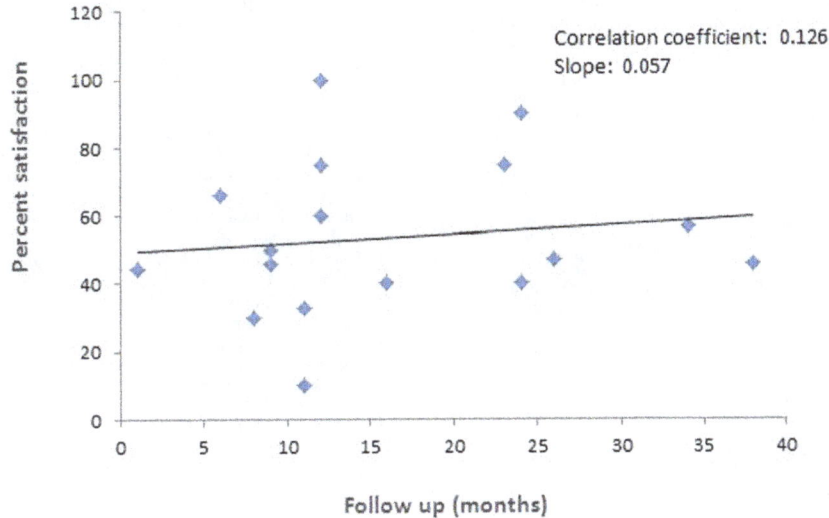

Figure 5. Scatter plot showing relationship between percent satisfaction of the subjects of percutaneous resolution procedures and follow-up duration in months.

It seems that the success rate of percutaneous resolution procedures will increase with the improvement in decision-making information and advancement in technology and skill training and exposure. However, of much importance is the availability of results of a few or a bigger, multi-center randomized controlled trial/s with adequate power to assess the success rate as well as the predicting factors for percutaneous resolution procedure selection. Without which as pointed out by Arnold et al. [43], patient is presented with the coin flip odds for percutaneous vs surgery choice.

Conclusion

By analyzing all available evidence pertaining to the efficacy of percutaneous cyst resolution procedures the present study finds this therapeutic regimen as an alternative to surgical interventions but is unable to identify subgroup/s of patients that can be benefited more reliably with this technique and therefore urges to conduct comparative studies with longer follow-up periods.

Author Contributions

Conceived and designed the experiments: JGT SXH. Performed the experiments: SXH FS JLZ DFR ZC. Analyzed the data: FS SXH JLZ DFR ZC JGT. Wrote the paper: FS SXH.

References

1. Epstein NE, Baisden J (2012) The diagnosis and management of synovial cysts: Efficacy of surgery vs cyst aspiration. Surg Neurol Int 3: 157–66.
2. DePalma MJ (2009) Driving the lane: a clearer view of facet joint cyst intervention. Spine J 9: 921–3.
3. Shipley JA, Beukes CA (1998) The nature of spondylolytic defect. Demonstration of a communicating synovial pseudoarthrosis in the pars interarticularis. J Bone Joint Surg Br 80: 662–4.
4. Alicioglu B, Sut N (2009) Synovial cysts of the lumbar facet joints: a retrospective magnetic resonance imaging study investigating their relation with degenerative spondylolisthesis. Prague Medical Report 110: 301–9.
5. Budris DM (1991) Radiologic case study, intraspinal lumbar synovial cyst. Orthopedics 14: 618–20.
6. Gheyi GY, Uppot RN, Flores C, Koyfman YU (1999) Unusual case of lumbar synovial cyst. Clin Imaging 23: 394–6.
7. Boviatsis EJ, Staurinou LC, Kouyialis AT, Gavra MM, Stavrinou PC, et al. (2008) Spinal synovial cysts: pathogenesis, diagnosis and surgical treatment in a series of seven cases and literature review. Eur Spine J 17: 831–7.
8. Abdullah AF, Chambers RW, Daut DP (1984) Lumbar nerve root compression by synovial cysts of the ligamentum flavum. Report of four cases. J Neurosurg 60: 617–20.
9. Kurz LT, Garfin SR, Unger AS, Thorne RP, Rothman RH (1985) Intraspinal synovial cyst causing sciatica. J Bone Joint Surg Am 67: 865–71.
10. Ayberg G, Ozveren F, Gok Yazgan A, Tosun H, Seçkin Z, et al. (2008) Lumbar synovial cysts: experience with nine cases. Neurol Med Chir 48: 298–303.
11. U.S. Department of Health & Human Services.Quality Assessment Tool for Observational Cohort and Cross-Sectional Studies. Available: http://www.nhlbi.nih.gov/health-pro/guidelines/in-develop/cardiovascular-risk-reduction/tools/cohort.htm. Accessed 2014 March.
12. Allen TL, Tatli Y, Lutz GE (2009) Fluoroscopic percutaneous lumbar zygapophyseal joint cyst rupture: a clinical outcome study. Spine J 9: 387–95.
13. Amoretti N, Huwart L, Foti P, Boileau P, Amoretti ME, et al. (2012) Symptomatic lumbar facet joint cysts treated by CT-guided intracystic and intra-articular steroid injections. Eur Radiol 22: 2836–40.
14. Bjorkengren AG, Kurz LT, Resnick D, Sartoris DJ, Garfin SR (1987) Symptomatic intraspinal synovial cysts: opacification and treatment by percutaneous injection. AJR Am J Roentgenol 149: 105–7.
15. Boissière L, Valour F, Rigal J, Soderlund C (2013) Lumbar synovial cyst calcification after facet joint steroid injection. BMJ Case Rep 2013. pii: bcr2012008029.
16. Braza DW, Dedianous D, Peterson B (2005) Lumbar synovial cyst. Am J Phys Med Rehabil 84: 911–2.
17. Bureau NJ, Kaplan PA, Dussault RG (2001) Lumbar facet joint synovial cyst: percutaneous treatment with steroid injections and distention—clinical and imaging follow-up in 12 patients. Radiol 221: 179–85.
18. Cambron SC, McIntyre JJ, Guerin SJ, Li Z, Pastel DA (2013) Lumbar facet joint synovial cysts: does T2 signal intensity predict outcomes after percutaneous rupture? AJNR Am J Neuroradiol 34: 1661–4.
19. Carrera GF (1980) Lumbar facet joint injection in low back pain and sciatica: preliminary results. Radiol 137: 665–7.
20. Casselman ES (1985) Radiologic recognition of symptomatic spinal synovial cysts. AJNR Am J Neuroradiol 6: 971–3.
21. Chang A (2009) Percutaneous CT-guided treatment of lumbar facet joint synovial cysts. HSS J 5: 165–8.
22. Foley BS (2009) Percutaneous rupture of a lumbar synovial facet cyst. Am J Phys Med Rehabil 88: 1046.
23. Gishen P, Miller FN (2001) Percutaneous excision of a facet joint cyst under CT guidance. Cardiovasc Intervent Radiol 24: 351–53.
24. Hong Y, O'Grady T, Carlsson C, Casey J, Clements D (1995) Percutaneous aspiration of lumbar facet synovial cyst. Anesthesiol 82: 1061–2.

25. Imai K, Nakamura K, Inokuchi K, Oda H (1998) Aspiration of intraspinal synovial cyst: recurrence after temporal improvement. Arch Orthop Trauma Surg 118: 103–5.

26. Kozar S, Jeromel M (2014) Minimally invasive CT guided treatment of intraspinal synovial cyst. Radiol Oncol 48: 35–9.

27. Lim AK, Higgins SJ, Saifuddin A, Lehovsky J (2001) Symptomatic lumbar synovial cyst: management with direct CT-guided puncture and steroid injection. Clin Radiol 56: 990–3.

28. Lin TL, Chung CT, Lan HH, Sheen HM (2014) Ultrasound-guided facet joint injection to treat a spinal cyst. J Chin Med Assoc 77: 213–6.

29. Lutz GE, Shen TC (2002) Fluoroscopically guided aspiration of a symptomatic lumbar zygapophyseal joint cyst: A case report. Arch Phys Med Rehabil 83: 1789–91.

30. Martha JF, Swaim B, Wang DA, Kim DH, Hill J, et al. (2009) Outcome of percutaneous rupture of lumbar synovial cysts: a case series of 101 patients. Spine J 9: 899–904.

31. Melfi RS, Aprill CN (2005) Percutaneous puncture of zygapophysial joint synovial cyst with fluoroscopic guidance. Pain Med 6: 122–8.

32. Ortiz AO, Tekchandani L (2013) Improved outcomes with direct percutaneous CT guided lumbar synovial cyst treatment: advanced approaches and techniques. J Neurointerv Surg doi: 10.1136/neurintsurg-2013-010891.

33. Parlier-Cuau C, Wybier M, Nizard R, Champsaur P, Le Hir P, et al. (1999) Symptomatic lumbar facet joint synovial cysts: clinical assessment of facet joint steroid injection after 1 and 6 months and long-term follow-up in 30 patients. Radiol 210: 509–13.

34. Rauchwerger JJ, Candido KD, Zoarski GH (2011) Technical and imaging report: fluoroscopic guidance for diagnosis and treatment of lumbar synovial cyst. Pain Pract 11: 180–4.

35. Sabers SR, Ross SR, Grogg BE, Lauder TD (2005) Procedure-based nonsurgical management of lumbar zygapophyseal joint cyst-induced radicular pain. Arch Phys Med Rehabil 86: 1767–71.

36. Sauvage P, Grimault L, Ben Salem D, Roussin I, Huguenin M, et al. (2000) Lumbar intraspinal synovial cysts: imaging and treatment by percutaneous injection. Report of thirteen cases. J Radiol 81: 33–8.

37. Schulz C, Danz B, Waldeck S, Kunz U, Mauer UM (2011) Percutaneous CT-guided destruction versus microsurgical resection of lumbar juxtafacet cysts. Orthopade 40: 600–6.

38. Shah RV, Lutz GE (2003) Lumbar intraspinal synovial cysts: conservative management and review of the world's literature. Spine J 3: 479–88.

39. Shin KM, Kim MS, Ko KM, Jang JS, Kang SS, et al. (2012) Percutaneous aspiration of lumbar zygapophyseal joint synovial cyst under fluoroscopic guidance - A case report. Korean J Anesthesiol 62: 375–8.

40. Slipman CW, Lipetz JS, Wakeshima Y, Jackson HB (2000) Nonsurgical treatment of zygapophyseal joint cyst-induced radicular pain. Arch Phys Med Rehabil 81: 973–7.

41. Deyo RA, Weinstein JN (2001) Low back pain. N Engl J Med 344: 363–70.

42. Kennedy DJ, Dreyfuss P, Aprill CN, Bogduk N (2009) Paraplegia following image-guided transforaminal lumbar spine epidural steroid injection: two case reports. Pain Med 10: 1389–94.

43. Arnold PM (2009) Efficacy of injection therapy for symptomatic lumbar synovial cysts. Spine J 9: 919–20.

24

A 35-Year Trend Analysis for Back Pain in Austria: The Role of Obesity

Franziska Großschädl[1]*, Wolfgang Freidl[1], Éva Rásky[1], Nathalie Burkert[1], Johanna Muckenhuber[2], Willibald J. Stronegger[1]

1 Medical University of Graz, Institute of Social Medicine and Epidemiology, Graz, Austria, 2 University of Graz, Institute of Sociology, Graz, Austria

Abstract

Background: The prevalence of back pain is constantly increasing and a public health problem of high priority. In Austria there is a lack of empirical evidence for the development of back pain and its related factors. The present study aims to investigate trends in the prevalence of back pain across different subpopulations (sex, age, obesity).

Methods: A secondary data analysis based on five nationally representative cross-sectional health surveys (1973–2007) was carried out. Face-to-face interviews were conducted in private homes in Austria. Subjects aged 20 years and older were included in the study sample (n = 178,818). Obesity was defined as BMI ≥ 30 kg/m^2 and adjusted for self-report bias. Back pain was measured as the self-reported presence of the disorder.

Results: The age-standardized prevalence of back pain was 32.9% in 2007; it was higher among women than men (p < 0.001), higher in older than younger subjects (p < 0.001) and higher in obese than non-obese individuals (p < 0.001). During the investigation period the absolute change in the prevalence of back pain was +19.4%. Among all subpopulations the prevalence steadily increased. Obese men showed the highest increase of and the greatest risk for back pain.

Conclusion: These results help to understand the development of back pain in Austria and can be used to plan controlled promotion programs. Further monitoring is recommended in order to control risk groups and plan target group-specific prevention strategies. In Austria particular emphasis should be on obese individuals. We recommend conducting prospective studies to confirm our results and investigate causal relationships.

Editor: Rasheed Ahmad, Dasman Diabetes Institute, Kuwait

Funding: The authors have no support or funding to report.

Competing Interests: The authors have declared that no competing interests exist

* Email: franziska.grossschaedl@medunigraz.at

Introduction

Back pain represents an extremely common public health problem [1–3] and is especially widespread in Western countries [4]. A systematic review investigating the global prevalence of activity-limiting low back pain among adults estimated a point prevalence to range from 1.0% to 58.1% (mean 18.1%) and a 1-year prevalence from 0.8% to 82.5% (mean 38.1%). Back pain has a negative impact at the individual level, e.g. through strong pain and activity limitations [2], and at the social level, e.g. through absenteeism, the need for disability pension [5–7], a high utilization of health care resources, and other financial aspects [5,8,9]. Given the high total economic costs of back pain, even a small reduction in the incidence of back pain would have a sustained economic impact [10]. A whole range of environmental and personal factors must be considered when investigating back pain as a disorder. Studies have found e.g. age [7,11,12], sex [2,7,12] and BMI [13] to present a significant association with the risk of suffering from back pain.

An association between obesity and the presence of back pain has been reported [10,14–17]. Compared to individuals with normal weight, subjects with obesity more often self-report a poorer health status [18]. It has been observed that the morbidity and mortality risk increase with increasing body mass index (BMI kg/m^2) [19]. While the prevalence of obesity increased strongly worldwide over the last decades, there was also a clear parallel upward trend in the prevalence of different obesity-associated diseases and disorders, such as type 2 diabetes mellitus, cardiovascular diseases, malignant tumours or back pain [20]. A large Austrian population-based study showed a strong upward trend in the mean BMI and the prevalence of obesity among adult women and men. At present the age-standardized obesity prevalence is estimated to be 14.5% and seems to be rising among Austrian adults [21].

There is a lack of information regarding the development of back pain in Austria and its relation to obesity. Evidence-based confirmation is still lacking. A representation of existing long-term trends for back pain could demonstrate the extent of this problem in Austria and the investigation of subgroups would furthermore allow to identify the factors behind back pain-affected populations and detect special risk groups [22]. This would facilitate the planning of target group-specific preventive measures and reduce the number of people affected by back pain. In addition, the monitoring of secular back pain trends can be utilised to evaluate prevention strategies.

The purpose of this study was to demonstrate the changes in back pain trends among the Austrian adult population in the period 1973 to 2006–07. Long-term trends in the prevalence of back pain were to be presented for Austria as a whole and for different subpopulations (based on sex, age, and obesity). This study also aimed to identify possible risk groups by assessing the associations of back pain with collected variables.

Methods

Data source and sampling

Data were derived from representative cross-sectional health surveys carried out in Austria using comparable methodology. Since 1973, five nationwide health surveys have been conducted at irregular time intervals. Health data were collected through the Austrian Microcensus in 1973, 1983, 1991 and 1999. The last health survey – titled Austrian Health Interview Survey (AT-HIS 2006–07) – was conducted in 2006–07 instead of the former Microcensus on health as part of the European Health Interview Survey (E-HIS; http://www.euhsid.org), an important high-quality survey. The Microcensus and the AT-HIS are surveys conducted by the federal statistical office 'Statistik Austria'. Statistics Austria (http://www.statistik.at/web_en/) is the owner of the data and makes them available. The Microcensus data are chargeable and the data for the ATHIS are free.

For the AT-HIS 2006–07 a random sample was drawn from the Austrian population register. For the sake of representation, the sample was stratified by the 32 administrative Austrian districts. For the four Microcensus surveys the sampling was made by a stratified selection of addresses by federal states. The selection framework for the Microcensus sampling was the housing census revised by the current housing statistics in Austria.

In all five surveys data were obtained through standardised face-to-face interviews by trained interviewers of 'Statistik Austria' questioning individuals aged 15 years and older in their private homes or long-term care facilities (such as nursing homes), using interviewer questionnaires. While a household sample was selected for the Microcensus surveys (this means that data from all household members were collected), a sample of the respective individuals was interviewed for the AT-HIS 2006–07. Another difference between Microcensus and AT-HIS is that in the AT-HIS, the participants were questioned by computer-assisted personal face-to-face interviews (CAPI), which allows direct data entry. To ensure that interviews were conducted in the same way, interviewers of all five surveys had to participate in trainings where they were instructed on how to conduct the interviews. In all five surveys participants had to give full information for the baseline survey portion. The raw data were screened for errors from 'Statistik Austria'.

The participation rates were quite large for the Microcensus surveys, especially in 1973, and relatively low in the AT-HIS 2006/07. This is due to the fewer number of questions asked in the first surveys. The questionnaire applied in the AT-HIS was much more extensive in comparison with the questionnaires of the earlier surveys. However, each survey sample was weighted

according to sex, age and region to ensure representativeness of the Austrian population distribution.

Data analysis for this study was limited to adults. Subjects aged 20 years and older were included since the AT-HIS survey rather concerned entire age groups (5 year intervals) than exact age levels. Therefore, the data of 64,052 subjects were excluded since they were younger than 20 years at the time of the survey. Furthermore, cases with missing data regarding gender and BMI were not included (n = 29,709). Cases with implausible BMI values (BMI≤10 kg/m^2, BMI≥75 kg/m^2) were also removed from the data base. This reduced the total sampling frame to 178,818 individuals. The proportion of individuals included in the analysis was 63% in total. 53.7% of the participants were female. The mean±SD age of the individuals was 47.7±17.5 years, which refers only to the first four surveys. The subjects included in this study were between 20 and 99 years old.

Ethical approval

The consent procedure and the conductance of this study were approved by the Ethics Committee of the Medical University of Graz (EK-number: 23–172 ex 10/11). The study was carried out in compliance with the principles laid down in the Helsinki Declaration. No minors or children were included in the study sample. Data were collected anonymously. Verbal informed consent was obtained from all subjects, witnessed, and formally recorded for every survey.

Variables and measurement

Demographic and socioeconomic characteristics, as well as health data were collected in each health survey. In every survey the presence of back pain was queried. When collecting the data in the Microcensus surveys (1973, 1983, 1991, 1999) participants were asked if they suffered from back pain at the time of the survey In the AT-HIS 2006–07 data for back pain were collected by asking the participants if they suffered from the disorder within the last 12 months. The surveys used different definitions for identifying back pain. In the last survey the 12-month prevalence of back pain was collected, while in the first four Microcensus surveys the point prevalence was measured. Despite the different collection methods in the Microcensus and the AT-HIS it was reported that back pain is often chronic [2] and that there is no great difference in the prevalence for back pain at the time of the survey or rather within the 12 months before. Besides, the data for back pain from the AT-HIS 2006–07 did not seem conspicuous and were similar and corresponded roughly to the data of the Microcensus surveys. Hence, the effect of different definitions is probably minimal and only accounts for a small change in the back pain prevalence during the study period. For measuring obesity, the participants were asked to indicate their body height (without wearing shoes) in centimetres and their body weight (without wearing clothes) in kilograms. The BMI for each subject was calculated by dividing body weight in kilograms by the square of body height in meters (kg/m^2). According to the WHO [20], obesity was defined as a BMI greater than 30 kg/m^2. To stratify the outcomes by age, adult subjects were categorized into the following four age groups: 20–34 years, 35–54 years, 55–74 years and 75 years and older.

Correcting for self-report bias

Self-reported data on weight and height may lead to a misclassification of BMI values and may induce bias in measuring obesity [23]. Therefore, based on the results of a preliminary validation study among Austrian residents [24], BMI correction factors were applied only to subjects 45 years and older given that variations between self-reported and measured BMI significantly increased only in older women and men. Correction factors for women: 45 to 59 years old: +0.41 kg/m^2, 60 years and older: + 1.09 kg/m^2. Correction factors for men: 45 to 59 years old: + 0.50 kg/m^2, 60 years and older: +0.54 kg/m^2.

Self-reported information about the presence of disorders is more valid when it comes to chronic illnesses. Health surveys based on self-reported data have thus been considered as a good instrument for measuring the prevalence of diseases or disorders [25]. Therefore, no correction for self-reported presence of back pain was made in this study.

Data analysis

Selected variables from all five surveys were fed into a common database. Crude prevalence and age-standardized prevalence were calculated, using the new European standard population for direct standardization in accordance with WHO guidelines [26]. Prevalence calculations were stratified by sex, age, and obesity. Chi-square tests were carried out for the whole study population and for subgroups, thereby analysing the statistical significance for the survey period. Figures representing the course of the prevalence of back pain, stratified by sex and obesity between 1973 and 2006–07, were created using Microsoft Office Excel 2007. To quantify trends in the prevalence of back pain, the percentages of absolute change (AC) were assessed. The aetiologic fraction (AF), a ratio measure, was computed to represent the subgroup with the greatest relative obesity risk. The AF denoted the percentage portion of the disease risk. To calculate the AC and AF, the prevalences of the first and last year (Pf and Pl, respectively) estimated by binary logistic regression models, were used. Binary logistic regression analyses were calculated for the whole study period with the dichotomous variable of back pain as dependent variable and the survey period as predictor. The correction variable for regression was age (in intervals of 5 years). The AC was defined as AC = Pl−Pf, and the AF was defined as AF = (Pl−Pf)/Pl. The precise formulas are presented in Figure 1. Statistical tests were two-sided and a p<0.05 was considered statistically significant. All statistical analyses were conducted using IBM SPSS Statistics for Windows version 21.0 (IBM Corp., Armonk, New York) and Stata/SE for Windows version 11.2 (StataCorp., College Station, TX, USA).

Results

Table 1 shows that in 2006–07 the age-standardized prevalence of back pain was 32.9% among the general adult population in Austria, with the highest prevalence among obese subjects (36.2%). Overall, the prevalence was slightly higher in women than in men. Considering female and male adults in different age groups, the oldest group (≥75 years) suffered the most from back pain. Nearly half of the women in that age category reported back pain in the last survey. Among men the prevalence of back pain in 2006–07 was highest for those aged 55 to 74 years. When stratifying the outcomes of the most recent survey by age and obesity, we observed the highest prevalence of back pain in obese female (51.8%) and obese male (48.6%) adults aged 55 to 74 years. Among the non-obese the prevalence was highest for women aged 75 years and older (48.7%), and for men aged 55 to 74 years (43.4%) (Table 1).

In the period 1973 to 2006–07 the prevalence of back pain increased steadily across all subgroups (Table 1). Figure 2 illustrates how the age-standardized prevalence of back pain rose from survey to survey, among women and men and among obese and non-obese subjects. Overall, obese subjects were still the most affected by back pain during the study period. The continuous increase in the prevalence of back pain among obese and non-obese women and men is also illustrated in Figure 2. The outcomes for obese women demonstrated the highest prevalence across all surveys with an approximation in the prevalence of back pain among obese men in 2006–07. In the period 1999 to 2006–07 the prevalence of back pain strongly increased among women not suffering from obesity.

For the whole study population the increase in the prevalence of back pain represented by the absolute change (AC) was 19.4%. Obese subjects showed the highest growth between 1973 and 2006–07. Overall, the strongest AC was calculated for obese men (25.6%) and the lowest for non-obese men (16%). The greatest risk for back pain presented by the aetiologic fraction (AF) was found for obese men (61.8%). The lowest AF was observed among obese women (50%) (Table 2).

Discussion

According to the age-standardized prevalence, about one third of the Austrian adult population suffered from back pain in 2006–07. Similar rates were found in a comparable study. A Greek

$$AC = 1 / (1 + \exp[-(B0 + B * T)]) - 1 / (1 + \exp[-B0])$$

$$AF = (RR - 1) / RR$$

B = Regression coefficient

B0 = Intercept

T = Time period in years

RR = Relative risk = $(1 + \exp[-(B0)]) / (1 + \exp[-(B0 + B * T)])$

Figure 1. Formulas for computing the absolute change (AC) and the aetiologic fraction (AF).

Table 1. The prevalence of back pain in five health surveys in Austria stratified by sex, obesity and age.

Sex (n) Age group (n)	P value[a]			1973 (n=55,814)			1983 (n=38,835)			1991 (n=35,093)			1999 (n=34,731)			2006–07 (n=14,318)		
	Total	Obese	Non-obese	Total %	Obese %	Non-obese %	Total %	Obese %	Non-obese %	Total %	Obese %	Non-obese %	Total %	Obese %	Non-obese %	Total %	Obese %	Non-obese %
Total (178,818)	p<0.001	p<0.001	p<0.001	14.8	19.1	14.2	16.7	21.2	16.2	19.2	24.4	18.7	25.0	33.7	23.7	34.3	42.8	32.8
Total age-standardized	p<0.001	p<0.001	p<0.001	13.9	16.3	13.6	16.5	18.5	16.4	19.0	22.0	19.0	24.3	28.7	23.5	32.9	36.2	32.2
20–34 (50,509)	p<0.001	p<0.001	p<0.001	7.0	10.9	6.9	7.6	11.2	7.5	9.8	18.3	9.5	14.6	19.6	14.3	18.6	23.9	18.2
35–54 (64,666)	p<0.001	p<0.001	p<0.001	15.5	17.3	15.2	19.3	22.4	19.0	22.3	23.5	22.2	26.0	30.7	25.4	33.6	38.0	32.9
55–74 (49,112)	p<0.001	p<0.001	p<0.001	19.3	22.0	18.7	22.1	21.1	22.3	25.6	25.2	25.7	33.0	38.8	31.4	45.8	50.4	44.4
≥75 (14,531)	p<0.001	p<0.001	p<0.001	19.8	22.0	19.5	21.7	27.9	21.0	23.9	31.9	23.0	29.6	39.1	28.1	46.4	48.4	46.0
Women total (96,017)	p<0.001	p<0.001	p<0.001	15.7	21.3	14.9	17.0	22.7	16.4	19.0	25.7	18.2	24.6	35.2	23.0	36.3	44.5	34.7
Women total age-standardized	p<0.001	p<0.001	p<0.001	14.2	18.3	13.8	16.4	20.0	16.1	18.5	22.0	18.2	23.6	29.0	22.6	34.3	35.7	33.7
20–34 (25,140)	p<0.001	0.444	p<0.001	7.1	14.2	6.9	7.3	11.8	7.2	9.4	15.5	9.2	13.6	18.0	13.6	19.7	17.4	19.9
35–54 (33,168)	p<0.001	p<0.001	p<0.001	15.3	18.8	14.3	18.8	23.8	18.2	20.7	25.0	20.3	24.7	30.9	23.9	34.9	39.4	34.3
55–74 (27,967)	p<0.001	p<0.001	p<0.001	20.4	23.3	19.7	22.5	22.2	22.6	25.4	25.6	25.3	32.6	40.1	30.2	47.0	51.8	45.2
≥75 (9,742)	p<0.001	p<0.001	p<0.001	22.1	25.0	21.7	22.7	28.9	21.9	25.4	34.5	24.2	30.5	39.9	28.7	49.3	51.2	48.7
Men total (82,801)	p<0.001	p<0.001	p<0.001	13.7	15.5	13.5	16.3	18.9	16.0	19.5	22.6	19.2	25.5	31.8	24.6	32.2	40.9	30.7
Men total age-standardized	p<0.001	p<0.001	p<0.001	13.2	13.5	13.2	16.5	16.3	16.6	19.7	21.0	19.8	24.9	28.0	24.5	31.2	35.6	30.5
20–34 (25,368)	p<0.001	p<0.001	p<0.001	6.9	8.7	6.8	8.0	10.7	7.9	10.2	20.3	9.8	15.3	21.1	15.0	17.5	30.4	16.5
35–54 (31,498)	p<0.001	p<0.001	p<0.001	15.6	15.5	15.6	19.8	21.0	19.7	24.0	22.1	24.2	27.4	30.5	26.9	32.3	36.8	31.5
55–74 (21,146)	p<0.001	p<0.001	p<0.001	17.7	18.9	17.5	21.6	18.9	22.0	25.9	24.2	26.1	33.4	36.7	32.7	44.6	48.6	43.4
≥75 (4,789)	p<0.001	p<0.001	p<0.001	15.1	11.8	15.3	19.5	23.1	19.4	20.8	23.1	20.7	27.7	36.2	26.7	41.0	38.0	41.2

[a] according to the Chi-square test of period effect.

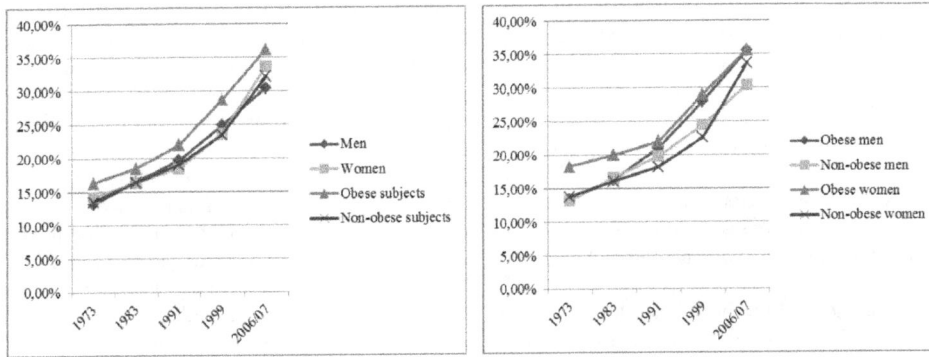

Figure 2. The age-standardized prevalence of back pain in Austria by sex and obesity in five health surveys.

population study estimated a self-reported 1-month prevalence to be 31.7% [7]. In Belgium the point prevalence of back pain was estimated to be 33% among adults. However, this study dates back to the early 1990ies [27]. Compared to other European countries the prevalence of back pain was quite high in this study [2,5,10,28]. Hoy et al. [2], in their meta-analysis of summarized evidence from 165 studies in 54 countries, stated a pooled estimate of the mean point prevalence of low back pain to be 11.9%.

Considering the overall trend, the prevalence of back pain in Austria was not always so high. A progression of back pain was observed and thus the prevalence rose with every survey. Data from cross-sectional surveys conducted over 40 years among English adults were investigated by Harkness et al. [28] They found a strong increase in the point prevalence of self-reported back pain. While the prevalence of low back pain was 9.1% for both women and men in 1956, it went up to 18.2% for women and 17.8% for men in 1995. Slightly higher rates than in the 1990ies were observed in our study. However, no other current studies were found that examined long-term trends in the prevalence of back pain. Therefore, comparisons for long-term back pain trends are not possible.

We believe that there is a series of factors that may have led to this strong increase in the prevalence of back pain in Austria. One reason is that the demographic has changed during the study period in Austria. There was a change in the age structure of the population in favor of the older age groups and the demographic aging has led to a more frequent occur of chronic diseases,

including back pain. Over the period, the work situation has also changed. Increased workload and increased sedentary activities may have contributed to a higher prevalence of back pain [29]. The increase in back pain is probably attributed partly to the rise of BMI and obesity prevalence. Among obese subjects an almost linear trend in the increasing prevalence is discernible from 1991 onwards [21]. Another reason could be that there was an increase of subjects with mental disorders, which causes future episodes of pain [30]. An assumption is also that the willingness to report pain symptoms increased. This may be due to cultural factors as changes in the attitudes to report their disorders [29], which is also noticeable by increased sickness reporting [13]. Furthermore an increased awareness of pain symptoms by patients and health professionals could have been contributed to the rise in the prevalence of back pain. It is unclear if the high prevalence in the most recent surveys indicates a true increase or represents a rise in unclear diagnosis [29]. Overall, the evidence suggests that the real increase in back pain is likely to be somewhat lower than the self-reported figures.

The analysis of subgroups in this study showed interesting results. The literature indicates back pain is more common among female and older persons [5,2,7,17,27,31]. In line with earlier studies, women showed a higher prevalence of back pain than men [32,33]. Results from a systematic review also showed that back pain worldwide more often concerns women than men [2]. Possible underlying reasons for the gender difference were investigated in Germany [31]. When investigating different factors

Table 2. Absolute changes (AC) and aetiologic fractions (AF) of the prevalence of back pain for the period 1973 to 2006–07 in Austria by sex and obesity (adjusted for age).

Predictor	AC back pain in %	AF back pain in %	P value*
Total	19.4	54.6	<0.001
Obese	25.0	53.7	<0.001
Non-obese	18.4	53.9	<0.001
Women	19.7	52.6	<0.001
Obese	23.3	50.0	<0.001
Non-obese	19.5	52.4	<0.001
Men	17.3	58.0	<0.001
Obese	25.6	61.8	<0.001
Non-obese	16.0	57.1	<0.001

*p value for period effect (from logistic regression analyses).

related to back pain (e.g. BMI, age) it was not possible to reduce or explain the gender difference. They recommended exploring rarely investigated constructs, such as anxiety and considering anatomic differences in muscle strength. While the prevalence of back pain was highest among women in Austria, the strongest increase and the greatest risk were found for men. In Bulgaria the risk of getting back disorders was also higher in men [34]. This could be due to the fact that women paid more attention to a healthy lifestyle, including back exercises, in the last decades as social norms generally make women more cautious about their body.

Considering different age groups the prevalence for back pain increases with age, with the highest incidence in the third decade [11,28]. In the oldest age group the prevalence decreases [1,35], which was also true for this study. There are a whole range of factors behind this phenomenon: decreased pain perception or increased pain tolerance, existence of other health problems with higher priority, increasing influence of mental health problems and the exclusion from studies of older individuals living in nursing homes [1]. It is striking that in young obese men the prevalence is already very high in contrast to young obese women. The latest survey showed one third of all 20–34 year old obese men to suffer from low back pain, while the same applies to only half of the non-obese peers. Lean body mass is found more often in younger than in older subjects. Therefore, the lower back pain prevalence among young men with a high BMI may be due to increased muscle mass [36]. However, it should be noted that the women are clearly catching up at a later age, which is why the overall prevalence of low back pain is generally somewhat higher among women.

Studies reported that obesity is associated with a higher prevalence of low back pain [10,15,34,37], which is more pronounced in women [18,32,38]. Study results showing higher prevalence of back pain for obese than for non-obese subjects are in accordance with our findings. We observed the highest prevalence among obese women, however the increase of and the greatest risk for back pain were highest among obese men. Therefore, special emphasis should be placed on obese individuals when planning low back pain prevention strategies. A moderate level of physical activity is recommended to prevent back pain [17,18].

Strengths and Limitations

One limitation was that only self-reported data were available for Austria. This disadvantage was compensated by correcting the self-reported BMI [24]. Another limitation was due to the fact that the last survey used a different definition for identifying back pain. This restriction is described in more detail in the Method section. Furthermore, the literature showed that low back pain is more

often associated with obesity [17,18]. In our study only data concerning general back pain was available for analysis. In addition the data concerning back pain did not include any information on the severity and frequency of the pain. More precise data would be needed in order to develop an appropriate therapeutic approach.

When interpreting the prevalence of diseases, it is recommended to standardize crude rates since populations may differ in their age composition. However, consideration should be given to the fact that age-adjusted rates are partially derived from a reference population, so they do not precisely describe the study population. It is a strength that crude and age-standardized prevalence was mentioned in this study. Another strength comprises the unique database with a large number of subjects included, enabling us to obtain statistically reliable data in subgroups. Examination over such a long investigation period allowed an accurate assessment of the development of this public health problem, which does represent a major advantage.

Conclusion

In conclusion, back pain strongly increased in the last decades and currently represents a widespread public health problem in Austria. The outcomes further indicate that there was an increase in the prevalence of back pain among all investigated subgroups, with the highest prevalence among obese women. However, obese men showed the highest increase of and the greatest risk for back pain during the study period. Our findings confirm the effect of a high BMI as a risk factor for back pain in the general adult population. The link between obesity and back pain underlies the importance of promoting preventive measures to reduce the incidence of obesity. We recommend that this worrying trend be monitored throughout the Austrian population and that preventive measures be implemented for specific target groups, as obese subjects. The results could be used to plan controlled promotion programs among adults suffering from back pain.

It should be noted that this study did not identify the nature of the stated relationships. The precise process leading to the relationship between low back pain and investigated variables should be clarified through further studies in order to combine our epidemiologic results with the processes leading to the genesis of back pain. Prospective studies are needed to confirm our results and investigate causal relationships.

Author Contributions

Conceived and designed the experiments: FG WS. Performed the experiments: FG WS. Analyzed the data: FG WF WS. Contributed reagents/materials/analysis tools: WF ÉR NB JM. Contributed to the writing of the manuscript: FG WS. Corrected the manuscript: ÉR NB JM WF WS. Supported the data analysis: WF ÉR.

References

1. Dionne CE, Dunn KM, Croft PR (2006) Does back pain prevalence really decrease with increasing age? A systematic review. Age Ageing 35: 229–234.
2. Hoy D, Bain C, Williams G, March L, Brooks P, et al. (2010a) Global prevalence of low back pain. Arthritis Rheum 64: 2028–2037.
3. Hoy D, March L, Brooks P, Woof A, Blyth F, et al. (2010b) Measuring the global burden of low back pain. Best Pract Res Clin Rheumatol 24: 155–165.
4. Buchbinder R, Blyth FM, March LM, Brooks P, Woolf AD, et al. (2013) Placing the global burden of low back pain in context. Best Pract Res Clin Rheumatol 27: 575–589.
5. Carmona L, Ballina J, Gabriel R, Laffon A on behalf of the EPISTER Study Group (2001) The burden of musculoskeletal diseases in the general population of Spain: results from a national survey. Ann Rehum Dis 60: 1040–1045.
6. Leijon M, Hensing G, Alexanderson K (2004) Sickness absence due to musculoskeletal diagnoses: association with occupational gender segregation. Scand J Public Health 32: 94–100.
7. Stranjalis G, Tsamandouraki K, Sakas DE, Alamanos Y (2004) Low back pain in a representative sample of Greek population: analysis according to personal and socioeconomic characteristics. Spine 29: 1355–1360.
8. Luo X, Pietrobon R, Sun SX, Liu GG, Hey L (2004) Estimates and patterns of direct health care expenditures among individuals with back pain in the United States. Spine 29: 79–86.
9. Thelin A, Holmberg S, Thelin N (2008) Functioning in neck and low back pain from 12-year perspective: a prospective population-based study. J Rehabil Med 40: 555–561.
10. Nilsen TIL, Holtermann A, Mork PJ (2011) Physical exercise, body mass index, and risk of chronic pain in the low back and neck/shoulders: longitudinal data from the Nord-Trondelag Health Study. Am J Epidemiol 174: 267–273.
11. Kopec JA, Sayre EC, Esdaile JM (2004) Predictors of back pain in a general population cohort. Spine 29: 70–77.
12. Volinn E (1997) The epidemiology of low back pain in the rest of the world. A review of surveys in low- and middle income countries. Spine 22: 1747–1754.

13. Waddell G, Aylward M, Sawney P (2002) Back pain, incapacity for work and social security benefits: an international literature review and analysis. London: Royal Society of Medicine Press.

14. Hershkovich O, Friedlander A, Gordon B, Arzi H, Derazne E, et al. (2013) Associations of body mass index and body height with low back pain in 829,791 adolescents. Am J Epidemiol 178: 603–609.

15. Melissas J, Volakakis E, Hadjipavlou A (2003) Low back pain in morbidly obese patients and the effect of weight loss following surgery. Obes Surg 1: 389–93.

16. Shiri R, Solovieva S, Husgafvel-Pursiainen K, Telama R, Yang X, et al. (2013) The role of obesity and physical activity in non-specific and radiating low back pain: the Young Finns study. Semin Arthritis Rheum 42: 640–650.

17. Shiri R, Karppinen J, Leino-Arjas P, Solovieva S, Viikari-Juntura E (2010) The association between obesity and low back pain: A meta-analysis. Am J Epidemiol 171: 135–154.

18. Ali SM, Lindstroem M (2006) Socioeconomic, psychosocial, behavioural, psychological determinants of BMI among young women: differing patterns for underweight and overweight/obesity. Eur J Public Health 16: 324–330.

19. Adams KF, Schatzkin A, Harris TB, Kipnis V, Mouw T, et al. (2006) Overweight, obesity, and mortality in a large prospective cohort of persons 50 to 71 years old. N Engl J Med 355: 763–778.

20. World Health Organization (2014). Obesity and overweight. Available: http://www.who.int/mediacentre/factsheets/fs311/en/index.html. Accessed on February 6, 2014.

21. Großschädl F, Stronegger WJ (2013) Long-term trends in obesity among Austrian adults and its relation with the social gradient: 1973–2007. Eur J Public Health 23: 306–312.

22. van der Windt DA, Dunn KM (2013) Low back pain research – future directions. Best Pract Res Clin Rheumatol 27: 699–708.

23. Shiely F, Perry IJ, Lutomski J, Harrington J, Kellehr CC, et al. (2010) Temporal trends in misclassification patterns of measured and self-report based body mass index categories – findings from three population surveys in Ireland. BMC Public Health 10: 560.

24. Großschädl F, Haditsch B, Stronegger WJ (2012) Validity of self-reported weight and height in Austrian adults: sociodemographic determinants and consequences for the classification of BMI categories. Public Health Nutr 15: 20–27.

25. Espelt A, Goday A, Franch J, Borrell C (2012) Validity of self-reported diabetes in health interview surveys for measuring social inequalities in the prevalence of diabetes. J Epidemiol Community Health 66: e15.

26. World Health Organization (1993) World Health Statistics Annual. Geneva: WHO.

27. Skovron ML, Szpalski M, Nordin M, Melot C, Cukier D (1994) Sociocultural factors and back pain. A population-based study in Belgian adults. Spine 19: 129–137.

28. Harkness EF, Macfarlane GJ, Silman AJ, McBeth J (2005) Is musculoskeletal pain more common now than 40 years ago?: two population-based cross-sectional studies. Rheumatology 44: 890–895.

29. Airaksinen O, Brox JL, Cedraschi C, Hildebrandt J, Klaber-Moffett J, et al. (2006) Guidelines for Chronic Low Back Pain. Chapter 4. European guidelines for the management of chronic nonspecific low back pain. Eur Spine J 15: 192–300.

30. Demyttenaere K, Bruffaerts R, Lee S, Psada-Vill J, Kovess V, et al. (2007) Mental disorders among persons with chronic back or neck pain: results from the world mental health surveys. Pain 129: 332–342.

31. Schneider S, Randoll D, Buchner M (2006) Why do women have back pain more than men? A representative prevalence study in the federal republic of Germany. Clin J Pain 22: 738–747.

32. Shiri R, Solovieva S, Husgafvel-Pursiainen K, Taimela S, Saarikoski LA, et al. (2008) The association between obesity and the prevalence of low back pain in young adult. The cardiovascular risk in young Finns study. Am J Epidemiol 167: 1110–1119.

33. Wijnhoven HA, de Vet HC, Picavet HS (2006) Prevalence of musculosetal disorders is systematically higher in women than in men. Clin J Pain 22: 717–724.

34. Kostova V, Koeva M (2001) Back disorders (low back pain, cervicobrachial and lumbosacral radicular syndromes) and some related risk factors. J Neurol Sci 192: 17–25.

35. Fejer R, Leboeuf-Yde C (2012) Does back and neck pain become more common as you get older? A systematic literature review. Chiropr Man Ther 20: 27.

36. Hunter GR, Lara-Castro C, Byrne NM, Zakharkin SO, Onge MP, et al. (2005) Weight loss needed to maintain visceral adipose tissue during aging. Int J Body Compos Res 3: 55–61.

37. Lake JK, Power C, Cole TJ (2000) Back pain and obesity in the 1958 British birth cohort. Cause or effect? J Clin Epidemiol 53: 245–250.

38. Han TS, Schouten JSAG, Lean MEJ, Seidell JC (1997) The prevalence of low back pain and associations with body fatness, fat distribution and height. Int J Obes 21: 600–607.

Permissions

The contributors of this book come from diverse backgrounds, making this book a truly international effort. This book will bring forth new frontiers with its revolutionizing research information and detailed analysis of the nascent developments around the world.

We would like to thank all the contributing authors for lending their expertise to make the book truly unique. They have played a crucial role in the development of this book. Without their invaluable contributions this book wouldn't have been possible. They have made vital efforts to compile up to date information on the varied aspects of this subject to make this book a valuable addition to the collection of many professionals and students.

This book was conceptualized with the vision of imparting up-to-date information and advanced data in this field. To ensure the same, a matchless editorial board was set up. Every individual on the board went through rigorous rounds of assessment to prove their worth. After which they invested a large part of their time researching and compiling the most relevant data for our readers.

The editorial board has been involved in producing this book since its inception. They have spent rigorous hours researching and exploring the diverse topics which have resulted in the successful publishing of this book. They have passed on their knowledge of decades through this book. To expedite this challenging task, the publisher supported the team at every step. A small team of assistant editors was also appointed to further simplify the editing procedure and attain best results for the readers.

Apart from the editorial board, the designing team has also invested a significant amount of their time in understanding the subject and creating the most relevant covers. They scrutinized every image to scout for the most suitable representation of the subject and create an appropriate cover for the book.

The publishing team has been an ardent support to the editorial, designing and production team. Their endless efforts to recruit the best for this project, has resulted in the accomplishment of this book. They are a veteran in the field of academics and their pool of knowledge is as vast as their experience in printing. Their expertise and guidance has proved useful at every step. Their uncompromising quality standards have made this book an exceptional effort. Their encouragement from time to time has been an inspiration for everyone.

The publisher and the editorial board hope that this book will prove to be a valuable piece of knowledge for researchers, students, practitioners and scholars across the globe.

List of Contributors

Cherie Wells
Faculty of Health, University of Canberra, Bruce, Australian Capital Territory, Australia
School of Science and Health, University of Western Sydney, Campbelltown, New

Gregory S. Kolt and Paul Marshall
School of Science and Health, University of Western Sydney, Campbelltown, New South Wales, Australia

Bridget Hill
Epworth HealthCare, Richmond, Victoria, Australia

Andrea Bialocerkowski
Griffith Health Institute, Griffith University, Gold Coast, Queensland, Australia

In-Hyuk Ha
Jaseng Medical Foundation, Jaseng Hospital of Korean Medicine, Seoul, Republic of Korea
Graduate School of Public Health & Institute of Health and Environment, Seoul National University, Gwanak-ro, Gwanak-gu, Seoul, Korea

Jinho Lee
Jaseng Medical Foundation, Jaseng Hospital of Korean Medicine, Seoul, Republic of Korea
Department of Herbology, Graduate School of Korean Medicine, Kyung Hee University, Seoul, Republic of Korea

Me-riong Kim, Hyejin Kim and Joon-Shik Shin
Jaseng Medical Foundation, Jaseng Hospital of Korean Medicine, Seoul, Republic of Korea

Stefan Schandelmaier, Susan C. A. Burkhardt, Wout E. L. de Boer and Regina Kunz
Academy of Swiss Insurance Medicine, University Hospital Basel, Basel, Switzerland

Shanil Ebrahim and Gordon H. Guyatt
Department of Clinical Epidemiology and Biostatistics, McMaster University, Hamilton, Ontario, Canada

Thomas Zumbrunn
Clinical Trial Unit, University Hospital Basel, Basel, Switzerland

Jason W. Busse
Department of Clinical Epidemiology and Biostatistics, McMaster University, Hamilton, Ontario, Canada
Department of Anesthesia, McMaster University, Hamilton, Ontario, Canada

Pavel Vostatek and Daniel Novák
Department of Cybernetics, Czech Technical University in Prague, Prague, Czech Republic

Tomas Rychnovský and šarka Rychnovská
AVETE OMNE Physiotherapy Center, Filmarska 19, Prague, Czech Republic

Aida Ferreiro-Iglesias, Eva Perez-Pampin, Marisol Porto-Silva and Antonio Gonzalez
Research Laboratory 10 and Rheumatology Unit, Instituto de Investigacion Sanitaria – Hospital Clinico Universitario de Santiago, Santiago de Compostela, Spain

Antonio Mera-Varela and Juan J. Gómez-Reino
Research Laboratory 10 and Rheumatology Unit, Instituto de Investigacion Sanitaria – Hospital Clinico Universitario de Santiago, Santiago de Compostela, Spain
Department of Medicine, University of Santiago de Compostela, Santiago de Compostela, Spain

Eric Manheimer and Brian M. Berman, Lixing Lao
University of Maryland School of Medicine, Center for Integrative Medicine, Baltimore, Maryland, United States of America

Claudia M. Witt
University of Maryland School of Medicine, Center for Integrative Medicine, Baltimore, Maryland, United States of America
Charité University Medical Center, Institute for Social Medicine, Epidemiology and Health Economics, Berlin, Germany

Richard Hammerschlag
Research Department, Oregon College of Oriental Medicine, Portland, Oregon, United States of America

Rainer Lüdtke
Carstens Foundation, Essen, Germany

Sean R.Tunis
Center for Medical Technology Policy, Baltimore, Maryland, United States of America

Hugh MacPherson
Department of Health Sciences, University of York, York, United Kingdom

Emily Vertosick and Andrew J. Vickers
Memorial Sloan-Kettering Cancer Center, New York, New York, United States of America

George Lewith
Faculty of Medicine, Primary Care and Population Sciences, University of Southampton, Southampton, United Kingdom

Klaus Linde
Institute of General Practice, Technische Universität München, Munich, Germany

Karen J. Sherman
Group Health Research Institute, Seattle, Washington, United States of America

Claudia M. Witt
Center for Complementary and Integrative Medicine, University Hospital Zurich, Zurich, Switzerland
Institute for Social Medicine, Epidemiology and Health Economics, Charité - Universitätsmedizin, Berlin, Germany

Maria M. Wertli and Manuela Schöb, Johann Steurer
Horten Center for Patient Oriented Research and Knowledge Transfer, Department of Internal Medicine, University of Zurich, Zurich, Switzerland

Florian Brunner
Department of Physical Medicine and Rheumatology, Balgrist University Hospital, Zurich, Switzerland

Valéria Martinez
Anesthésiologie-Réanimation, Hô pital Raymond-Poincaré , Garches, France
INSERM U-987, Centre d'Evaluation et de Traitement de la Douleur, CHU Ambroise Paré , Boulogne-Billancourt, France

Nadine Attal and Didier Bouhassira
INSERM U-987, Centre d'Evaluation et de Traitement de la Douleur, CHU Ambroise Paré, Boulogne-Billancourt, France
Université Versailles-Saint-Quentin, Versailles, France

Bertrand Vanzo
General Practitioner, Athis Mons, France

Eric Vicaut
Unité de Recherche Clinique - Hô pital Fernand Widal, Paris, France

Jean Michel Gautier
Réseau InterCLUD Languedoc Roussillon, CHRU Montpellier, Montpellier, France

Michel Lantéri-Minet
CHU de Nice, Centre d'Evaluation et Traitement de la Douleur, Nice, France
INSERM/UdA, U1107, Neuro-Dol, Universite´ de Clermont-Ferrand, Clermont-Ferrand, France

Tobias Consmü ller and Daniel Weinland
Epionics Medical GmbH, Potsdam, Germany

Antonius Rohlmann, Georg N. Duda and William R. Taylor
Julius Wolff Institute, Charite´ – Universitätsmedizin Berlin, Berlin, Germany

Claudia Druschel
Center for Musculoskeletal Surgery, Charité–Universitätsmedizin Berlin, Berlin, Germany

Steven Z. George
Department of Physical Therapy and Center for Pain Research and Behavioral Health, University of Florida, Gainesville, Florida, United States of America

John D. Childs, Deydre S. Teyhen, Alison C. Wright and Jessica L. Dugan
U.S. Army- Baylor University Doctoral Program in Physical Therapy (MCCS-HGE-PT), Army Medical Department Center and School, Fort Sam Houston, Texas, United States of America

Samuel S. Wu
Department of Biostatistics, University of Florida, Gainesville, Florida, United States of America

Michael E. Robinson
Department of Clinical and Health Psychology and Center for Pain Research and Behavioral Health, University of Florida, Gainesville, Florida, United States of America

Roland Zemp, Renate List, Turgut Gü lay, William R. Taylor and Silvio Lorenzetti
Institute for Biomechanics, ETH Zurich, Zurich, Switzerland

Jean Pierre Elsig
Spine Surgery, Küsnacht, Switzerland

Jaroslav Naxera
Röntgeninstitut Zurich-Altstetten, Zurich, Switzerland

Xue-Qiang Wang, Jing Liu and Pei-Jie Chen
Department of Sport Rehabilitation, Shanghai University of Sport, Shanghai, China

Jie-Jiao Zheng, Yi Chen, Yu-Jian Pan, Guo-Hui Xu and Zhuo-Wei Yu
Department of Rehabilitation Medicine, Huadong Hospital Affiliated to Fudan University, Shanghai, China

Xia Bi
Department of Rehabilitation Medicine, Shanghai Gongli Hospital, Shanghai, China

Shu-Jie Lou
Department of Exercise and Sport Science, Shanghai University of Sport, Shanghai, China

Bin Cai
Department of Orthopaedics and Rehabilitation, Ninth People's Hospital Affiliated to Shanghai Jiaotong University Medical School, Shanghai, China

Ying- Hui Hua
Department of Sport Medicine, Huashan Hospital Affiliated to Fudan University, Shanghai, China

Mark Wu
Department of Rehabilitation and Ancillary Services, Gleneagles International Medical and Surgical Center, Shanghai, China

Mao-Ling Wei
Chinese Evidence-based Medicine, West China Hospital of Sichuan University, Chengdu, China

Hai-Min Shen
Department of Orthopaedics and Trauma Surgery, Huadong Hospital Affiliated to Fudan University, Shanghai, China

Raymond W. McGorry and Jia-Hua Lin
Liberty Mutual Research Institute for Safety, Hopkinton, Massachusetts, United States of America

Ingo Froböse
Institute of Health Promotion and Clinical Movement Science, German Sport University Cologne, Cologne, Germany

Sven Karstens
Institute of Health Promotion and Clinical Movement Science, German Sport University Cologne, Cologne, Germany
Department of General Practice and Health Services Research, University Hospital Heidelberg, Heidelberg, Germany

Katja Hermann
Department of General Practice and Health Services Research, University Hospital Heidelberg, Heidelberg, Germany

Stephan W. Weiler
Audi Medical Services, Audi, Ingolstadt, Germany
Department of Occupational Medicine, University Medical Center Schleswig-Holstein, Campus Luebeck, Luebeck, Germany

Lars L. Andersen, Thomas Clausen and Andreas Holtermann
National Research Centre for the Working Environment, Copenhagen Ø, Denmark

Hermann Burr
Federal Institute for Occupational Safety and Health (BAuA), Berlin, Germany

Saad M. Alsaadi
Department of physiotherapy, King Fahd Hospital of the University, The University of Dammam, Khobar, Saudi Arabia

Pelvic Girdle Pain, 118, 122

Penetrating Needles, 65-67, 69-71

Physical Disability, 119, 145

Pilates Exercise, 1-14

Portable Instruments, 145, 147, 149-151

Postsurgical Nerve, 82

Postural Function, 36-37, 39, 41, 43, 45-48

Psychological Distress, 100-102, 105-106, 146-147, 151

R

Radiculopathy, 82, 134, 162, 186, 196, 198, 200-203

Rheumatoid Arthritis, 49, 51, 53-54, 132, 134-138, 151

S

Sacroiliitis, 49-54

Sciatica, 15, 18-19, 22, 47, 56, 118, 138, 146, 181, 184-187, 189-191, 193, 195-197, 201-202, 205

Skeletal Kinematics, 109, 115

Skin Marker, 109, 114-116

Sleep Disturbance, 145-147, 149, 151

Spinal Cord Injury, 82

Spinal Flexion, 93-95, 97, 99, 115

Spinal Pathology, 93-94, 146

Spinal Stenosis, 171, 173-176, 182, 184-186, 194, 196-198, 203

Spine Disorders, 36

Spondylarthrosis, 36

Strain Gauge, 94

Surgical Treatment, 93-94, 172, 175

Systolic Blood Pressure, 15-18, 21, 178

T

Thoracic Curvature Angles, 109, 112, 115

Thoracic Segments, 109, 111-112, 114

Thoracolumbar, 38, 93-94, 99

Transcutaneous Electric Nerve Stimulation, 66

Trunk Muscles, 47-48, 101, 118-119

Tumor Necrosis, 53, 185-187, 189, 191-197

V

Vertebrogenic Diseases, 36

Michael E. Robinson
Department of Clinical and Health Psychology and Center for Pain Research and Behavioral Health, University of Florida, Gainesville, Florida, United States of America

Roland Zemp, Renate List, Turgut Gü lay, William R. Taylor and Silvio Lorenzetti
Institute for Biomechanics, ETH Zurich, Zurich, Switzerland

Jean Pierre Elsig
Spine Surgery, Küsnacht, Switzerland

Jaroslav Naxera
Röntgeninstitut Zurich-Altstetten, Zurich, Switzerland

Xue-Qiang Wang, Jing Liu and Pei-Jie Chen
Department of Sport Rehabilitation, Shanghai University of Sport, Shanghai, China

Jie-Jiao Zheng, Yi Chen, Yu-Jian Pan, Guo-Hui Xu and Zhuo-Wei Yu
Department of Rehabilitation Medicine, Huadong Hospital Affiliated to Fudan University, Shanghai, China

Xia Bi
Department of Rehabilitation Medicine, Shanghai Gongli Hospital, Shanghai, China

Shu-Jie Lou
Department of Exercise and Sport Science, Shanghai University of Sport, Shanghai, China

Bin Cai
Department of Orthopaedics and Rehabilitation, Ninth People's Hospital Affiliated to Shanghai Jiaotong University Medical School, Shanghai, China

Ying- Hui Hua
Department of Sport Medicine, Huashan Hospital Affiliated to Fudan University, Shanghai, China

Mark Wu
Department of Rehabilitation and Ancillary Services, Gleneagles International Medical and Surgical Center, Shanghai, China

Mao-Ling Wei
Chinese Evidence-based Medicine, West China Hospital of Sichuan University, Chengdu, China

Hai-Min Shen
Department of Orthopaedics and Trauma Surgery, Huadong Hospital Affiliated to Fudan University, Shanghai, China

Raymond W. McGorry and Jia-Hua Lin
Liberty Mutual Research Institute for Safety, Hopkinton, Massachusetts, United States of America

Ingo Froböse
Institute of Health Promotion and Clinical Movement Science, German Sport University Cologne, Cologne, Germany

Sven Karstens
Institute of Health Promotion and Clinical Movement Science, German Sport University Cologne, Cologne, Germany
Department of General Practice and Health Services Research, University Hospital Heidelberg, Heidelberg, Germany

Katja Hermann
Department of General Practice and Health Services Research, University Hospital Heidelberg, Heidelberg, Germany

Stephan W. Weiler
Audi Medical Services, Audi, Ingolstadt, Germany
Department of Occupational Medicine, University Medical Center Schleswig-Holstein, Campus Luebeck, Luebeck, Germany

Lars L. Andersen, Thomas Clausen and Andreas Holtermann
National Research Centre for the Working Environment, Copenhagen Ø, Denmark

Hermann Burr
Federal Institute for Occupational Safety and Health (BAuA), Berlin, Germany

Saad M. Alsaadi
Department of physiotherapy, King Fahd Hospital of the University, The University of Dammam, Khobar, Saudi Arabia

James H. McAuley and Chris G. Maher
The George Institute for Global Health, Faculty of Medicine, The University of Sydney, Sydney, Australia

Julia M. Hush
Department of Health Professions, Faculty of Human Sciences, Australian School of Advanced Medicine, Macquarie University, Sydney, Australia

Delwyn J. Bartlett and George C. Dungan II
The Woolcock Institute of Medical Research, The University of Sydney, Sydney, Australia

Ronald R. Grunstein
The Woolcock Institute of Medical Research, The University of Sydney, Sydney, Australia
Department of Respiratory and Sleep Medicine, Royal Prince Alfred Hospital, Sydney, Australia

Zoe M. McKeough
Clinical and Rehabilitation Sciences, The University of Sydney, Sydney, New South Wales, Australia

Svetlana Solovieva, Johanna Kausto, Rahman Shiri and Kirsti Husgafvel-Pursiainen
Centre of Expertise for Health and Work Ability, Finnish Institute of Occupational Health, Helsinki, Finland
Disability Prevention Centre, Finnish Institute of Occupational Health, Helsinki, Finland

Tiina Pensola
Centre of Expertise for Health and Work Ability, Finnish Institute of Occupational Health, Helsinki, Finland

Eira Viikari-Juntura
Disability Prevention Centre, Finnish Institute of Occupational Health, Helsinki, Finland

Markku Heliövaara
National Institute for Health and Welfare, Helsinki, Finland

Alex Burdorf
Erasmus MC, University Medical Center Rotterdam, Rotterdam, The Netherlands

Benjamin Luchting, Banafscheh Rachinger-Adam, Julia Zeitler, Lisa Egenberger, Patrick Möhnle, Simone Kreth and Shahnaz Christina Azad
Department of Anesthesiology and Pain Medicine, Ludwig-Maximilians University Munich, Munich, Germany

Pekka Kuittinen
Department of Neurosurgery, Kuopio University Hospital, Kuopio, Finland and Institute of Clinical Medicine, University of Eastern Finland, Kuopio, Finland

Petri Sipola
Department of Clinical Radiology, Kuopio University Hospital, Kuopio, Finland and Unit of Radiology, Institute of Clinical Medicine, University of Eastern Finland, Kuopio, Finland

Ville Leinonen
Department of Neurosurgery, Kuopio University Hospital, Kuopio, Finland and Unit of Neurosurgery, Institute of Clinical Medicine, University of Eastern Finland, Kuopio, Finland

Tapani Saari
Department of Clinical Radiology, Kuopio University Hospital, Kuopio, Finland

Sanna Sinikallio
Institute of Public Health and Clinical Nutrition, University of Eastern Finland, Kuopio, Finland

Sakari Savolainen
Department of Neurosurgery, Kuopio University Hospital, Kuopio, Finland

Heikki Kröger
Department of Orthopaedics and Traumatology, Kuopio University Hospital
and Bone and Cartilage Research Unit, University of Eastern Finland, Kuopio, Finland

Veli Turunen
Department of Orthopaedics and Traumatology, Kuopio University Hospital, Kuopio, Finland

Olavi Airaksinen
Department of Physical and Rehabilitation Medicine, Kuopio University Hospital, Kuopio, Finland

Timo Aalto
Health Center Ikioma OY, Mikkeli, Finland

Ingrid Heuch
Department of Neurology and FORMI, Oslo University Hospital, Oslo, Norway

Ivar Heuch
Department of Mathematics, University of Bergen, Bergen, Norway

Knut Hagen
Department of Neuroscience, Norwegian University of Science and Technology, and Norwegian National Headache Centre, Department of Neurology, St. Olavs Hospital, Trondheim, Norway

John-Anker Zwart
Department of Neurology and FORMI, Oslo University Hospital, Oslo, Norway
Faculty of Medicine, University of Oslo, Oslo, Norway

Yun Fu Wang, Li Li Xu, Song Lin Wang, Jie Luo and Guang Jian Liu
Department of Neurology, Taihe Hospital Affiliated to Hubei University of Medicine, Shiyan City, Hubei Province, China

Ping You Chen
Medical Imaging Center, Taihe Hospital Affiliated to Hubei University of Medicine, Shiyan City, Hubei Province, China

Wei Chang
Department of Spine Surgery, Taihe Hospital Affiliated to Hubei University of Medicine, Shiyan City, Hubei Province, China

Fi Qi Zhu
Department of Neurology, Yuebei People's Hospital Affiliated to Shantou University Medical College, Shaoguan City, Guangdong Province, China

Li Ying Chang
Department of Neurology, Xiangyang Center Hospital Affiliated to Hubei University of Arts and Science, Xiangyang City, Hubei Province, China

Shu-Xun Hou, Jia-Liang Zhu, Dong-Feng Ren, Zheng Cao and Jia-Guang Tang
Department of Orthopaedics, The First Affiliated Hospital of General Hospital of Chinese PLA, Beijing, China

Feng Shuang
Department of Orthopaedics, The First Affiliated Hospital of General Hospital of Chinese PLA, Beijing, China
Department of Orthopedics, The 94th Hospital of Chinese PLA, Nanchang, China

Franziska Großschädl, Wolfgang Freid, Éva Rásky, Nathalie Burkert and Willibald J. Stronegger
Medical University of Graz, Institute of Social Medicine and Epidemiology, Graz, Austria

Johanna Muckenhuber
University of Graz, Institute of Sociology, Graz, Austria

Index

A

Acupuncture, 55-56, 58-72, 76, 78, 80-81, 122, 132

Analgesics, 61, 68, 90, 132, 134, 136, 162, 198

Angular Velocity, 93, 95-96

Ankylosing Spondylitis, 49, 53-54

B

Back Pain, 1-3, 5, 7-22, 26-27, 29, 34-38, 45-53, 55-56, 58, 60-64, 66-70, 72-74, 76-78, 80-82, 84, 88-90, 92-94, 96, 99-109, 115-119, 121-139, 141-145, 147, 149, 151-152, 154-155, 157-163, 165, 167, 169-177, 179-184, 187-188, 190, 193-194, 196-197, 199-200, 202-203, 205-213

Back Pain Episode, 124-125, 127, 129-131

Back Pain Functional Scale, 126, 131

Breathing Cycle, 36, 46-47

C

Cardiovascular Disease, 15-16, 18-19, 21-22, 152, 159, 182-183

Chronic Low Back Pain, 1, 3, 5, 7-9, 11-17, 19-22, 26, 34-37, 46-48, 55-56, 63-64, 72-73, 76, 108, 117, 119, 121-123, 131, 137-138, 151, 161-163, 165, 167, 169-170, 177, 179, 181, 183, 213

Conventional Exercise, 118

Core Stability Exercise, 117-123

Curvature, 44, 93-95, 99, 109-116

D

Depression, 24, 26, 29, 73, 80, 84, 92, 101, 103, 106, 108, 145, 147-148, 152, 154-155, 157-160, 169-170, 172-174, 176, 187

Diaphragm Function, 36-37, 46

Dichotomous, 24, 134, 140, 173, 200, 209

Doppler Signal, 49-53

E

Electrical Silence, 124-125

Electromyography, 36, 77-78, 131

Enthesitis, 49-54

Epionics Spine, 93-95, 99

Erector Spinae, 101, 124-126, 130

Exercise Therapy, 13-14, 117-118, 122-123, 136, 138, 145, 151

Expiratory Position, 36

F

Flexion Phase, 124, 126, 128

Functional Capacity, 93-94, 96, 98

Functional Kinematics, 93, 98

G

Gastroenterology, 36

General Exercise, 10, 12, 14, 107, 117-123

L

Lbp Symptoms, 124-125, 127

Long-term Sickness Absence, 23, 139-144

Lordosis Angle, 93-99, 115

Lower Limbs, 36-37, 42-46

Lumbar, 1-2, 4, 10, 12-13, 15, 18-19, 22, 34, 36-37, 47, 50, 56, 80, 93-94, 96, 99-100, 107, 109-116, 122, 124-125, 128-131, 134, 154, 161, 170-177, 181-184, 186, 196-199, 201-203, 205-206

Lumbar Motion Monitor, 93, 99

M

Madrid Sonography Enthesitis Index, 49

Magnetic Resonance Imaging, 22, 36-37, 39, 41, 43, 45-47, 50, 116, 171-172, 176, 198, 205

Medical Interventions, 55

Mri Processing, 38

Multiple Sclerosis, 82

Muscle Fatigue, 124, 131

Musculoskeletal Disorders, 26, 34, 138-139, 143, 183

N

Neoplastic Disease, 125

Neuropathic Pain, 82-92, 161, 170, 197

Nicotine Consumption, 132

O

Obesity, 15, 18, 22, 47, 168, 170, 181, 207-213

P

Pain Intensity, 4, 8-10, 38, 44-46, 66, 84, 100-102, 104, 106, 108, 118-119, 121, 134-136, 139-143, 146-148, 162-163, 170, 173, 177, 179, 183, 186

Pain Pathology, 93

Pain Symptoms, 37, 90, 125, 130, 169, 171, 211

www.ingramcontent.com/pod-product-compliance
Lightning Source LLC
Chambersburg PA
CBHW082047190326
41458CB00010B/3477